MODERN HEALTH

JAMES H. OTTO

CLOYD J. JULIAN

J. EDWARD TETHER

JANET ZHUN NASSIF

HOLT, RINEHART AND WINSTON, PUBLISHERS

NEW YORK   TORONTO   MEXICO CITY   LONDON   SYDNEY   TOKYO

AUTHORS

JAMES H. OTTO was head of the Science Department of George Washington High School, Indianapolis, Indiana.

CLOYD J. JULIAN is a former principal of George Washington High School, Indianapolis, Indiana, and a classroom teacher of health, as well as a former consultant in Health, Safety, Physical Education, and Athletics for the Public Schools of Indianapolis. Presently, he is a teacher of health education at Wood High School of Continuing Education, Indianapolis, Indiana.

J. EDWARD TETHER, M.D., F.A.C.P., is Associate Professor of Neurology, Indiana University Medical Center and School of Medicine, Indianapolis, Indiana, a member of the American Medical Association and the American Academy of Neurology, and a Fellow of the American College of Physicians.

JANET ZHUN NASSIF holds a Master of Public Health degree in health education from Columbia University. She is an active member of the American School Health Association and the American Public Health Association. She is an associate of the National Center for Health Education and a director for New Healthways. She has served as coordinator of Community Health Promotion, National Health Council. She also has served as a consultant and high school faculty member for the New York City Board of Education.

Cover photo credits
Center: Richard Hutchings; Photo Researchers
Top Left: Nadeau; The Stock Market
Top Right: Walker Iooss Jr.; Image Bank
Bottom Left: M M Productions; Image Bank
Bottom Right: Ken Lax; The Stock Shop

Acknowledgments and photo credits appear on pages 578, 579

ISBN 0-03-071902-X
45678 032 987654321

PREFACE

In recent years there has been an increased emphasis on health promotion and disease prevention. The new edition of *Modern Health,* while maintaining the comprehensiveness of past editions, also reflects this wellness focus in health education. Throughout, the edition emphasizes student self-awareness for better health and the development of personal skills for health improvement.

The first unit, "Help Yourself to Health," explores the importance of developing good health habits and taking personal responsibility for health. Topics covered include the importance of life-style, decision-making, good nutrition, the structure and function of bones and muscles, and the basics of a fitness program. Students are encouraged to develop their own personal fitness programs for healthier life-styles.

Unit 2, "Your Personality," begins with a chapter on appearance, since personality is often reflected in how we look and feel. A chapter on behavior examines human behavior from a nature-nurture perspective. A chapter on emotions includes a description of human emotions and a new section on marriage, the family, and human-relations skills.

Unit 3, "Personality Under Stress," often elicits high interest since most teenagers experience emotional turmoil and are keenly interested in understanding themselves. A chapter on stress describes how stress affects your health and how to manage stress. A chapter on defensive mechanisms explains defensive behavior, using anecdotes to illustrate each mechanism. In a chapter on mental disorders, anecdotes and case studies also are used to make this information more interesting and understandable. A chapter on psychotherapy gives a brief history of how mental disorders have been viewed, describes the purpose of therapy, and lists some sources of help today for the personality in trouble.

Unit 4, "Substance Use and Abuse," presents timely, detailed and practical information on drugs, alcohol, and tobacco. The information is presented without the use of scare tactics and sensationalism. Decision-making skills are emphasized in these chapters since many teenagers are subjected to strong peer pressure to try drugs, alcohol, and tobacco.

Units 5 and 6 explore human anatomy and physiology. The wellness theme runs thoughout these chapters. Information on prevention and treatment of common disorders of each system is detailed.

Unit 7 begins with a new chapter on heredity that gives students an introduction to genetics, some common genetic disorders, and prenatal care. A chapter on today's leading causes of death also follows the wellness approach. Information is provided on the risk factors, symptoms, causes, prevention strategies, and latest medical treatments for these diseases. In a new section, aging and death are described as natural parts of life. The chapter on infectious diseases includes up-to-date descriptions of the causes of diseases, some disease problems (including sexually transmitted diseases), how the immune system works, and autoimmunity.

Unit 8, "Safeguarding Your Health," begins with a chapter on public health and the environment. This chapter has been revised to reflect timely issues such as sources of pollution, the effects of pollution on health, and what the individual can do to minimize risks. Other chapters in the unit provide practical consumer information on getting health care, the basics of safety and accident prevention, and a brief introduction to first aid procedures.

Several medical and educational authorities read and offered suggestions for chapters in their fields of specialty. The authors are indebted to these authorities.

The new **Modern Health** textbook has the following features:

- Colorful, contemporary photographs and illustrations help clarify and reinforce concepts in the text.
- **Objectives** at the beginning of each chapter identify learning outcomes and skill performances that are expected at the end of each chapter.
- A **Motivational Story** introduces each chapter.
- A **Summary** at the end of each chapter summarizes the key concepts in the chapter.
- Technical vocabulary, in boldface with phonetic spelling, is included in each chapter to aid students in identifying and pronouncing words.
- **Health in History** marginal notes are interesting historical facts related to health.
- **Health Tips** marginal notes provide practical, consumer-oriented advice on health care.
- **Health Action** marginal notes enable students to apply material learned to practical situations.
- **Careers** provides information on responsibilities, requirements, and where to get further information concerning the health professions.
- **Focus on Health** describes interesting recent developments in the health field.
- **Wellness Watch** self-tests help students determine whether or not they are following good health habits.
- **Words at Work** helps students review chapter vocabulary.
- **Review Questions** provides immediate reinforcement and a self-test of chapter material.
- **Discussion Questions** presents higher-level questions that challenge students to think.
- **Investigating** activities are easy and fun to perform. They enhance the learning process and make health education come alive in the classroom. They also engage the student in an active learning process.

CONTENTS

1

HELP YOURSELF TO HEALTH

YOUR PERSONALITY

PERSONALITY UNDER STRESS

SUBSTANCE USE AND ABUSE

YOUR CONTROL SYSTEMS

YOUR SUPPLY SYSTEM

7

HEALTH PROMOTION AND PROTECTION

SAFEGUARDING YOUR HEALTH

UNIT 1

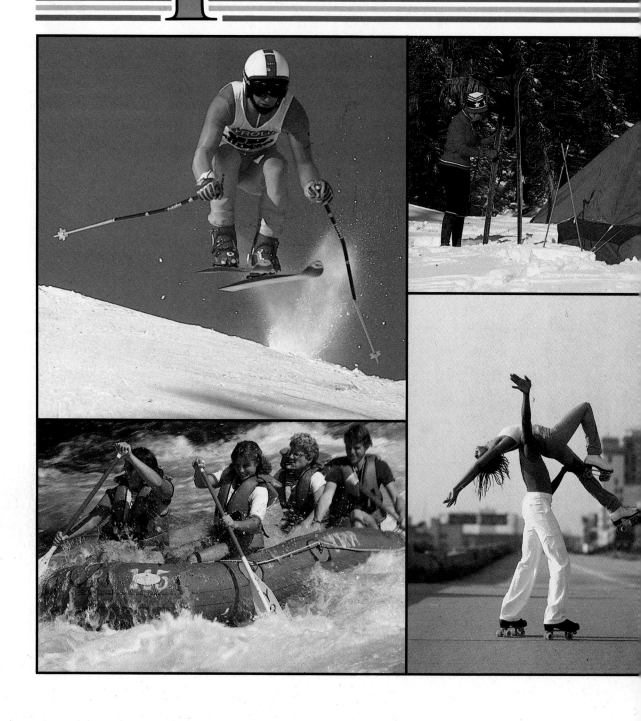

Help Yourself to Health

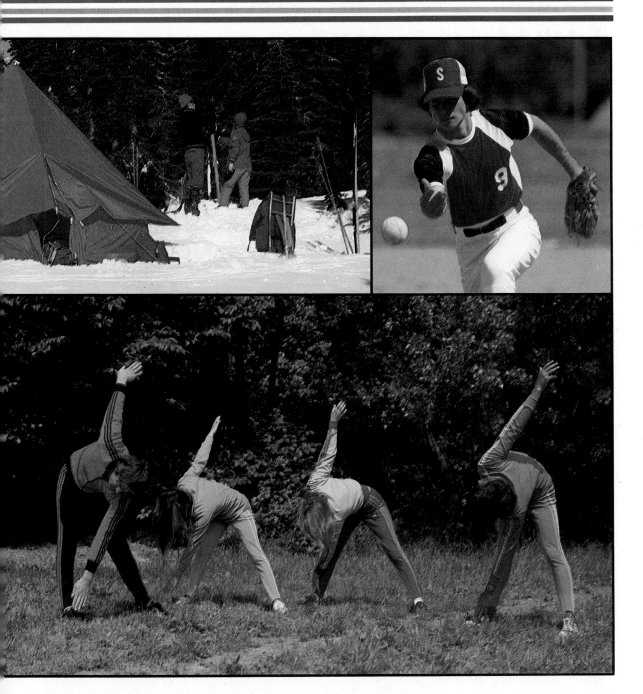

CHAPTER 1

A Life-Style for Wellness

OBJECTIVES

- EXPLAIN why the new focus in health is on life-style and wellness
- IDENTIFY the factors that make up health and a positive life-style
- OUTLINE factors that affect health behavior
- NAME the steps involved in good decision-making and be able to APPLY these steps to real-life situations

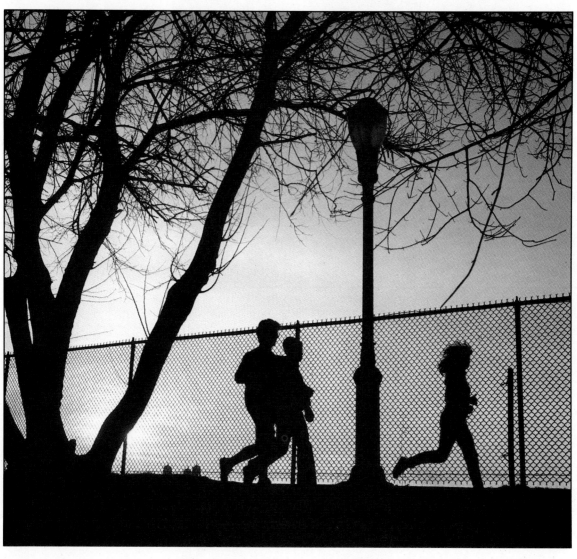

Monday morning Mike was up early. He jogged his usual two miles, showered, ate a good breakfast, and flossed and brushed his teeth. Gosh, he thought, I feel ready for anything today!

After school he met his friend Tom. "You look beat Tom," Mike exclaimed, "What's wrong?" "Aw, nothing," Tom replied, "just my usual Monday blahs. Too much weekend partying, I guess." Tom had only had four hours of sleep the night before and had awakened late feeling dead tired. He skipped breakfast and ate a candy bar on the way to school for energy. "I need a cigarette to rev me up. Want to join me?" asked Tom. "Hey, Tom, you know I don't smoke. Why don't you forget the cigarette and come running with me instead," Mike suggested. "I always feel better after some exercise. Keeps me healthy." Tom laughed, "You know that's not for me Mike. I get plenty of exercise just walking to class and changing the TV channels. And I'm healthy, too. Besides there's always Doc Williams to take care of me if I run into problems. Don't try to turn me into a 'health nut'!" Mike shrugged and laughed. "You're impossible Tom. You're the real 'health nut.' "

Obviously, Mike and Tom have different ideas about health and the way they choose to live. Do they each have a valid point of view?

YOUR HEALTH IS UP TO YOU

What does good health mean to you? Would you say that being in good health is the same as not being sick? What about days when you feel tired or out-of-sorts? Are you in good health then, too? Health means different things to different people. The World Health Organization has defined **health** as a "state of complete physical, mental, and social well-being, not merely the absence of disease." In other words, your health involves your whole being and the environment in which you live. A healthy body is strong, fit, energetic and well-nourished. A healthy mind is one that has a positive attitude toward life. Together, a healthy mind and body provide the basis for social well-being. You can enjoy all aspects of your environment, including your school, family, and friends.

YOUR HEALTH HERITAGE

No generation of Americans has as many opportunities to enjoy good health as you have. **Infectious diseases,** great killers of the past, have been brought under control through better sanitation, housing, and nutrition. Immunization and

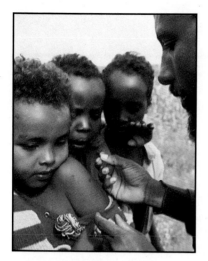

1–1. Some infectious diseases, like smallpox, have been wiped out through worldwide vaccination programs.

Table 1–1

improved medical care have also helped win the battle against these diseases. You need not worry about epidemics of smallpox, typhoid, or diphtheria as Americans once did. In fact, you probably take your health for granted as long as you are not feeling sick.

PAST AND PRESENT. At the beginning of this century, the health picture was very different. One out of ten babies born did not survive infancy. Babies who lived could expect an average life span of only 47 years. Table 1-1 shows the leading causes of death in 1900. As you can see, they were infectious diseases such as pneumonia, influenza, and tuberculosis.

TEN LEADING CAUSES OF DEATH	
1900	1980
Flu and pneumonia	Diseases of the heart
Tuberculosis	Cancer
Inflammation of parts of the digestive tract	Circulatory diseases of the brain, including strokes
Diseases of the heart	Accidents
Circulatory diseases of the brain, including strokes	Chronic lung diseases, including bronchitis and emphysema
Kidney disease	Pneumonia and flu
Accidents	Diabetes mellitis
Cancer	Liver diseases, including cirrhosis
Certain diseases of infancy	Artherosclerosis
Diphtheria	Suicide

HEALTH IN HISTORY

Infectious diseases did not become a serious health threat to civilization until about 10,000 years ago. Up to then, humans lived like nomads in small groups and had an adequate food supply. Once they settled in specific areas, the population expanded more quickly than the food supply. Weakened by hunger and malnutrition, people easily fell prey to infectious diseases, which thrived up to the twentieth century.

Today most children live to adulthood. A baby born in the 1980's can look forward to an average life expectancy of nearly 74 years. This is more than a 50% increase in life span! Look at the table again. What were the leading causes of death in 1980? The three leading causes of death were **chronic diseases:** heart disease, cancer, and circulatory diseases. Why do you think that the major causes of death have shifted away from infectious diseases? Now that infectious diseases have been conquered, people are living longer. So chronic diseases, which usually take a long time to develop, are finally taking their health toll.

Since the rise of chronic diseases, medicine has been hard at work to cure or control them. Major progress has been made. We now have new drugs, miracle operations, and other amazing techniques to combat chronic diseases. Many lives have been saved through such medical marvels.

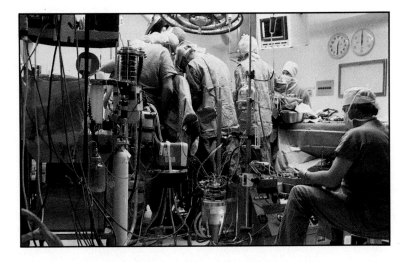

1–2. The techniques of modern surgery can correct some modern health problems, but a life-style directed toward wellness is a better safeguard for your health.

Yet for too many Americans this help comes too late. Chronic illnesses often rob them of a normal life and cause premature death. Despite advanced technology, modern medicine has not overcome the leading causes of death today. Why not?

Yesteryear's killers were largely caused by microorganisms. Once identified, specific public health measures could be developed to conquer them. The causes and effects of diseases were clear. Today the answers are not so clear-cut. Research shows that many factors, not a single cause, contribute to our present pattern of illness and death. Most of these factors relate to the way we live. Here modern medicine has little influence. Each individual, not the doctor, now has the key role in determining health.

HEALTH RISKS

Would you expect to do well in school without studying? Certainly your chances of getting good grades improve when you prepare for your classes properly. Not studying poses a risk if you want to be a good student. This is a risk factor you can control.

Good health depends on many **risk factors.** These factors can be grouped into three major areas: heredity, environment, and life-style.

HEREDITY.   At birth, we do not all have the same chances of developing various health problems. We inherit certain traits from our parents that may increase or decrease our chances of developing different diseases. For example, a

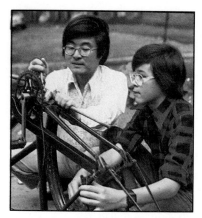

1–3. Heredity determines a variety of traits including the tendency for certain health problems. For example, it is more likely that you will have weak eyes if your parents do.

baby whose family has a history of heart disease has a greater than average chance of developing this same problem later in life. Whether you were born a boy or a girl makes a difference too. Some diseases, such as breast cancer, generally affect only females. Males have a higher chance of developing other life-threatening health problems.

Heredity is a risk factor that you cannot control. You must work with the biological potential that you have inherited. However, a family history of certain health problems does not mean that you will automatically develop these problems. Much depends on your environment and life-style.

ENVIRONMENT. The total environment in which we live, including physical, social, and economic factors, can also affect our health. Risks within the physical environment may include exposure to radiation, unsafe consumer products, and the quality of air, water, and food. Your social environment includes your family and your friends. The support of a caring family eases the stress of living that can jeopardize health. Factors within your economic environment, such as whether or not your community has adequate medical services or good housing, can also affect health.

You can control some environmental risks. For example, you can limit your exposure to unnecessary radiation and choose consumer products wisely. Other environmental risks are generally beyond an individual's control. For the most part you cannot change the availability of medical services in your neighborhood or affect the quality of the air you breathe. To reduce these risks requires broader community action.

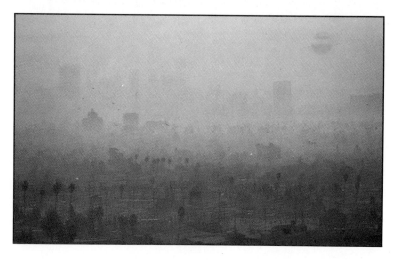

1–4. Heavy smog in some urban areas can create respiratory problems for many people.

LIFE-STYLE: THE KEY TO GOOD HEALTH. Your *life-style,* which is the way you live, has the greatest affect on health. Statistics show that seven out of ten leading causes of death are related to personal habits and behavior. In other words, what you eat, what you drink, whether or not you smoke or use drugs, your mental attitude and how you handle daily stress all affect your health.

Let's use your age group as an example. In your age group the leading cause of death and disability is accidents, mostly automobile accidents. Can you think of any personal habits or behavior that might lead to accidental deaths and injuries? Speeding, drinking while driving, and not wearing seat belts are a few examples of how teenagers' actions can increase their risks of accidents.

Let's now focus on adults. The leading cause of adult deaths overall is heart disease. The risk of heart disease increases with factors such as smoking, the amount you are overweight, and the lack of exercise. These risk factors are related to the way people live.

So at any age good health is not the result of luck or fate. Nor is it just a matter of medical care. Your health today and in the future depends a great deal on your life-style.

WELLNESS: THE NEW HEALTH FOCUS

The expression "an ounce of prevention is worth a pound of cure" is certainly true about health. By following positive health habits, you decrease your health risks and increase your chances for a long life. Most important, you also improve the quality of your life from day to day. The new focus on health is not just avoiding sickness in the future, but achieving total wellness today. When you are totally well, you enjoy life to the fullest. Of course, you are sick less often. You also feel good and look your best. You have more energy and endurance, sleep better, and feel more confident. Your body is in good shape, your eyes are clear, and your skin and hair are healthy. You are more enthusiastic about life. This positive sense of well-being extends to your relationships with family, friends, and others.

To achieve total wellness requires a **holistic** (whole-**iss**-tic) approach to health. This means that your body, mind, and spirit are key factors in your total health. The environments in which you live, work, and play contribute to total wellness, too. Do you think total wellness is a goal worth striving for?

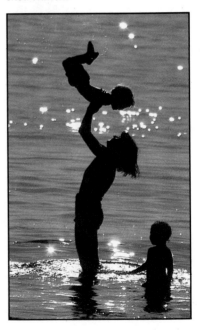

1–5. The holistic model of health includes your mental and physical well-being as well as your environment.

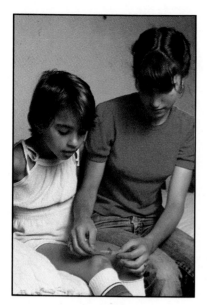

1–6. Young adults are role models for children.

WHAT INFLUENCES HEALTH HABITS

Why do some people live an unhealthful life even though they know the difference between good and poor health habits? For example, why do people still smoke when they know it greatly increases their risks of getting cancer and heart disease?

Health behavior, like all human behavior, is not easily explained. There are many interacting factors that can influence a person's behavior. Let's use Tom and Mike, whom you met at the chapter's opening, as an example. If you discussed smoking with each of them you would learn more about why each behaves differently. They have different attitudes, values, perceptions, beliefs, and backgrounds, which all influence their behavior. Their responses are shown in Table 1-2. Can you think of another reason why Tom might smoke? Once any habit is formed, the behavior pattern is hard to change. So achieving wellness depends on avoiding poor habits and building positive health habits. This requires becoming aware of your habits and learning to make responsible decisions about your health behavior each day.

DECISION-MAKING SKILLS

Each day throughout life you have to make your own decisions not only on matters that concern your health, but on other matters as well. Many people make decisions on impulse or from habit, without much thought. They do not consider the consequences of their decisions. Whether you make decisions carefully or without much thought, the decisions you make will affect your behavior, your life-style, and your health.

What are some key decisions you will face in the future? You will have to make decisions about your life-style, education, career, and marriage. What are some decisions that you may face now that can have a major impact on your life? These might include decisions about whether or not to use alcohol, drugs, and tobacco. You may also have to make decisions about dating, who your friends will be, and how to use your leisure time. Good **decision-making skills** can help you reach your full health potential not just in terms of physical health but in other aspects of your life as well. These skills help you develop an awareness of who you are today and who you can become.

Here are some steps that you can take to make better decisions.

1. Define the decision that you must make.
2. Get as much reliable information as possible on the matter in question.
3. Identify all the other possible choices.
4. Examine the probable negative and positive effects of each choice.
5. Identify your goals (what you want to achieve) and your values (the aspects of life, such as friendship, money, and self-respect, which are important to you).
6. Evaluate and rank all choices.
7. Develop and implement your plan of action.
8. Assess the results of your action.

Table 1–2

MAJOR FACTORS IN HEALTH BEHAVIOR USING SMOKING AS AN EXAMPLE

	Tom	Mike
KNOWLEDGE (What do you know about the issue?)	"In health class I learned that smoking causes cancer."	"My parents told me about the dangers of smoking and I also studied about it in health class."
ATTITUDES AND BELIEFS (What do you feel and believe about the issue?)	"I feel very adult when I smoke. I know that smoking is supposed to cause cancer but I don't completely believe it. Not every smoker gets cancer."	"I don't need to smoke to feel mature. I believe smoking causes cancer. Scientific evidence is impressive."
VALUE OF HEALTH (What value do you place on your health?)	"I'm almost never sick so why should I pay attention to my health?"	"I want to look and feel good so being fit and healthy is important to me."
PERCEIVED RISK (What personal risk do you associate with the issue?)	"You have to smoke a long time before you get cancer. I've got a greater chance of getting killed crossing a street."	"My family has a history of heart disease and cancer. I don't need any unnecessary risks."
PERCEIVED CONTROL AND RESPONSIBILITY (What control can you exercise over the issue?)	"Whether or not you get cancer is a matter of luck. I can't do anything about it, so why worry?"	"I like being in charge of my life. I know my chances of getting lung cancer are slim if I don't smoke."
AVAILABILITY (How available are related products or services?)	"I always carry a pack of cigarettes with me but if I run out there's always a vending machine or store where they are available."	"Cigarettes are widely available so I know it's hard for some teens to resist smoking."
SKILLS (Do you have the decision-making, consumer health, or other skills necessary for positive health action?)	"I never really made a real decision to smoke. I just started smoking now and then. Now it's a habit."	"I know I can smoke if I want to but I thought about the pros and cons. I've decided it's not for me."
SOCIAL ENVIRONMENT (What support does your environment provide?)	"My parents smoke. So do most of my friends. Those cigarette ads are very appealing."	"My parents are proud that I don't smoke, They gave it up themselves. Tom's the only friend I have who smokes. I wish he'd quit."

1–7. Each year, thousands of people run in marathons.

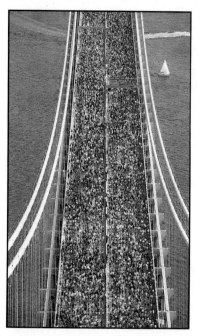

You can use these steps for all important decisions that you must make, including decisions about alcohol, tobacco, drugs, and personal relationships. You may have to consider what is most important to you, such as feeling good about yourself or guilty about your actions; doing what you know is right or conforming to the crowd; and weighing popularity against being your own person. Sometimes writing down all of your possible choices and their possible outcomes can help you to make the right decision. (See the "Decision-Making Tree" in the Appendix.) Are you ready to make your own decisions carefully and take responsibility for yourself?

YOUR HEALTH DECISIONS

Are you conscious of all the decisions you make each day that affect your health? In today's world more people are becoming aware of their health and are making conscious decisions to improve their own health habits and life-styles. Just think about it for a moment. Joggers are now a common sight. This was not true 20 years ago. Aerobics and body-building for men and women are just two of the many kinds of exercises that are popular today. Think of all the health and exercise clubs that have sprung up overnight. People are more conscious of what foods they eat. There are many available groups to help people stop smoking, lose weight, or form other more positive health habits. People are also growing more interested in their mental well-being. Many are learning how to manage the stress in their lives naturally without alcohol, tobacco, or drugs. They are seeking ways to realize their full human potential and achieve total wellness. Why have health and wellness become so important to so many people? What personal payoffs does it hold for you?

EVALUATING YOUR OWN HEALTH HABITS AND LIFE-STYLE

Is your life-style on target for wellness? You do not have to live a rigid, restrictive life. Some basic changes in the way you live can make an important difference. Physical fitness tones and trims the body so that you can actively enjoy life. As little as thirty minutes of exercise three times a week can help keep you fit. Good nutrition gives you the energy you need for work and play. If you eat breakfast regularly, consume *more* fresh vegetables and fruit, and eat *less* sugary, fatty, and salty foods, your diet will improve. Stress control prevents the tension of daily life from wearing down physical and mental health. Everyone needs a relaxing break each day. Good communication with family and friends and community participation ease stress too. If you avoid alcohol, tobacco and drug use, you reduce unnecessary health risks. Why not enjoy life naturally? Good safety habits and wise medical care safeguard your health so you can enjoy the benefits a healthful life brings. The wellness test on page 12 can help you evaluate your health habits.

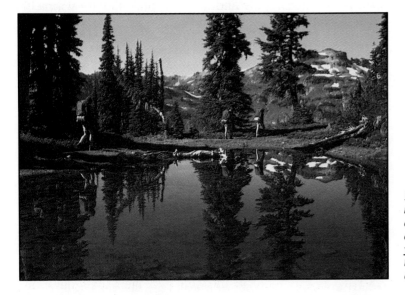

1–8. You will need to make many decisions during your life that will affect your health. How you spend your leisure time is one of these decisions.

SUMMARY: Health is not merely the absence of disease. It involves your whole being and the total environment in which you live. Infectious diseases, the major killers of the past, were overcome by improved sanitation, housing, nutrition, and medical care. The leading causes of death and ill health today are accidents and chronic diseases. Heredity and the environment pose health risks, but life-style plays a major role in these problems. The new focus in health is not just on curing sickness or avoiding it, but on helping people achieve total wellness through positive health habits and life-style. This includes physical fitness; nutrition; stress control; avoiding alcohol, tobacco, or drug use; practicing good safety habits; and using medical care wisely. Wellness begins with the individual's taking responsibility for health and using decison-making skills to make better life-style choices.

On a sheet of paper, answer each of the following questions with *almost always, very often, sometimes,* or *almost never.*

WELLNESS TEST

HEALTH AND SAFETY HABITS

1. I wear a seat belt while riding in a car.
2. I avoid riding with someone who drives while under the influence of alcohol or other drugs.
3. I am careful when using potentially harmful products or substances (such as poisons, and electrical devices).
4. I avoid drinking alcohol.
5. I read and follow the label directions when using prescribed drugs.
6. I avoid smoking cigarettes and using other forms of tobacco.
7. I brush and floss my teeth every day.
8. I avoid illegal drug use.
9. I practice monthly self-examination for cancer (girls, breast; boys, testicles).
10. I know when to seek professional care for mental and physical problems and do not delay treatment.

NUTRITION

1. I do not eat fast food more than twice a week.
2. I eat breakfast daily.
3. I eat a fresh fruit or vegetable each day.
4. I avoid eating sweets, including sugary breakfast cereals, and I drink fewer than five soft drinks a week.
5. I limit the amount of beef and pork in my diet and eat fewer than four eggs per week.
6. I avoid fried or fatty foods.
7. I avoid foods with aritificial colors and flavors.
8. I do not snack between meals on sweet or salty foods.
9. I taste my food before salting.
10. I maintain a healthful body weight, avoiding being overweight and/or underweight.

STRESS

1. I find time to enjoy relaxing activities each day.
2. I participate in group activities such as religious, school, or community events or hobbies that I enjoy.
3. I can fall asleep within 20 minutes when I go to bed and enjoy 7-8 hr of rest each night.
4. I do not rely on alcohol, tobacco, or drugs.
5. I find it easy to relax and to feel and express emotions.
6. I recognize and prepare for events or situations that are likely to be stressful to me.
7. I am generally healthy and free of symptoms of illness.
8. I have close friends or relatives whom I can talk to about personal matters and call on for help.
9. I avoid procrastination.
10. I am satisfied with my life and have an enthusiastic outlook.

FITNESS

1. When practical, I walk or bike rather than ride in a motor vehicle.
2. When practical, I use the stairs instead of escalators or elevators.
3. I enjoy physical activity.
4. I engage in exercise each day.
5. I do vigorous exercise such as running, swimming, or brisk walking for 15-30 minutes at least three times a week.
6. I do exercises that enhance my muscle tone such as stretching, yoga, or calisthenics for 15–30 minutes at least three times a week.
7. I do warm-up and cool-down exercises as part of my fitness activity.
8. I engage in sports or other fitness-related leisure activities such as bicycling that I can continue to participate in throughout my life.
9. I avoid vigorous exercise for at least two hours after eating.
10. I have enough energy for daily exercise, work, and play.

NUTRITION

I eat whatever and whenever I want, without regard to good nutrition. 1-12

I practice good eating habits if it is convenient. 13-26

I practice good eating habits with conscious effort. 27-39

Good eating habits are a part of my lifestyle. 40-50

GENERAL LIFE-STYLE

I live my life without regard to health risks such as smoking, drugs, alcohol, and safety risks. 1-12

I practice risk-reducing habits if convenient. 13-26

I usually practice risk-reducing habits. 27-39

Risk-reducing habits are a way of life. 40-50

FITNESS

I lead an inactive life and rarely get exercise. 1-12

I exercise if it is convenient or if I'm in the mood. 13-26

I exercise often, but not regularly and not for total fitness. 27-39

I exercise regularly for total fitness. 40-50

STRESS

I do not take time to enjoy relaxing activities and I'm bothered by stress-related symptoms. 1-12

My lifestyle is too hectic to enjoy relaxing activities each day and I may be

No matter how busy, I find time to relax each day. 40-50

I usually find time to relax each day. 27-39

I enjoy relaxing activities regularly. 13-26

To find out how healthful your life-style is, score your answers as follows:

Almost always = 5
Very often = 3
Sometimes = 1
Almost never = 0

Add up your scores in each of the four areas to see how healthful your life-style is.

CHAPTER REVIEW

words at work

Use the words below to fill in the blanks. DO NOT WRITE IN THIS BOOK.

In the past, _____ were the major cause of most deaths. Today, _____ such as cancer, heart disease, and stroke, claim most lives. Factors that increase a person's chances of accidents, death, or illness are known as _____. _____ is one risk factor that we cannot control. We can control certain risk factors in our _____. The new focus on health is _____. It involves taking a _____ approach to health and making positive changes in _____.

risk factors	holistic
environment	life-style
infectious diseases	heredity
wellness	chronic diseases

review questions

1. Give the World Health Organization's definition of health.
2. Contrast the leading causes of death today to those at the turn of the century.
3. Explain the meaning of the term *life-style*.
4. Name three risk factors that affect health.
5. Does heredity determine whether you will develop certain diseases? Explain your answer.
6. Explain how the leading cause of teenage death is related to life-style.
7. Cite three factors that comprise a positive life-style.
8. Define the first step toward achieving a wellness life-style.
9. Outline five factors that can affect health behavior.
10. Explain the role of self-responsibility in the decision-making process.
11. Define the first step in the decision-making process.

discussion questions

1. Do you think that our society promotes a positive wellness life-style? Give evidence to support your answer.
2. Higher income tax rates for smokers have been suggested, since society bears the cost for increased poor health. Do you think such measures should be sanctioned? Why or why not?
3. Discuss the statement "an ounce of prevention is worth a pound of cure" in relation to today's health problems.
4. How important are decision-making skills? Cite examples to support your position.
5. In your opinion, what are the major problems people encounter in trying to change poor health habits?

investigating

PURPOSE:
To evaluate your health habits, devise a plan to improve them, and follow the plan for one month.

MATERIALS NEEDED:
Paper and pencil.

PROCEDURE:
A.   Take the wellness test on page 12.
    1.   What are your scores for general life-style, stress, nutrition, and fitness?
B.   Look over the questions on page 12. Think about a positive health habit that you would like to establish.
    2.   In one sentence, state the positive health habit you would like to work on. For example, you may want to increase your exercise or quit smoking.
C.   Develop a plan of action for the next month to help you establish your chosen health habit.
    3.   State what you will do and when you will do it. For example, you may state, "Each day I will eat breakfast, fewer sweets and fatty foods, and at least one fresh fruit."
D.   Make a calendar for one month. Keep a record of your progress on your calendar. For example, if you have decided to increase your physical activity, write down how much you exercise each day.

CHAPTER 2

Nutrition

OBJECTIVES

- NAME the basic nutrients and outline their functions in the human body
- EXPLAIN the principles of the U.S. dietary guidelines and necessary diet changes to reach them

- COMPARE foods for their nutritional value
- APPLY the principles of nutrition to eating habits and maintenance of desirable body weight
- DESCRIBE consumer issues in nutrition

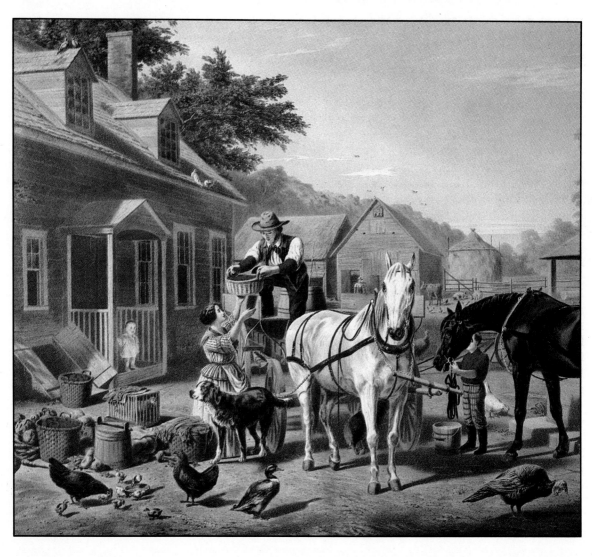

Marcia and her brother George were rushing to get dressed for school. As George quickly buttoned his shirt, he glanced in the mirror. "Why am I so skinny?" he sighed.

Marcia was in her room tugging at her skirt. "Have I gained weight?" she wondered. "This skirt fit perfectly last month. Now it seems snug."

At breakfast Marcia gulped some coffee and then announced, "No oatmeal for me. It's too fattening." "I won't have any either," George said as he raced out of the house. "I'll just eat a doughnut on the way to school."

Do their decisions make good nutritional sense?

FOOD: FOUNDATION OF LIFE

Do you know if your diet is a healthy one or not? Everyone should be concerned about their diet. The stakes are high. Total fitness can be achieved only if the body gets proper nourishment. Food supplies the energy you need for studying, playing sports, and doing all of your other activities. Food also supplies the **nutrients** (**new**-tree-ents) your body needs to grow and repair itself. Food, in part, determines how you develop and whether or not you reach your full physical and mental potential.

Beyond health, food adds pleasure to life. Can you imagine a party without something good to eat or a traditional holiday without special foods? Eating with family and friends gives you a chance to relax, talk, and share experiences and feelings.

Clearly there is a strong and growing interest in nutrition in our country. Health food stores, diet books, vitamin ads and "natural" foods are just a few signs of this. But, you need solid knowledge of the subject to separate food facts from fads and sound nutrition from nonsense. In this chapter you will learn the basics of good nutrition. You will also learn how you can apply the knowledge and skills to your own diet decisions.

THE AMERICAN DIET: PAST AND PRESENT

Since the early 1900's, the American diet has undergone major changes. Around 1910, the typical American diet included a lot of flour and whole grains such as rye, barley,

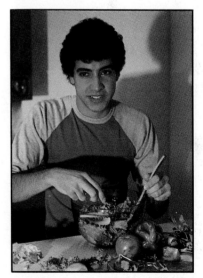

2–1. Food can be a pleasure to prepare as well as to eat. Do you enjoy cooking?

and corn. Fresh potatoes were plentiful. People relied on fresh or canned fruits or vegetables because frozen foods were unknown. They consumed little red meat and few sweets, such as soft drinks.

This is not true today. The average American diet today consists of over 30 percent more red meat than its 1910 counterpart. Today, Americans eat fewer whole-grain products and fresh potatoes. On the other hand, they do eat more fruits and vegetables.

Why has there been such a great shift in our diet and food habits? A changing food industry and American life-style have affected our eating habits. Convenience and fast foods, which are often high in sugar and fats, have grown in popularity. Today, highly sugared soft drinks have replaced milk as the preferred beverage of Americans. In 1982 the average American drank almost 40 gallons of soft drinks.

The American diet has also changed due to a lack of understanding of nutrition. For example, people often shun flour and whole-grain products such as bread. Why? Many people have the mistaken belief that they are fattening.

DIETARY HEALTH RISKS AND GUIDELINES.　These diet changes have had an impact on our health as a nation. Today, many of the leading causes of death are linked to dietary habits, as well as other life-style practices.

Look at Table 2-1. These government guidelines are based on scientific research about diet and disease. These guidelines cannot guarantee health. But together with other good health habits, such as exercise, they can improve your health and reduce your risk of developing chronic diseases.

GOOD NUTRITION

How would you define good nutrition? Good nutrition provides the body with all the nutrients it needs. Nutrients are chemical substances that the body requires for energy, the growth and repair of tissues, and the regulation of functions. Over 55 different nutrients have been discovered. They are divided into six major groups: **carbohydrates, fats, proteins, minerals, vitamins,** and **water.** *All* of these key nutrients are needed in varying amounts. Different foods provide different amounts of the key nutrients. No one food supplies them all. Therefore, good nutrition begins with the first dietary guideline: *eat a variety of foods.*

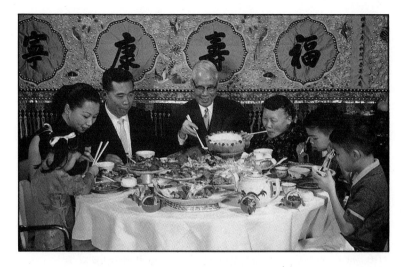

2–2. There are many enjoyable ways to add variety to your diet.

Table 2–1

DIETARY GUIDELINES

1. Eat a variety of foods.
- Include selections from fruits; vegetables; milk, cheese, yogurt; meats, poultry, fish, eggs; and legumes (dry peas and beans), whole-grain and enriched breads, cereals, and grain products.

2. Maintain ideal weight.
- To improve eating habits: eat slowly; prepare smaller portions; avoid "seconds."
- To lose weight: increase physical activity; eat less fat and fewer fatty foods; eat less sugar and fewer sweets; avoid too much alcohol.

3. Avoid too much fat, saturated fat, and cholesterol.
- Choose lean meat, fish, poultry, dry beans, and peas as your protein sources.
- Moderate your use of eggs and organ meats (such as liver).
- Limit your intake of butter, cream, hydrogenated margarines, shortenings, and coconut oil, and foods made from such products.

4. Eat foods with adequate starch and fiber.
- Substitute starches for fat and sugar. Select foods that are good sources of fiber and starch, such as whole-grain breads and cereals, fruits and vegetables, beans, peas, and nuts.

5. Avoid too much sugar
- Use less of all sugars, including white sugar, brown sugar, raw sugar, honey, and syrups.
- Eat fewer foods containing these sugars, such as candy, soft drinks, ice cream, cake, and cookies.
- Select fresh fruits or fruits canned without sugar or with light syrup rather than heavy syrup.
- Read food labels for clues on sugar content: if the names sucrose, glucose, dextrose, lactose, fructose, or corn syrup appear first, there is some sugar.
- Remember, how often you eat sugar is as important as how much sugar you eat.

6. Avoid too much sodium.
- Learn to enjoy the unsalted flavors of foods.
- Cook with only small amounts of added salt.
- Add little or no salt to food at the table.
- Limit your intake of salty foods, such as potato chips, pretzels, salted nuts and popcorn, condiments (soy sauce, garlic salt), cheese, pickled foods, and cured meats.
- Read food labels carefully to determine the amounts of sodium in processed foods and snack items.

7. If you drink alcohol, do so in moderation.

Source: *Nutrition and Your Health: Dietary Guidelines for Americans,* U.S. Department of Agriculture and U.S. Department of Health, Education & Welfare.

ENERGY VALUE OF FOODS

Your body digests the food you eat by breaking it down into nutrients. These nutrients are carried to the cells by the bloodstream. At the cell level, some of them are further broken down to produce energy. Food scientists measure the amount of energy in foods in *kilocalories*, more commonly referred to as **Calories** (**kal**-lor-rees). A Calorie is the amount of heat required to raise the temperature of one kilogram (35 oz) of water one degree centigrade. Foods vary in Calorie content. For example, a slice of bread provides about 70 Calories of energy. Spread a tablespoon of peanut butter on the bread and you add 85 more Calories.

PROTEIN

The term *protein* is derived from the Greek word meaning *primary* or *holding first place.* This nutrient is aptly named, since it accounts for many vital body functions. Protein supplies about 4 Calories of energy per gram. It also builds, repairs, and maintains the body. The texture of your hair and nails and the structure of your muscles depend on protein. Protein is found in *hemoglobin*, the substance that transports oxygen to the cells, and in *enzymes*, which control body processes.

The building blocks of protein are known as **amino acids.** The body can make some amino acids. The other amino acids, known as the *essential amino acids*, must be supplied by the food we eat. *High-quality proteins* supply a large amount of these essential amino acids. Animal foods, such as milk, eggs, meat, and fish, provide high-quality proteins. *Low-quality proteins* are low in certain essential amino acids. Plant foods, such as beans, peas, and cereal grains, provide low-quality proteins. However, do not discount their value. When different plant foods are combined, high-quality protein results. For example, combining rice and beans can supply the same protein value as a steak. Also, when plant foods are combined with a small amount of an animal food, the overall protein value of a dish improves. For example, macaroni and cheese or milk and cereal are protein-rich combinations. Are you concerned about getting enough protein in your diet? Don't be. Most Americans eat *twice* the protein the body requires. About 12 percent of the Calories in a typical daily diet are supplied by protein. Far too much of the protein consumed comes from animal sources. They are higher in saturated fats than plant foods.

HEALTH IN HISTORY

Have you ever heard the term "limey" used to describe a British sailor? When sailors lived for months at sea, eating nothing but canned foods, they developed a disease called "scurvy." Its symptoms were bleeding gums, aching joints, infections, and skin bruising. Many sailors died. By accident it was discovered that eating limes cured this disease. Thereafter, sailors ate a lot of limes and acquired the nickname limeys. It was actually vitamin C (contained in all citrus fruits) that cured the illness.

CARBOHYDRATES

If you are interested in having ample energy for sports or fuel to power your brain, pay attention to this nutrient. Carbohydrates come from plant foods. The name *carbo* (carbon) *hydrate* (water) explains their chemical composition. Plants use the sun's energy to put carbon dioxide and water together to form carbohydrates. During digestion, carbohydrates are broken down into **glucose,** the body's primary fuel. The bloodstream carries glucose to the cells, where it is broken down to produce energy. Carbohydrates provide 4 Calories per gram. Glucose not needed right away for energy is either stored in the liver and muscles as a starch called **glycogen** (**glie-**koe-jen), or it is stored as body fat.

SIMPLE AND COMPLEX CARBOHYDRATES. Plants provide either *simple* or *complex carbohydrates.* Simple carbohydrates are sugars that are present naturally in fruits, vegetables, and milk products. Refined sugars (such as cane or beet sugar) or processed sugars (such as corn syrups, molasses or honey) are also simple carbohydrates. Complex carbohydrates are starches found in foods such as bread, pasta, and cereals.

Some plant matter called **dietary fiber** cannot be digested. Fruits, vegetables, and whole grains are good sources of fiber. Though fiber does not supply energy, it is needed in the diet. Fiber provides roughage, or bulk, that aids normal function of the digestive tract.

Look at the dietary guidelines on page 119. Which ones concern carbohydrates? The guidelines recommend that you eat more carbohydrates as starches rather than sugars and that you avoid too much sugar altogether. Most people rely too much on sugar and "empty" Calorie foods to meet daily energy needs. These foods have few nutrients such as vitamins and minerals. They are also low in fiber and promote dental disease. To meet the dietary guidelines, cut back on sweets such as soft drinks and candies. Eat more vegetables, fresh fruits, and whole grains. These foods provide vitamins, minerals, and fiber, as well as energy. A diet rich in complex carbohydrates and fiber is very healthful. Complex carbohydrates keep blood glucose levels more constant which helps reduce fatigue and may also help prevent diseases such as diabetes. Increased dietary fiber helps prevent constipation. Many scientists state that fiber can also reduce the risk of colon cancer and other intestinal problems.

2–3. Would a snack like this appeal to you? What nutrients does it provide?

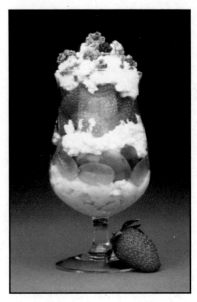

Table 2–2

PERCENTAGE OF TOTAL CALORIES FROM FAT IN SELECTED FOODS
over 50%
peanuts and peanut butter, weiners, most cheese, fried chicken, ground beef, pork (loin, butt), granola
30–50%
ice cream, whole milk, cottage cheese, pork (ham and shoulder), beef, lamb, roast chicken and turkey (including dark meat)
20–30%
beef (heel of round, pot roast), liver, fish (bass, salmon), roast chicken (white meat, no skin)
20% or less
most fish and shellfish, most peas and beans, most breakfast cereals, bread, skim milk

Adapted from *"NutriScore,"* Sabary, Fermes, 1976.

FATS

Name some fatty foods. Did you think of butter, margarine, oil, or perhaps french fries? As you can see in Table 2-2, many foods we consume have a high fat content. Fats are a more concentrated source of energy. Every gram of fat provides 9 Calories. A teaspoon of sugar contains 15 Calories whereas a teaspoon of butter has 35 Calories.

Fats digest more slowly than carbohydrates or proteins. Fatty foods fill you up faster and remain in your body for a long time. Some vitamins, such as vitamins A and E, are dissolved and transported in fats. Fats also add flavor to foods. Some fat is needed in the diet. But research suggests that a high fat diet increases the risks of **obesity** (oh-**bee**-sit-tee), heart disease, and cancer.

SATURATED AND POLYUNSATURATED FATS	
Kind of fatty acid	**Examples**
Saturated 	Butter Cheese Chocolate Milk Poultry
Monounsaturated 	Avocado Olives and olive oil Peanuts and peanut oil Peanut butter
Polyunsaturated 	Almonds Corn oil Fish Margarine (most) Mayonnaise Safflower oil Sunflower oil Walnuts

Table 2–3

Adapted from *Jane Brody's Nutrition Book,* Jane Brody. (New York: Bantam Books, 1982) p. 63

CHOLESTEROL AND SATURATED FATS. Advertising has made **cholesterol** (koh-**les**-ter-rol) and **saturated** (**sach**-yur-ray-ted) and **polyunsaturated** (pahl-ee-un-**sach**-yur-ray-ted) fats household words. But what do these terms really mean? Cholesterol is *not* a fat. It is a waxy substance produced by the body or found in animal foods. Egg yolk and organ meats such as liver and kidney are very high in cholesterol. Plants contain no cholesterol. Some cholesterol is necessary for good health. But high blood levels of cholesterol can build waxy deposits inside the walls of the blood vessels. In time, these deposits may clog the blood vessels of the entire body including those of the heart. Blood flow decreases and blood pressure rises. Heart disease may develop. High cholesterol levels in the blood greatly increase the risk of heart attack.

To understand the terms *saturated, monounsaturated,* and *polyunsaturated*, picture a chain bracelet with charms dangling from it. Fats are partly made of carbon chains with hydrogen attached (see Table 2-3). Saturated fats have no room for any more hydrogens. Monounsaturated fats have room or two or three more hydrogens. Polyunsaturated fats have room for at least four more hydrogens.

Saturated fats are solid at room temperature. Animal foods such as whole milk, butter, cream, and most cheeses are high in saturated fats. Only a few vegetable products, such as solid shortening, palm oil, coconut oil, cocoa butter, and chocolate, are high in these fats.

Polyunsaturated fats are liquid. Safflower, corn, cottonseed, and soybean oils are high in polyunsaturated fats.

Why are cholesterol and fats often discussed together? Saturated fats raise cholesterol levels in the blood. Polyunsaturated fats have a lowering effect. Monounsaturated fats neither raise nor lower cholesterol levels.

Is your diet high in and saturated fats? Cholesterol build-up can begin in adolescence. To meet the third dietary guideline you do not have to cut out meat or eggs. Just eat leaner meat and more poultry, fish, and beans. Decrease your fat intake by replacing high-fat with low-fat products. For example, drink skim milk instead of whole milk. Use polyunsaturated margarine and oils. Avoid eating a lot of deep-fried foods. Eggs, while high in cholesterol, are rich in vitamins and minerals. A low cholesterol diet can include three or four eggs a week. Scientists suggest eating less of *all* fats to reduce the risk of cancer.

MINERALS

It may surprise you to learn that the body contains many of the same minerals found in the earth's crust. Minerals are needed (1) for formation of bones and teeth; (2) for growth

HEALTH TIP

Many people are unable to digest milk and milk products, and experience gas, bloating, and cramps when they drink more than a small amount of milk. This problem, called *lactose intolerance,* can be overcome by using "sweet acidophilus" milk available in many stores. Another solution is to add 3 to 4 drops of a product called Lact-Aid to milk, which is available in many health food stores and pharmacies.

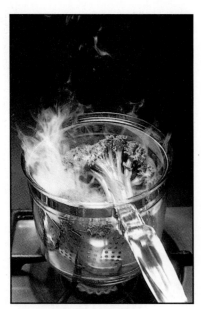

2-4. Use a steamer when cooking vegetables to preserve their vitamin content. This way, vitamins are not lost in the cooking water.

HEALTH TIP

You can add minerals and vitamins to your diet without using pills. For example, you can add small but valuable traces of iron to your diet by cooking in noncoated heavy iron skillets and pots.

Vitamin C is easily destroyed. To keep as much as possible in foods, (1) refrigerate vegetables, or store them in a dark, cool place; (2) cook vegetables in large pieces without peeling them; (3) cook vegetables rapidly in as little water as possible, and serve them immediately; and (4) omit baking soda when cooking vegetables.

of body cells, especially blood cells; and (3) for the essential components in various body fluids. Table 2-4 outlines the key facts about minerals. Make a special note of calcium and iron. These are likely to be low in the diets of teenagers, especially girls.

Do you salt your food *before* tasting it? This practice can add excess sodium and iodine to your diet. Reducing sodium intake is another dietary guideline. Excess sodium is a risk factor for high blood pressure. High blood pressure makes the heart work harder. Iodine, too much as well as too little, causes a condition called *goiter*. When you cook, cut down on salt by using herbs for flavor instead. Avoid processed foods such as ham, bacon, prepared lunch meats, and crackers. These foods have a very high salt content. Finally, taste your food BEFORE salting.

VITAMINS

The function of vitamins is often misunderstood. Vitamins are needed to promote growth and other body activities. They do not provide Calories or extra pep. Do you need vitamin pills to ensure good health? The answer to this question is no. Vitamins are found in rich supply in a nutritious diet. Yet the benefits of vitamin pills have been widely advertised. Vitamin C is reported to prevent colds if taken in huge doses. Vitamin E in large doses is supposed to prevent heart disease and other ailments. Yet careful research has not proved these claims. High dosages of these vitamins may have long-term effects on the body. However, it is known that large doses of vitamins A and D can seriously damage the body. For safety's sake, take vitamin pills only when they are prescribed by a doctor. Rely on a sound diet to get the vitamins you need. Just drinking a 150 millimeter (5 oz) glass of juice each day provides all the daily vitamin C you need. Table 2-4 gives an overview of vitamins. Pay close attention to vitamins A and C. They are often low in the diets of teenagers, especially girls.

WATER

You can live without food for weeks at a time, but without water you would die within days. This is why water is called a nutrient. Water is the basic part of blood and tissue fluids. About 60 to 75 percent of your body is made of water. It is the medium in which foods are transported in the blood for use throughout the body. Water helps remove waste products through the kidneys. It also cools the body as you perspire and as it evaporates from the lungs. Excessive water loss from the body is called **dehydration** (dee-hie-**dray**-shun). When you are dehydrated you feel thirsty. Five or six glasses of water are needed daily.

MAKING DIET DECISIONS
WHAT CAUSES HUNGER AND APPETITE?

Hunger is the physiological device that helps ensure survival. When you are hungry you feel hunger pangs. When your stomach is empty, its muscular walls contract. This irritates nerves that relay the message "hunger" to the brain. After eating, the stomach is stretched, the muscular walls relax, and the nerves are no longer stimulated. You then feel satisfied. In short, hunger tells you of your physical need for food.

Have you ever eaten a full meal, then walked by a bakery a short time later? Even though your physical need for food had just been met, you probably found yourself feeling hungry again. Why? Your **appetite** comes from a desire to repeat a pleasant experience associated with the foods you see.

Many factors control appetite. Foods presented in an attractive way are more appetizing. Do you lose your appetite when you feel excited or upset? Stress may quickly change your appetite. Social customs and situations can affect appetite, too. For example, do you ever eat more when you eat with friends? Eating habits also influence appetite.

YOUR EATING HABITS

Al often eats chicken for breakfast, pancakes for dinner, and a sandwich before bed. Wanda skips breakfast, eats only salad for lunch, and has more salad and a steak for dinner. Henry lives on fast foods and snacks such as soda, potato chips, pretzels, and candy. Sharon eats only nuts, seeds, vegetables and fruit. Are your eating habits close to any of these? Many teenagers skip meals or adopt nontraditional eating habits.

Eating habits first develop in childhood. Parents control what and when children eat. During adolescence, those habits often change. Teenagers often decide when, where, and what they will eat. These decisions are important. During the

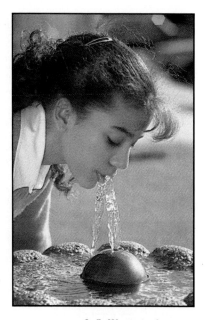

2–5. Water is the most essential ingredient in our diet. Do you drink at least 5 glasses a day?

ESSENTIAL VITAMINS AND MINERALS

Vitamin	Best Sources	Needed For	Deficiency Disorders	Risks of Megadose
A	liver, eggs, fortified milk, orange and dark green vegetables, and fruit	healthy teeth, bones, skin, eyes	night blindness, poor growth, rough skin	blurred vision, headaches, fatigue, damage to liver and nervous system
D	fortified milk, eggs; made by skin when exposed to sun	strong bones and teeth	rickets in children, softens bones in adults	kidney stones; high blood pressure, deafness
E	vegetable oils, whole grain foods, green vegetables	formation of red blood cells and other tissues	unknown	unknown
K	green leafy vegetables, peas, potatoes; made by intestinal bacteria	blood clotting	bleeding problems	skin yellowing in infants; adult risk unknown
B_1 (Thiamin)	pork, liver, oysters, whole grain foods	use of carbohydrates, healthy heart and nerves	beriberi (muscle weakness, heart and nerve damage)	unknown
B_2 (Riboflavin)	milk, meat, green vegetables, whole grains, eggs,	use of nutrients, healthy skin and mucous membranes	skin disorders, eyes sensitive to light	unknown
B_3 (Niacin)	meat, tuna, eggs, whole grain foods, beans	use of protein, energy production	pellagra (skin scaling, diarrhea)	ulcers, abnormal liver function
B_6 (Pyridoxine, Pyridoxol, Pyridoxamine)	whole-grains, liver, spinach, bananas, fish, meats, nuts, potatoes	use of nutrients, formation of red blood cells, healthy nervous system	skin disorders, anemia, convulsions	high doses produce dependency
B_{12} (Cobalamin)	in animal foods, such as meat, fish, eggs, milk; nutritional yeast	formation of red blood cells, healthy nervous system	pernicious anemia (severe reduction of red blood cells, muscle weakness)	unknown
Folacin (Folic acid)	liver, leafy vegetables, wheat germ, dried beans	formation of hemoglobin	anemia, enlarged blood cells, diarrhea	unknown
Pantothenic Acid	all foods; also made by intestinal bacteria	use of nutrients, formation of hormones	unknown	may cause B_1 deficiency
Biotin	egg yolk, liver, green vegetables; made by intestinal bacteria	use of carbohydrates, B_{12}, and folic acid	unknown	unknown
C	citrus fruits, melon, green pepper, potatoes, dark green vegetables	maintains connective tissue; healthy bones, skin	sore gums, poor healing, scurvy (muscle loss, brown, tough skin)	high doses cause dependence, diarrhea

Mineral	Best Sources	Needed for	Deficiency Disorders	Risks of Megadose
Calcium	milk products, canned fish, dark green leafy vegetables, citrus fruits, dried beans	strong bones and teeth, heart and nerve action, blood clotting	rickets in children (bowed legs, stunted growth), osteoporosis in adults	severe fatigue, calcium deposits in body tissues
Phosphorus	meat, poultry, fish, eggs, dried peas and beans, milk products	strong bones and teeth, energy release from nutrients	appetite loss, fatigue	calcium deficiency
Magnesium	raw green leafy vegetables, nuts, seeds, whole grains	strong bones and muscle, nerve action	muscle weakness, irregular heart beat	disorders in nervous system
Sodium	naturally present in most foods and water, table salt	internal water balance, transmission of nerve impulses	muscle cramps and weakness, nausea, diarrhea	high blood pressure in some people
Potassium	oranges, bananas, meats, bran, dried beans, potatoes	fluid balance in cells, transmission of nerve impulses	abnormal heart action, fatigue	muscle paralysis, abnormal heart beat
Sulfur	beef, wheat germ, dried beans and peas, peanuts	formation of body cells	unknown	unknown
Chloride	table salt	regulation of body fluids	upsets acid-base balance in body fluids	upsets acid-base balance in body fluids
Iron	red meats, egg yolk, leafy vegetables, beans, molasses, whole grains	formation of red blood cells	anemia, fatigue	toxic buildup in liver, pancreas, heart
Copper	oysters, nuts, cocoa powder, liver, kidneys, dried beans	formation of red blood cells	unknown	violent vomiting and diarrhea
Iodine	seafood, iodized salt, sea salt	thyroid gland function	goiter (enlarged thyroid)	a different form of goiter
Fluoride	fish, animal foods, fluoridated water	strong teeth, bone strength	excess dental decay	mottling of teeth, toxic in large doses
Magnesium	nuts, whole grains, vegetables and fruits	healthy nervous system and bones	unknown	slurred speech, muscle spasm
Selenium	seafood, whole grains, meat, eggs, milk, garlic	prevents breakdown of body chemicals	unknown	unknown
Zinc	meat, liver, eggs, poultry, seafood, milk, whole grains	enzyme formation	delayed wound healing, loss of taste, stunted growth	nausea, vomiting, anemia, stomach bleeding

Table 2–4

RECOMMENDED SERVINGS PER DAY FROM THE FIVE FOOD GROUPS	
Milk; cheese	Children: 2–3 servings Teens: 4 Adults: 2
Meat; fish; poultry; beans	2 servings
Vegetable; fruit	4 servings
Bread; cereal	4 servings
Fats; sweets; alcohol	none

Table 2–5

2–6. For good nutrition, select nutrient-dense foods from these food groups. Limit servings from the fats, sweets, and alcohol group.

teen years, rapid growth occurs. Eating habits may become part of a life-style and set the stage for health or disease in later life. Are your eating habits geared toward health?

HOW CAN YOU PLAN A NUTRITIONALLY BALANCED DIET?

A "well-balanced" diet means one that contains all the key nutrients and enough Calories for daily activity. To guide diet planning, the Food and Nutrition Board of the National Academy of Sciences has devised a list of Recommended Daily Allowances (RDAs) for nutrients. The guide is organized into five basic food groups. A diet based on proper servings from four food groups meets the U.S. RDA guidelines (see Figure 2-6).

Look at Table 2-5. Notice that the recommended servings of the milk group varies. Growing children, teenagers, and pregnant and nursing mothers have increased nutritional needs, as well as people who are sick or recovering from injuries such as broken bones or burns. Can you explain why?

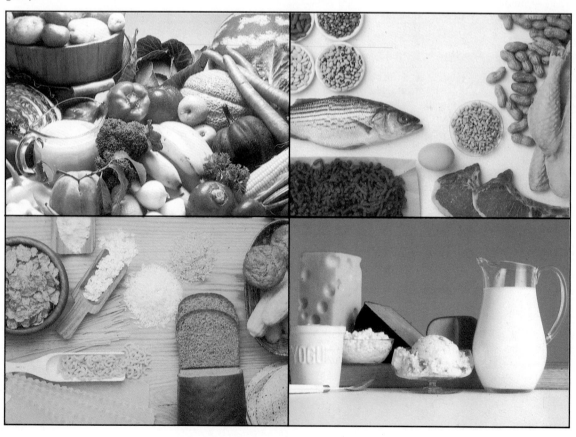

Calorie needs also vary with age, sex, weight, body build, and activity. How many Calories do you need daily? A teenage male needs about 2,700 to 2,800 Calories a day. This averages to 20 to 25 Calories per .45 kilogram (1 lb) of body weight. A teenage female needs 2,100 to 2,200 or about 18 to 23 Calories per .45 kilogram. After 18 years of age, your Calorie needs will level off to about 16 to 18 Calories per .45 kilogram per day. After age 55, Calorie needs decrease again. However, in planning Calorie needs, you must consider your daily activities (see Table 2-6).

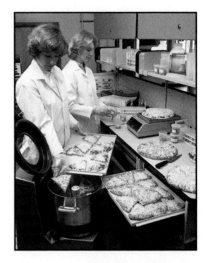

2–7. The calorimeter scientifically measures the Caloric content of foods.

CALORIES EXPENDED PER HOUR IN VARIOUS ACTIVITIES					
	WEIGHT IN POUNDS				
Activity	*100*	*120*	*140*	*160*	*180*
Bicycling	112	134	157	179	202
Dancing (vigorous)	352	423	493	564	634
Dishwashing	45	54	63	72	81
Driving	40	48	56	64	72
Eating	18	22	25	29	32
Piano Playing	63	75	88	100	113
Running (medium speed)	314	376	439	502	564
Skating	157	188	220	251	282
Tennis	218	261	305	348	392
Walking (5 m.p.h)	372	446	521	596	669
Writing	18	22	25	29	32

Table 2–6

CHOOSING FOODS. When you buy something for yourself, do you shop for the best value for your money? You can apply the concept of smart shopping to choosing the foods you eat. When you spend your daily Calories on foods high in energy but low in nutrients, you get poor food value.

When you choose foods, consider their **nutrient density.** This is the ratio of nutrients to Calories that a food provides. Foods high in nutrient density offer good food value. They provide Calories packed with vitamins, minerals and other key nutrients. Which foods shown in Figure 2-8 offers the best value? The nutrient-dense baked potato is the food bargain. The high fat content of potato chips and french fries dilutes the nutrient density of their Calories. In order to get the same nutrients that the baked potato provides, you would have to eat a lot more potato chips and fries. You would also be eating extra fat and salt. Would this be healthful? Too much fat and sodium in the diet increases the risk of heart disease.

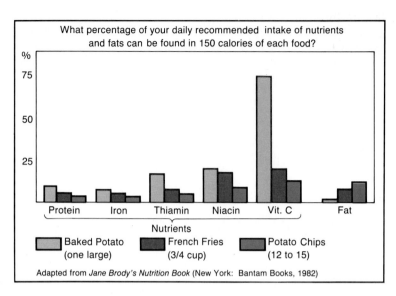

What percentage of your daily recommended intake of nutrients and fats can be found in 150 calories of each food?

Nutrients: Protein, Iron, Thiamin, Niacin, Vit. C, Fat

Baked Potato (one large) · French Fries (3/4 cup) · Potato Chips (12 to 15)

Adapted from *Jane Brody's Nutrition Book* (New York: Bantam Books, 1982)

2–8. *Compare these three foods for their nutrient density.*

NUTRITION INFORMATION PER SERVING

SERVING SIZE 1 OZ. (28.4 g ABOUT 1 CUP) CEREAL ALONE OR WITH ½ CUP VITAMIN D FORTIFIED WHOLE MILK.
SERVINGS PER PACKAGE. 15

	1 OZ.	WITH ½ CUP WHOLE MILK
CALORIES	110	190
PROTEIN	2 g	6 g
CARBOHYDRATE	25 g	31 g
FAT	1 g	5 g
SODIUM	125 mg	185 mg

PERCENTAGE OF U.S. RECOMMENDED DAILY ALLOWANCES (U.S. RDA)

	1 OZ.	WITH ½ CUP WHOLE MILK
PROTEIN	2	10
VITAMIN A	25	30
VITAMIN C	25	25
THIAMIN	25	30
RIBOFLAVIN	25	35
NIACIN	25	25
CALCIUM	*	15
IRON	25	25
VITAMIN D	10	25
VITAMIN B₆	25	30
FOLIC ACID	25	25
PHOSPHORUS	2	15
MAGNESIUM	2	6
ZINC	25	30
COPPER	4	4

*CONTAINS LESS THAN 2% OF THE U.S. RDA OF THIS NUTRIENT.

INGREDIENTS: SUGAR, CORN, WHEAT AND OAT FLOUR; PARTIALLY HYDROGENATED VEGETABLE OIL (ONE OR MORE OF COTTONSEED, COCONUT, SOYBEAN AND PALM); SALT; ARTIFICIAL COLORING; SODIUM ASCORBATE (C); ASCORBIC ACID (C); NIACINAMIDE; ZINC OXIDE; REDUCED IRON; NATURAL ORANGE, LEMON, CHERRY WITH OTHER NATURAL FLAVORINGS; VITAMIN A PALMITATE; PYRIDOXINE HYDROCHLORIDE (B₆); RIBOFLAVIN (B₂); THIAMIN HYDROCHLORIDE (B₁); FOLIC ACID; AND VITAMIN D. BHT ADDED TO MAINTAIN PRODUCT FRESHNESS.

CARBOHYDRATE INFORMATION

	WITH ½ CUP WHOLE MILK
STARCH AND RELATED CARBOHYDRATES	12 g
SUCROSE AND OTHER SUGARS	13 g
TOTAL CARBOHYDRATES	25 g

(STARCH AND RELATED CARBOHYDRATES: 12 g; SUCROSE AND OTHER SUGARS: 19 g; TOTAL CARBOHYDRATES: 31 g with ½ cup whole milk)

2–9. *How many servings are in this container? How many Calories are in one serving? How many grams of simple and complex carbohydrates are in one serving?*

When your Calories come from foods with low nutrient density it is harder to get all the nutrients you need each day. The diets of teenagers, especially girls, often lack enough Calories, iron, and vitamins A and C.

READ THE LABEL! One way to learn about food value is to read and compare food labels. As you can see in Figure 2-9 a food label provides information on a product's contents. Ingredients are listed in order, based on the amount present by weight, from most to least. Therefore this product contains more sugar than flour. The label also lists the U.S. RDAs for certain nutrients, as required by law. Some labels provide extra information such as sodium, cholesterol or fiber content.

When you compare food labels, do not look just at the protein, vitamin, and mineral content. Look at the sugar, fat, and salt content, too. See if they are high on the ingredient list. Remember that sugar comes in many forms. Even if foods have added vitamins, a high sugar and fat content decreases their worth as healthful foods. Also note the water content and net weight of the product.

IS BREAKFAST IMPORTANT?

If you sometimes feel listless in class at midmorning, your eating habits may be the cause. A poor or skipped breakfast can impair mental and physical performance. This is why breakfast is called the most important meal of the day. After

30

fasting through the night your body has used about half its stored glycogen supply. Unless replaced through a nutritious breakfast, the rest of this stored energy is used by midmorning. This leaves you fatigued.

A good breakfast need not take a lot of time to fix. Leftovers from soup to spaghetti can serve as a quick, healthful breakfast. When you have little time for breakfast, why not switch from sugary breakfast foods to whole grain muffins, or a sandwich made with whole grain breads? You can make these ahead of time and then eat wisely while on-the-run.

WHAT ABOUT FAST FOODS AND SNACKS?

Have you ever noticed that a fast food shake is not usually called a *milkshake*? You may think you are sipping a calcium-rich milkshake made from milk and ice cream. What you really get is a mixture of sweeteners, artificial colors and flavors, salt, vegetable oils, and dried milk products. This is just one example of the pitfalls of a fast food diet. On the whole, fast foods are low in calcium, iron, vitamins A and C, certain B vitamins, and fiber. They are high in Calories, sugar, salt, and fat. The same is true for most popular snack foods.

If you enjoy fast foods and snacks, learn to choose your foods more wisely. Curb the number of fast food meals you eat to three or fewer per week. Substitute milk or juice (not a fruit-flavored drink) for sodas and shakes. Limit the extra pickles, salt, ketchup, and other salty sauces on your foods. Add lettuce and tomatoes to burgers. When available, eat coleslaw or salads instead of french fries. Remove part or all of the crusty skin from fried chicken. Avoid smaller fried foods such as chicken tidbits. They contain more fat than larger fried foods such as a chicken breast. When you eat a fast-food meal, pay close attention to the rest of your diet that day. Include extra fruit, milk, green vegetables, and whole grains to make up for the nutrients lacking in your fast-food "feast."

When it comes to snacking, munch on the nutrient-dense foods like those shown in Figure 2-10. Cut back on potato chips, candy, and other traditional snack foods.

IS A VEGETARIAN DIET HEALTHFUL?

For varying reasons about 10 million Americans choose a **vegetarian diet.** Some are strict vegetarians, who eat only plant foods. However, most vegetarians do consume eggs,

2-10. Assorted raw vegetables served with a tangy cottage-cheese dip is a quick, easy, and nutritious snack.

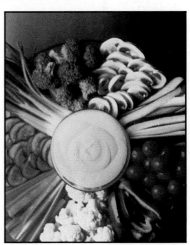

SAMPLE MODIFIED VEGETARIAN MENUS
Breakfast: skim milk, grapefruit sections, whole grain toast, margarine, shredded wheat cereal
Lunch: egg salad sandwich, lettuce and tomato
Snack: yogurt, sesame bread sticks
Dinner: macaroni and cheese, apple-raisin-nut salad, collard greens, whole grain bread and margarine

Table 2–7

milk, cheese or other dairy products.

If well planned, these diets are not harmful and can even benefit health. Vegetarian diets reduce the risks of cancer, heart disease, and obesity due to their lower fat and cholesterol contents and higher fiber content. Also, vegetarians eat more dark green and deep yellow vegetables. Research shows this may have a cancer prevention effect.

Most vegetarians can meet their nutrient needs by eating dishes that combine plant proteins or have added milk or eggs. They should also eat a variety of fruits, vegetables, whole grains, beans, nuts, and seeds. Without dairy foods or eggs, strict vegetarians may not get needed nutrients. Since their diets often lack enough vitamins B-12 and D, iron, and calcium, these supplements are often needed. Their diets should provide an extra measure of soy products with added vitamin B-12, beans, peas, peanuts and leafy dark green vegetables. Table 2-7 shows sample menus for healthful vegetarian eating.

WEIGHT CONTROL

BODY IMAGE

The human body has always been admired for its symmetry and beauty. But the image of the ideal physique has varied throughout history and among cultures. What is your ideal body image? Does it reflect health as well as appearance? The healthy male or female body has a proper balance between muscle tissue and fat; thus, it is neither obese nor underweight. Good nutrition and a fitness program are the keys to a healthful, more attractive self-image.

OBESITY AND HEALTH

The second dietary guideline stresses weight control for the sake of health, not appearance. Obesity increases the risk of both heart disease and strokes. Can you imagine carrying a 13.5-kilogram (30-lb) backpack with you everywhere you go? A person who gains 13.5 kilograms adds this burden to the body. The body adjusts to carrying this extra load as best it can, but there are dangers. Blood pressure increases and the heart enlarges. Too often the body gives up long before it would if proper weight were maintained. Obesity also increases the risks of diabetes, kidney, gallbladder, joint diseases, and posture problems.

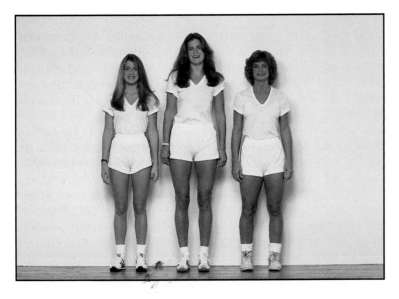

2–11. These three teenagers each have a different body type, yet they are all physically fit and at their ideal weights.

WHO IS OBESE?

WHO IS OBESE? Weight charts can help people determine if they are obese. However, these charts can sometimes be misleading. Muscle tissue weighs more than fat. Active, well-muscled people may exceed their so-called "ideal" body weight by as much as 20 percent, and yet not be obese. Obese people are "over-fat." They have an excess of body fat compared to leaner, heavier muscle tissue. People can even weigh in at an ideal weight, yet still be obese. If inactive, they may have too much fat and too little muscle tissue. One simple way of measuring whether you have too much fat is the pinch test shown in Figure 2-12.

There is one basic cause for being overweight. The body takes in more Calories (energy) than it burns. Just 15 extra Calories a day (the Calories in a teaspoonful of sugar) can add .68 kilograms (1.5 lb) to a person's weight each year. At this rate, how much weight would a person slowly gain between the ages of 18 and 38?

HOW DO YOU OVERCOME OBESITY?

Do obese teenagers eat more food than their leaner peers? Surprisingly, the answer is generally no. Most obese teenagers gain extra weight from being inactive and eating the wrong foods. The secret to overcoming obesity does not lie in any strange diet. The secret for sensible weight loss is simple: Get more exercise and make each Calorie count nutritionally.

2–12. Skin fold thickness for teenage boys should be less than 3/5 inch. Skinfold thickness for teenage girls should be less than 1 inch.

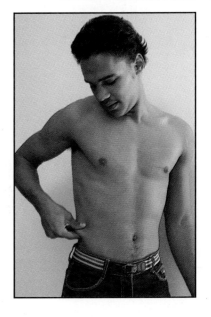

To lose weight your body must draw on its stored energy supply, fat. Your body taps this energy supply when you eat fewer Calories than you use, by either cutting Calorie intake, increasing activity, or both. To lose .45 kilogram of fat your body must burn 3,500 Calories of energy. If you use 500 more Calories a day than you eat, you will lose this amount in a week. When cutting Calories, it is crucial to still get the essential nutrients. You can cut Calories without cutting food intake by simply making better food choices. For example, you can cut Calories by eating a baked potato (without butter or sour cream) instead of eating french fries.

If you combine exercise with diet, you will lose weight more quickly. In fact, extra activity is often all that is needed to control weight sensibly. For example, if you burn just 200 more Calories a day through extra activity (the equivalent of a 20-minute walk twice a day) you can lose 20 pounds in a year. Exercise also builds muscle tissue and decreases fat tissue. Muscle tissue requires more Calories to maintain itself than does fat. As your muscle to fat balance improves, you can eat more Calories than before without gaining weight. This is every dieter's dream! Do not worry that exercise will increase your appetite, thus making weight loss harder. Exercise generally reduces appetite.

A DIET PROGRAM. Before you begin a diet, examine your eating and exercise habits. Do you eat nutrient rich foods? Do you eat slowly and avoid seconds? Do you get enough exercise? Are you overeating out of loneliness or boredom? If so, try sharing activities with friends. Perhaps even diet with a friend. Outline a program for balanced nutrition, reduced Calorie intake, and increased exercise. Then discuss your diet plan with a doctor or school nurse. Once you reach your ideal weight, keep the weight off by proper diet, regular exercise, and good eating habits.

DIET FADS. Are there any quick ways to lose weight? Heavy perspiration removes water and salts from your body, causing quick weight-loss. However, this weight is just as quickly regained. Diet pills reduce appetite, but they can be harmful since they are addictive drugs. Many fad diets are dangerous to health. Fasting is particularly harmful to adolescents. Not eating regularly during these crucial years can prevent proper growth.

How can you evaluate a diet for its potential risks to your health? Review the food groups on page 28. Sound diet menus are based on the basic food groups. By eating nutrient-dense foods from every food group, you can reduce your Calorie intake. Risky diets, such as high-protein or fruit diets, often limit your choice of foods. Unless you are under a doctor's care for weight loss, avoid prepared diet liquids that replace normal meals. Although these liquids may contain enough nutrients, they do not provide fiber. Some liquid diets have been linked to severe illness and even death. The major problem with most diet fads is that they do not change eating habits. Unless eating habits change, weight loss is usually followed by weight gain.

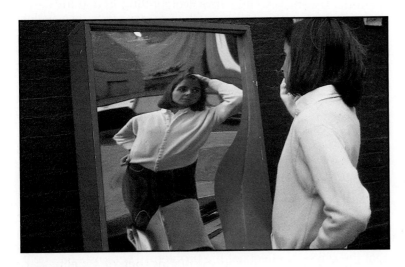

2–13. People suffering from anorexia and bulimia have a distorted picture of themselves and are obsessed with the fear of becoming fat.

DIETING DANGERS: ANOREXIA AND BULIMIA

Lois is 16.25 centimeters (5 feet 5 inches) tall and weighs only 45 kilograms (100 lb). To others, she looks thin and malnourished. But when Lois looks at herself in the mirror she sees the image of an overweight teenager. So she continues her starvation diet. After every meager meal she exercises a lot to burn the Calories just consumed.

Carol's weight is normal, but she, too, worries about her weight. She started a strict diet but severe hunger made her lose control. She ate several hamburgers, a box of cookies, five candy bars, and a quart of ice cream: over 5,000 Calories at a single meal. Right after this eating binge, Carol felt guilty. To ease her conscience, she induced vomiting to purge herself of all that food. Soon this binge-purge cycle of eating became an out-of-control habit. As the habit took control of her life, she withdrew from her family and friends.

Lois's condition is called **anorexia** (an-or-**ex**-see-ah); Carol's problem is called **bulimia** (byou-**lee-**mee-ah). Both of these problems can become life-threatening. These conditions can trouble anyone, but young women are more prone to them.

As the anorexia-dieter starves the body, muscle tissues waste away. The skin dries and yellows and the hair thins and falls out. Blood pressure drops, menstruation ceases, and weight drops drastically. A young woman of average height may weigh only 31.75 kilograms (70 lb), yet she will continue dieting. At this low weight, brain damage and death often occur.

In bulimia, the dieter seldom wastes away. Still the binge-purge cycle takes its health toll. Vomiting upsets the body's fluid balance, which can cause irregular heart action and sometimes sudden death. Habitual vomiting of strong stomach acids can cause severe tooth decay and a constant sore throat. When laxatives are used for purging, constipation becomes a regular problem. Just as life-threatening is the huge volume of food consumed, which can severely stretch and even rupture the stomach.

What causes these conditions? Doctors disagree. Many think that these problems stem from the overconcern with thinness in our society. Dieters, such as Lois and Carol, become obsessed with a fear of becoming fat. Professional help is available for people with these disorders. Physicians treat the physical effects of the problem. Therapists can help dieters change their dangerous habits. However, change cannot begin until the dieter sees that there is a problem and wants to overcome it.

HOW DO YOU GAIN WEIGHT?

If you are underweight, defined as 10 percent or more below ideal weight, you may be worried about your appearance and your health. A doctor's visit can rule out health problems. A sound weight-gain plan can help improve your appearance.

First review your habits. Are you really eating enough food each day? Underweight people often skip meals or eat less food at meals than they think they do. Are you getting enough rest? Staying up late or rising very early burns extra Calories. Are you getting enough exercise? Proper exercise can help you relax so you don't waste Calories as nervous energy. But do not overdo it. Do you smoke or drink lots of caffeine beverages? This decreases appetite and may promote nervous activity.

Second, review your diet. Add about 500 Calories to your diet each day. Eat healthful higher Calorie snacks, about 2 to 3 hours before meals so you won't dull your appetite. For example, snack on peanut butter sandwiches, creamed soup, or fruit-flavored yogurt. If you seem to get filled up fast at mealtimes, eat smaller but more frequent meals.

If you can't seem to gain weight, you can still improve your appearance. Learn more about fashions and hairstyles that can make you appear heavier . For example, avoid dark-colored clothes that will make you look thinner.

CONSUMER ISSUES IN NUTRITION

ARE PROCESSED FOODS HEALTHFUL?

Because of food technology more than half of our diet now consists of **processed** foods. The benefits and drawbacks of processed foods must be individually weighed.

We hardly think of some of the foods we consume today as being "processed." Most milk, for instance, is first *pasteurized* to destroy the bacteria in it. Next, the milk is *homogenized* to break up the fat in it. This prevents the cream and milk from separating. Finally, vitamin D is usually added to milk. Processing milk has many benefits. The reduction

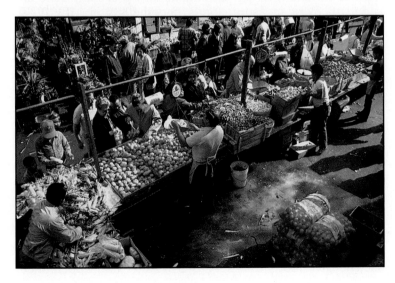

2–14. Because more people prefer eating fresh rather than processed foods, city green markets and food cooperatives are becoming more common.

of bacteria decreases the risk of infection. The milk stays fresher, longer. The added vitamin D prevents a childhood disease called *rickets* that affects bone growth and may cause bowed legs. Homogenizing milk makes it more appealing to consumers. More people are apt to drink milk and get needed calcium in their diets.

WHAT ARE FOOD ADDITIVES?

Calvin always makes his spaghetti sauce from scratch. "No food **additives** for me," he says. "I don't want to eat chemicals." He uses fresh tomatoes and special herbs and salt to make his sauce. His homemade sauce does taste better and is cheaper than commercial sauce. But in truth Calvin's sauce contains many food additives. An additive is any substance that is added to foods. His sauce contains chemicals, too. Food is really nothing more than a complex of chemical compounds.

Some additives creep into foods indirectly when they are processed, packaged, or stored. For instance, chemicals from plastic packaging may seep into foods. Most additives are put directly into foods for special purposes.

Have you ever noticed the words "vitamin-enriched" or "fortified" on food products? Additives are used to maintain or improve food value. When vitamins are lost during food processing and then replaced, those foods are then called **enriched.** For example, bread, flour, and cereals are usually vitamin enriched. When vitamins already present in food are added in extra measure, foods become vitamin **fortified.** Certain drinks may be fortified with vitamin C. Fortification has helped reduce or eliminate certain diet-related diseases in our country.

Additives also help maintain food freshness and safety. In fact, our food supply is one of the safest world-wide. *Preservatives* reduce food spoilage caused by bacteria or molds. *Antioxidants* bind to oxygen. They prevent fats and other foods from turning stale upon exposure to air. Without such additives, you would have to purchase foods frequently and in smaller amounts. There would be more waste since foods would spoil more quickly. This would decrease the food supply and raise food costs.

Finally, additives are used to make foods more convenient and appealing to consumers. Frozen pizza, cake mixes, and other easy-to-fix foods require additives. Some additives are used to give foods a better taste, texture, and appearance.

For example, what would a gelatin desert be like without the texturing, coloring, and flavoring agents?

But additives have drawbacks, too. Salt, sugar, and sweeteners are the most common food additives. What health drawbacks do they have? The practice of adding vitamins to so many foods concerns consumer advocates. They point out that vitamin deficiencies are rare in our country. Yet consumers often think that "more is better" and are willing to pay for it. As a result, food companies may add vitamins needlessly to some foods such as breakfast cereals. By adding just a penny's worth of vitamins, they can charge much more for the product. In fact, advertising foods as "vitamin-packed" often boosts sales. Adding nutrients to foods such as bread is important. But this practice can be misleading. Consumers may be misled into thinking that all nutrients lost during processing have been replaced. For example, enriched white bread does not contain fiber and trace minerals that are lost during processing.

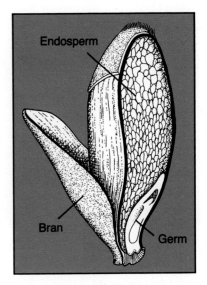

2–15. Refined white flour is pure endosperm. The nutrient-rich germ and bran (containing protein, fiber, vitamins, and trace minerals) are lost.

THE SAFETY ISSUE: BENEFITS VERSUS RISKS.

For most consumers, the major issue in additive use is safety. At present about 2,800 substances may be added to foods. How many of these additives are safe? How many are really necessary? Where safety is concerned, the terms *natural* and *synthetic* mean little. Many substances found naturally in foods are toxic. Uncooked rhubarb, for example, contains trace amounts of a poisonous acid. Many synthetic additives are safe. The synthetic additive EDTA binds with metals. Doctors use EDTA injections to treat cases of metal poisoning. In foods, it helps prevent products from getting stale.

The Federal Food and Drug Administration (FDA) governs the use of additives in foods. Before the FDA approves an additive for use, it must be tested for safety. For example, experiments must prove that the additive does not cause cancer in humans or animals. Some additives once thought safe were later found to cause cancer in animals. The artificial color Red Dye No. 2 and *cyclamate* were withdrawn from foods for this reason.

Sodium nitrate and *sodium nitrite* are controversial preservatives used today. They are added to hot dogs, bacon, ham, lunch meats, and smoked fish. They give many processed meats their red color. They also prevent the growth of a bacteria that causes a deadly form of food poisoning called **botulism** (**bot-**you-liz-em). However, research has found that in lab animals nitrates and nitrites combine with other compounds in the body to form cancer-causing

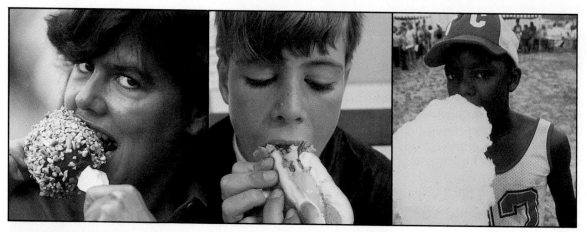

2–16. Foods containing artificial colors and flavors can be eaten occasionally, but should not be a regular part of your diet.

substances. When the FDA moved to ban these additives, controversy arose. Consumer advocates supported the ban. They felt that safer preservatives should be used. Food companies objected that without coloring, foods would not appeal to consumers. They also argued that without these preservatives constant refrigeration would be needed. Some scientists also argued against the ban. They pointed out that nitrates occur naturally in foods like beets and lettuce. Also, nitrites are found in human saliva. They concluded that their cancer risk must be small. After much debate over benefits and risks, these preservatives were not banned. However, the FDA ordered lower levels in some foods and in others, complete removal.

Controversial additives remain in use today. Many scientists believe that some widely used artificial colors pose needless health risks. Their potential hazards range from allergic reactions to cancer. Their *only* benefit is the improvement of a food's appearance. Would you choose a naturally dull food over a rosy, artificially colored product? Many consumers would. In order to meet consumer demand, companies are starting to make products with fewer additives. But, such pressure does not always produce positive changes. For consumer appeal, some bakers no longer add the preservative *calcium propionate* to bread and pastries. They can then state their products are "preservative-free." Yet this additive prevents the growth of harmful molds, and it also provides some calcium. It is found naturally in swiss cheese and is added to foods only in small amounts. One slice of swiss cheese contains as much of this additive as two loaves of bread.

What is the answer to the additive issue? As a consumer you must weigh the benefits and risks of additives. Try to learn more about additives in order to make wiser choices. The table of food additives in the appendix can help you make better diet decisions. Reading food labels can help you make better decisions. You can also reduce your additive-related risks through better eating habits. Eat more fresh foods whenever possible. Cut back on your intake of artificially flavored or colored products.

ARE HEALTH FOODS REALLY HEALTHFUL?

What are "health foods," "natural foods," and "organic foods"? At present there are no laws that define these terms. Hence, their meaning varies widely from one food company to another. Some people think that certain "magic health foods," such as brewer's yeast, will keep them healthy, no matter what else they eat. Others think that anything sold in a health food store is healthful. This is not necessarily true. Kelp tablets, a common supplement, may contain high levels of arsenic; bone meal may have high levels of lead. As with any foods, consumers should use common sense when buying "health foods." Read labels carefully. Avoid supplement use, unless recommended by a doctor.

People assume that "natural" foods mean unrefined and unprocessed. However, fruit drinks with artificial color may claim they have "natural" flavors. Potato chip bags may state that the chips have been "made the natural way." The word *natural* may be added to products just to boost sales.

What about the claims made for "organic" foods? Many people think that since organic foods are grown without pesticides, they are more nutritious. In fact, these foods often contain pesticide traces despite their organic labels. There is no monitoring program that ensures how these foods are grown. So far, studies have not shown organic foods to be more nutritious than foods grown with commercial fertilizers and pesticides.

WHAT ABOUT IMITATION AND LIGHT FOODS?

Imitation foods lack enough of the major ingredient, like cheese or meat, to qualify as the real thing. A meat-*flavored* sauce lacks enough meat to be a real meat sauce. A "cheese food" does not contain enough butterfat to be a real cheese.

HEALTH ACTION

Few food advertisements are devoted to healthful products. Write a television commercial or a newspaper or magazine advertisement to sell a healthful food, such as your favorite fresh fruit or vegetable. Design any packaging to make the product appealing. Remember to include the nutritional value of the food.

FOCUS ON HEALTH

EATING AND ATHLETICS

Paul and Frank, football teammates, each enjoyed their pre-game breakfast at home. Paul sat down to a plate of steak, eggs, and home-fried potatoes. Frank had a bowl of cereal, skim milk, and fruit. Who had the breakfast of champions? The experts say Frank's meal was best for sports performance. Many myths persist about eating and athletics.

What should athletes eat to compete? Athletes do not need extra protein, vitamins, yeast, or other proclaimed aids in their diet. These do not build muscle or increase strength and endurance. Athletes *do* need extra Calories to meet the increased demands of sports. They also need water before, during, and after sports. Too many athletes still restrict water intake, yet dehydration *reduces* performance by 20 to 30 percent.

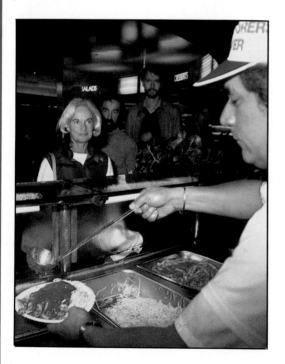

Besides the normal daily intake, drink 1 to 2 glasses of water 15 minutes before sports. During events, don't rely on thirst to tell you when you should drink more. Drink another glass of water about every 20 minutes. Weigh in and out after sports to determine how much water your body has really lost during events. For each pound lost, drink two glasses of water for replacement.

Special beverages *are not* recommended. Plain, cold (and cheap) water is best. Never use alcohol as a water replacement. Salt tablets, even in hot weather, are not needed and can be harmful. Don't believe the myth about not drinking milk before events. A dry "cottonmouth" comes from the natural stress and excitement of competition, not milk.

Eat a diet rich in complex carbohydrates, such as breads or pasta 2 or 3 days before *endurance* sports (bicycling, long-distance running, etc.). The marathon runners in the photo are eating a spaghetti dinner to help them prepare for the New York marathon. The foods will be digested and stored as glycogen in the liver and muscles. Glycogen is the energy source you need for endurance events. At the same time, to increase glycogen storage, avoid exercise and rest the muscles. For *nonendurance* sports such as football or tennis, eat a light, high-starch, low-fat pre-game meal, like Frank's, 3 to 4 hours before the sport event. A heavy, high-fat, high-protein diet, like Paul's, digests slowly. It does not provide fuel for sport's events.

If you work out before digestion is completed (2-3 hr), nausea or cramps may occur. Do not eat sugary foods for quick energy before events. This practice speeds exhaustion and can cause stomach upset.

In brief, if you really want to eat to compete, avoid fasting and drying out. Eat a sensible diet. Drink lots of fluids. Do this and you will be off to a winning start!

There are many so-called "light foods" on the market for dieters. Most light foods have a lower sugar or fat content. A typical light food is salad dressing made mostly with water instead of oil.

Light and imitation food prices are often high. Some of these foods, like those with reduced fat, may be lower in Calories. However, many of these foods also lack trace minerals and other key nutrients. Some of these products, like nondairy creamers, may be high in saturated fats. Others may be high in sodium.

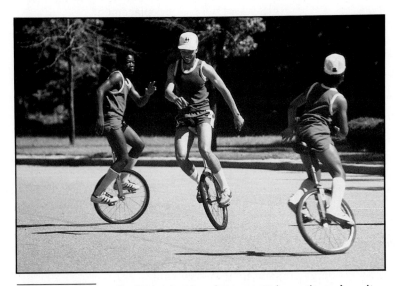

2–17. A healthful diet is the foundation for a wellness life-style.

SUMMARY: Carbohydrates, fats, protein, minerals, vitamins, and water are essential nutrients. They furnish energy, are needed for growth and repair of body tissues, and act as regulators of body processes. Medical researchers believe that improper diet can increase the risk of chronic disease. A well-balanced diet contains all of the key nutrients and enough Calories. It can be achieved by eating the proper number of servings daily from the basic food groups and choosing foods from the groups according to the U.S. dietary guidelines. Good eating habits, which include a daily breakfast and limiting sugary, fatty, and salty foods and snacks, are also important. A healthy body is neither obese nor underweight. Weight loss or weight gain requires changing the normal caloric intake and/or the Calories used through activity. Food additives are substances that are added to foods. Consumers must evaluate *all* foods, additive-free or not, for their diet benefits and potential risks.

CHAPTER REVIEW

words at work

Find the word in the left column that fits one of the definitions in the right column. DO NOT WRITE IN THIS BOOK.

a. Calories
b. dietary fiber
c. anorexia
d. fats
e. amino acids
f. botulism
g. cholesterol
h. dehydration

1. Most concentrated source of energy
2. A deadly form of food poisoning
3. Made by body or found in animal foods
4. Building block of protein
5. A measure of energy in foods
6. Indigestible plant matter
7. Excessive water loss from body
8. Dangerous dieting

review questions

1. Define the term "nutrient," distinguishing it from a food.
2. Why is variety in the diet important?
3. Define the term "Calorie" and give an example to illustrate its use.
4. Name the nutrients that provide energy and cite their energy value.
5. Contrast simple and complex carbohydrates. Give an example of each.
6. Contrast high-quality and low-quality proteins. Give an example of each.
7. Define the term "cholesterol" and explain how an excess of it affects the body.
8. What are vitamins and minerals? Which of these nutrients may be low in a diet?
9. Why is water considered a nutrient?
10. What diet changes can help meet U.S. dietary guidelines for carbohydrate intake?
11. Why do the dietary guidelines recommend avoiding fats and saturated fats?
12. Name five common food sources of sodium in a typical diet.
13. List five factors that determine the Calorie needs of an individual.
14. Define the term "well-balanced diet."
15. What is nutrient density? How can this concept help you in food selection?
16. Name the number of daily servings recommended from each food group.
17. List five ways to improve nutrition when dining on fast foods.
18. Outline a program for sensible weight loss and weight gain.
19. Contrast anorexia and bulimia. Why are these dieting practices dangerous?
20. Define food additives. Name their major functions in the diet.
21. What are "imitation" and "light" foods? Cite an example of each.

discussion questions

1. Overall, do you think advances in food technology have improved or hurt the American diet? Why or why not?
2. Discuss whether, and to what extent, consumers shape the manufacturing decisions of the food industry or the food industry shapes consumers' diet decisions.
3. A friend tells you that he or she has decided to adopt a vegetarian lifestyle. What advice would you give?
4. Discuss teen eating habits and their motiviation. Do you think most teens eat a nutritionally sound diet? Why or why not?
5. It takes several pounds of grain to produce a pound of beef. In light of this fact and worldwide hunger, discuss the high consumption of beef as part of the traditional American diet.
6. In your opinion, should television advertising of sugary breakfast cereals or nutrient-poor snack foods be banned from prime-time children's hours (for example, Saturday morning)? Why or why not?

investigating

PURPOSE:
To compare foods by applying the concept of nutrient density.

MATERIALS NEEDED:
Food packages to compare; graph paper; colored pencils or pens.

PROCEDURE:
A.   Bring to class at least four different food labels that list U.S. RDA percentages. As a class, group everyone's food labels into food groups.
B.   Choose two food labels from each food group to compare. For example, from the fruit and vegetable group you could compare two different fruits or two different vegetables. Or you could compare frozen versus canned peas or beans. From the bread and cereal group you could compare two different kinds of cereal, or white versus whole wheat bread. From the milk group you could compare yogurt and ice cream or milk.
C.   Make a graph, showing U.S. RDA percentages, from 0 to 100 percent, along the vertical axis and the nutrients protein, vitamins A and C, thiamine (B-1), riboflavin (B-2), niacin, calcium, and iron along the horizontal axis.
D.   Draw a graph for U.S. RDA percentages per serving from your food labels. Plot the information from each label in a different color.
   1.   Which foods are the most nutrient-dense for each nutrient?
E.   Make one graph comparing the Calorie content per serving for each of your food labels and one showing the percentage of Calories derived from sugars and fat.
   2.   Which foods contain the most Calories? Do these foods contain empty Calories or do they also contain other nutrients?

CHAPTER 3

Bones, Muscles, and Fitness Fundamentals

OBJECTIVES

- DESCRIBE the structure and function of bones
  DESCRIBE the composition of bone tissue
  DESCRIBE the structure and function of
- muscles

- STATE some common bone, muscle, and joint problems, and their prevention and care
- DESCRIBE how exercise improves the overall fitness of bones and muscles

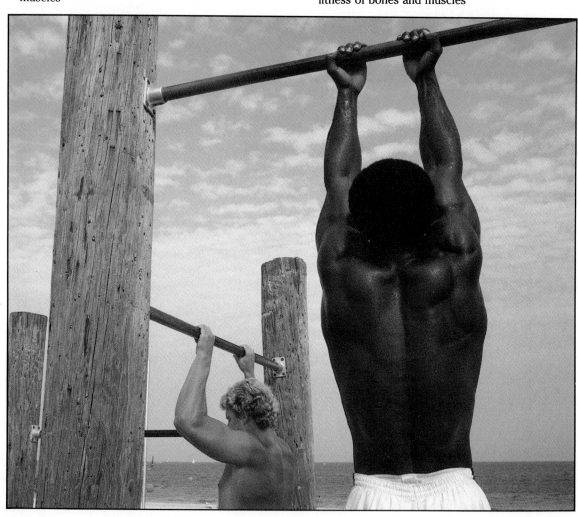

Suppose you are an architectural engineer and your assignment is to build a movable framework that is as strong as iron but fifteen times lighter. It has to last a century and be resistant to water. The framework also has to move freely and repair itself in case of a break. This structure should not wear out with use, but should actually strengthen with use.

What an assignment! Impossible, you say? Yet, your bones and muscles are such a system. Bones provide a strong framework capable of repairing itself. Exercising bones and muscles actually strengthens them. No engineer can build a machine to duplicate the intricate structure and function of your bones and muscles.

THE STRUCTURE AND FUNCTION OF BONE

Bones serve many important functions. Without bones, you would not be able to walk, talk, or lift objects. There would be little protection for your brain and internal organs. Nor would you have blood. In fact, without bones, you would be a formless blob. Bones serve the following functions:

1. They form the supporting framework of the body.
2. They provide areas for muscles to attach and function in the movement of the body.
3. They protect vital internal organs that lie under them.
4. They serve as the storehouse for essential minerals.
5. They function as centers for the production of red blood cells and certain kinds of white blood cells.

COMPOSITION OF BONE TISSUES

Your bone is a living organ that is richly supplied with blood. It requires oxygen and nourishment so that it can continually grow and repair itself. Living bone cells constantly remove nutrients from the blood and form new bone tissue.

Bone tissue is composed of living cells and hard mineral matter. Look at the magnified cross section of bone tissue in Figure 3-1. As you can see, bone tissue is made up of units of concentric rings. The light-colored core of each unit is a canal, through which blood vessels and nerves pass. The concentric rings are made up of mineral matter, mainly cal-

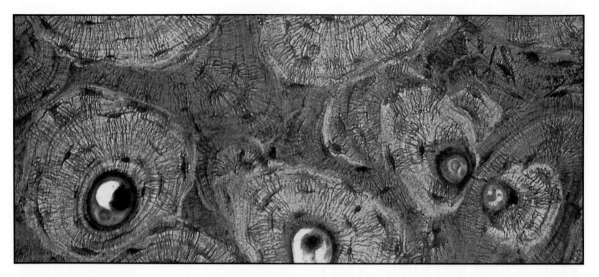

3–1. A cross-section of living bone tissue (magnified 162 times).

cium phosphate and calcium carbonate. About two thirds of the bone substance in an adult is mineral matter. The small dark areas scattered between the rings are living bone cells. The numerous thin dark lines running outward from the central canal are ducts through which fluids diffuse.

STRUCTURE OF BONE

The diagram in Figure 3-2 shows a thighbone cut lengthwise. At its upper end, the ball-shaped head of the thighbone fits into the socket of the hipbone. The point at which two bones meet is called a **joint.** For example, the thighbone joins the lower leg bone at the knee joint.

Have you ever seen the thin, pink, tough membrane covering the outside of a bone? This is the **periosteum** (pear-ee-**ahs**-tee-um), a tough, living membrane that covers all of the bone except the ends. This living membrane is richly supplied with blood vessels. The blood vessels branch into the bone at various openings. The periosteum is necessary for nourishing the bone and for producing bone cells. It also works at repairing injuries.

The ends of the bone are covered with *articular cartilage*, a form of permanent cartilage. This provides a smooth surface so that two bones can glide over each other.

As you can see in Figure 3-1, bones are not solid. Because the bone tissue near the joints is loose or spongy, it has the ability to absorb mechanical shock. This area is referred to as *spongy bone*. There are many cavities in spongy bone,

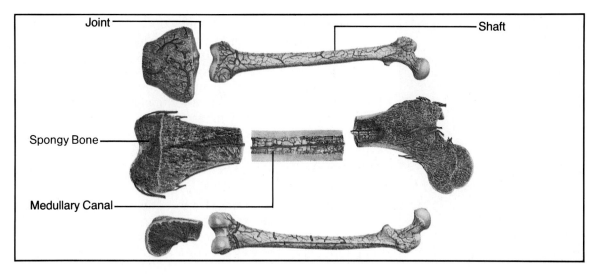

Joint — Shaft

Compact Bone — Periosteum

Medullary Canal — Vein and Artery

3–2. The femur, or thighbone, cut lengthwise.

which contain mostly *red marrow*. Red marrow produces the red blood cells and most of the white blood cells.

Between the joint ends, the bone narrows into the more slender area called the *shaft*. At the center of the shaft is a broad **medullary canal** (me-**dull**-lar-ree ka-**nal**), filled with yellow marrow. Most of the cells in this marrow are fat cells. One of the main functions of yellow marrow is to store fat. In addition, the yellow marrow contains many blood vessels and a few cells that form white blood cells.

Beneath the periosteum is a hard bony layer. This layer, formed by the periosteum, thickens as the bone grows in diameter. There is a network of canals running throughout the bony layer. These canals, called **Haversian** (ha-**ver**-zhun) canals, contain blood vessels that supply nourishment to the bone cells.

The body framework is made up of both cartilage (a semi-isoft substance) and bone. The skeleton of a baby contains a lot of cartilage. As the bones grow older, cartilage cells are replaced by bone cells and minerals. The process is called *ossification* (os-si-fik-**kay**-shun). Ossification involves the deposit of calcium between bone cells. This makes the bones stronger. Ossification continues through childhood and into early adult life. The bones become harder and capable of bearing more weight, but they also become more brittle. This explains why bones fracture more easily in an adult than in a young person. By old age, much of the organic matter and some of the mineral matter in bones has disappeared. As a result, bones become very brittle.

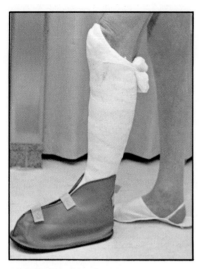

3–3. This cast will allow this woman to walk on her broken leg. How will walking help it to heal faster?

Some parts of the body's framework are composed of permanent cartilage. Examples are the outer ears, the end of the nose, the larynx (voice box), the rings of the trachea (the windpipe), the rib cartilages, the disks between the vertebrae, and the disks that cushion the leg bones at the knee joint. Permanent cartilage gives form without being hard and rigid. Think of how many times you would fracture an ear or the end of your nose if they were bone instead of cartilage!

BUILDING BONE TISSUE

Living bone cells constantly tear down old bone tissue and replace it with new tissue. Three conditions are necessary for growth and hardening of bone. *First*, an adequate supply of minerals, like calcium and phosphorus, is essential to bone formation. There is a *second* equally important requirement for bone formation. Certain chemical substances must be present for bone cells to make use of minerals in the diet. One of these is vitamin D, found in egg yolk, fortified milk, and fresh vegetables. *Third*, certain hormones are essential for proper growth and maintenance of bones.

Bones store the body's supply of calcium and phosphorus. If there is enough calcium and phosphorus in the diet, then the body does not use the deposits in the bones. However, if there is a lack of these minerals in the blood, the muscles, or the nerves, the body will use the supply in the bones. The result, of course, is a weakening of the skeleton with increased danger of bone fractures.

Bones become stronger with use. Bones that anchor strong muscles thicken to bear the stress. Weight-bearing bones develop heavy mineral deposits. If you had to spend most of your life in bed, you would lose much of the mineral deposits in your leg bones, weakening them. Minerals would be deposited in a bone fracture slower if you stopped using a broken leg for a while. If the fractured bone is supported by a brace or cast, and you continue using it, the healing process is speeded up. This is the principle of a *walking* cast.

THE STRUCTURE OF THE SKELETON

The skeleton in an adult consists of about 206 separate bones of many sizes, shapes, and functions. The bones of your skeleton range in size from the tiniest bones of the middle ear to the largest bones of the upper leg. The shapes of bones also vary. Some are long and cylindrical, and others are flat and platelike.

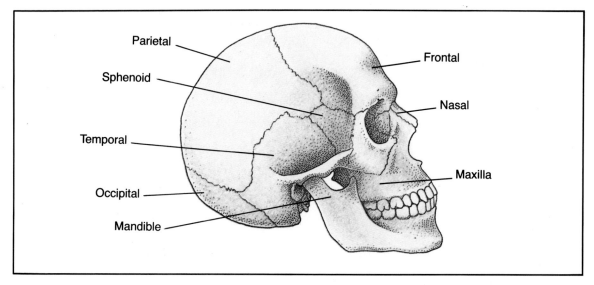

Parietal

Sphenoid

Temporal

Occipital

Mandible

Frontal

Nasal

Maxilla

BONES OF THE SKULL

To better understand the structure of the skull bones, we will divide the skull into various regions. Beginning with the cranium, eight immovable and interlocking **cranial** (**kray**-nee-al) bones form a firm case enclosing the brain. These bones join along zigzag lines known as **sutures** (**sue**-churs) (see Figure 3-4).

Three tiny ear bones form a flexible chain across the middle ear. They perform a special function in transmitting sound vibrations.

Fourteen **facial** (**fay**-shul) bones form the face. Thirteen of them are interlocking and immovable. The fourteenth, the lower jawbone, moves up and down and sidewise when you speak and chew food. A small **hyoid** (**hi**-oid) bone lies at the base of the tongue as support. The teeth are not bones but grow out of soft tissues that line their bone sockets.

The bones on each side of the cranium contain air cavities called **sinuses** (**sigh**-nuss-sez). The sinuses open into the nasal passages. The exact function of the sinuses is not known. They may serve to lighten the weight of the skull.

THE SPINAL COLUMN

Thirty-three small bones, called the **vertebrae** (**ver**-teh-bray), form the "backbone," or spinal column. The spinal cord is located inside the spinal column. Run your hand along your backbone. Each bump you feel is a vertebra.

3–4. Except for the jaw bone, the bones of the skull are fused together to form a single unit.

FRONT VIEW OF BONES AND MUSCLES

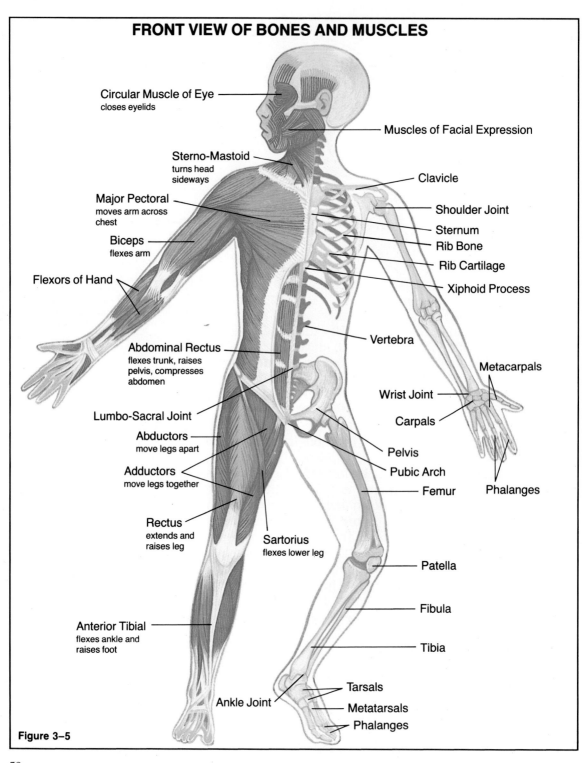

Circular Muscle of Eye
closes eyelids

Muscles of Facial Expression

Sterno-Mastoid
turns head
sideways

Clavicle

Major Pectoral
moves arm across
chest

Shoulder Joint

Sternum

Rib Bone

Biceps
flexes arm

Rib Cartilage

Flexors of Hand

Xiphoid Process

Vertebra

Abdominal Rectus
flexes trunk, raises
pelvis, compresses
abdomen

Metacarpals

Wrist Joint

Lumbo-Sacral Joint

Carpals

Abductors
move legs apart

Pelvis

Pubic Arch

Adductors
move legs together

Femur

Phalanges

Rectus
extends and
raises leg

Sartorius
flexes lower leg

Patella

Fibula

Anterior Tibial
flexes ankle and
raises foot

Tibia

Tarsals

Ankle Joint

Metatarsals

Phalanges

Figure 3–5

BACK VIEW OF BONES AND MUSCLES

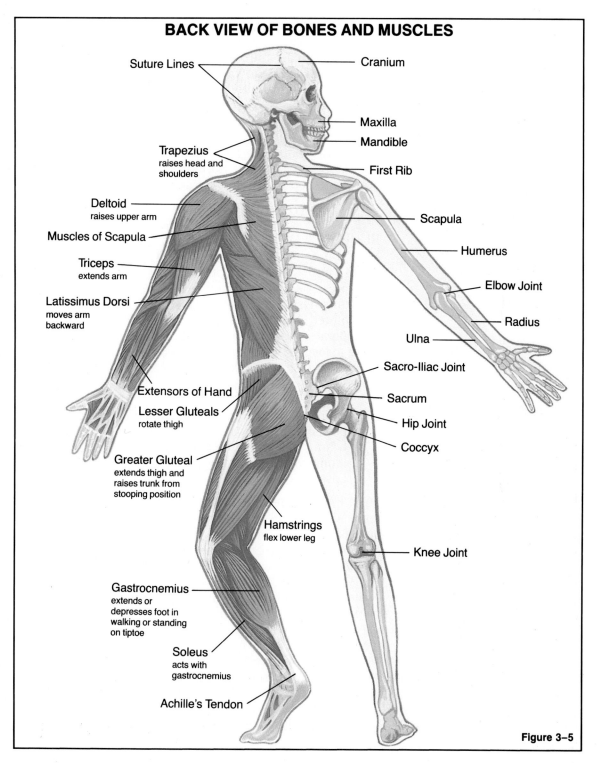

Suture Lines

Cranium

Maxilla

Mandible

Trapezius
raises head and
shoulders

First Rib

Deltoid
raises upper arm

Scapula

Muscles of Scapula

Humerus

Triceps
extends arm

Elbow Joint

Latissimus Dorsi
moves arm
backward

Radius

Ulna

Sacro-Illiac Joint

Extensors of Hand

Sacrum

Lesser Gluteals
rotate thigh

Hip Joint

Coccyx

Greater Gluteal
extends thigh and
raises trunk from
stooping position

Hamstrings
flex lower leg

Knee Joint

Gastrocnemius
extends or
depresses foot in
walking or standing
on tiptoe

Soleus
acts with
gastrocnemius

Achille's Tendon

Figure 3–5

Each of the vertebrae is cushioned by cartilage disks. The spinal column is divided into five regions (see Figure 3-5). Seven **cervical** (**ser-**vih-kul) vertebrae form the neck. Twelve **thoracic** (tho-**ras-**ik) vertebrae lie in the chest region. The first ten vertebrae in this region contain sockets to which the ribs are fastened. The five **lumbar** (**lum-**bar) vertebrae of the abdominal region are the largest and heaviest. In the pelvic region, five vertebrae are fused to form the **sacrum** (**say-**krum). The last four vertebrae are fused to form the tailbone, or **coccyx** (**kock-**siks). The coccyx is a functionless region of the spinal column.

SPINAL PROBLEMS

RUPTURED DISKS.   The cartilage disks between vertebrae have soft, jellylike centers that, under stressful back movements, may rupture out of their disks. These centers may then press on spinal nerves. This causes pain with tingling and numbness, which may reach all the way to the foot.

Ruptured disks are usually treated with bed rest, traction to separate the vertebrae, and certain exercises. Should these measures fail, surgery may be necessary. Recently, injecting the disk with a substance that dissolves the jellylike material seems successful in some cases. To prevent ruptured disks, one should:

1. Exercise to strengthen the abdominal muscles and promote better posture.
2. Learn to lift with a straight back by "squatting" and lifting with the more powerful leg muscles.
3. Lose excess weight.

SCOLIOSIS: Lateral Spinal Curvature.   The spine is normally slightly curved. The *forward* curve in the lumbar region is the most pronounced. However, some people have *lateral* curvatures, called **scoliosis,** which may occur during puberty. When observing the spine of a person with scoliosis, his or her spine appears "S-shaped." One shoulder is higher than the other. In more severe cases, one shoulder blade is more prominent than the other. If not corrected during puberty, scoliosis may cause serious deformity in later life.

The usual treatment is a special brace designed to gradually correct the scoliosis. In some cases, surgery is required to correct the curvature. A newer experimental treatment consists of electrical stimulation of certain back muscles to pull the spine into a more normal alignment.

3–6. When lifting heavy objects, squat and use your leg muscles, not your back muscles.

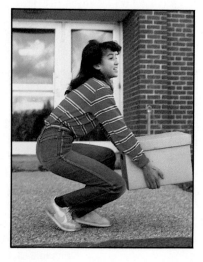

UNIT 1   HELP YOURSELF TO HEALTH

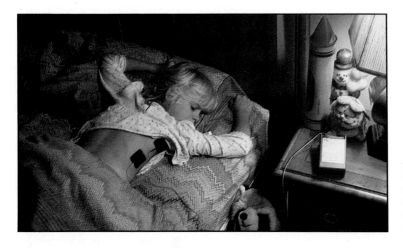

3–7. This child is being treated for scoliosis while she sleeps. Mild electrical stimulation of her back muscles brings her spine into proper alignment.

THE EXPANDABLE CHEST

The bones of the chest form a cone-shaped cage that encloses the heart and lungs. The flat *sternum*, or breastbone, lies in the middle and in front of the chest. The rib cage is an expanding framework. When the chest cavity expands, the lungs fill with air. Put your hands around your rib cage, and feel how it expands as you take a deep breath.

Twelve pairs of *ribs* arch around the chest cavity. Counting from the top down, the first seven pairs of ribs are the *true ribs*. They are called true ribs because they are fastened to the sternum by flexible cartilages at the front. This allows the chest to expand and contract during breathing movements. The cartilages of the next three ribs are called *false ribs*, since they are not directly attached to the sternum. These are attached in a group to the pair of true ribs above them. The last two pairs of ribs are shorter than the others and are not attached to the sternum. These are the so-called *floating ribs*.

BONES OF THE PECTORAL GIRDLE

The **pectoral girdle** (**pek-**tore-al **gir-**dl) is formed by two pairs of bones called the shoulder bones. The **clavicles** (**klav-**eh-kulz), or collarbones, extend from the breastbone to the points of the shoulders. The tip of each clavicle joins a **scapula** (**skap-**you-lah), or shoulder blade, forming the socket for the bone of the upper arm. You can easily feel your collarbone, from your breastbone to your shoulder. Can you feel where it joins your shoulder blade?

BONES OF THE ARM AND HAND

The upper arm contains a single bone called the **humerus** (**hue**-mer-us). The upper end of the humerus is a ball that fits into the socket of the scapula. In the elbow, the humerus joins the two bones of the lower arm. Turn the palm of your hand toward the front. The bones of the lower arm are side by side with the arm in this position. The **ulna** (**ul**-nah) is on the same side as the little finger. The **radius** (**ray**-dee-us) is on the thumb side.

Eight small **carpal** (**kar**-pal) bones form each wrist. These small, angular bones are arranged in two rows. Their placement allows movement in all directions. Five **metacarpals** (met-ah-**kar**-palz) extend through the hand. Each finger contains three short bones, or *phalanges*. The thumb has two phalanges. This makes 14 phalanges in each hand. Altogether, you have 30 bones in each hand and in each arm.

BONES OF THE PELVIC GIRDLE

The hip bones form a strong arch called the **pelvic** girdle. These bones carry the weight of the body, anchor the legs, and partly enclose the pelvic organs. The **sacroiliac** joint, which joins the pelvic bones to the spine, is well known because it is often the center of lower back pain.

The **ilium** (**ill**-ee-um) is the broad, flat portion of the pelvic girdle to which powerful back, hip, and thigh muscles are attached. The **ischium** (**is**-key-um) bones arch downward from the ilium forming a base that supports the body in a sitting position. The **pubic** bones arch toward the front and join in the midline of the pelvis. Since all of these bones are tightly fused, they are usually grouped as a pair of pelvic bones. The pelvic girdle is broader in women than in men, making childbearing possible.

BONES OF THE THIGH, LEG, AND FOOT

The bone structure of the leg and foot is similar to that of the arm and hand. The **femur** (**fee**-mur), or thighbone, is the largest bone of the body. Its upper end, or head, is a ball, which fits into the socket of the pelvic girdle. The broadened lower end of the femur joins the bones of the lower leg at the knee joint. This large joint is protected by a flat, triangular bone called the kneecap, or **patella** (pah-**tell**-lah). The **tibia** (**tib**-bee-ah) is the larger of the two

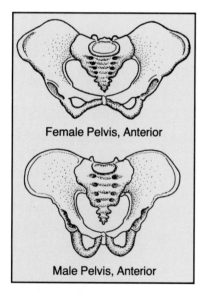

Female Pelvis, Anterior

Male Pelvis, Anterior

3–8. The pelvic girdle is broader in women to make childbearing possible.

bones of the lower leg. The smaller **fibula** (**fib**-you-lah) toward the outside of the leg gives added support for muscle attachments.

The foot contains 26 bones. The seven ankle bones, including the heel, form the principal weight-bearing part of the foot. Five **metatarsals** (met-ah-**tar**-salz) and 14 toe bones and their ligaments provide spring to cushion the shock involved in walking.

FOOT PROBLEMS

FALLEN ARCHES. The **longitudinal** (lengthwise) **arch** extends from the heel to the toes. The **transverse arch** runs across the foot where the toes join them.

If the transverse arch weakens, you usually develop a telltale callus on the sole of your foot. A weakened or fallen longitudinal arch causes a *flat foot*. This forces the body weight to shift to the inside, throwing the ankle and leg out of line. Pain in the arch, the ankle, and the calf muscles are common symptoms of *fallen arches*.

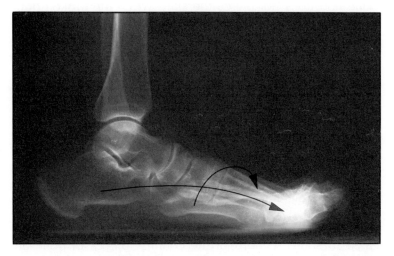

3–9. The longitudinal arch extends from the heel to the toes. The transverse arch runs across the foot.

3–10. Bunions, such as these, can only be corrected through surgery.

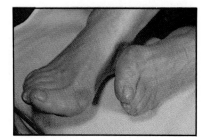

BUNIONS. A **bunion** is a painful, bony enlargement of the joint between the big toe and the first metatarsal. The big toe bends inward at the tip and outward where it joins the metatarsal bone. The inflamed joint at the base of the big toe develops a bunion. As the bunion increases in size, it may become painful to wear any shoes. In its early stages, a bunion can be helped by getting wider shoes. In later stages, an operation may be necessary.

CORNS. **Corns** are hard, thickened areas of epidermis. They develop from pressure and friction of shoes that do not fit well. They usually form on the toes or between them. Pain is caused by pressure of the hardened corn on the tender tissues beneath it. Paring corns with an instrument is dangerous because it can carry bacteria into tissues, causing infection. Pads may be used to relieve pressure on corns. If, after several weeks, a corn has not improved, a doctor should be consulted.

BONE FRACTURES

Any **fracture** is a break in a bone, which may be partial or complete. A child whose bones are flexible may bend a bone enough to break some of the fibers without breaking the whole bone. This is called a *greenstick fracture*. It doesn't usually need setting and heals rapidly. In a *closed fracture*, also called a *simple fracture*, a bone may be partially or completely broken. A fracture is closed when the bone end does not pierce the skin. When the broken bone pierces the skin, the break is an *open fracture*, or *compound fracture*. This is more serious because the ends are torn apart and the bone is exposed to infection.

The first step in healing is swelling and inflammation around the break. The blood supply around the break is increased. A sticky substance from the blood oozes around the fracture, forming a bony deposit called a *callus*. This aids in holding the broken bones together. The periosteum deposits new bone cells in the callus, and a deposit of new minerals begins. As the callus hardens, the bone ends are cemented together as they repair.

Through the miracles of bone surgery, fractured bones can be united with pins. Crushed bones are repaired by grafting bone onto the destroyed section. In bone banks, located in some sections of the country, pieces of bone are available for bone surgery. This bone tissue can serve as a framework until it is absorbed by the body and replaced with new bone.

Some fractures, especially of the tibia, fail to heal. This is called *non-union*. It has been found that certain kinds of electrical current will bring about healing in about 80 percent of such fractures.

Table 3-1 summarizes some of the most common bone injuries and their prevention and treatment.

3–11. Fractures of the left femur bone; a) a greenstick fracture; b) a closed fracture; c) a crushed femur bone fragment penetrated, producing an open fracture.

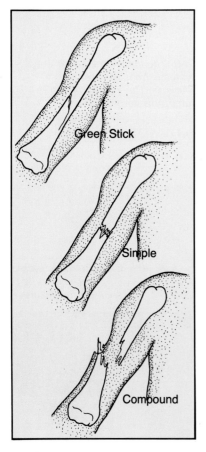

Green Stick

Simple

Compound

PREVENTION AND TREATMENT OF MUSCLE, BONE AND JOINT INJURIES

Injury	Cause	Common Sites	Symptoms	Prevention	Remedy
Dislocations	Tearing of ligaments that keep 2 bones in place	Fingers, thumbs, knees, hips, shoulders, jaw	Pain, swelling, stiffness	Exercises for strength and flexibility	Never try to push bones back into place, support damaged joint and seek medical help
Sprains	Damage to ligaments	Ankles, knees, back, wrists	Swelling and tenderness	Warm-up and cool-down exercises	Rest, use a cold compress for first aid; firm support; see a doctor
Strains	Stretching of muscles or tendons without tearing their fibers, (e.g., taking a wrong step)	Muscles in the neck, lower back, arm, wrist, leg, and ankle	Sudden sharp pain, without bruising or swelling	Regular exercise; warm-up and cool down exercises; do not use back muscles to lift	Rest, heat
Cramp	Muscle fibers contract but don't relax, often caused by muscle fatigue (not enough O_2 to muscle)	Diaphragm muscles, calves	Pain and tightening of muscle	Avoid large meals before exercise	Stretch & squeeze muscle; if it occurs often, see a doctor
Shin splints	Inflamed tendon that has been partly separated from the bone	Shins	Pain over shin area	Avoid running on hard surfaces, use proper running shoes	Stop strenuous exercise, do stretching exercises
Muscle tears	Tearing of many or all fibers	Lower back, arm, leg	Sudden disabling pain	Regular exercise; do not use back muscles to lift	Stop using muscle at once; see a doctor
Pulled muscles	Misstep, sudden stop or burst of activity	Hamstrings (back of thigh), calf muscles	Immediate or delayed soreness	Warm-up, avoid over-training, strengthening and stretching exercises	Stretching exercises; linament
Fractures	Cracks or complete breaks in bones	Long bones	Very painful swelling, loss of movement	Regular exercise to strengthen bones	Immobilize injured part, seek medical attention
Tendinitis	Inflamed tendon	Knees, elbows, Achilles tendon	Pain, usually worse in morning	Avoid strain; regular exercise	Rest; see a doctor
Torn knee cartilage	Tearing of cartilage in knee joint	Knees	Pain, Swelling Unable to move	Strengthen muscles and joints through exercise	Part or all of cartilage may need to be removed
Bursitis	Inflammation of the bursa (small sacs near a joint)	Knees, shoulders	Pain in the joints affected	Do not irritate joints by overusing	Rest, heat, aspirin; see a doctor, if persistent

Table 3–1

JOINTS: YOUR MOVABLE HINGES

STRUCTURE OF JOINTS

The point at which two bones meet is called a *joint*. Joints allow movement of the body framework. The ends of some bones are covered by thin membranes. Others are cushioned with layers or pads of cartilage. Strong, flexible **ligaments** bind bones together to form a sheath, or capsule, enclosing the movable joints. A joint capsule is lined with a membrane that secretes **synovial** (sigh-**no**-vee-al) **fluid,** a lubricating substance.

Generally, we classify joints as *freely movable*, *partially movable*, or *immovable*. These types of joints are shown in in Figure 3-12. Some allow freedom of movement. In other joints, movement is reduced to increase support. There are also joints that fuse bones together so that they form a protective shield or cover, and no movement can take place (such as the cranial bones).

Table 3-2 shows the kinds of joints in the body and their locations, structures, and uses.

3–12. These six types of joints represent the varieties found in the human body.

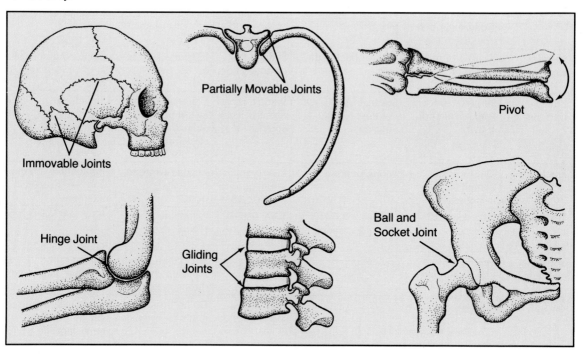

Immovable Joints

Partially Movable Joints

Pivot

Hinge Joint

Gliding Joints

Ball and Socket Joint

JOINTS OF THE BODY

Kind of Joint	Location	Structure	Use
Freely movable ball and socket	Shoulder, hip	A ball on one bone turns in the socket of another	Freedom of motion
Hinge	Elbow, knee, finger	Bone ends fit into each other and allow movement in one direction only	Strong support
Pivot	Head on spine, junction of radius and of humerus (lower arm)	Bone rotates in a ring or ring rotates around a bone	Turning or rotating movement
Gliding	Carpal bones of wrist and tarsal bones of ankle	Two nearly flat surfaces glide across each other	Limited movement, strong support
Partially movable	Cervical, thoracic, and lumbar vertebrae, pelvic bones and sacrum	Vertebrae separated by cartilage disks, pelvic bones and sacrum separated by coverings of cartilage	Varying degress of motion
Immovable	Bones of adult cranium	Bones joined along interlocking jagged lines	Protection

Table 3–2

JOINT INJURIES

SPRAINS.   A *sprain* results when a joint is moved too far. During a slight sprain, ligaments or tendons are stretched. In severe cases, they are torn loose, causing a painful and slow-healing injury. Swelling in a sprain is caused by increased fluid pouring into the joint from the surrounding membrane. The cause of a sprain is usually a sudden twist or an excessive pull. Since a sprain may be confused with a fracture, treatment should be prescribed by a doctor. There may also be damage to associated blood vessels or muscles.

DISLOCATIONS.   A *dislocation* is more severe than a sprain. The bone ends are moved out of place at the joint, and the ligaments holding them are severely stretched or torn. A dislocation must be set into a normal position and held during healing with a bandage or cast as support.

BURSITIS.   A *bursa* is a small sac situated near a joint. There are 52 in the body. Bursas lie between tendons that rub on each other, or between tendons and bones, to relieve friction between these structures. There is a large bursa at the kneecap and several around the knee joint; others are found at the elbow and the ankle. The bursa in the shoulder is situated near the ball of the humerus. A bursa may become inflamed due to injury, arthritis, or infection. The inflammation is very painful and is known as *bursitis*. It is most common in the shoulder and knee.

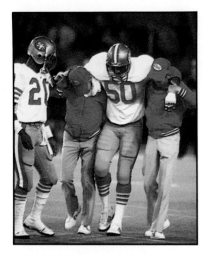

3–13. The cartilage pads in the knees are frequently torn in football.

TORN KNEE CARTILAGE. The cartilage pads in the knee joints are frequently torn in sports, especially football. They may then become loose and cause pain, swelling, and obstruction to free movement. It is estimated that about 200,000 Americans need surgical removal of part or all of one or both cartilage pads in their knees. This is usually done by opening the knee joint. A new method involves using an *arthroscope*, a slim viewing instrument that can be inserted, along with tiny surgical instruments, through small holes into the joint. In contrast to an open-knee operation, after use of an arthroscope a patient may leave the hospital on the same day, and walk within 24 hours. However, the procedure does require an experienced operating surgeon with a high level of skill. Table 3-1 summarizes some common joint injuries and their prevention and treatment.

MUSCLES

Without our muscles, our bones and joints would be useless. Bones cannot move by themselves. Moving, breathing, and swallowing would be impossible without muscles.

There are three kinds of muscles: (1) *skeletal muscle*, also known as *striated* or *voluntary*; (2) *smooth* or *involuntary muscle*, which forms the muscle layers of the digestive tract and other internal organs; and (3) *cardiac* or *heart muscle* (see Figure 3-14). In this chapter, we will concentrate only on *skeletal muscles*, so called because they are attached to the bones. They are under voluntary control, as opposed to smooth muscle and cardiac muscle, which are not.

3–14. These are cross-sections of the three types of muscles: skeletal, smooth, and cardiac (magnified 250 times).

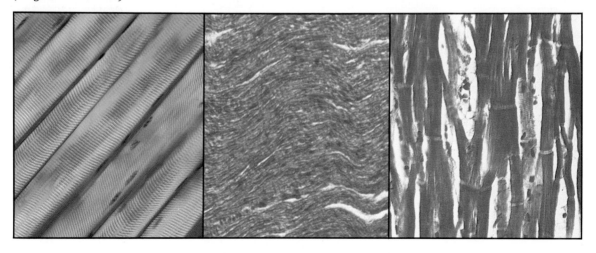

A skeletal muscle consists of a mass of muscle fibers grouped together. If you look at Figure 3-14, you will see that the fibers look like strands of a cable. Individual muscle cells make up the fibers. Notice the stripes (striations) running across them. This is why we refer to the skeletal muscles as **striated** (**strye**-ate-ted).

Muscle fibers have the power of shortening, called **contraction.** Each muscle fiber is connected to a nerve ending. When the brain sends a message to a muscle fiber, it contracts. But muscle fibers do not contract singly. The brain sends impulses to groups of fibers. The combined contraction of many muscle fibers shortens an entire muscle. The more muscle fibers that are stimulated in a muscle, the greater the force exerted. For example, more muscle fibers in your arm contract when you lift a heavy object than when you lift a light object.

MUSCLES WORK IN PAIRS

Muscles exert opposing pulls to bend and straighten joints by contracting. They cannot exert pushes. You can see how this works in your arm muscles (see Figure 3-15). The muscle on the front of your upper arm is your **biceps** muscle. When you contract this muscle, what happens? Your lower arm is pulled up. Your biceps muscles are attached to the shoulder bones by a pair of tendons. The shoulder bones, which are points of attachment that do not move, are called **origins.** The other end of the biceps attaches to one of the lower arm bones (the radius). This bone, the point of attachment that moves, is called the **insertion.**

3–15. The arm is straightened by contraction of the triceps muscle. In this position, the biceps muscle is relaxed. When the arm is bent, the action of the muscles reverses.

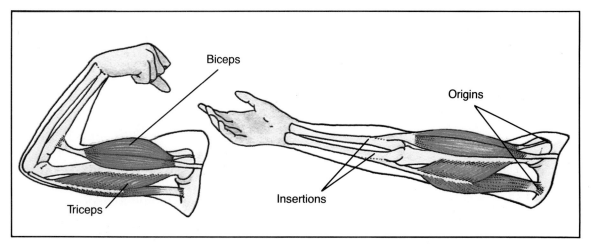

Biceps

Origins

Triceps

Insertions

Place your hand around your upper arm. Bend and straighten your arm several times. Do you feel the biceps contract when you bend your arm? What do you feel when you straighten your arm? The muscle on the backside of your upper arm, called the **triceps,** contracts when you straighten your arm. This pulls your arm down. The triceps has its origin in the shoulder. It has its insertion on the ulna of the lower arm. Muscles that bend joints are called **flexors.** Muscles that straighten joints are called **extensors.** Can you find the flexors and extensors for your knee joints?

ENERGY FOR MUSCLES

A muscle is like an engine. It cannot operate without fuel and oxygen. What do muscles use for energy? The principle raw fuel for muscles is *glucose* (blood sugar). Glucose is transported to the muscles through the bloodstream. The bloodstream also carries oxygen from the lungs to muscle fibers. Oxygen burns glucose for energy. Carbon dioxide and water, waste products of this reaction, are carried away by the bloodstream. When you exercise vigorously, you begin to breathe faster and your heart beats faster. This is because your muscle cells need more energy, and thus more oxygen and glucose. If you really exert yourself, your bloodstream may not be able to bring an adequate supply of oxygen to your muscle cells. Then your muscle cells begin to break down glucose for energy without oxygen. The same amount of glucose does not yield as much energy as it would if oxygen were present. Also, if oxygen is not present, the glucose breaks down into lactic acid, rather than carbon dioxide and water. This lactic acid can build up in muscle cells. After exercising, the lactic acid that has built up must be broken down, which requires oxygen. Deep breathing or panting continues after exercising so that oxygen is supplied for this. If too much lactic acid builds up, the muscles are irritated. Have you ever experienced aching muscles after vigorous exercising? Lactic acid buildup is what caused it.

MUSCLE INJURIES

Muscle strain is the most common muscle injury. Usually, no permanent damage is done. A hot bath and a good rest will relieve the soreness. A *torn muscle* is more serious. As a result of heavy lifting or a sudden pull, a tendon may rupture at some point or be torn loose from its bone anchorage. Surgery may be necessary to repair the tendon. A *muscle bruise* results from a blow on the muscle body. The muscle may be ruptured, allowing blood to escape around it. This causes a black-and-blue spot and painful swelling.

MUSCLE CRAMPS. If you exercise a muscle vigorously without warm-up exercises, you may experience a painful cramp. That is, the muscle contracts and will not relax. Rubbing a muscle will help it relax. If you can keep working it, the cramp will go away. Muscles may cramp during strenuous exercise due to lactic acid buildup. This is a constant danger while swimming. A victim may panic rather than simply work out a severe cramp. For this reason, you should avoid swimming alone.

RUPTURE OR HERNIA. The abdominal cavity is supported by sheets of muscle, ligaments, and tendons. The muscle tone holds the internal organs in their normal positions. However, there are weak places in the abdominal muscles, especially in the region of the navel and the lower groin area. A sudden pressure in the abdominal cavity during a hard cough or a strain while lifting causes a tear in the muscle layer at a weak place. This allows the intestine to press through the opening, causing a bulge. The condition is called a rupture, or *hernia*. Ordinary hernias may be relieved by wearing a support, but surgery is usually necessary to correct the condition.

Hernias are most common during childhood before the abdominal muscles have strengthened fully. During old age, the abdominal muscles weaken and lose tone. This change may allow a hernia to develop.

Table 3-1 summarizes some common muscle injuries and their prevention and care.

MUSCULAR DYSTROPHY

Muscular dystrophy is a disease that affects muscles. It is estimated that about 200,000 people have this disease. Muscular dystrophy occurs mostly in young children and is characterized by a gradual, progressive destruction of muscle fibers. As a result, the limbs may become useless. Its cause is unknown, but it is hereditary. No effective cure has yet been discovered. However, there are medicines that slow down the loss of protein from muscles. Also, exercise and physical therapy help people with this disease to retain the use of their limbs. The Muscular Dystrophy Association funds research to find the cause and a cure for this disease.

HEALTH TIP

If you suffer from backache, follow these measures unless otherwise advised by your doctor: sleep on a firm mattress; sit on hard, straight-backed chairs; and most important, do exercises to improve the strength and flexibility of the muscles in your back and stomach.

KEEPING BONES AND MUSCLES HEALTHY

Hippocrates, the father of medicine, observed that the parts of the body that are used are strengthened and those parts that are not used waste away. This is certainly true of your bones and muscles. Many people do not get enough exercise. As a result, muscles grow soft and weak, and bones grow brittle and break easily. People who exercise regularly keep their muscles strong and healthy. Exercise also strengthens bones and joints, so that they are less liable to be injured.

Totally fit muscles have four important characteristics. They are strong, flexible, well-coordinated, and can endure exercise over a long period of time. In this chapter, you will take a closer look at what happens to your muscles and bones when you exercise. In Chapter 4 you will learn more about how to put your bones and muscles to work to improve your overall fitness.

STRENGTH

What happens when muscles are exercised for strength? Muscles are a mix of two distinct types of muscle fibers. There are light-colored fibers and dark reddish brown fibers. The light-colored fibers can contract very quickly, but they also tire very quickly. The dark-colored fibers contract more slowly, but they also tire more slowly. When you exercise muscles to improve their strength, the light-colored muscle fibers increase in size. The overall number of muscle fibers remains the same. With strengthening exercises you can also contract more light muscle fibers at one time. Sprinting short distances and lifting weights are exercises that improve strength.

The light-colored muscle fibers in males can grow much bigger than those in females. This is because males have more of the hormone testosterone in their bodies, which is necessary for developing large muscles.

ENDURANCE

Muscle endurance is the ability of a set of muscles to repeat the same movement or exert the same pressure over a long period of time. For example, endurance is needed for swimming long distances. Exercises for endurance improve the dark-colored muscle fibers. They do not increase in number, but they do become more efficient. Do you remember what happens when you exercise? More oxygen and glucose are needed by your muscle cells for energy. If the bloodstream cannot supply sufficient oxygen, muscle cells break down glucose without it, and lactic acid builds up. With regular exercise, your body becomes more efficient in supplying oxygen and glucose to muscle cells. The heart becomes more efficient at pumping blood to supply more of both oxygen and glucose to the muscle cells. Blood vessels also become more efficient. As a result, oxygen and glucose reach dark-colored muscle fibers more quickly. Lactic acid does not build up as quickly and the muscles do not tire as readily.

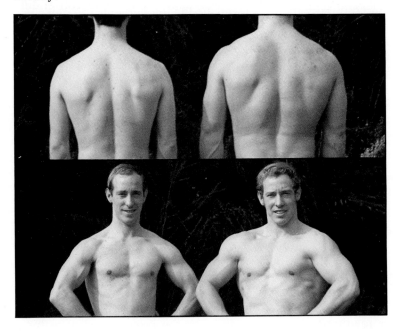

3–16. These two people are twins. Notice the difference in muscle development. What type of exercise do you think each one does?

Exercises for endurance also improve *muscle tone*. Let us imagine that you have a rope fastened to a wagon. The rope is a tendon, and the wagon is a movable bone. When you pull on the rope, the wagon moves toward you. If the rope is lying on the ground, you have to pull it tight before the wagon moves. But if the rope is already tight, the wagon moves as soon as you pull. Dark-colored muscles "keep their ropes tight" by being slightly contracted even when they are not pulling. This is what we mean by *tone*.

FLEXIBILITY

Muscles are grouped into muscle bundles. Surrounding these bundles is a tough tissue called *fascia.* Some of these fascia extend beyond the muscle bundles, becoming ligaments and tendons that attach the muscle to other muscles or to joints. If the fascia, ligaments, and tendons are inflexible, then movement is restricted. Doing stretching exercises lengthens and loosens them, which allows for more freedom of movement.

MOTOR SKILLS

Motor skills include skills that make it possible to move with more ease, speed, and grace. This involves the ability of the nervous system to coordinate the movements of muscles. The more you practice certain skills, the better coordination becomes. Muscular coordination is different for different sports. For example, different coordination is needed for bicycle riding than for swimming. With practice, nerve pathways are learned. Also, nerve cells at the muscles develop additional nerve endings.

POSTURE

Good posture means that the various parts of your body are in balance with one another. Look at the two people in Figure 3-17. The person with good posture stands so that you can draw a straight line through the neck, shoulders, lower back, pelvis, hip joints, knee joints, and ankle joints. Check your own posture in a mirror. Always try to remember to walk tall and sit tall.

In good sitting posture, the hips and back of the thighs support the weight. The feet should be flat on the floor. If the legs are crossed, they should be crossed at the ankles. Spreading the knees tends to let the body slump. The hips should be well back in the chair. The back of the chair is designed to give support to the lower part of the back.

When walking, start in the ideal standing posture. The heels of the leading leg should contact the ground first. Then immediately shift to the outer borders of the foot and forward. Swing your weight and your legs freely and easily from the hips to minimize jarring on contact. Maintain balance without twisting by allowing an easy arm swing from the shoulder. When you walk for exercise, try to work up a brisk pace and stay with it.

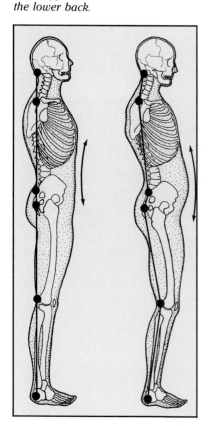

3–17. Strong abdominal muscles help to keep the posture aligned. Weak abdominal muscles cause an exaggerated curve in the lower back.

Good posture is important, not only because of appearance. Poor posture can cause backaches, poor circulation, and cramping of internal organs. Weak, inflexible muscles are the most common cause of poor posture. Doing exercises to increase strength, tone, and flexibility of your muscles is the best way to improve your posture. For example, exercises that build strength and tone in the abdominal muscles will improve overall posture. When abdominal muscles sag, the pelvis rotates downward and backward. The resulting swayback and potbelly throws the whole spine out of line. This causes strain on the muscles and ligaments, which may result in low backache, neckaches, and aching leg muscles.

Stand with your back to a wall, with every part of your upper body against it. You should not be able to get your fingers in back of your lower spine. To do this you must rotate your pelvis, which is accomplished by tightening your abdominal muscles. Here are two simple exercises to strengthen your abdominal muscles:

1. Lie on your back. With your knees bent and your hands clasped behind your head, curl up until half of your back is off the floor. Hold this position, then curl back down. Do 10 curls first; then gradually increase.
2. Tighten your abdominal muscles as though you were about to receive a blow there. Hold them tight 30 seconds and relax. You can do this exercise several times during the day, for example, while combing your hair or just walking down the street.

SUMMARY: Bones are made of living cells and hard mineral matter. Bone tissue is constantly being replaced. Good nutrition and exercise are essential for this process. The skeleton consists of 206 separate bones of many sizes and shapes. The point at which two bones meet is called a joint. There are three types of muscles: smooth, cardiac, and skeletal. Skeletal muscles, which are under voluntary control, are striated.

There are many different types of bone, muscle, and joint injuries. Many can be avoided by exercising properly to strengthen the body. Exercises for strength, endurance, flexibility, and motor control are essential to keep bones and muscles healthy. Good posture means the various parts of the body are in balance with one another. Good posture is important, not only for appearance, but also for overall health.

HEALTH IN HISTORY

Leonardo da Vinci (1452-1519), the great Renaissance artist, participated in dissection of the human body in order to learn more about the body to make his paintings and drawings more realistic. During this period, public dissections were also held to demonstrate the parts of the human body to medical students. The dissections were called "anatomies." Da Vinci is reported to have performed thirty dissections. Da Vinci originated a technique of medical illustration that is still in use today: the presentation of four views of an object so that the observer could, in effect, "walk around it" while looking at his drawing.

CHAPTER REVIEW

words at work

Find the word in the left column that fits one of the definitions in the right column. *DO NOT WRITE IN THIS BOOK.*

a. bursa
b. callus
c. corn
d. femur
e. longitudinal arch
f. ossification
g. periosteum
h. scoliosis
i. sinus
j. synovial fluid

1. The large bone in the upper leg
2. The fibrous membrane that covers a bone
3. A sac found near certain joints
4. The replacement of cartilage with bone
5. The lubricating substance in joint capsules
6. A deposit formed in the repair of a fracture
7. The arch that extends from the heel to the base of the toes
8. Abnormal lateral curvature of the spine
9. Hard, thickened area resulting from abnormal pressure on the toe
10. An air-filled cavity in facial bone

review questions

1. List five different functions of the bones of the body.
2. Identify the living parts of bone.
3. Describe ossification.
4. List three requirements for building bone.
5. What is a ruptured disk?
6. Describe the rib structure of the chest.
7. Describe the bone structure of the pectoral (shoulder) girdle.
8. Describe the bone structure of the arm and hand.
9. Locate the sacroiliac joint.
10. What causes flat feet?
11. What causes corns?
12. Classify fractures on the basis of the nature and extent of bone and tissue damage.
13. Name six kinds of joints and give an example of each.
14. Distinguish a sprain from a dislocation.
15. Name and identify three kinds of muscles.
16. Explain how flexor and extensor muscles work in pairs.
17. What is muscle tone?

18. What causes a muscle to contract?
19. What serious disease results from gradual destruction of the muscle fibers?
20. Define: muscle strain, torn muscle, and a muscle bruise.
21. What is the best way to handle a muscle cramp?
22. Describe what happens to dark and light muscle fibers when you exercise.
23. What is the best way to improve posture?
24. Describe what changes take place in the body when you exercise for flexibility.

discussion questions

1. Discuss how the structures of various bones, muscles, and joints are related to their functions.
2. Discuss the importance of posture.
3. Discuss what you would do for different muscle, bone, and joint injuries.
4. Discuss how the body changes in response to exercising for strength, endurance, flexibility, and motor skills.

investigating

PURPOSE:
To evaluate the strength of your leg and abdominal muscles.

MATERIAL NEEDED:
Tape measure.

PROCEDURE:
A. Wear comfortable, loose-fitting clothes and rubber-soled shoes for these exercises. Get a partner to work with you. Do not try these tests if you know you have a health problem.
B. To test abdominal strength, do bent knee sit-ups. Lie on your back with knees flexed, feet about 1 foot apart. Grasp your fingers together and hold behind your head. Your partner should hold your ankles so that your heels stay in contact with the floor. Curl up, beginning with your head. Touch one elbow to your opposite knee, then roll back down to the floor. Curl up again, and touch your other elbow to the other knee. Do as many sit-ups as you can in one minute. To pass the Youth Fitness Test, girls should do about 40 curls, and boys should do about 50.
C. To test the strength of your leg muscles, do a standing broad jump. Lay a measuring tape flat against the floor. Stand with your toes just behind the takeoff line. To prepare for the jump, swing your arms backward and forward. When ready to jump, swing your arms forcefully forward and upward, taking off from the balls of your feet. Allow three trials. Measure the longest jump from the take-off line to the nearest place where any part of the body hit the floor. Measure to the nearest inch. To pass the Youth Fitness Test, girls should jump at least 180 cm (6ft), and boys should jump over 210 cm (7ft).

CHAPTER 4

Exercise and Rest

OBJECTIVES

- STATE the mental and physical benefits of exercise
- DESCRIBE fitness tests and exercises for flexibility, strength, agility, and capacity of the heart and lungs
- DESCRIBE the factors that should be considered when planning a fitness program
- DEVISE a complete workout for total fitness
- DESCRIBE why sleep is needed and STATE some common causes of fatigue

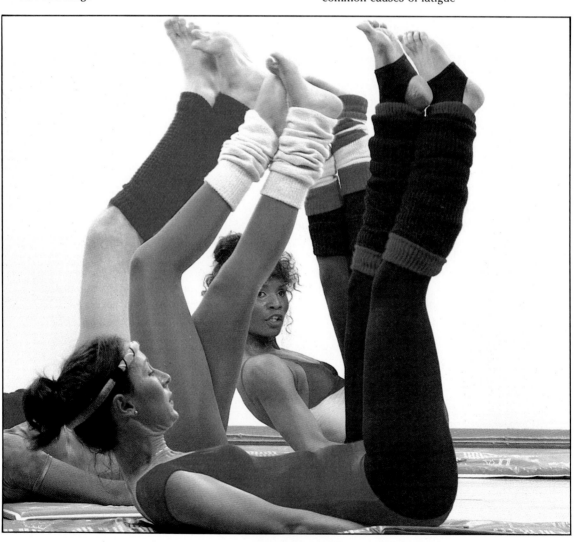

Less than a century ago life was very different in this country. Work was mostly done by human labor. Cars had not yet been invented, nor was there electricity to run labor-saving devices such as washing machines, dishwashers, can openers, and sewing machines.

Today, most people sit all day at work, drive everywhere rather than walk, and spend a lot of time in front of the television set.

Human inventions are wonderful for saving time and avoiding dreary tasks. However, the human body is built for moving. For these reasons, exercising for fitness is more important today than ever before.

THE IMPORTANCE OF PHYSICAL FITNESS

What is **physical fitness?** Physical fitness is the ability to carry out daily tasks comfortably with ample energy left over to meet unexpected emergencies. The more physically fit a person is, the greater is his or her energy reserve throughout the day. Can you complete your work at school, and then have energy left to pursue other activities, such as sports or hobbies? If so, you have achieved a minimal level of fitness. Fitness is not something that can be obtained without effort. It requires physical conditioning through an exercise or sports program. Total fitness also requires a commitment to live a life-style that includes good health habits, such as good nutrition, avoidance of harmful drugs and cigarettes, wholesome management of stress, and sufficient rest and sleep. It also includes good medical and dental care.

BENEFITS OF A FITNESS REGIME

You may be asking yourself, "Does exercise pay?" If you consider the beneficial physical and mental effects of exercise, then the answer is yes. Exercise helps you to look good and feel better. Different exercises can tone different areas of your body. Exercise can flatten the abdomen, remove excess fat, and improve posture.

Have you ever felt relaxed and exhilarated after a good workout? It has been proved that exercise is one of the best ways to reduce stress. Expending physical energy by hitting or throwing balls or running or doing other types of exercise

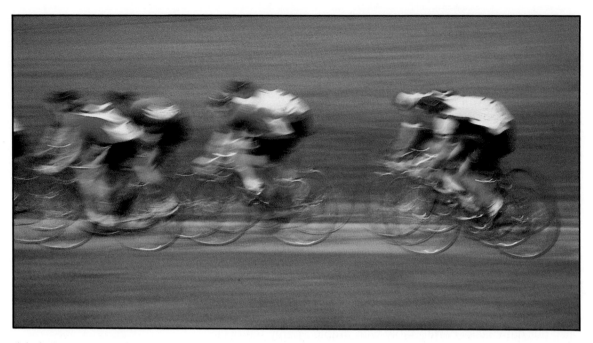

4-1. Active sports can keep you fit and relieve tension as well.

Table 4-1

SOME BENEFITS OF EXERCISE
Improved appearance
Improved circulation and respiration
Reduced susceptibility to injury
Improved alertness
Increased strength and endurance
Helps you lose weight
Improved self-esteem
Reduced risks of heart disease
Reduced risks of infections
Reduced stress
Helps you stop smoking

is a good way to get rid of frustrations and bothersome thoughts. Also, exercise increases the circulation of blood to the brain so that thinking becomes clearer.

Exercise can improve your physical health as well. As muscles, bones, and joints become stronger and more flexible, they are less susceptible to injury. Other complaints such as backaches and flat feet can also be reduced. But the most important benefits of exercise are its effects on the cardiovascular system (heart and blood vessels) and the respiratory system. Stamina can be increased by doing regular exercises that make the heart beat faster over long periods of time. The body can be trained to use oxygen more efficiently. During rigorous exercise, your body is forced to make changes that will supply extra oxygen to the muscle cells. The heart enlarges and the red blood cells, which carry oxygen from the lungs, also increase in number. In this way, each beat of the heart carries more oxygen. Increased stamina has beneficial effects on the rest of the body as well. The digestive, excretory and respiratory systems all benefit, too. A well-conditioned person can more easily fight off infectious diseases. It has been proved that exercise can also reduce the risks of developing chronic diseases, such as heart disease. Table 4-1 summarizes some of the benefits of exercise.

The President's Council on Physical Fitness was organized in 1956. Its purpose is to promote physical fitness in schools. The council recently conducted fitness tests on over 40 million students. Fifty-seven percent of these students were found to be physically unfit. Even more surprising was the fact that many of these young people were overweight and had high blood cholesterol. Their risks of developing high blood pressure and heart disease are very high. These are risk factors that doctors had believed appeared only later in life. Now is the time to begin a lifelong fitness program!

TAILORING A FITNESS PROGRAM FOR YOU

Fitness programs should be "tailor-made" for each individual. First of all, exercise programs should be based on the general condition and health of the participant. Thus, it is important to get a medical evaluation before beginning a fitness program. Many schools have medical examinations or screening procedures for all students participating in physical education programs. Before individuals begin personal fitness programs on their own, they should consult with a physician. A doctor may be able to help evaluate how much and how often to exercise.

HOW FIT ARE YOU?

You can do the following tests for endurance, flexibility, strength, and agility to rate your current level of fitness. However, do not be overly concerned about your ratings. What is most important is to find out where you are and where you want to be. These tests can also be used to measure improvement during a regular exercise program. People who have a history of cardiovascular problems should not take the test without medical approval.

RECOVERY INDEX TEST. The Youth Physical Fitness program sponsored by the President's Council on Physical Fitness recommends the *recovery index test*. This is a method of determining an individual's response to moderately strenuous exercise. Specifically, this test measures how efficient the respiratory and circulatory systems are. The more efficiently the lungs, heart, and circulatory system work, the slower the heart beats during and after exercise.

Great sages of the past knew the benefits of exercise. In about 100 B.C., Cicero observed that "exercise and temperance can preserve something of strength in our old age." Aristotle believed in exercise to "maintain a healthy mind in a healthy body." Thomas Jefferson advised people to "habituate yourself to walk fast without fatigue."

The test consists of stepping up and down on a platform about 16 inches high, 30 times a minute, for 4 minutes. At the signal "up," step up on the platform. Then immediately step down again. Step up and down every 2 seconds to the count of "Up, two, three, four." After sitting down for one minute, count your pulse for 30 seconds. Two minutes after the exercise, count your pulse for another 30 seconds. Three minutes after the exercise, do another 30-second count. Total the three counts. If the total is 132 or less, your rating is "excellent;" 133 to 149 is "very good;" 150 to 170 is "good;" 171 to 198, "fair;" 199 or more is considered "poor." Try the test and see how well you do.

FLEXIBILITY TEST. Another test for assessing fitness is the *flexibility test* for muscles. Sit on the floor with legs extended in front of you. Reach forward, as far as you can. If you can touch your toes, you have average muscular flexibility. If you can reach seven inches beyond your toes, you have excellent flexibility. If you fail to reach your toes by as much as seven inches, you are out of shape.

STRENGTH TESTS. The bent-knee sit-up and the standing broad jump described on page 71 can be used to measure abdominal and leg strength. The flexed-arm hang for girls and pull-ups for boys measure arm and shoulder strength. To do the flexed-arm hang, use an overhand grip on a sturdy bar. Hang free from the bar with elbows flexed and chin above the bar. Hold for as long as possible without moving your legs. To pass, girls should be able to hang for three seconds. To do pull-ups, hang from a sturdy bar. When pulling up, the chin should be above the bar. When lowering the body, the arms should be fully extended. To pass, boys age 14 should be able to do two pull-ups; age 15, three; age 16, four; and age 17, five.

AGILITY TEST. Can you change direction quickly while moving at full speed? If so, you have **agility.** The squat thrust can be used to measure agility. This is done in four counts. Start standing erect. On count one, bend your knees and place your hands on the floor in front of your feet; on count two, thrust your legs back so that your body is perfectly straight in a push-up position; on count three, return to the squat position; on count four, return to the standing position. To pass, girls should be able to do three squat thrusts in ten seconds. Boys should be able to do four in ten seconds.

HEALTH TIP

You can adapt your daily activities to help yourself achieve fitness. For example: walk, don't ride; roll your head and stretch your arms backward, forward, and up during the day; use the stairs rather than the elevator. In general, take the more physically difficult way whenever possible.

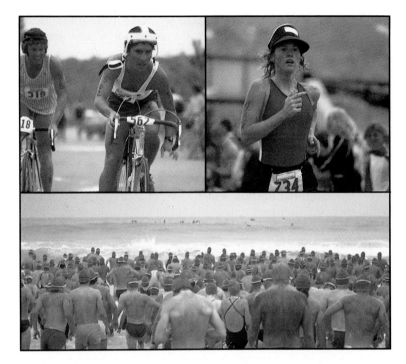

4-2. In triathlon competitions, contestants must swim 2 miles, run 20 miles, and bicycle 100 miles! This requires an incredible amount of endurance.

A BASIC FITNESS PROGRAM

There are some basic principles that you should consider when planning a fitness program. These include **intensity, duration, frequency,** and **type.**

How hard and for how long should you exercise? Intensity (how hard you work out) and duration (how long you work out) depends on how physically fit you are. An exercise program should be started slowly and increased gradually. Many people over-exercise at the beginning of a fitness program. Exercise should make you feel fresh and alive. If it makes you feel overly tired and sore, then cut down.

During an exercise program, muscles should be given a workout that exceeds normal demands. This is called **overload.** Strengthening of muscles does not take place unless the overload principle is followed. For example, if you can easily do twenty sit-ups, than push yourself to do five more. When twenty-five sit-ups become easy, do thirty. However, do not strain too much. If it hurts, something is wrong.

Frequency, or how often you exercise, is also important to consider. To be effective, exercises must be done on a regular basis. Hit and miss exercising may be worse than none. Conditioning occurs only if exercise is regular. Suddenly over-exercising an unconditioned body puts excess stress on the muscles, bones, and cardiovascular system. This is likely to result in injuries and illness. What type of exercise program should you begin? A fitness program should be fun. Choose activities that are enjoyable to you. In this way, you will be more likely to continue exercising.

SAFETY PRECAUTIONS

Although exercise entails some risks of being injured, most accidents and injuries can be prevented by following these simple rules:

1. Get a medical examination before beginning an exercise program.
2. Avoid steroid drugs that are used to build up muscles. They can have dangerous side effects, such as disrupting the normal development and function of the reproductive system.
3. Stop exercising if there is any problem, such as chest pain, dizziness, or shortness of breath.
4. Choose activities wisely for your fitness level. Make sure your body is in shape for the stresses involved.
5. Always learn and follow the proper techniques for the exercises of your choice.
6. Wear comfortable clothes that do not restrict circulation. Make sure you use the proper equipment, especially footwear. Remove jewelry, which may become snagged on immovable objects.
7. Drink plenty of water before, during, and after exercise. During vigorous exercise the body loses a lot of water through perspiration.
8. Always do warm-up exercises before and cool-down exercises after a work out to help prevent muscle pulls and muscle soreness.
9. Follow the preventive measures and treatments for muscle, bone, and joint injuries.
10. If you are exercising near traffic, be very careful. When bicycling, follow all traffic rules.
11. When you are outdoors exercising on a hot day, reduce the duration and intensity and drink extra water. On cold days, outdoors, wear several layers of clothing, but do not overdress since excess sweating can lead to chilling. Wear a hat and mittens.

EXERCISES FOR ENDURANCE

Exercises to improve your endurance are the most beneficial for overall health. These exercises are called **aerobics** (air-**roe**-bics). Aerobic means using air or oxygen. Aerobic exercises require the heart, lungs, and blood vessels to deliver oxygen and fuel to muscle cells over long periods of time. Jogging, swimming, bicycling, cross-county skiing, and aerobic dancing are good examples of aerobic exercises.

The harder you exercise, the faster your heart beats. To get the maximum benefits from exercise, you should exercise until you reach your **target heart rate.** This is 60 to 90 percent of your **maximum heart rate.** Maximum heart rate is the number of times your heart beats per minute when you have been running as far, as fast, and as long as possible. It can be estimated by subtracting your age from 220. Target heart rate is maximum heart rate multiplied by .75 and .85.

Halfway through a workout, stop and measure your heart rate. Find your pulse in your wrist or your neck. (See Figure 4-3.) Count the beats you feel for 10 seconds. Multiply that number times six to find your heart rate per minute. If your heart rate is below 75 percent, increase the intensity of your exercise. If it is above 85 percent, decrease the intensity of your exercise. As you improve, your heart rate should slow up. This will not happen immediately, but, if you stay on a good exercise program, you will see improvement.

Table 4-2 lists how often and for how long different aerobic exercises should be done for a minimum level of fitness.

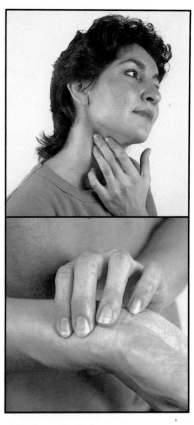

4-3. Can you find your pulse in your wrist and in the left side of your neck? Use your fingers, not your thumb, since your thumbs also have a pulse.

EXERCISE NEEDED FOR MINIMUM AEROBIC FITNESS				
Activity	Days per Week			
	6 days	5 days	4 days	3 days
Running	1 mi in 8 min	1 mi in 6.5 min	1.5 mi in 12 min	2 mi in 16 min
Swimming	600 yd in 15 min	800 yd in 20 min	1000 yd in 25 min	1,200 yd in 30 min
Cycling	5 mi in 20 min	6 mi in 24 min	8 mi in 32 min	10 mi in 40 min
Basketball or handball		40 min	50 min	70 min

Table 4-2

Adapted from *Choosing for Health*, O'Connor. (New York: Sanders College) p. 433.

JOGGING. Over 40 million Americans are now jogging to improve their health. It is one of the most beneficial kinds of aerobic exercise. If you start a jogging program, it is important to start slowly and gradually increase your speed and distance. Table 4-3 is a training schedule recommended by the President's Council on Physical Fitness and Sports.

When you jog, it is also important to pay attention to your form. Watch an expert runner. The whole body moves in perfect rhythm. The toes are pointed straight ahead. The body leans slightly forward from the hips. The arms swing loosely straight forward and back, never from side to side. The distance runner holds his forearms nearly parallel with the ground. When you jog, remember to hold your head up. Keep your back straight. Avoid looking at your feet. Bend your elbows and hold your arms away from the body. The foot lands on the heel, not on the ball of the foot. If you become tired, slow down and walk. Then begin again.

Wear loose, comfortable clothes. Select a pair of shoes with firm soles, good arch supports, and pliable tops. Wear well-fitted socks.

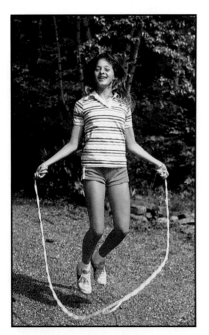

4-4. Jumping rope is an excellent aerobic exercise. It not only exercises the legs, but the wrists and arms as well.

BOYS' 12-WEEK JOGGING SCHEDULE

Distance	Week											
	1	2	3	4	5	6	7	8	9	10	11	12
660 yd	XX	XX	X	X								
880 yd	XXX	XX	XX	X	X	X	X					
1320 yd		X	XX	X	XX	X	X	X		X	X	X
1 mi				XX	X	XX	X	X	X	X	X	X
1¼ mi					X	X	XX	X	XX	X	X	X
1½ mi								XX	X	X	X	X
1¾ mi										X	X	X

GIRLS' 12-WEEK JOGGING SCHEDULE

Distance	Week											
	1	2	3	4	5	6	7	8	9	10	11	12
440 yd	XX	XX	X									
660 yd	XXX	XX	XX	X	X	X	X					
880 yd		X	XX	X	XX	X	X	X	X	X	X	X
1100 yd				XX	X	XX	X	X	X	X	X	X
1320 yd					X	X	XX	X	X	X	X	X
1 mi								XX	X	X	X	X
1¼ mi										X	X	X

Table 4-3

Adapted from *Youth Physical Fitness,* President's Council on Physical Fitness and Sports. (Washington, D.C.: U.S. Government Printing Office) p. 67.

Running tracks, grass fields, and parks are good places to jog. Try different routes to make your program more interesting. Try to avoid running on hard surfaces, since this tends to cause muscle, tendon, and joint injuries. Beware of traffic. The time of day when you jog is not important, although it is best not to jog until two hours after eating. Try to develop a regular schedule.

There are many excellent books on running. Some of these books will emphasize the fitness aspects of running; others will explain techniques such as speed and agility.

SWIMMING.   Swimming is one of the most beneficial exercises. All of the major muscle groups of the arms, legs, and trunk are used. It is also an excellent aerobic exercise if done steadily and vigorously. Swimming can also strengthen a weak back or loosen stiff joints.

Everyone should know how to swim, not only for exercise and enjoyment, but also in case of emergencies. You should not venture out into water alone unless you can swim well enough in case of an emergency. Only strong swimmers can rescue themselves and, if necessary, aid someone else. Instructions from an expert will help you to develop proper form for distance and speed strokes. If you get tired easily while swimming, get instruction to develop endurance and learn the proper techniques for swimming.

EXERCISES FOR MUSCULAR STRENGTH

Exercises to improve muscular strength should also be included in a program for total physical fitness. Muscular strength is the amount of force a muscle or group of muscles can exert when they contract. There are basically two types of exercises for muscular strengthening and toning. These are **isometric** and **isotonic** exercises. Isometric exercises contract muscles, yet they do not move the joints. Muscles do not increase in length, hence the term "isometric," which means "same length." One group of muscles exerts pressure on another group of muscles or on an immovable object. For example, contract your upper arm muscles and hold the contraction for ten seconds, or push against the door jamb for ten seconds. Isometric exercises can be practiced almost anyplace. Isotonic exercises are primarily for strengthening various parts of the body. They involve lifting or moving a weight through the complete range of movements of a particular joint or joints. Weight lifting and calisthenics are the most popular isotonic exercises.

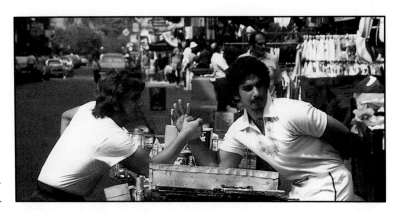

4-5. Arm wrestling is an isometric exercise. Muscles contract but joints do not move.

WEIGHT TRAINING. Weight training consists of a series of weight exercises designed to promote physical development and conditioning. Weight training, when performed properly, contributes to most aspects of physical conditioning, but especially to strength. Weight training also contributes to posture and appearance. Body measurement can be reapportioned and sagging contours can be firmed up through weight training.

Many schools have set up weight-training programs for both boys and girls. The program is not only for athletes. Everyone can profit from a weight-training program. Women should not fear that these exercises will cause them to develop bulky, mannish, overly muscular bodies. This occurs only during intensive, competitive weight-training programs.

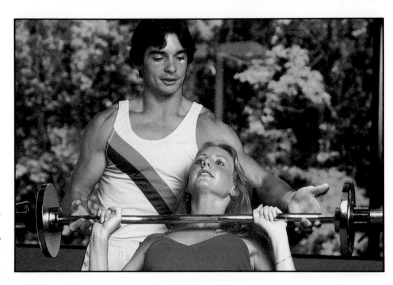

4-6. Weight training, for girls as well as boys, can improve strength and endurance and trim the body.

Women do not have enough of the male hormone testosterone, which naturally builds larger muscles in men. Through weight training, girls, as well as boys, can develop strength and muscle tone and have the added benefit of trim, well-formed figures.

One word of caution is in order. More harm than good can be done by improperly using a weight program to develop fitness. It is crucial that participants start slowly and gradually increase their workload. The size and physical condition of the participant should determine the amount of weight lifted. A weight-training program should always be under the direction of someone familiar with the rules of weight training. The following are rules for weight training:

1. Warm up before lifting and cool down after.
2. Never lift weights that are too heavy for your ability.
3. Lift weights slowly rather than swinging them, through a full range of motion.
4. Be sure to execute the return slowly.
5. The frequency of the workout should require time for recovery of worn-out tissue. Improvement can best be achieved by working three days per week for a half hour each time.

EXERCISES FOR FLEXIBILITY

Flexibility refers to the range of movement in joints and muscles. It is achieved by slowly stretching the joints and muscles to a desired point and then holding the stretch for 10 to 20 seconds. Flexibility reduces the risk of injury and helps prevent muscle soreness. Do not stretch muscles abruptly or bounce while stretching. This sets off a stretch reflex, which causes the muscles to contract and even be torn. Stretching exercises should begin and end every exercise program.

EXERCISES FOR MOTOR SKILLS

Exercises for motor skills are especially important if you wish to participate in sports. Practice improves the ability of muscles and nerves to work together. It is important to practice the *correct* techniques. Faulty techniques result in many athletic injuries, such as pulled muscles, strained ligaments, and bursitis. All sports involve the same basic skills, but different sports emphasize different skills. For example, a basketball player requires jumping ability, a baseball player needs striking power, and a place kicker needs to develop special skills in kicking.

THROWING. Consider three things when you practice throwing: stance, delivery, and follow-through. Your stance is the position from which you throw. Your delivery may be overhand, side arm, or underhand. The follow-through adds both power and control. You add power by putting your body behind the throw.

STRIKING. Striking with an object, such as a bat, hockey stick, tennis racket, or a golf club, is a basic part of many sports. Your striking power depends on the position of your feet and your ability to get your body behind the blow.

KICKING. A football kicker's combination of power and rhythm takes years of practice. The kicker kicks with the tip of the toe, the top of the foot, or the side of the foot. The soccer player controls the ball with the inside of the foot.

JUMPING. A jump combines a spring from your feet and the sudden force from straightening your legs. Your body weight supplies momentum. In certain sports, like basketball and rope jumping, timing a jump is of utmost importance. In high jumping, timing and form are essential. In long jumping, speed and drive are the greatest assets.

HEADING, PUSHING, AND PULLING. Heading means striking a ball with the head. It is used in soccer. Pushing and pulling are power skills. The climber and the wrestler use them. The person at an oar of a racing shell has a highly developed pulling skill.

4-7. Timing and form are essential in high jumping.

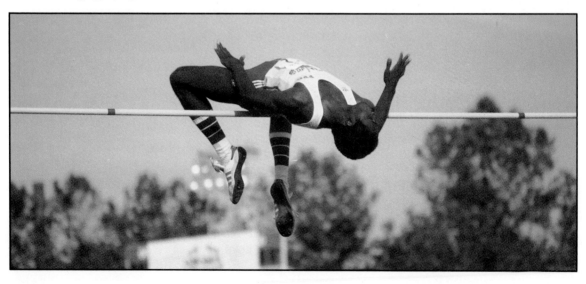

UNIT 1   HELP YOURSELF TO HEALTH

THE COMPLETE WORKOUT
FOR TOTAL FITNESS

A very efficient way of improving your overall fitness is to set up and follow a regular exercise program. The program should include all of the following phases.

THE WARM-UP. The **warm-up** gradually prepares the body for a more strenuous workout. The warm-up helps to prevent muscle injuries and soreness. If you plunge cold, tight muscles into vigorous exercise, you are asking for trouble. The warm-up also prepares the cardiovascular system for more strenuous work. You may choose not to do aerobic or isotonic exercises, but never skip the warm-up. The warm-up should continue for at least five to ten minutes and include several stretching exercises and some aerobic activity done at a reduced level. When you feel warm all over you will know that your body is ready for more strenuous work.

THE AEROBIC PHASE. The main purpose of this phase is to improve the capacity of the circulatory and respiratory systems. During aerobic exercises, large muscle groups are used in a rhythmic way. Remember that the aerobic workout needs to keep the body working continuously at your target heart rate for 20 to 30 minutes.

THE MUSCULAR STRENGTHENING AND TONING PHASE. Isotonic exercises, such as calisthenics and weight lifting, should be included for improving muscle strength and endurance. Although they are important, they should not be substituted for aerobic activities. The Isotonic phase includes exercises for major muscle groups and joints. The exercises should shift from one muscle group to another. This gives the muscles a chance to relax.

FLEXIBILITY PHASE. Stretching exercises are necessary to improve and maintain the range of movement in muscles and joints. When the muscles are completely warmed up, they stretch more effectively, and flexibility can be improved.

THE COOL-DOWN. The purpose of the cool-down is to return the body to a nonexercising state. Always include stretching exercises in the cool-down. This will help prevent muscle soreness. It usually takes about 10 minutes, depending on your degree of fitness. During the cool-down, gradually slow down your activity. For example, cool down by walking after jogging.

4-8. Exercise is important at any age.

STARTING A LIFELONG FITNESS PROGRAM

Now that you know some basic principles about fitness, you can better plan a lifelong fitness program. What do you enjoy more: individual or team sports? Are there sports that you enjoy during every season of the year? Participating in team and individual sports is an excellent way to maintain your physical fitness throughout life. Which sports you participate in is a matter of personal choice. Sports can be a means of socializing with others. Many friendships are formed through sports. Participating in team sports tests your ability to get along with others. You learn to depend on others, and others learn to depend on you. You learn the value of rules and the penalties for breaking them, and you take part in building team strategy. Although team sports are of great value, they have limitations. More space, more equipment, more players, and more supervision are necessary than for individual sports. In individual sports, you can compete against yourself or against others. You can progress at your own rate and choose opponents of similar ability.

Table 4-4 lists the fitness values of a variety of sports. In general, the more vigorously you exercise, the more calories you will burn and the more you will increase your endurance. For example, jogging at 5 mph will burn about 600 calories per hour, whereas running at 8 mph will burn 1000 calories per hour.

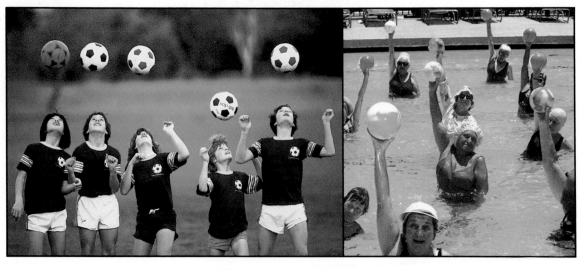

FITNESS VALUES OF SPORTS

Activity	Heart and Lung Capacity	Muscular Endurance	Strength	Flexibility	Calories Burned Per Hr
Baseball	low	medium	none	none	280
Basketball*	high	high	none	none	360-660
Bicycling*	high	high	medium	none	240-660
Bowling	none	low	none	none	240
Calisthenics	medium to high	medium to high	low	medium to high	360-600
Football	medium	high	medium	none	700
Golf	medium	none	none	none	300
Handball*	medium	medium	none	none	600
Jogging* (5 mph)	medium to high	medium to high	none	none	600
Skating (ice or roller)	low to high	low to high	none	none	420-700
Rope skipping*	medium to high	medium to high	none	none	300-800
Running* (8 mph)	high	medium to high	none	none	1000
Skiing downhill	low to high	low to high	low to medium	low	600
Skiing,* cross-country	medium to high	medium to high	low to medium	low	700-1000
Swimming*	low to high	low to high	low	none	360-1000
Tennis (singles)	high	medium	none	none	360-480
Tumbling	none	medium	medium	high	300
Volleyball	low to medium	low	none	medium	300-450
Walking (briskly)	medium	medium	none	medium	360
Weight training	none	low	medium to high	medium	480
Wrestling	medium to high	medium to high	low to medium	medium to high	900

*Aerobic exercises

Table 4-4

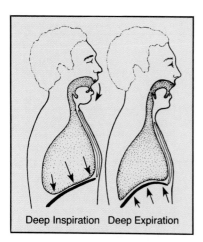

Deep Inspiration   Deep Expiration

4–9. Yawning is an involuntary reflex that is caused by fatigue, boredom, lack of oxygen, or seeing someone else yawn. Once a yawn starts, it is almost impossible to stop.

4–10. Drinking milk before bedtime can help you sleep. This is because it contains tryptophan, a natural sedative.

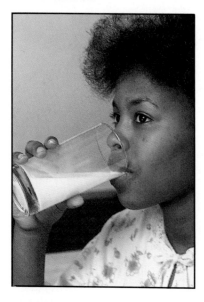

REST

Getting the proper rest is as important as getting enough exercise. Why must we sleep? Sleep is necessary to support human life. If the body is deprived of sleep, certain changes take place, such as personality disturbances and loss of coordination and the ability to concentrate.

Regular periods of sleep refresh the whole body. Many body changes take place during sleep that are not fully understood. Breathing changes noticeably when a person goes to sleep; it slows down and often becomes irregular. Heart action slows as much as 10 to 25 beats, which lowers the blood pressure. The rate at which the body tissues use food for energy decreases. Muscles lose much of their tone. Even the eyes relax, turning upward and outward under the closed eyelids. During deep sleep, growth hormones are released into the blood, which are necessary for the growth and maintenance of a healthy body. In children these hormones are needed for growth and repair. In adults they function only to restore tissue.

After a good night's sleep, a person feels a sense of well-being. The mind is alert, the muscles are relaxed, digestion functions properly, and appetite is healthy.

SLEEP REQUIREMENTS

CONDITIONS FOR SLEEP.   During sleep you lose nearly all sensory contact with your surroundings. This is easy to do if your surroundings are pleasant. A comfortable bed is essential. If your mattress has a lump in it, sensory nerves may bombard your brain with impulses all night long. A soft mattress may feel delightful when you first lie on it, but by morning you may wonder if you went to bed at all. Such a mattress will sag, causing tension on your back muscles. Some people believe that a very hard mattress is most healthful, but tests show that you sleep best on a medium-hard mattress, because it offers better support. Select a mattress and springs that are comfortable but that also provide support.

Quiet surroundings make it easier to sleep. Unusual noises during the night may not wake you but will disturb your sleep. However, a person who lives close to an airport becomes accustomed to the roar of jet planes. In this case, the brain learns to disregard the sound. A cool room is better than a hot one for sleeping. However, this does not mean

FOCUS ON HEALTH

RESEARCH ON SLEEP

What happens when you go to sleep? Sleep can be studied by measuring the electrical activity of the brain. Many thousands of volunteers have slept "wired up" to give researchers a picture of a typical night's sleep. Tiny electrodes are attached to different areas of the scalp. The electrical signals picked up by these electrodes are recorded on an electroencephalogram (EEG). EEG's show that there are four different depths, or stages, of sleep. Each of these stages has a different pattern of brain waves. During the night the depth of sleep increases and decreases in cycles. During a typical night's sleep, about four or five cycles occur, each about 90 minutes long. The cycles gradually become less deep until you awaken in the morning. The figure below shows the brain waves recorded during each stage of sleep and the sleep cycles.

When you go to bed, the rapid brain waves of the waking state are gradually replaced by the slow brain waves of light sleep. Then you sink into the second and third stages of sleep, marked by greater muscle relaxation and even slower brain waves. Next you slip into Stage IV sleep, which is the deepest sleep state. In this state, you are difficult to arouse and would be confused if awakened. After 70 minutes of Stages III and IV sleep, you drift into a lighter sleep and begin to

move restlessly. The eyes begin to move rapidly under closed lids, which is why this stage is called "rapid eye movement," or REM, sleep. People awakened from this stage of sleep report that they were dreaming. After ten minutes of REM sleep, you begin to drift back down into the deeper sleep stages, which marks the end of the first sleep cycle. The sleep cycle repeats itself about four more times during the night. With each repetition, REM periods lengthen and Stages III and IV periods shorten.

Many different sleep experiments have been performed. In dream laboratories, researchers wake the subjects after each period of REM sleep. The subjects then recount their dreams. Sleep deprivation experiments show that sleep is a necessity. After two or three nights without sleep, subjects lose their ability to perform routine tasks.

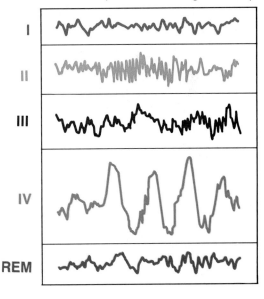

Brain wave patterns of 5 stages of sleep

that a bedroom should be too cold for comfort. Humidity is important, too. On warm, sticky nights you perspire heavily. A relative humidity of about 45 percent is ideal for sleeping comfort.

PERIOD OF REST. Individuals vary in the amounts of sleep they need. Regularity is more important than length of time. If you wake up in the morning refreshed and ready to go, undoubtedly you are getting enough sleep. The amount of sleep needed varies with age groups. A baby usually sleeps sixteen to twenty hours a day. During childhood the sleep period is reduced to ten to fourteen hours a day. The average adolescent or adult sleeps seven to nine hours, but needs vary with each individual. Some people require only five or six hours of sleep a day, while others need nine or ten hours. Older people require less sleep, often fewer than five to seven hours.

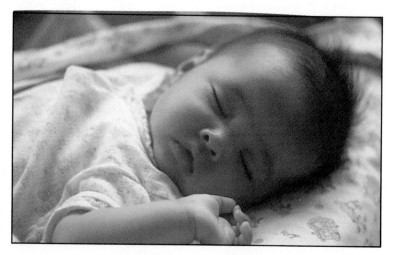

4–11. Babies require far more sleep than adults since they are growing rapidly.

SLEEP DISORDERS

Do you know how it feels to be completely worn out and yet you can't fall asleep? When the lights go out in your community tonight, more than one in twenty people will begin a period of restless tossing and worrying because they cannot go to sleep. In the morning they will get up tired and grouchy. Tomorrow night they will probably worry more because they lost sleep the night before. The inability to sleep is called **insomnia** (in-**sahm**-nee-ah). Insomnia can become a vicious circle. Worry and tension bring on insomnia, and worrying about insomnia increases sleeplessness.

For some people stimulants, such as nicotine and caffeine, as well as other drugs, such as alcohol, cause insomnia. Anxiety and depression are other causes of insomnia. Many people keep themselves awake worrying. If lack of sleep due to depression or anxiety continues, it may be necessary to seek help or to learn how to handle stress more effectively. Physical exercise during the day can also help you fall asleep at night. Don't learn to rely on sleeping pills. Over $100 million a year is spent on prescription sleeping pills. Yet sleep experts claim that most of these pills are a total waste of money. They usually lose their effectiveness within two weeks.

Occasional insomnia is common. If you should ever have insomnia, remember that your body benefits just by lying quietly in bed. That thought should prevent panic about loss of sleep. It is also important to realize that the body will take over and force you to sleep if lack of sleep becomes serious. Whatever you do, don't try to fall asleep. Try to distract your attention by counting sheep or by reading a boring book. In Chapter 8 you will learn about some progressive relaxation techniques that can also help you fall asleep.

Remember "Sleepy," one of the seven dwarfs? You probably know many people who tend to fall asleep in class. But there are some who fall asleep talking to others, or even when driving a car, resulting in serious accidents. These people may have a condition called **narcolepsy** (**nar**-coh-lep-see). Some victims of severe narcolepsy may experience brief attacks of paralysis after laughing or talking. The cause of narcolepsy is unknown, but it may be due to overactivity of the parts of the brain that induce sleep. There are certain medications that will control this condition and give its victims a chance to live a more normal life.

FATIGUE: A SYMPTOM WITH MANY CAUSES

Fatigue is the most common symptom any doctor hears. It is also more frequently heard in conversation with others than even the weather. There are many causes for fatigue, which include the amount of stress involved in daily living, exercise, diet, and sleep habits. More seriously, physical illnesses can be a cause of fatigue.

FATIGUE DUE TO PHYSICAL EXHAUSTION. Fatigue is usually a protective device. It is a warning that the body needs rest. During mental and physical exertion, the body oxidizes foods and releases energy to the tissues. Energy

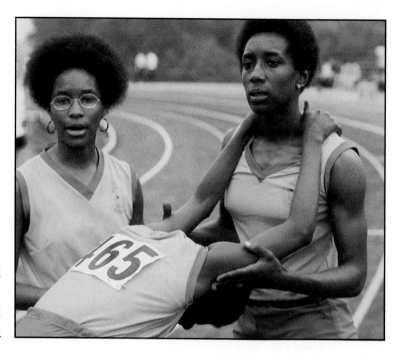

4–12. Exhaustion is a warning sign that you need to rest until wastes, such as carbon dioxide and lactic acid, can be eliminated from the body.

supplies power for all body activities. The greater the activity, the greater the demand for energy. Waste products, mainly carbon dioxide and lactic acid, are produced during the production of energy by body cells. Removal of these wastes is necessary for continued body activity. Our waste-removal system cannot keep up with an active body. As a result, waste products gradually build up and act as fatigue poisons. The poisonous waste products lower physical and mental activity, creating a feeling of exhaustion. This is your body's warning that fatigue has set in and that you need to rest until wastes have been eliminated. If you ignore the warning and push your body too far, you place it under strain.

FATIGUE DUE TO ILLNESS.   A sore throat, flu, a cold, or a bad sinus infection may leave one with an exhausted feeling. Often an infection can bring on fatigue in a few hours. Many kinds of infections produce poisons or toxins that are poured into the body tissues. The blood carries these poisons to all parts of the body. Bed rest is essential when these toxins cause general weakness and fatigue.

Anyone who has been in bed for several days during an infection remembers the physical fatigue that follows. The body has expended a great amount of energy fighting the infection. Also, muscles that were not worked have lost strength and tone. It can take several days for muscles to recover. It is important to take it easy after an illness to prevent a relapse.

FATIGUE DUE TO EMOTIONAL PROBLEMS.   Stan had been feeling tired and listless for the last several months. Even though he slept late on weekends and always went to bed early, he felt so tired that he could barely lift his feet when he walked. Recently he had lost a lot of weight. Yet the doctor could find nothing physically wrong with him. But upon questioning, the doctor discovered that Stan had been disappointed a number of times over the last year. His parents had separated and just after that his girl friend had left him. Stan had been severely depressed. He was so busy distracting himself and worrying about his fatigue, that he did not even recognize his depression.

Emotional conflicts, such as Stan's, are by far the most common causes of prolonged fatigue. When feelings are not expressed openly they often come out as physical symptoms. Fatigue is the most common symptom of repressed feelings.

When Stan realized what the real problem was, he was on the way to recovery. He began to talk about his feelings openly with a therapist. He also started exercising, which helped to relieve his anxiety. He quickly regained weight and soon he was back to his old self.

WHAT TO DO ABOUT FATIGUE.   If the cause of fatigue is lack of rest, the solution is simple. Get more rest. Get to know yourself better. Some people need more sleep than others. How much sleep do you need each night to feel your best? At what point during the day do you feel more energetic? Each person has his or her own inborn energy cycle, sometimes referred to as *biorhythm*. Some people are tired in the morning and gain momentum as the day goes along. They do their best work in the afternoon and evening and tend to go to bed late. Others arise early and are immediately wide awake. They do their best work in the morning and begin to wear down in the late afternoon. Try to schedule your activities around your own energy patterns.

Sometimes diet may be the cause of fatigue. What do you eat for breakfast? A low-sugar, high-protein diet in the morning will provide you with energy all morning. A doughnut or other sweets will give you a boost, but will quickly leave you feeling more tired than you were to begin with.

HEALTH ACTION

Construct a graph using time and energy levels as variables. Start with the hour you rise in the morning and mark the graph every two hours until bedtime. Use a range of 1 to 5 for the energy level. The number 1 indicates a low energy level. Do this for three days to determine your most productive period.

Today doctors report that tiredness is more likely a consequence of not enough physical activity, rather than too much. As you learned, regular exercise increases your body's ability to handle a greater workload. You get tired less quickly because your capacity is greater. Exercise also has a tranquilizing effect. It makes you feel pleasantly tired at the end of the day. It helps you to sleep soundly during the night.

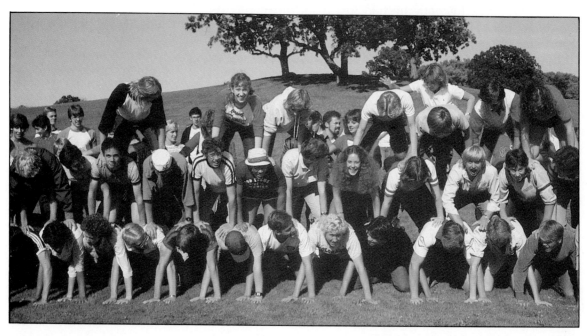

4–13. Proper rest and exercise are essential for optimal health.

SUMMARY: Physical fitness is the ability to carry out daily tasks with ample energy left over to meet emergencies. The benefits of exercise include improved appearance, self-esteem, strength and endurance, circulation and respiration, and general physical and mental health. The four factors that should be considered when planning a fitness program are frequency, duration, intensity, and type. For total fitness, an exercise program should include exercises for endurance, muscular strength, and flexibility. Rest is as important as exercise. Regular sleep refreshes the whole body. People's sleep requirements and energy cycles vary. There are many causes of fatigue, including physical and mental exhaustion, sickness, emotional problems, and diet.

CHAPTER REVIEW

words at work

Find the word in the left column that fits one the definitions in the right column. DO NOT WRITE IN THIS BOOK.

a. aerobic
b. warm-up
c. fatigue
d. insomnia
e. physical fitness
f. narcolepsy
g. cool-down
h. agility
i. target heart rate
j. overload

1. Exercises to return the body to a resting state
2. An abnormal tendency to fall asleep
3. Activities that require the use of a lot of oxygen
4. The ability to carry out daily tasks comfortably with ample energy left over
5. A warning that the body needs rest
6. Inability to sleep
7. Exercises to prepare the body for a more strenuous workout
8. Ability to change direction quickly while moving at full speed.
9. 75 to 85 percent of your maximum heart rate
10. A workout that exceeds normal demands

review questions

1. Define physical fitness.
2. List several benefits of exercises.
3. Define or explain isometric, isotonic, anaerobic, and aerobic types of exercises.
4. Make a list of several activities that have aerobic value.
5. List three major benefits of aerobic exercise.
6. What type of exercise would you recommend for increasing strength? Endurance?
7. Describe the recovery index test.
8. Explain how to determine your target heart rate.
9. Define intensity, frequency, and duration as they relate to exercise.
10. Explain the principle of "overload" as it applies to exercise.
11. Explain the importance of the warm-up and the cool-down periods.
12. List the basic athletic skills.
13. Describe the ideal form for jogging or running.
14. List some safety precautions to take when exercising.
15. List at least six training rules to follow in a weight-lifting program.
16. How does exercise relieve fatigue?

17. What is the best way to relieve fatigue caused by the general body weakness that usually follows an illness?
18. Account for the fact that some persons do their best work in the morning and others do their best work at night.
19. Why is sleep necessary?
20. Make a list of ideal conditions for sleeping.
21. What causes insomnia and how can it best be controlled?
22. List some common causes of fatigue.

discussion questions

1. Discuss the advantages and disadvantages of running for fitness.
2. Discuss the strengths and weaknesses of the physical education program in your school.
3. Is it true that older people are more fitness-conscious than high school students? Why or why not?
4. How can people make total fitness a way of life?

investigating

PURPOSE:
To devise an exercise program for total fitness that meets your needs.

MATERIALS NEEDED:
Paper and pen.

PROCEDURE:
A. Evaluate your fitness level, using the test described on pages 75-76.
　　1. What were your results on the recovery index test, the flexibility test, the strength test, and the agility test?
B. Calculate your target heart rate, as described on page 79.
　　2. What is your target heart rate?
C. Devise a weekly exercise program for total fitness. Include three to five exercise sessions that last 20 to 30 minutes each. Include exercises for endurance, flexibility, and strength. Decide what days and what time of day you will exercise.
　　3. Write down your exercise plan. Make a calendar for the week and record when and how you will exercise.
D. Follow your exercise schedule for one week. Keep track of your progress on the calendar. Measure your heart rate halfway through each exercise session to make sure you are within your target rate. Each time your exercise, record it on your calendar. At the end of the week, evaluate your exercise program.
　　4. Did you follow your exercise plan? Does the plan suit your needs, or does it need to be revised in some way? If so, how?
E. You can continue to exercise for total fitness. At the end of each month, check your progress by taking the fitness tests.

HEALTH
CAREERS

DIETITIAN

Educating consumers on how to get the most food value and nutrition for their dollar is just one way dietitians help improve our health. Dietitians also help fight sickness. This is because diet is an important factor in many health problems, such as diabetes, high blood pressure, and heart attack. When illness does strike, the dietitian must evaluate the patient's nutritional needs and then design a diet suited to those needs. Dietitians also help industry to

research, develop, and test new food products. They help restaurants, schools, and other food services to provide the best nutrition and quality. They help special groups, such as expectant mothers or aged people, get the nutritional advice they need. Having an interest in food and nutrition is the first requirement for this career. Science courses are important because dietitians must understand what happens to food after it enters the body: how it is broken down and how it is

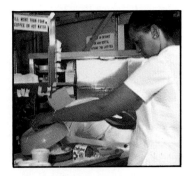

used by the body. For information, write to the American Dietetic Association, 430 North Michigan Avenue, Chicago, Illinois 60611.

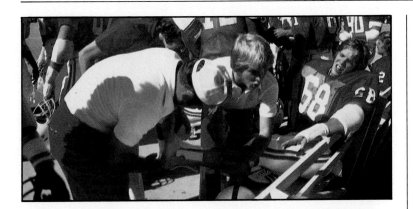

PHYSICAL EDUCATION TEACHER/ATHLETIC TRAINER

Athletic trainers are an important and growing part of physical education and team sports. They are responsible for preventing injuries and giving immediate first aid. They help carry out

treatment and rehabilitation prescribed by a physician who knows sports medicine. A four-year approved college program in athletic training includes courses in anatomy and physiology, nutrition, remedial exercise, and first aid and safety. If you enjoy sports and physical activities,

you may also want to consider a career as a physical education teacher. This job requires a college degree in physical education. Physical education teachers must have studied many subjects, including health education, sports, gymnastics, recreation, and first aid. They may teach health and physical education, or lead recreational programs. Explore these career choices. For information, contact the National Athletic Trainers Association, P.O. Box 1865, Greenville, North Carolina 27834; and the Alliance for Health, Physical Education and Recreation, 1201 Sixteenth Street, N.W., Washington, D.C. 20036.

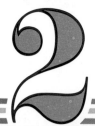

UNIT 2

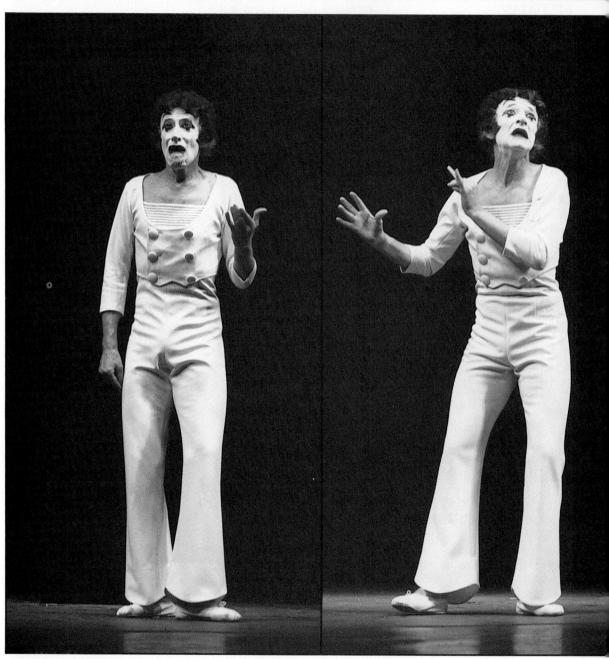

98

Your Personality

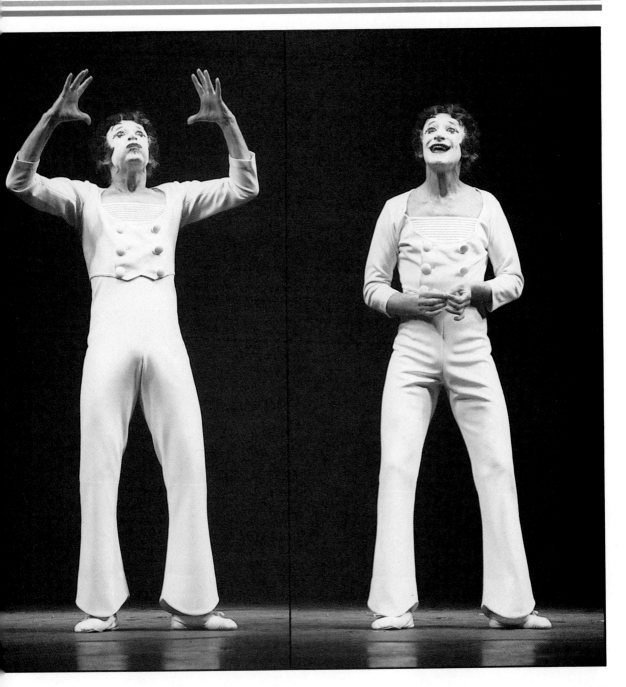

CHAPTER 5

Appearance

OBJECTIVES

- DESCRIBE the structure and function of the skin
- DISCUSS common skin problems and their treatment

- TRACE the development of tooth decay, tooth loss, and other dental problems
- OUTLINE and APPLY the principles of good skin, hair, nail, and dental care

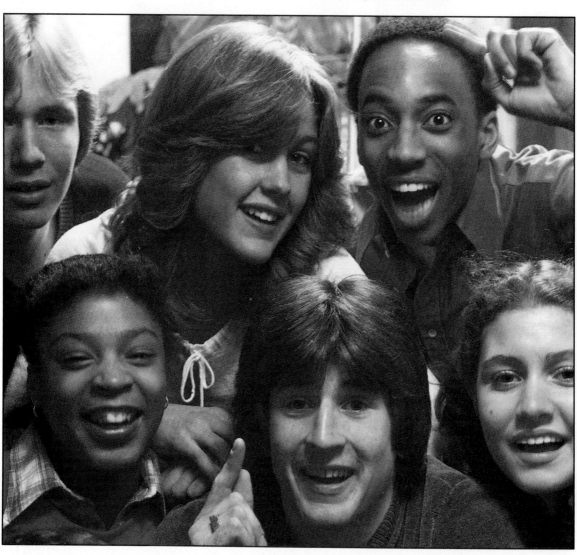

Gail was excited about her blind date with Jack. Her girl friend had told her all about him. Jack was tall and good-looking, a senior, and on the football team. He had a sense of humor and liked to dance.

Gail took extra care that night while getting ready for her date. She carefully pressed her best dress. Then she showered and polished her nails. She even fixed her hair in a new style.

When the bell rang, Gail finally met Jack. He was tall and handsome. But he was dressed in a rumpled shirt and badly worn jeans. His hair looked as if he had just run his fingers through it. He was unshaven and his nails were dirty. He needed deodorant. "Hi, Gail," he said. "Are you ready to go?" Who made the better impression?

YOUR FIRST IMPRESSION

When you meet people for the first time, what do you notice? Chances are you notice their appearance. You don't just see their physical features; you also see how they take care of their skin, hair, nails, and teeth. You may also notice their clothes, facial expressions, and posture. When others meet you, what impressions do they form? Do you make the best impression that you can?

Learning more about the structure and function of your skin, hair, nails, and teeth will help you take better care of yourself. Better personal health care will make you feel better about yourself. Others will feel better about you, too.

YOUR SKIN

The skin is the body's largest and most visible organ. It measures over 19,000 square centimeters (3,000 square inches). Therefore, the condition of the skin is an important part of your appearance. Do you know how to keep your skin looking its best? If you understand the structure and function of the skin, then you can apply the basics of proper skin care.

STRUCTURE AND FUNCTION OF THE SKIN

Most people assume that the skin is just a smooth body covering. However, if you look at a cross section of the skin under a microscope, you will see three distinct layers: the *epidermis*; the *dermis*; and the *subcutaneous layer*.

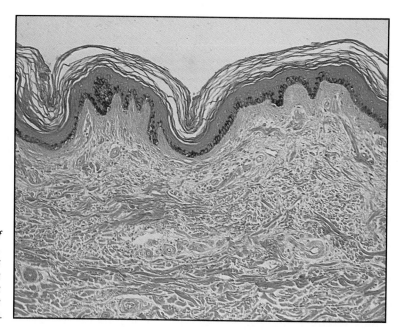

5–1. A cross section of skin, magnified 86 times. The solid purple is epidermis with the keratin layer on top. The black dots are melanin, and the rest is dermis.

THE EPIDERMIS. The **epidermis** (ep-eh-**der**-mis) is the outer skin layer. As you can see in Figure 5-1, the skin's surface has many ridges and valleys. These ridges, called **papillae** (pah-**pill**-a), form a complex design on the fingertips. The eye can detect small openings in the skin surface called **pores.** Look at Figure 5-2. Trace the route of the pores from the skin's surface to oil or sweat glands.

The top coat of the epidermis is composed of dead cells. This cell layer shields the body from sun, wind, harmful chemicals in the environment, and injuries. It also prevents moisture from leaving the body and forms a natural germ barrier. Beneath this surface, the inner cell layers of the epidermis are alive and active.

Do you know what gives the skin its particular color? A pigment called **melanin** (**mell**-ah-nin) is made in the inner layers of the epidermis. Dark-skinned people have more melanin than light-skinned people. Melanin protects the skin against the harmful ultraviolet rays of the sun. When exposed to the sun, the skin produces more melanin and tans. Freckles are small patches of melanin.

Cells at the bottom layer of the epidermis reproduce constantly. As new cells divide, older cells are pushed slowly to the surface. As they journey upward, they produce **keratin** (**care**-ah-tin). Keratin is a transparent, waterproof substance.

102

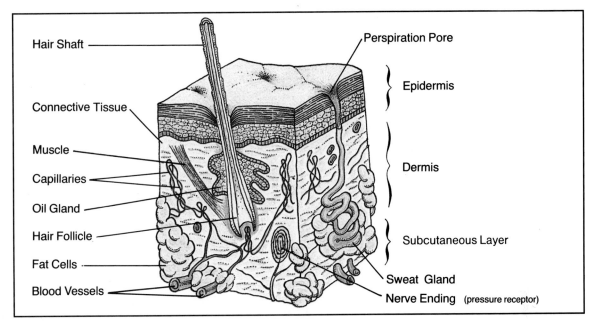

Labels on figure:
Hair Shaft — Perspiration Pore — Epidermis — Connective Tissue — Dermis — Muscle — Capillaries — Oil Gland — Hair Follicle — Fat Cells — Sweat Gland — Nerve Ending (pressure receptor) — Blood Vessels

5-2. A cross section of skin showing its structures

By the time these cells reach the surface, they are dead and completely formed of keratin. Water from the cells below helps keep the keratin layer moist and soft, making the skin look smooth. When moisture is lost, the keratin begins to crumble. Cells break apart and skin becomes dry and flaky.

THE DERMIS. A deep cut in the skin causes bleeding. Exercise causes perspiration. If the skin is pinched, it bounces back. These are all reactions of the **dermis,** the middle layer of skin. The dermis is called the true skin because it houses the skin's vital structures.

The dermis contains a dense network of blood vessels. Within the dermis are five types of nerve endings that carry sensations of touch, pain, pressure, heat and cold. Protein fibers called *collagen* run through the dermis, giving the skin strength and elasticity.

Oil glands and sweat glands are found in the dermis. (See Figure 5-2.) The glands found around hair shafts secrete an oil, **sebum.** Sebum moves up through the duct around the hair shaft and out of the pore at the surface of the skin. It coats and lubricates the keratin layer of the epidermis. This makes the skin more waterproof and helps prevent water loss from the body.

Sweat glands secrete perspiration, ridding the body of excess water, salt, and other waste products from the blood.

As perspiration evaporates from the skin surface, it cools the body. The perspiration flow varies with conditions inside and outside the body. How do exercise and emotions affect perspiration? How does an increase in temperature affect perspiration?

Perspiration is often blamed for body odor. But it is not the actual culprit. Body odor is caused by bacteria acting on perspiration. Thoroughly washing your skin daily will retard bacterial growth and control body odor. There are more sweat glands under the arms and around the mammary glands and genitals. These areas should be washed with soap. Antiperspirants help reduce odor and perspiration. They contain chemicals that close the pores. Deodorants contain chemicals that counteract odor but do not close the pores. Neither product is a substitute for washing.

THE SUBCUTANEOUS LAYER. The deepest of the skin layers is the **subcutaneous** (sub-kew-**tain**-ee-ous) layer. The body's supplies of fat deposits are in this layer. Everyone—male or female, fat or thin—has fat cells in the subcutaneous layer. This bottom layer naturally insulates the body against heat and cold. It also acts as an inner cushion to protect the body against injuries. As the body ages, some fat is lost from this layer. The skin shrinks unevenly and causes creases and wrinkles.

COMPLEXION COMPLAINTS

Are you bothered by skin problems? Skin problems are among the most common complaints of adults and teenagers. Proper care can help correct various skin problems.

ACNE. Acne is one of the most common complexion complaints, especially among teenagers. Why does this problem occur so frequently during the teen years?

During adolescence, sex glands increase the secretion of hormones, and this produces many body changes. There is a noticeable growth spurt and an increase in body hair. A child's figure changes into that of an adult. At the same time, these hormones stimulate the oil glands to produce more sebum. This extra oil causes the acne problem.

What exactly is acne? A *dermatolgist*, a physician specializing in skin disorders, will say that acne is a *group* of skin conditions. Blackheads, pimples, and boil-like cysts are all characteristics of acne. Acne often appears on the face, neck, shoulders, and back.

Blackheads are not caused by dirt. They form when ducts and pores around hair follicles become blocked with sebum and dead cells. The dark color results from a chemical reaction between sebum and melanin.

If oil ducts become infected by bacteria, blackheads can develop into pimples. White blood cells rush to the infection site and attack the infecting bacteria. As this happens pus forms and a pimple swells up. The infecting bacteria can destroy skin tissues, leaving deep scars. Should bacteria invade deeper areas within the dermis, the tissue forms a wall around the infected area to prevent further spread of infection. A hard, red, raised, boil-like cyst appears.

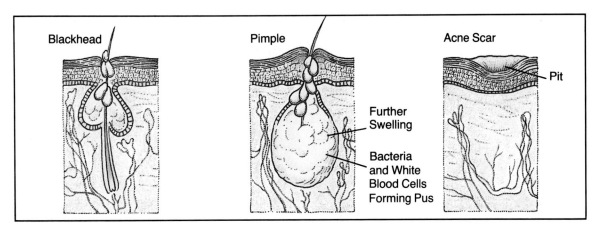

Blackhead

Pimple

Further
Swelling

Bacteria
and White
Blood Cells
Forming Pus

Acne Scar

Pit

5–3. When a pore becomes clogged, a blackhead may form. If bacteria infect the pore, a pimple develops. An acne scar is an area of dead skin tissue.

CONTROLLING ACNE.   Can acne be prevented? No, but it can be controlled to some extent. In most cases, acne clears by itself after the teen years. But don't allow an "I'll-grow-out-of-it" attitude to stop you from getting help.

Although you may be tempted, never squeeze blackheads, pimples, or cysts. Squeezing can damage the skin and promote infection. Pus from squeezed pimples can get into other pores and cause more pimples. Be careful not to touch acne blemishes around the nose or upper lip. Blood vessels in these areas can take the infection directly to the brain. A device called a *comedo extractor*, available in pharmacies, can safely remove blackheads. Gently wash your skin several times a day with hot water and soap. This will reduce skin bacteria and excess oil. This will also help dry the skin and cause it to peel. Peeling helps loosen blackheads. Avoid scrubbing the skin. This does not decrease blackheads and can irritate the skin and spread infection. A mild astringent can be used after washing to help prevent oil buildup. An **astringent** (as-**strin**-gent) is a drying lotion that contains alcohol. Avoid using oily creams and cosmetics. Completely remove all cosmetics at night.

You may wonder whether exercise or rest can affect acne. Also, you may wonder if eating chocolate, french fries, or other sweet and fatty foods causes acne. Research shows that diet does not cause or control acne. Nevertheless, practicing positive health habits, such as a well-balanced diet, proper exercise, and rest, is important for general good health, including the health of your skin. When you are healthy, your body can more easily fight infections, including those that cause acne.

Many teenagers spend money on advertised acne creams and lotions. Do these products work? Products containing *sulfur, resorcinol,* and *salicylic acid* may help mild acne. These chemicals mildly inflame the skin, causing it to peel. However, if the skin becomes overly irritated or dry, stop using these products. Seek medical advice.

MEDICAL TREATMENT. Doctors may drain pus from cysts and use antibiotics to control infection. They may also prescribe ointments that promote skin peeling. In certain severe acne cases, doctors may prescribe a newer drug called *Accutane.* As Figure 5-4 shows, *Accutane* treatment can be very effective. This drug is only prescribed in certain cases, since there are dangerous side effects. Pregnant women should not take it.

Early medical treatment can help prevent permanent acne scarring. If scarring does occur, treatments are available that may help to improve the skin's appearance. However, these

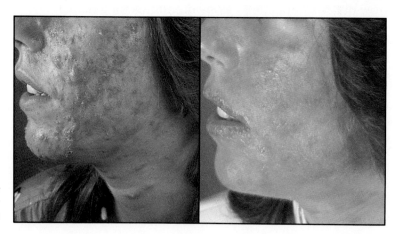

5-4. Before and after accutane treatment for severe acne

treatments do not always work and are not always advisable. In the newest treatment available, liquid protein is injected into the skin around acne pits and scars in order to fill these areas. As a rule, these results are not permanent but may last for several years. How long the treatment lasts varies from one person to the next.

Permanent results can sometimes be produced by treating the skin surface. In *dermabrasion* or *dermaplaning,* the skin is first frozen. Then, a motor-driven brush or plane removes the epidermis surgically. In *chemabrasion,* chemicals are applied to the skin to remove the epidermis. After these treatments, the skin heals and acne scars are less noticeable. Only a doctor with special training can apply these treatments.

BOILS. A deep, serious infection that invades all layers of the skin is called a **boil.** Boils can occur alone or in groups anywhere on the body. Like pimples, boils should *never* be squeezed. Boils require medical attention. A doctor can drain pus from the boil and use antibiotics to control infection. Frequent or numerous boils can be a sign that the body has lost its ability to fight infection. Diabetes or other disease may be the cause of the problem.

WARTS. Often warts appear as raised growths on the skin. Warts are caused by a virus that can be picked up anywhere. At present there is no drug that will prevent warts.

Warts can grow anywhere but are most common on the face and hands. Warts can spread from one person to another, or from one area to another on the same person's body. They usually disappear spontaneously. However, if warts are irritating or if they begin to multiply rapidly, a doctor can remove them by a simple and painless procedure.

The word *plantar* means on the sole of the foot. *Plantar warts* grow only on the sole of the foot. Plantar warts cannot grow out from the skin because your weight puts pressure on the soles of your feet. If they grow into nerves, plantar warts can be very painful. They can penetrate deeply and can be easily infected. They should be immediately treated by a doctor.

SKIN SPOTS. White spots, called **vitiligo** (vih-**till**-eh-go), are patches where the skin fails to produce melanin. The cause is unknown. Prescription drugs are available to treat this disorder. However, it may be easier and more practical to cover vitiligo with cosmetics.

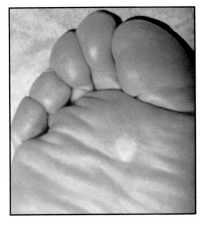

5–5. Because the plantar wart grows inward and can possibly affect nerves, it should be treated as soon as possible.

5–6. Vitiligo is a harmless condition that can be covered with make-up if it occurs on the face.

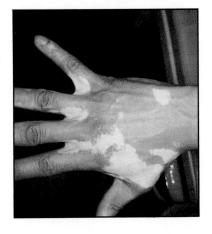

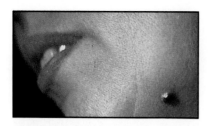

5–7. A darkened mole, such as this one, may be a sign of cancer.

Moles are slight overgrowths of skin with excess pigment. Most brown moles range in color from light to dark brown. These moles are usually harmless. However, black or blue-black moles can be dangerous. They can develop into a deadly skin cancer at any time. Skin growths that grow rapidly, change color, or bleed should be checked at once. Of course, if you have any unusual skin condition, see a doctor.

CHAPS AND MINOR BURNS. If you are outdoors you should avoid getting skin chaps and burns. Chaps and windburns are caused by overexposure to wind and cold. This overexposure dries the epidermis, causing it to become red and irritated.

To help prevent chapping and windburn, rub the skin with cream, lotion, or oil before going outside. Also apply these products after exposure to soothe dry areas. Frostbite is a much more serious problem. It needs proper first aid and medical attention (see Chapter 28).

What causes sunburn? Sunburn is caused by the sun's ultraviolet rays. These rays can even penetrate clouds and burn you on a cloudy day. Sunburning causes small blood vessels in the skin to expand. Then more blood goes to the skin, and it gets red. Although you may think a suntan is attractive, it is unwise to expose the skin to the sun for a long time. Besides causing premature aging of the skin, too much exposure can cause skin cancer. How can you protect the skin from the sun's damaging effects? Wear protective clothes, and use protective skin lotions, especially when the sun is most intense. Sunblocks offer the greatest protection against burning. They contain *para-amino benzoic acid* (abbreviated PABA), which effectively blocks the sun's ultraviolet rays. *Some* tanning preparations also contain PABA, but in smaller amounts. Hence they are less effective in preventing sunburn.

5–8. Over exposure to sun ages the skin and may cause cancer.

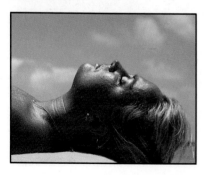

SEVERE BURNS. Did you know that burns are rated by degrees? You may have experienced a first-degree burn, which reddens the skin (such as mild sunburn). In a second-degree burn, blisters appear (such as acute sunburn), which is a sign of more serious skin damage. Blisters form when fluids seep from injured cells in the dermis. The most severe burn is a third-degree burn, which causes skin charring. With this burn, most skin structures have been destroyed and tissue damage extends to the deepest skin layer.

Do you recall the skin's major functions? If so, you will understand why extensive second- and third- degree burns pose a serious danger to health. When the skin is severely damaged, vital body fluids are rapidly lost. This upsets the delicate balance of the circulatory system and can place the body in a state of shock. The body also loses its natural germ barrier and infection becomes a constant danger.

Second- and third- degree burns require immediate attention. Apply first aid as described in Chapter 28. Second-degree burns over more than 130 square centimeters (20 square inches) of skin are considered extensive and should be treated by a doctor. Also consult a doctor in cases of smaller second-degree burns on the face and hands. Improper self-care can increase skin scarring, and may even result in partial loss of hand function. *All* third-degree burns need prompt medical care.

SKIN SCALES. **Psoriasis** (soar-**rye**-eh-sis) is a skin disease that appears as patches of red, raised skin and silver scales of dead skin. It is most common on the scalp, elbows, knees, and outer surfaces of the arms and legs. It can last a short or a long time, and it can occur in cycles. Psoriasis seems less severe in summer than in winter. This is because the sun's ultraviolet rays are stronger in the summer. Ultraviolet light seems to improve this condition. The exact cause of psoriasis is unknown. There is no cure, but medical treatment can control this condition.

ALLERGIES

Does contact with poison ivy make you itch? Does a certain food make your skin break out? These are examples of common allergic reactions. An **allergy** is a reaction of the body to a certain substance. Allergies are highly individual. For example, strawberries can be a dessert delight for one person and the cause of an allergy for another.

An allergic reaction can occur when allergy-causing substances are eaten, inhaled, or touched. The list of allergy-causing substances is nearly endless. Pollen, chocolate, and pets are common causes of allergies.

Allergic reactions range from mild to severe. In a mild reaction the skin and the soft tissues around the eyes and nose can become itchy, red, and swollen. Nausea, vomiting, and diarrhea can also be allergic reactions. Severe allergic reactions can cause swelling of the throat, collapse of the circulatory system, heart failure, and even death.

Most allergies develop gradually. When the body is first exposed to the substance, an allergic reaction does not

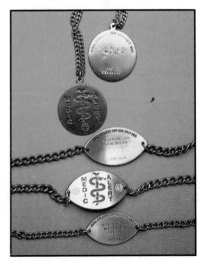

5–9. Special medic alert identification tags should be worn by people who are allergic to penicillin or other drugs.

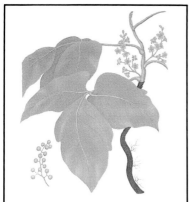

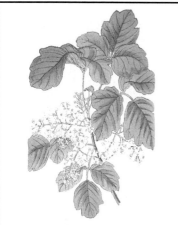

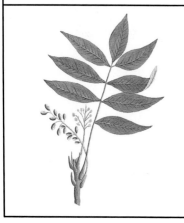

5–10. These plants are (from top to bottom) poison ivy, poison oak, and poison sumac.

usually occur. With repeated exposures, the body may develop a **sensitivity.** This means that there will probably be an allergic reaction each time the substance contacts the body. If sensitivity increases, the reactions become more severe.

Some people are highly allergic to penicillin or other drugs. Tell your doctor about any reaction that occurs after taking a drug. You may be allergic to the drug. People who are highly allergic to certain drugs should wear special identification tags that list these drugs. This information is vital in an emergency.

ECZEMA. Many people refer to **eczema** (**egg**-zeh-mah) as a specific disease. But it is really an allergic reaction. Many substances can produce eczema, but the reactions to each one are similar. The skin becomes red, swollen, crusty, and scaly. Small blisters also form and ooze a clear fluid.

Eczema often results when certain substances contact the skin directly. This condition is called *contact dermatitis.* Do you know the plants shown in Figure 5-10? Their oils can cause contact dermatitis. Chemicals found in detergents, soaps, cosmetics, perfumes, hair dyes, and synthetic fibers can also cause this condition.

HIVES. Red, raised areas on the skin are an allergic reaction called **hives.** Hives vary in size and depth and are usually very itchy. When severe reactions occur, giant hives sometimes appear. These are deeper and less defined than ordinary hives. They can form on the skin and membranes of the lips, mouth, throat, and larynx. Giant hives in the throat and larynx can be very dangerous. They can block the airway and cause death by suffocation. The victim needs immediate medical attention.

Causes of hives are numerous and hard to determine. Hives are often caused by foods and other substances, such as sulfa drugs and aspirin. Hives can also be caused by emotional states. (See Chapter 8.)

Allergic reactions are not limited to those just described. Hay fever and asthma, discussed in Chapter 19, are also allergic reactions.

TREATMENT OF ALLERGIES. Why do some people have allergies while others do not? This is still unknown. The body's natural defense system, discussed in Chapter 22, may be responsible. Heredity also plays a part. How can a suspected allergy be checked? Family doctors can sometimes tell the cause of contact dermatitis just by examining the rash. When an allergy's cause is more difficult to detect, it may be necessary to go to an *allergist*. This is a doctor who specializes in the diagnosis and treatment of allergies. Allergists conduct special *scratch tests*. The allergist applies a drop of the suspected substance to the skin or injects it just below the skin surface. Later, the allergist observes the effects of the substance on the skin where it was applied. Skin swelling or redness indicates an allergic reaction.

How are allergies treated? Avoiding the irritating substance is often the recommended and simplest solution. Drugs can help relieve allergy symptoms. In severe cases a series of injections can be given that reduce sensitivity. This decreases and sometimes eliminates the allergic reaction.

HAIR
STRUCTURE OF HAIR

Hair is a special structure of the skin. Hair is formed by epidermal cells that line a pocket called a **follicle** (**foll**-eh-kul), which lies deep within the dermis. The outside layer of the hair and skin are both composed of transparent *keratin* cells. If you look at Figure 5-11, you will see that these cells overlap like scales on a fish. When these cells lie flat they reflect light giving hair its shine. The melanin pigment gives hair as well as skin its color. Whether hair is curly or straight depends on the angle of the hair follicle and the shape of the hair shaft. Curly hair has a flat shaft; straight hair has a round one. Hair fullness depends on the number of shafts and the diameter of each one.

HAIR CARE

Do you admire shiny hair? Proper hair brushing and washing can help make hair shine. Using a rounded-bristle brush, gently stroke the hair from the back of your neck forward to the ends of your hair. No more than twenty-five strokes are needed daily. Brushing hair helps remove dirt and film and distributes natural scalp oil along the hair shaft. Oil then coats the overlapping keratin cells and creates a smoother hair surface. This smoother surface reflects more light, adding luster to the hair. When dirt attaches itself to the hair shaft, it creates an uneven hair surface, which poorly reflects light. The hair then appears dull and stringy.

Hair oil, spray, gel, or lotion makes the hair sticky. Then dirt can easily stick to the hair. Harsh hair-coloring, waving,

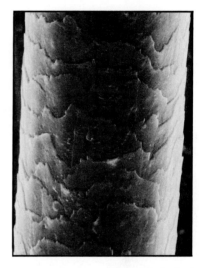

5–11. A hair shaft magnified 100 times. Notice the overlapping scales.

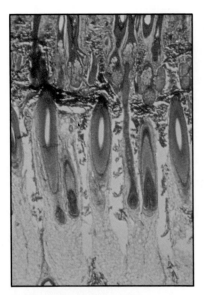

5–12. A cross section of the scalp magnified 300 times. Notice each hair growing out of its own follicle in the dermis.

and straightening products can also dull hair by marring its reflective surface.

Washing the hair removes oil, dirt, dandruff, and other residue that clings to the hair and scalp. How often should hair be washed? Unless your hair is dry or damaged, frequent washings keep hair looking its best.

Despite the variety of shampoos available, they all contain soap or detergents that dissolve oil and grime. Some shampoos also contain oils such as lanolin and conditioners. Trial and error is the only way to find the shampoo that works best for you.

After rinsing, gently blot the hair dry. Wet hair should be combed, never brushed. Use caution when blowing hair dry. Do not pull the hair, hold the dryer too close, or use excessive heat. This can make the hair brittle and dry.

Treat your hair as carefully as anything else that is important to you. Remember, your hair is your personal statement. Make it a good one.

HAIR PROBLEMS

DANDRUFF. The normal flaking of the outer cells of the epidermis on the scalp causes dandruff. It is easily noticed because the flakes cling to the hair. Ordinary dandruff is not an infection, nor is it carried from one person to another. Simple shampooing and brushing the scalp usually controls this normal condition. For unknown reasons, excessive dandruff can sometimes develop. Special dandruff shampoos can help control this condition.

In some cases what appears to be dandruff is actually a scalp infection that can cause severe soreness and scaling. *Seborrheic dermatitis* is another condition that is more serious and difficult to control. Red, oozing patches appear on the scalp that can spread to other areas, especially if scratched. This condition can also occur on the skin of the eyelids, cheeks, ears, and chest. Regular dandruff shampoos cannot control this condition. See a doctor for proper diagnosis and care.

RINGWORM. If you buy a pair of shoes or slacks, you may return them to the store. A new hat may not be returned. Public health laws do not permit the exchange of items that contact the head, like head scarfs and combs. This prevents the spread of contagious scalp infections such as **ringworm.** Ringworm is caused by a skin fungus. Its name comes from the distinct, raised circular areas that characterize the infection. These areas are caused by a fungus growth in the scalp tissues. The infection starts when the fungus invades the scalp at the base of a hair shaft. As the fungus spreads, spotty and ragged bald spots appear on the scalp. Ringworm can also infect the face, neck, and other areas. Scratching the infected area generally spreads the infection. Ringworm is most common in young children. Doctors treat ringworm with antifungal drugs. Washing with soap and then thoroughly drying also prevents the growth of ringworm.

PROBLEM PARASITES.   Can you identify the insect in Figure 5-13? What you see are *headlice* and *nits.* These insects suck blood from the scalp, which causes irritation and itching. Another species of louse lives in hair in the pubic region. A third species lives in clothes and body hair. Any invasion of lice is called **pediculosis** (peh-**dick**-kew-low-sis). Head lice are a common problem among school age children. When checking for head lice, use a magnifying glass. Look for the eggs, called nits, on the hair shafts next to the scalp.

Lice and nits are carried easily from one person to another through direct body contact or through use of infected articles, such as clothes, linen, and combs. Infection does not have anything to do with cleanliness or hair style. A doctor or pharmacist can recommend special shampoos that will kill lice but not nits. Therefore the shampoo must be reapplied one week later. Fine tooth combs can be used to pull nits off the hair. Any infected clothing and bedding should be machine washed in water hotter than 52°C (125°F).

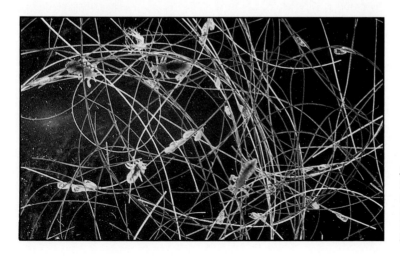

5–13. Head lice and nits on hair. If you suspect an infection, look for the nits with a magnifying glass. They are more abundant than mature lice.

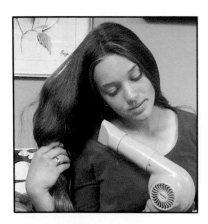

5–14. A blow dryer can be used to style hair. It is not harmful to the hair and scalp when properly used.

HAIR LOSS. Hair has a life cycle all its own. It grows for two to six years, followed by a three-month resting period. During the resting phase, replacement hair forms in the hair follicle and the old hair falls out. These are the hairs seen after you wash, comb, or brush the hair. Each day about sixty to two hundred hairs are lost. This loss is perfectly normal. Because the growth phase of individual hairs is staggered, the hair remains full. Thinning occurs when normal loss exceeds the rate of new growth.

What causes baldness? You may inherit the tendency for baldness or **alopecia** (al-low-**pee**-she-ah). This is much more common in males, but females can inherit it, too. Some diseases, medical treatments, drugs, malnourishment, and severe emotional or physical stress can cause temporary baldness. In most cases, hair regrowth occurs naturally within months when the root cause of the baldness is corrected.

One form of hair loss is preventable. It occurs when hair is excessively brushed or tightly pulled into braids and pony tails, or stretched over curlers. If these practices are stopped, hair will grow back. However, if hairs are repeatedly pulled, hair loss may be permanent.

UNWANTED HAIR. When excess hair appears where there is usually little growth, the condition is called **hirsutism** (**her**-suit-izm). Like baldness, this tendency is usually inherited. Sometimes, however, a hormone imbalance or

5–15. Split ends, such as these, can be caused by improper hair care. Do not brush hair when it is wet. Holding a hair dryer too close or overuse of chemicals, such as bleach, can cause split ends.

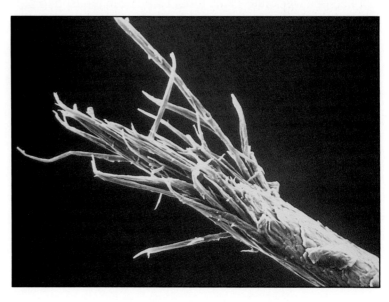

certain drugs cause extra hair growth. In these cases medical treatment can usually correct the problem. Shaving removes excess hair safely and simply. *Waxing* is another method. Warm, melted strips of wax are placed on the skin. When the wax cools and hardens, it is quickly peeled off, removing the hair. Chemical creams or sprays, called **depilatories,** also remove hair. They chemically break down the structure of the hair but may also irritate the skin. Hair regrowth occurs with all these methods. Only the hair at the skin's surface is removed. The hair follicle is still alive.

Electrolysis removes hair permanently. A fine needle is inserted into each hair follicle and an electric current is passed through it. Several treatments may be necessary before a follicle dies. This method can be expensive and painful. It is used mostly on small skin areas such as the upper lip. *Only* a beautician experienced in electrolysis should administer this treatment. Improper electrolysis can leave scars.

NAILS

Your nails are another special structure of the skin. The hard part of a nail is made of dead skin tissue. The nail grows from the epidermal cells below it. The skin around the nail forms a hardened margin, called the *cuticle.*

Good nail care is important for everyone. Dirty, broken, and bitten nails and cuticles are unattractive and can lead to painful and serious infections. A neatly manicured hand can prevent infections and improve appearance and can also help break a nail-biting habit.

Basic nail care is not difficult. Use a nail file or emery board to shape nails (see Fig. 5-16). File them before washing when they are hard and firm. Soak nails in soap and water to soften them. When they are soft, gently push back the cuticles with a manicuring stick. This will prevent hangnails from forming. A *hangnail* is a sliver of cuticle that has separated along the edge of the nail. If you do get a hangnail, never pull it as this will tear the skin. Clip it as close to the cuticle as possible. Nails can become brittle and break when exposed to detergents such as dishwashing liquids. Using gloves can protect your nails.

Toenails should be trimmed straight across to prevent painful *ingrown toenails.* This condition occurs when pressure on the nail forces it to grow toward the nail base.

5–16. You can shape nails with a nail file or emery board. Start at the sides and stroke in one direction towards the center of the nail.

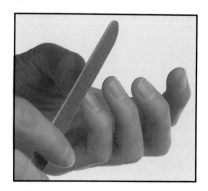

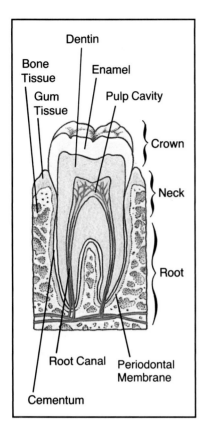

Dentin

Bone
Tissue

Enamel

Gum
Tissue

Pulp Cavity

Crown

Neck

Root

Root Canal

Periodontal
Membrane

Cementum

5–17. A cross-section of a healthy tooth, cut lengthwise.

TEETH

Your teeth play an obvious role in appearance. They also have other important functions. Teeth are helpful for clear speech. Certain sounds, such as "s" and "th," cannot be easily pronounced without front teeth. Teeth are also important for grinding food into small particles, so it can be more easily digested.

Teeth and gum problems can cause unpleasantness, ranging from bad breath to pain. If teeth become infected, the infection can be carried to other parts of the body. Do you give your teeth the attention they deserve?

STRUCTURE OF THE TEETH

The visible portions of a tooth are the neck and crown. Figure 5-17 shows a tooth cut lengthwise. Notice the crown appears above the gum and narrows to form the neck. A hard, white protective layer of *enamel* covers the crown and neck. The root of the tooth lies in a socket in the jawbone. Its outer covering is called *cementum*. The tooth is anchored firmly in the jaw by the fibrous periodontal membrane. Lying beneath the enamel layer is a softer substance called *dentin*. It forms the actual body of the tooth, and it houses the pulp cavity. Blood vessels and nerves lie inside the pulp cavity. They join the jawbone's larger nerves and blood vessels at the base of the roots.

PRIMARY TO PERMANENT TEETH. *Primary teeth*, commonly called the baby teeth, start arriving at about 6 months of age. They are lost gradually over a period of years, starting at about age 6. The first tooth is usually a front tooth, or *incisor*. By age two and one half, all twenty primary teeth have arrived.

Figure 5-18 shows *permanent teeth* that replace primary teeth in the jaw. Permanent teeth grow in the jaws beneath the roots of the primary teeth. When a permanent tooth's root is well developed, the tooth is ready to emerge. By then, the root of the primary tooth is absorbed. As a rule, only the crown and neck remain when the primary tooth is lost.

Adults have 32 teeth of four types. Each type performs a separate job. The upper and lower permanent incisors cut food. Directly behind there are four pointed *cuspid* or canine teeth (two in each jaw). They cut and tear food. There are eight *bicuspids*, two on each side of the upper and lower jaws. The bicuspids cut and crush food. Behind the bicus-

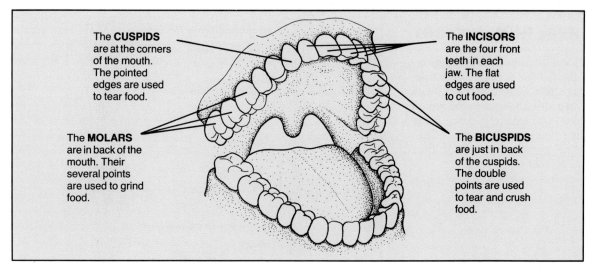

The **CUSPIDS** are at the corners of the mouth. The pointed edges are used to tear food.

The **INCISORS** are the four front teeth in each jaw. The flat edges are used to cut food.

The **MOLARS** are in back of the mouth. Their several points are used to grind food.

The **BICUSPIDS** are just in back of the cuspids. The double points are used to tear and crush food.

5–18. The types of teeth and their arrangement. In front, there are four incisor teeth. On each side of the jaw is a canine tooth, two premolar teeth, and three molar teeth.

pids are the *molars*, which grind food. If all the molars develop, there will be 12 altogether, three on each side of the upper and lower jaws. Molars first appear at age 6 or 7. They do not replace primary teeth; they grow behind them. At about age 12 the second molars develop behind the first ones. Third molars known as *wisdom teeth* usually appear sometime between ages 18 and 21. These teeth may cause problems. They may grow in on their sides or become wedged against the second molars. A dentist can tell you whether your third molars may harm adjacent teeth. If this happens, they should be removed.

DENTAL PROBLEMS

DENTAL DAMAGE.   **Dental caries,** known as tooth decay, is a common dental disease. This disease produces holes, called **cavities,** in teeth. Tooth decay can start close to the gum line, or between teeth or on the biting surface of the molar. Tooth decay is not a communicable disease. It is caused by bacteria that are always in the mouth. Bacteria, food residues, and saliva form a sticky colorless film on the teeth called **plaque** (plak). The bacteria in plaque use the sugars in foods to form acids and other byproducts that destroy tooth enamel and irritate gums.

Decay penetrates the enamel and spreads to the dentin. As the cavity grows toward the pulp, the tooth becomes more sensitive. When the decay reaches the pulp and exposes a nerve, a toothache starts. In the final stage of decay,

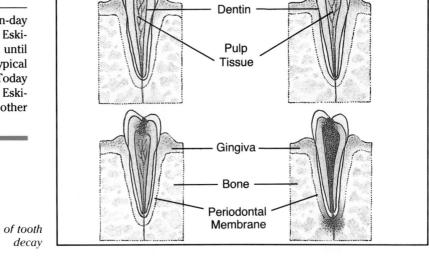

the bacteria in the nerve canal destroy the pulp. An abscess, or pus collection, forms at the base of the tooth. If not treated, the infection can spread to other parts of the body. A decayed tooth can be saved by cleaning, medicating, and filling the cavity.

When tooth decay penetrates deeply into the pulp, a tooth can often still be saved. *Endodontics*, commonly called root canal therapy, is required. The dentist removes the diseased nerve canal contents, cleans out the infection, and sterilizes and fills in the canal. If possible, teeth should always be saved. Although root canal therapy removes the nerve and blood vessels in the root canal, the tooth looks almost the same. However, it may become brittle due to the loss of its pulpal blood supply. For this reason, your dentist may crown the tooth with gold or porcelain to help protect it.

PERIODONTAL DISEASE.   Do you know what the major cause of tooth loss among adults is? The answer is **periodontal disease.** This disease, which can begin as early as age five, is mainly caused by plaque formation. When plaque is not removed daily, its harmful products collect along the gum line, irritating the gums. They become red, swollen or tender, and bleed easily. As plaque builds up, it hardens into a limelike substance called *tartar* (calculus) which pushes against the gums. Pockets form between the gums and teeth where more plaque can grow and further damage the tooth root. As periodontal disease spreads,

118

gums recede and pus forms. Eventually the bony structures supporting the teeth are destroyed. Then, teeth loosen and fall out.

How can you recognize periodontal disease? Warning signs are pointed out in Figure 5-20. The first sign is a pink toothbrush (bleeding gums). It indicates an inflammation of the gums called gingivitis.

5–20. Signs of periodontal disease.

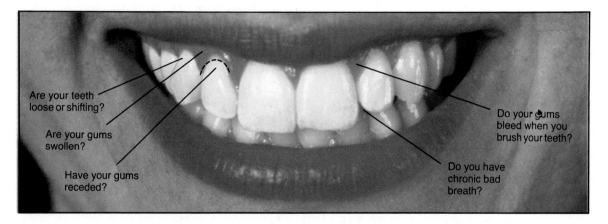

Are your teeth loose or shifting?

Are your gums swollen?

Have your gums receded?

Do your gums bleed when you brush your teeth?

Do you have chronic bad breath?

MALOCCLUSION.   More and more adults, teenagers, and young children are wearing braces because they look forward to the improvement that braces produce in the positioning of their teeth. Orthodontics is the dental specialty that corrects **malocclusion** (mal-oh-**clue**-shun), which is an irregularity in the position and bite of teeth.

Why does malocclusion occur? Sometimes malocclusion is inherited. The size of the jaw and teeth and missing permanent teeth are hereditary traits. Oral habits such as thumb sucking and fingernail biting can cause dental malocclusions. An abnormal bite can produce unhealthy chewing and speech defects and later periodontal disease.

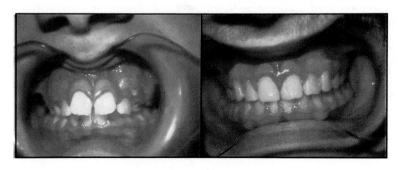

5–21. Malocclusion before and after treatment.

Wearing braces is often more pleasant today than it used to be. Slim tooth-colored plastic or metal attachments (brackets) can be glued to each tooth. A flexible wire track connects each attachment to gently move teeth. Special rubber bands act like pulley systems to help teeth move. In some cases, invisible braces can be used. Brackets are bonded to the inside instead of the outside of the teeth.

ORAL INJURY. Imagine that you are riding your bicycle on a slippery road. To avoid hitting a car, you suddenly slam on your breaks. The bicycle skids into the car. Luckily, you have no broken bones, but your front tooth has been knocked out. What should you do? If you act promptly the tooth can often be reimplanted in the jaw. Rinse the tooth gently in running water, but do not scrub the tooth. If possible, put the tooth back in its socket and hold for 3 to 5 minutes. If this cannot be done, place it in a glass of water or wrap the tooth in a clean, damp cloth. See a dentist *immediately*, within 30 minutes if possible. Cases of broken or loosened teeth also need immediate dental care.

Oral injuries can often be prevented. Figure 5-22 shows one way to prevent tooth loss. Can you suggest other means?

DENTAL CARE

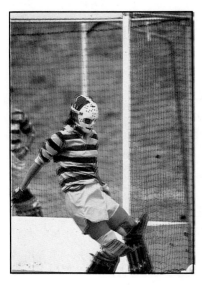

5–22. Protective headgear can protect your teeth and skull.

Half the Americans who are age 65 or older do not have any natural teeth. How many teeth do you expect to have at age 65? If you avoid dental disease by following the rules of basic dental care, your teeth should last a lifetime. Personal dental care can help prevent tooth decay, periodontal disease, and other dental problems. The guidelines below can help you develop your own personal dental-care program.

DIET FOR HEALTHY TEETH. Are soft drinks, chewing gum, cake, and candy a regular part of your diet? If so, you are paving the way for dental trouble. A diet that includes many sugary snacks encourages rapid bacterial growth and the formation of acids and plaque. Therefore, you should avoid sugary foods between meals. Instead of snacking on sweets, try snacking on fresh vegetables, cheese, or nuts. The longer sugar remains in the mouth, the greater the chances of tooth decay.

A proper diet is not only necessary for general health, it is essential for good oral health. It can help prevent tooth decay and periodontal disease. Milk and other dairy products provide vitamin D, calcium, and phosphorus, which are essential for healthy gums and the formation of tooth enamel. Until age eight, the enamel is still forming. Therefore, youngsters need adequate amounts of these important foods. A teenager's daily diet should contain about four servings of milk or dairy products. Vitamin C, commonly found in citrus fruits, and vitamin B complex are also necessary for normal, healthy gums.

In most cities **fluoride** is added to drinking water. Fluoride makes tooth enamel more resistant to acid attacks and reduces tooth decay. Water treated with the right amount of fluoride can reduce tooth decay in children by as much as 65 percent. Several fluoride toothpastes and mouth rinses with the seal of the American Dental Association have been proved effective. Some dentists treat the surface of teeth with a fluoride solution. Fluoride alone cannot fight tooth decay, but when it is used in combination with a healthy diet and proper oral hygiene habits, tooth decay can usually be avoided.

ORAL HYGIENE. Proper oral hygiene requires flossing and brushing the teeth each day. A thorough cleaning removes food particles and helps eliminate plaque before it hardens into tartar. This is why a thorough cleaning of the teeth at least once a day is essential.

Figure 5-23 shows why flossing is an essential oral hygiene practice. It removes plaque that brushing cannot reach. Flossing may seem difficult at first, but with practice it can be mastered. Use the method pictured in Figure 5-23.

After flossing, rinse the teeth thoroughly and then brush. To do a good job of brushing, you need the right equipment and techniques. Choose a toothbrush with soft, rounded bristles. The size and shape of the brush should allow you to reach every tooth. An electric toothbrush is helpful to

5–23. The recommended method for flossing. Use a 45 cm (18 in.) piece of unwaxed dental floss and wrap all but 8 cm (3 in.) around fingers of each hand. Use thumb and forefinger with a 2.5 cm (1 in.) piece of floss between them to guide the floss between the teeth. Floss should be held tightly so there is no slack. When floss reaches the gum line, curve it into a "c" shape against one tooth until resistance is felt. Never snap floss into gums. Hold floss tightly against tooth and move floss away from the gum by scraping the floss up and down against the sides of the tooth.

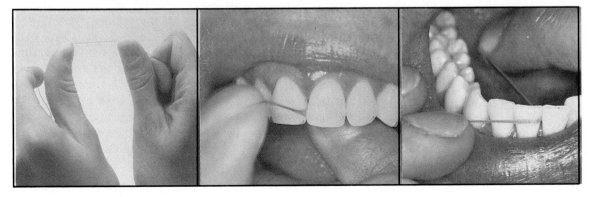

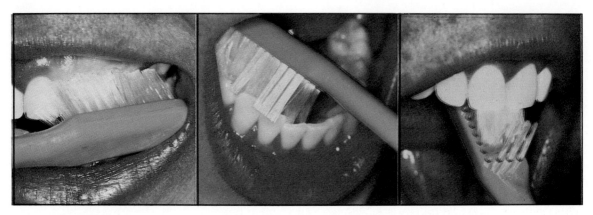

5–24. A recommended method of brushing teeth. Place side of brush against teeth with bristles pointing toward gums. Turn handle of the toothbrush toward teeth. While turning handle, pump toothbrush back and forth with short, quick movements. Turn brush toward the biting edge of the teeth while continuing the pumping movement. Brush inside and outside of all teeth, and the chewing surface.

5–25. X ray of a cavity

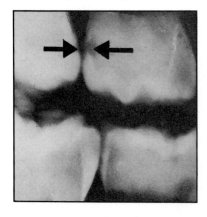

some people, especially those with physical handicaps. A worn-out toothbrush cannot clean your teeth properly. For proper brushing, use the method shown in Figure 5-24. Try to brush your teeth after every meal. When this is impractical, rinse with water to help remove food particles.

Dental devices such as rubber toothbrush-picks can be helpful, but they cannot replace flossing and brushing. Devices that shoot jets of water between and around teeth help remove trapped food but they cannot remove plaque. Toothpick-like devices, if properly used, can help control plaque. Before using dental devices, ask your dentist for advice. Faulty use of these devices can damage the gums.

PROFESSIONAL HELP.   Good dental care includes dental checkups at least twice a year. Most cavities develop over several months. Do not wait for a toothache before seeing a dentist. The dentist can spot problems before serious trouble develops. To prevent periodontal disease, a professional tooth cleaning called **prophylaxis** (pro-fi-**lax**-es) is usually needed. It removes tartar build up. The dentist may take an X ray of the teeth to locate hidden trouble. Figure 5-25 shows tooth decay that can be seen on an X ray, but is invisible to the naked eye. However do not expect your dentist to take X rays routinely. The American Dental Association recommends that dentists examine each patient and use X rays only as needed.

Do you know how to choose a dentist? Ask a family physician or a pharmacist, or check with hospitals that have dental services. Ask friends or neighbors for their recommendations. A local dental society or the American Dental Association can also provide the names of qualified dentists in your area.

THE FINISHING TOUCHES

People can form an instant impression from the way a person looks and dresses. How do you react to someone wearing dirty and wrinkled clothes? How do you react to someone whose clothes are always neat and clean? Your clothes make a personal statement about how you feel about yourself and others. One cannot say that any particular style or fashion in clothing is appropriate. Clothes are designed for every occasion, from sportswear to more formal attire. Styles change and, as far as possible, some people enjoy keeping up with the latest fashion. Each person should also consider what styles look best on him or her.

Did you ever hear the sound of your voice on a tape recorder? What impressions did you form? Good speech qualities include pleasant tone, clear enunciation, variation in volume, and natural accent. Mumbling, monotone, harshness, loudness, and affected accents detract from good speech qualities. Can a speech problem be corrected? Personal practice often helps. Speech therapy can also help. Local hospitals, a school nurse, or an English teacher can often recommend good professional help.

Body language, a person's posture and expression through movement, also affects the impression given to others. Poor posture detracts from an otherwise pleasing appearance. Regular exercise can improve posture. It strengthens muscles that hold the body in its proper position.

Finally, personality is a major factor that affects appearance. Individual attitudes are reflected when you smile or frown. In the chapters ahead you will learn how your personality can contribute to your appearance.

SUMMARY: The skin protects the body against injury, infection, and heat loss. It also helps regulate water and chemical balance in the body. Skin growths, infections, acne, and allergic reactions are common skin problems.

The hair and nails are structures related to the skin. Both are formed of keratin and grow from the epidermal layer of skin. Dandruff, hair loss, and excessive hair growth are frequent hair problems that affect appearance.

The teeth are not only important to appearance, but they also aid in speech and digestion. Dental caries and periodontal disease are major threats to oral health. However, they can be prevented by proper brushing, flossing, and dental care.

CHAPTER REVIEW

words at work

Find the word in the left column that fits one of the definitions in the right column. DO NOT WRITE IN THIS BOOK.

a. acne
b. allergy
c. dental caries
d. epidermis
e. follicle
f. fluoride
g. prophylaxis
h. papillae
i. melanin

1. Epidermal tissue from which a hair grows
2. A condition caused by an oversecretion of oil
3. A professional cleaning of the teeth and gums
4. A reaction of the skin and mucous membranes to pollens, various foods, and other substances
5. The outer layer of the skin
6. A mineral that helps prevent tooth decay
7. Determines pigmentation of skin
8. Tooth decay
9. The ridges and valleys on the surface of the skin

review questions

1. Explain the importance of the skin.
2. Describe the three layers of the skin and list their major functions.
3. What is melanin? How does it protect the skin?
4. Define *sebum*. What is its function?
5. Why is perspiration flow a necessary skin function?
6. What causes body odor?
7. Define *acne*. Why is acne more common during the teenage years?
8. Trace the development of blackheads, pimples, and acne cysts.
9. Outline a program to control acne.
10. When do boils require medical attention?
11. Describe first-, second-, and third-degree burns.
12. Define an allergy.
13. Give several examples of an allergic reaction.
14. Is eczema a disease? Explain your answer.
15. Outline a program for basic hair care.
16. List and identify the parts of a tooth.
17. Name the four types of teeth in the mouth and state their functions.
18. Give at least three warning signs of periodontal disease.
19. Define malocclusion. Why should malocclusion be corrected?
20. Explain the effects of diet on oral health.
21. Outline a program of basic oral hygiene.

discussion questions

1. Is it fair to base a strong first impression of a person only on appearance? State your reasons, pro or con.
2. Discuss the many factors that make up appearance.
3. Discuss whether professional help should be sought for various skin and hair ailments.
4. What should you consider when buying cosmetics, sun preparations, and home hair-care preparations?
5. Discuss a total program for improving appearance.
6. Discuss personal habits that affect oral health. What actions might encourage people to improve their oral hygiene?

investigating

PURPOSE:
To evaluate your dietary and oral hygiene habits.

PROCEDURE:
A. Make a log entitled "Dietary and Oral Hygiene Habits." Write the hours of the day down the left-hand side of a lined piece of paper. Start with the hour you arise in the morning, and end with the hour you retire at night. Make three of these logs for three different days.

B. For three days, record when and what you eat on your logs. Also record when you use floss and brush your teeth. Do not alter your current patterns during these three days. Pay special attention to the foods you eat that contain sugar. Many foods contain "hidden sugars." Look for ingredients such as honey, molasses, sucrose, fructose, dextrose, and corn sweeteners, which are all sugars. Circle the foods you eat that contain sugar.

C. After completing the logs, evaluate your dietary and oral hygiene habits.
   1. How many times a day did you eat sweets or foods with sugar in them?
   2. Most decay-causing acids form in the mouth and attack your teeth for at least 20 minutes after eating sugary foods. How many minutes each day were your teeth under acid attack? (Multiply the number of times you ate foods containing sugar each day times 20 minutes. Do not include the times you ate these foods if you brushed your teeth immediately after.)
   3. Did you eat dairy products and foods with vitamin C each day?
   4. Write up a plan on how you could improve your dietary and oral hygiene habits.

CHAPTER 6

Behavior

OBJECTIVES

- DISCUSS the role of heredity and environment on behavior
- DESCRIBE the biological bases for behavior
- DESCRIBE conditioning and cognitive learning;

DISTINGUISH between these two types of learning
- EXPLAIN the forces that affect behavior
- SUGGEST some skills for behavior change

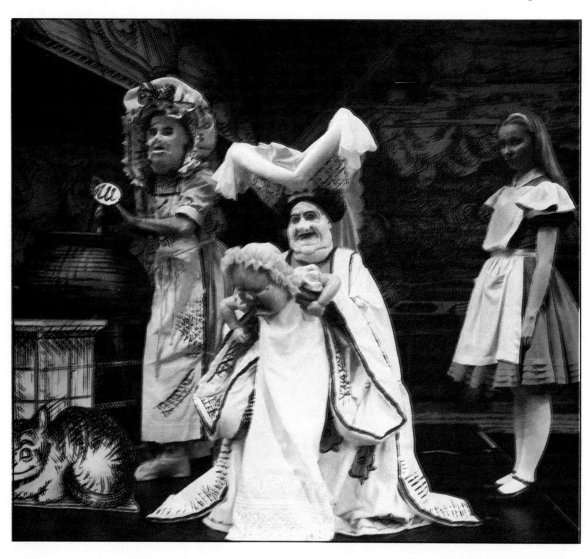

Many people tell Charles that he is just like his father. "Just a chip off the old block," or "Like father, like son," they always say. Charles does look a lot like his father. They talk the *same, walk the same, and even have a lot of the same mannerisms.*

Do you think Charles inherited these traits from his father, or did he learn them?

THE NATURE-NURTURE QUESTION

EVERYONE IS UNIQUE

Has anyone ever told you that you are just like your mother, or just like your father? You probably do have many traits in common with your parents. But there is really no one in this world exactly like you. Your appearance and your personality are unique. Think about yourself for a minute. In what ways are you unlike anyone else? Of course, you do not look exactly like anyone else. Nor is your personality like anyone else's. In this chapter, you will learn how two factors, what you inherited (nature) and what you learned (nurture), made you the unique individual that you are.

HEREDITY AND ENVIRONMENT

How much of your personality did you inherit and how much did you learn? Scientists have been trying to answer this question for many years. We know for certain that we inherit some of our physical traits from our parents. For example, eye color and hair color are traits that we inherit. Are behavioral traits inherited, too? To a certain extent, yes. But environment also plays a part in determining behavior. One way of looking at it is to regard inheritance as determining a person's potential for certain behavior patterns. Environment, including our life experiences, determines whether or not our potential is reached. For example, it is unlikely that a short person will ever become a star basketball player. Tall people may be born with the potential to become basketball players. But whether or not they do so depends on their total environment.

HEALTH ACTION

Investigate and compare general sociocultural customs and behavior between two groups (national, ethnic or age) or explore a single practice such as dating or child-rearing among four groups. Use books, articles, television, and interviews to obtain information. Report in class on your findings.

We are influenced by our environment each day. Every experience you have affects you in some way. No two persons except identical twins ever have the same heredity. No two people, not even identical twins, ever have the same life experiences. This explains why there never was, and never will be, another person exactly like you. It is impossible to tell just where the effects of heredity end and those of the environment begin. Our behavior is a complex combination of inherited and learned traits. Look at Table 6-1, which lists human traits. How do you think both the traits you have inherited and those you have learned effect your behavior?

HUMAN TRAITS	
Inherited	Learned
Blood type	Attitudes
Body structure	Concept of self
Eye color	Conscience
Facial features	Habits
Hair color and texture	Mannerisms
Instinct	Skills
Reflex reactions	Social customs
Skin color	Values
	Will power

Table 6-1

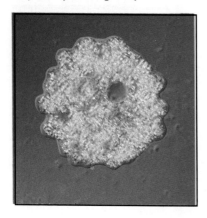

6–1. If you touch this one-cell animal (the ameba) with a probe, it would respond by moving away.

WHAT YOU INHERITED: THE BIOLOGICAL BASES OF BEHAVIOR

You can think of the biological bases of your behavior as a building. Each part of the building is a different aspect of your biological makeup. The foundation of the building is the *stimulus-response mechanism*, which makes all of your behavior possible. The first floor of the building is composed of your *reflexes*. These are very simple behavior patterns that you inherited. The second floor is made up of your *instincts*. These are also inherited behavior patterns, but they are much more complex than reflexes. The third floor contains your *emotional* capacity. You were born with the human capacity for emotions, but most of your emotions are learned. The fourth floor contains your *intelligence*. You are heir to an intelligence far beyond that of any other animal species. This makes very complex learned behavior possible.

128

THE STIMULUS-RESPONSE MECHANISM

How are human beings like all other living things? All living things, from plants to people, are made of living cells. All living cells are capable of receiving signals, called **stimuli,** from their environment. Living cells are also capable of responding to these stimuli. This stimulus-response mechanism is the basis for all behavior.

If you observe a one-celled organism such as an ameba under a microscope and touch it with a probe, what happens? The signal is received by the cell membrane and is then passed on to the protoplasm of the cell. The ameba responds by moving away from the probe.

If the same probe touched your hand, you would feel a sensation. You might respond by moving your hand away. In humans, the stimulus-response mechanism is much more complex. You are made of billions of cells. You receive signals from your environment through highly specialized nerve cells. These nerve cells perceive sensations of temperature, touch, sound, light, taste, smell, and pain. When the probe touches your hand, touch receptors in your skin receive the stimulus. They respond by sending messages, called impulses, to other nerve cells. The nerve cells receive the stimulus and in turn transmit the impulse to other nerve cells, until the impulse reaches your brain. The brain processes the message and then sends the command "move," by way of other impulses, to the motor nerve cells that control the muscles in your hand. In response, you move your hand away from the probe. This sequence of events is pictured in Figure 6-2. All human behavior is based on this stimulus-response mechanism.

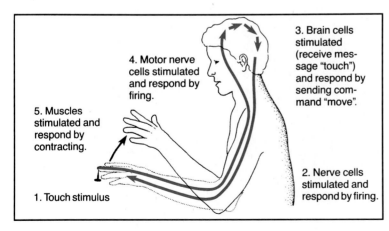

3. Brain cells stimulated (receive message "touch") and respond by sending command "move".

4. Motor nerve cells stimulated and respond by firing.

5. Muscles stimulated and respond by contracting.

2. Nerve cells stimulated and respond by firing.

1. Touch stimulus

6–2. All human behavior is based on the stimulus-response mechanism.

FOCUS ON HEALTH

TWIN RESEARCH

Twins have always captured people's attention and imagination. Throughout the ages, they have been the subject of ancient legends and literature. Among certain tribes, the birth of twins has been considered a great honor or a sign of good luck.

From a scientific viewpoint, identical twins offer a unique opportunity to examine the effects of heredity and environment. Studies have shown that identical twins have very similar personality traits. They are much more alike than non-identical (fraternal) twins or other brothers and sisters. Of course, you could argue that identical twins share not only the same heredity but the same environment while growing up. However, there are a few cases of identical twins growing up in different environments. Let's look at one such case studied at the University of Minnesota, a leading center for twin research.

Identical twin boys, born in Ohio, were adopted shortly after birth by two different families. By chance each family named its new son James. Thirty-nine years passed before Jim L. and Jim S. were reunited. The brothers discovered they had a lot in common. As children both twins had a dog they named Toy. In school, they both liked math but disliked spelling. As teens they had each gained and lost ten pounds. As adults, both Jims had been married twice to women named Linda and Betty. Each man had a son, James Allan and James Alan. Both twins had held similar jobs. They also had the same hobbies and sports interests. In regard to health, each had undergone the same operation and both Jims suffered from headaches.

What did scientists conclude from this case? Of course, they were amazed by the many coincidences. But conclusions can never be drawn from a single case. What can we learn from twin research? Scientists do not expect to solve the nature-nurture question. But more research will help us to understand better the interaction of heredity and environment and help us to develop ways to improve mental and physical health.

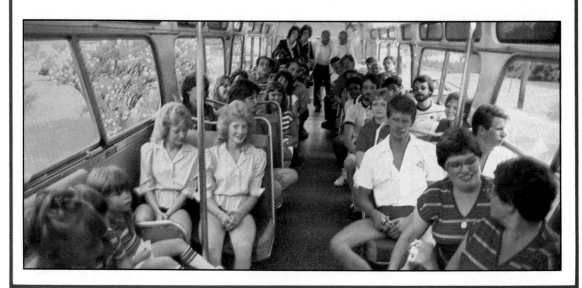

REFLEXES

Reflexes are the simplest behavior patterns in humans. When a bright light is shone into your eyes, your pupils immediately contract. That automatic response is called a *simple reflex*. A simple reflex is a response that does not involve thought processes. You don't have to learn the response, and you do not consciously control its action. Reflex behavior is inborn.

Why are simple reflexes important in behavior? Simple reflexes serve as protective devices. Have you ever touched a hot object? Before you could think, your hand instantly jerked away from the heat. The sudden withdrawal of your hand is called a *reflex action*. It protected you from getting burned. Blinking, sneezing, and coughing are other examples of simple reflexes.

INSTINCTS

Ants have a highly specialized civilization. The queen ant starts the colony by laying the eggs. Worker ants build the colony. They gather food and care for the eggs in the colony. Soldier ants guard the colony. Such complex behavior can easily be thought of as intelligent. However, ants do not learn these tasks. These actions are inborn behavior patterns called **instincts.** Instincts are more complicated than simple reflexes. They are usually made up of a complex series of actions that are directed toward specific goals, such as finding food, building nests, or taking care of the young. All animals of the same species perform tasks such as these in exactly the same way. This is why instincts are often referred to as *species-specific behavior.*

ANIMAL INSTINCTS. Although there are many different kinds of animal instincts, they can be grouped into two major categories: those for **self-preservation,** and those for **species preservation.**

Have you ever disturbed an ant as it was crawling along the ground? It does one of two things. It either runs away or bites you. This behavior illustrates the instinct for self-preservation. However, if you find an ant nest and expose it quickly, something different happens. The ants don't run away. Instead they carry their eggs and cocoons to safety. This is an example of the instinct for species preservation. Instincts for species preservation ensure reproduction and care of the young.

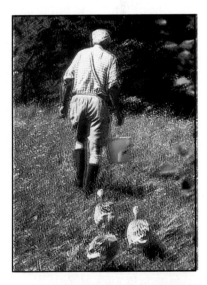

6–3. Ducklings instinctively follow the first moving object they see after hatching. Usually they first see the mother duck. These ducklings first saw Conrad Lorenz, a famous animal behaviorist.

Do these instincts oppose each other? Yes. One says, "Preserve the individual." The other says, "Sacrifice the individual to preserve the group." You might think this would produce conflict for the ants. It would if ants could think about it and be forced to make a decision. However, ants merely respond automatically to the stronger instinct, which is preservation of the species. The same instinct drives the Pacific salmon upstream to their spawning beds. After they reproduce, adult salmon die. A new generation comes downstream to the ocean, and later repeats the spawning behavior.

HUMAN INSTINCTS.   Do humans have instincts? It is hard to deny that some basic urge in us seeks self-preservation. However, very little human behavior can be considered purely instinctive. When we have the urge to act because of a basic instinct, we do not follow any set behavior pattern, as other animals do. Our instincts are modified by what we have learned.

Matthew was awakened in the middle of the night by the sound of a fire alarm. Half asleep, he rushed to the window of his dormitory room and saw flames shooting up from the floor below. He felt a desperate urge to save himself. He grabbed the doorknob and suddenly thought about what he had learned at a school fire drill. The doorknob felt hot. This indicated that the fire was near his door. He remained in control and returned to the window just in time to see the fire engines arrive. Some of Matthew's fellow students ran out of their rooms. As a result they had to be hospitalized for smoke inhalation. What guided Matthew's behavior? He felt the instinct to run in order to survive, but his behavior was also determined by what he had learned.

EMOTIONS

Feelings of pleasure or pain are called emotions. They play a vital part in determining personalities and they motivate much of our behavior. We are born with the capacity for emotions. Some psychologists believe that the basic emotions of love, anger, and fear develop from the basic instinct for self-preservation. Other psychologists believe that emotions stem from the basic urge to seek pleasure. You are attracted to the things that give you pleasure and make you feel secure. You *fear* the things that threaten you. You get *angry* at things that disturb your pleasure or interfere with the way you want things to be.

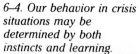

6–4. Our behavior in crisis situations may be determined by both instincts and learning.

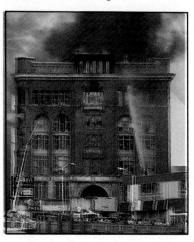

Emotions are physical as well as psychological feelings. Fear, for example, causes physical responses such as increasing heart rate and changing facial expressions. These physical reactions are controlled by your nervous system. You will be learning more about emotions in Chapter 7.

INTELLIGENCE

Intelligence is the capacity to learn, to solve problems, and to create new solutions to familiar problems. Most animals exhibit some degree of intelligence. For example, earthworms are capable of very simple learning. If food is placed at one end of a T-maze and an earthworm is placed at the other end, it will learn by trial and error which way to turn for the food. Higher animals such as chimpanzees are capable of more complex reasoning. (See Figure 6-5.)

But humans inherit reasoning abilities far beyond those of any other living species. No other animal species besides humans has the capacity to control its environment through science, language, and art. Humans alone have the ability to make critical decisions that influence their lives and the world around them.

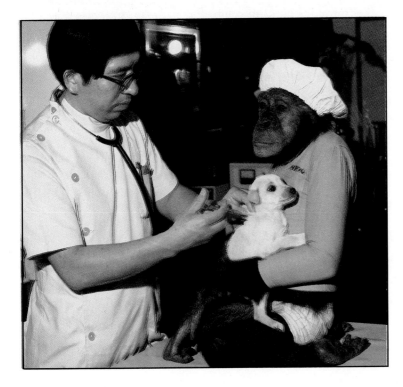

6–5. Chimpanzees are capable of more complex learning. This chimp has been trained to be a veterinarian's assistant.

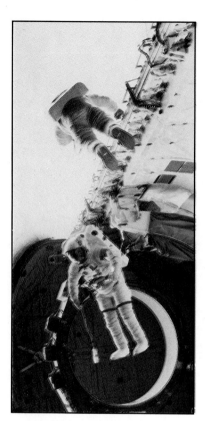

6–6. Human intelligence has enabled us to reach out beyond our planet.

LEARNED BEHAVIOR

Thus far you have learned how nature, that is, what you have inherited, affects behavior. At this juncture, you will understand why nurture, that is, your environment and everything you have learned, effects your behavior.

Human behavior is largely determined by learning. Learning begins during the first days of life, affecting your behavior in your new environment. As you grew, you learned to talk and walk. You learned customs, attitudes, beliefs, and values. In school and outside of school you acquired other knowledge and skills that broadened your world.

THE NATURE OF LEARNING

Learning is a *relatively permanent* change in behavior, which may be positive or negative. Learning occurs as a result of an *experience*. "Relatively permanent" and "experience" are key words in this definition. Not all changes in behavior can be attributed to learning. Physical growth and development affect human behavior. Temporary changes in behavior can also be due to illness, fatigue, or taking a drug.

Learning occurs through three basic functions of the brain: perception, memory, and association. **Perception** is the ability to receive stimuli, such as images and sound, from the environment. What we perceive depends on the sense organs we were born with. For example, our eyes can see colors only within the visible spectrum, from red to violet. Bees can see ultraviolet light, which is outside our visible range. Perception also depends on the stimuli we are paying attention to. For example, if you have a letter to mail, you will be more likely to notice a mailbox. Other times you would probably walk by one without even noticing it. **Memory** is the ability to recall past experiences. You use the memory of what you have learned to help you solve any problems encountered in the future. **Association** is the ability to draw conclusions from past experiences and relate these impressions to present situations. For example, you may have learned that a black animal with a white stripe down its back is a skunk. You may also have learned that skunks, when frightened, squirt a liquid that has a powerful odor. Should you see a skunk, you would first recall what you have learned. You would then associate what you know about skunks to your present situation. Then you would probably take a fast detour!

CONDITIONING

Have you ever wondered how circus animals are trained to perform amazing tricks? The circus animal is trained through a learning process called **conditioning.** Basic conditioning involves only simple degrees of memory and association. Conditioning uses rewards and punishments to get the desired behavior in response to a specific stimulus. If an animal is continually rewarded for a certain response, it will remember the reward and will associate it with the stimulus. Therefore, it responds to the same stimulus in the same way. Through repetition of the desired behavior, responses to the stimuli become automatic.

Can human behavior be shaped by conditioning? When a parent gives praise for a desired behavior, that behavior is likely to be repeated. Praise in this instance acts as the reward, which reinforces behavior. *Behavior modification* is a concept of behavior change based on conditioning. It can help people change habits and other behavior patterns such as emotional responses. In Chapter 11 you will learn how behavior modification can also be used to overcome mental and emotional disorders.

HEALTH IN HISTORY

Principles of classical conditioning were formulated in 1901 by Ivan Pavlov, Russian scientist and Nobel Prize winner. Pavlov taught dogs to salivate at the sound of a bell by first sounding the bell and shortly afterward presenting food to the animal. After the pattern had been repeated several times, the animal paired the sound of the bell with the food. Pavlov proved that learning by association had taken place because the dogs still salivated when the bell was sounded without receiving any food reinforcement.

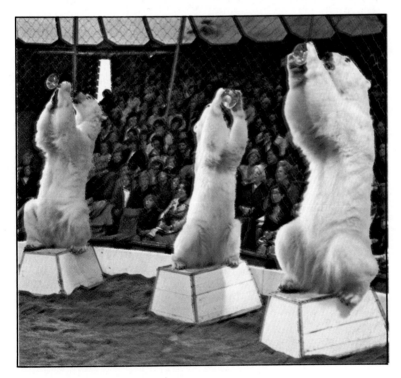

6–7. *How were these animals trained to perform this trick?*

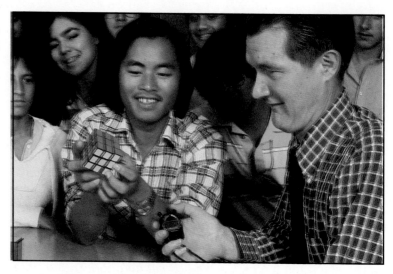

6–8. Solving a cube is an example of cognitive learning.

COGNITIVE LEARNING

Unscramble the anagram "IKTNH." Can a man marry his widow's sister? Who is buried in Grant's tomb? Solving these puzzles involves a complex mental process called **cognition.** Cognitive learning involves more complex degrees of perception, memory, and association than conditioning. When you read these questions, you first *perceived* the letters and words on the page. You understood their meaning because you were able to tap into your *memory* of the English language. To solve the riddles, your mind must put together in new ways many different kinds of information that you have learned in the past.

Cognitive learning involves all of the higher mental processes, such as thinking, reasoning, problem solving, and creativity. Cognitive learning is an unobservable activity that goes on in the privacy of our minds. Thoughts can range from using our imaginations to solving problems through logical thinking. Painting a picture, solving a math problem, and reading the words on this page are all examples of cognitive activities.

LEARNING AND INTELLIGENCE

How are learning and intelligence related? Intelligence can be defined as the capacity for learning. Intelligence tests are supposed to measure a person's potential performance. Achievement tests, on the other hand, measure actual performance in specific subject areas.

Most intelligence tests express intelligence in a *single* score. Therefore, people tend to think of intelligence as a single quality. However, intelligence tests measure a *range* of abilities. The results are usually expressed as an intelligence quotient (I.Q.). Studies have shown that intelligence is not a static quality. A person's environment, particularly in the early years, can significantly increase or decrease I.Q. Good nutrition, exposure to intellectual opportunities, and an emotionally stable environment help children achieve their full intellectual potential.

Are you familiar with the term *mental retardation*? The term *retardation* means a slowing or a delay. In mental retardation a person's ability to learn is slowed and learning capacity is limited. However, the mentally retarded person thinks and feels emotions and has the same basic needs for love and self-worth as other people. In this respect, most mentally retarded people function normally. Retardation stems from problems that occur before, during, or after birth. These problems are discussed in Chapter 21.

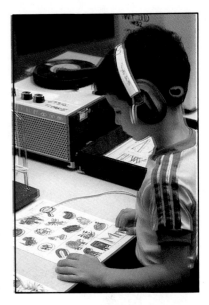

6–9. Special training can help children overcome learning disabilities.

LEARNING DISABILITIES

Neither ten-year-old Tom nor his parents could understand his problems with math and language arts. Tom was intelligent and applied himself to his schoolwork. What was wrong? Through special testing, Tom's problem was diagnosed as a *learning disability*.

Learning disabilities vary, but all are related to breakdowns in the way the brain processes information. In one common type of learning disability, students experience difficulties with language. Alphabet sounds may not be clearly distinguished. The letter "b," for example, may be substituted for the letter "d" when speaking. When words are written, spelled, or read, students may reverse letters. "WAS" becomes "SAW."

Problems with spatial relations and mathematical symbols are signs of another learning disability. Students may confuse left and right, up and down, or they may have trouble applying math to activities like making change for a dollar.

The cause of learning disabilities is not known. The problem can arise in any family. It is important to recognize and treat learning disabilities early since problems often intensify with age. Before the diagnosis is made, tests are performed to rule out vision, hearing, or other problems that could cause similar symptoms. Following diagnosis, special education classes can help overcome these learning problems.

What is the educational outlook for students with learning disabilities? Since most learning disabled students have average or above-average intelligence, their future need not be impaired. Proper professional help makes the important difference.

AUTOMATIC BEHAVIOR PATTERNS

MANNERISMS AND HABITS. Habits are learned behavior patterns that become automatic. How much of human behavior is habit? Consider the many things you do each day without thinking, for example, getting dressed in the morning, washing your face, and brushing your teeth. Through repetition you learned these behaviors. Now they are habits. Even behavior patterns that involve complex skills, such as driving a car or playing a sport, become automatic actions with practice.

Have you ever watched talented impressionists entertain? Even though they don't physically resemble the people they imitate, they can remarkably transform themselves into other people. Impressionists do this by imitating their subjects' mannerisms. Mannerisms are a type of personal habit. They are unique characteristics of an individual's speech and other behavior patterns. For example, some people move their hands often when they speak.

Mannerisms are also behavior patterns that become automatic. When they first occurred in response to a situation, they eased uncomfortable feelings or created a sense of well-being. This rewarded and reinforced the mannerism. Eventually these actions became fixed responses that were unconsciously performed.

FORCES AFFECTING BEHAVIOR

MOTIVATION AND NEEDS

Why does one student study several hours a day and another just enough to get by? What makes one person seek public office and another decide to take up a challenging sport? **Motivation** is the driving force behind behavior. In other words, our behavior is *motivated* by certain needs. Some of these needs, including food and protection from our environment, are vital, or essential. Other needs are not vital to physical survival, but can be powerful driving forces as well. For example, do you find that your friends exert a strong influence on the way you act? We all have the psychological need to belong and to feel accepted by others. This need may motivate you to go along with the crowd instead of exerting your independence.

One psychologist, Abraham Maslow, has formulated an interesting theory of personality based on the complexity of human needs. Look at the list of basic human needs shown in Figure 6-10. According to Maslow, each level of needs builds on the one below it, much like a pyramid. Until the lower needs are satisfied, the higher needs will generally not be reached. Have you ever skipped breakfast and then found it hard to think about anything else except food? According to Maslow's theory, your behavior was motivated by your hunger drive until the need for food was satisfied.

Figure 6–10

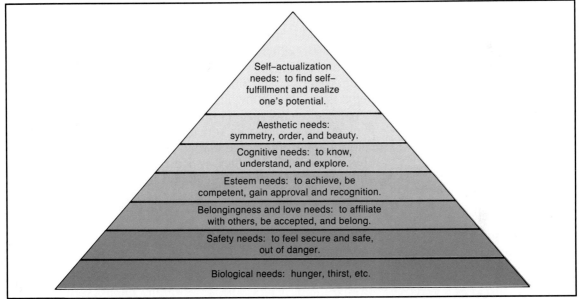

ATTITUDES AND BELIEFS: THE BASIS OF VALUES

Your reactions to life depend largely on your attitude. Attitude is the state of mind with which you approach daily situations. An *optimist* looks at life from a positive point of view, whereas the *pessimist* has a gloomy outlook on life. An optimist and a pessimist each looked at a bottle of milk. "The bottle is half empty," said the pessimist. "No," replied the optimist, "It is half full." Who do you think was right?

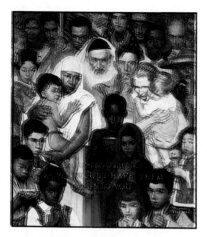

6–11. Norman Rockwell's painting entitled "Do unto others" depicts our conscience, one of the forces that motivates behavior.

6–12. What do children learn from grown-ups?

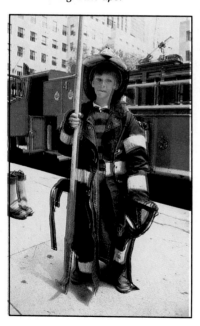

Your answer depends on your own attitude. Your attitudes can have a powerful effect on your behavior. Your appearance and your physical and mental states can be influenced by your attitude.

Your **conscience,** which is a moral attitude, also guides your behavior. Conscience directs you to perform actions that you think are right and to avoid those that are wrong.

Beliefs are closely related to attitudes. If you think certain facts or concepts are true, these beliefs can be reflected in your attitude. For example, if you believe that education is important to later success in life, you will probably have a more positive attitude toward schoolwork. How might this affect your behavior?

Attitudes, conscience, and beliefs are the basis of *values*. Values are personal standards that people live by. Self-respect, respect for others, and honesty are examples of values. Can you name others? One way to identify the values people hold is to observe what they do, not merely what they say. Inner conflict arises when behavior is not in harmony with one's values. Mature people have a well-developed value system based on experience and sound judgment. It helps them set worthwhile goals and lead productive lives.

Your value system was most likely formed by your family, your religion, and your education. As people grow and develop, they examine and clarify certain attitudes and beliefs. This evaluation of values is a process of personal growth. This growth process may lead you to adopt different values or strengthen your existing values.

SOCIAL ENVIRONMENT

Have you ever seen a child imitate a parent? The child observes the parent's actions and learns by example. Parents, brothers and sisters, and other family members usually act as the first role models for behavior. As children grow their social world and awareness expand. Teachers or others outside the home such as peers may serve as role models. Peers can affect behavior throughout life. But the influence of peers is particularly strong during adolescence. Can you suggest why?

Television, movies, and advertising are also recognized as outside influences that can foster social learning and promote certain behaviors. Today, there is growing concern among parents, educators, and psychologists over the effects of media on behavior. Children are exposed to television at very early ages, often for long periods of time. This practice may continue through adolescence and adulthood. What impact do you think television has on learning and behavior?

CULTURAL DIFFERENCES

Have you noticed that behavior may differ considerably among different nations, ethnic groups and age groups? These differences often arise from varying social customs that reflect differences in culture. *Customs* are practices that express social and cultural attitudes, beliefs, and values. Customs can have a powerful effect on the way people think and act. Do you shake hands when you are introduced to someone? This is a common custom taught to children in our country. In Japan a child is taught to bow politely to elders, whereas in India a child shows respect by touching the adult's feet.

The influence of culture is interwoven into many aspects of personal behavior. For example, there are different customs that are observed on occasions such as births, deaths, and marriage. Child-rearing practices, choice of food, and manner of dress are other examples of socially and culturally bound behaviors.

As the world changes, social and cultural systems may change, too. This, in turn, often changes behavior. Can you think of a behavior change that occurred this way?

HEALTH ACTION

Interview an older adult and obtain his or her oral biography. Ask about early life, learning experiences; important life events; and forces such as attitudes, values, and culture that your subject feels influenced his or her personal behavior. Take notes during the biography so all information is recorded. Share your biography in class and discuss similarities and differences among the people interviewed.

6–13. How do these Japanese, Tunisian, and Indian weddings differ from traditional American weddings?

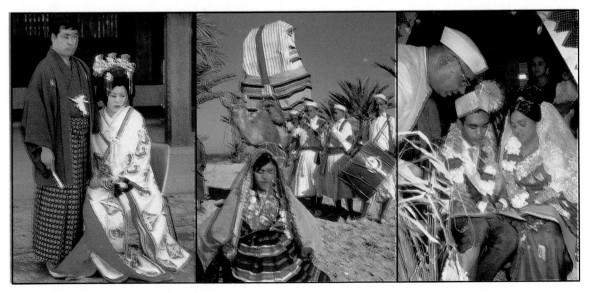

SELF-IMPROVEMENT SKILLS

Attitudes, habits, mannerisms, and other behavior patterns can be changed. It is not easy to do, but change can be accomplished with determination and effort.

CHANGING ATTITUDE

Changing behavior often involves first changing one's attitude. You can control attitudes so that they are a positive influence on your actions. Optimists International, a worldwide organization of positive people, offers the following suggestions for building an overall positive attitude.

1. Make friends feel that they are special in some way.
2. Try to look at the brighter side of things.
3. Think, work for, and expect only the best.
4. Be as enthusiastic about the success of others as you would be about your own.
5. Don't dwell on mistakes. Look to achievements.
6. Be cheerful and greet people with a smile.
7. Give time to improving yourself.

Besides adopting a generally positive attitude, self-improvement also requires building a sense of self-esteem. Self-esteem is the belief in one's own worth. What actions do you think indicate an attitude of self-worth? You can build self-esteem by turning your attention to your abilities and building on them.

DEVELOPING SELF CONTROL

Self-control requires using willpower. Willpower calls for action, or initiative, in some situations and restraint in other situations. *Initiative* is the ability to decide on an action and then carry it through. *Restraint*, on the other hand, means holding back from an action. One indicaton of willpower is the ability to forgo immediate satisfaction and look toward long-range goals. Can you think of an example of this?

CHANGING HABITS

Psychologists suggest these steps, which are based on learning principles, to help you gain control of and change your habits.

1. Analyze the habit or behavior you would like to change. Try to identify the environmental factors present when the behavior occurs. For example, does

142

it happen when you feel lonely, bored, or angry? Does it occur when you are with certain friends?

2. Set an achievable goal and develop a plan to reach it. Your plan might include substituting a new response for the old habit. For example, instead of biting your nails, use a nail file that you've kept handy. Or you might vary your routine to avoid falling into an old behavior pattern.

3. Work toward reaching your goal one day at a time. This helps prevent slipping back into familiar practices. However, don't be too hard on yourself when setbacks occur. These are a normal part of behavior change. Instead, analyze why the relapse occurred and then begin again.

Behavior change is often aided by participation in self-help groups. These groups are composed of people who are trying to make similar changes in their lives. Self-help groups are discussed in greater detail in Chapter 11. Why do you think these groups often make behavior change easier?

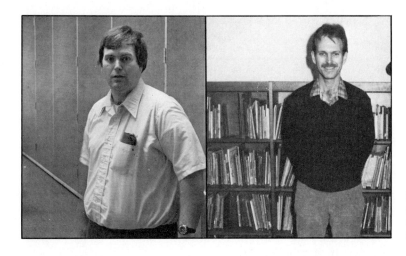

6–14. Gaining control of and changing habits can help you achieve goals such as this one.

SUMMARY: Heredity provides an inborn potential for behavior. Environment molds this potential into behavior patterns. The stimulus-response mechanism makes behavior possible. Reflexes, instincts, and intelligence are the inherited bases of behavior. Almost all human behavior is acquired through learning. Behavior is affected by many forces: motivation and needs, attitudes and beliefs, values, and culture. You can apply some principles of learning to accomplish desired changes in personal behavior.

CHAPTER REVIEW

words at work

Find the word in the left column that fits one of the definitions in the right column. DO NOT WRITE IN THIS BOOK.

a. behavior
b. emotions
c. heredity
d. attitudes
e. values
f. instincts
g. optimist
h. reflex

1. Love, fear, and anger
2. Passing on of traits to offspring
3. Looks at life from a positive perspective
4. Attitudes, conscience, and beliefs form their basis
5. Unlearned behavior responses
6. Is influenced by heredity and environment
7. The simplest behavior pattern in humans
8. Looks at life from a positive point of view

review questions

1. What is the nature-nurture question?
2. List three human characteristics that are learned and three that are inherited.
3. Compare reflexes and instincts.
4. Distinguish between the instinct for self-preservation and the instinct for species preservation.
5. Why is human behavior largely determined by learning?
6. Identify the basic emotions.
7. Describe three functions of the brain that are necessary for learning.
8. Explain how conditioning can affect animal and human behavior.
9. Give examples of a conditional response and of cognitive learning.
10. Describe how intelligence is measured and how intelligence can change.
11. Explain how social customs can affect behavior.
12. Give an example of how motivation affects behavior.
13. Explain how attitudes and beliefs affect behavior.
14. Describe how an optimist and a pessimist would look at the same situation.
15. Are habits useful? Give examples which support your viewpoint.
16. How do mannerisms affect appearance?
17. Outline a procedure for breaking or building habits.
18. How can you improve your self-esteem?
19. Give examples of when initiative should be used and when self-restrain should be used.

discussion questions

1. In your opinion, which contributes most to the total personality, appearance or behavior? If possible, give impersonal evidence to support your answer.
2. On more than one occasion you may have asked yourself, "What made me act that way?" Account for a situation such as this in terms of what you know about human behavior.
3. Discuss whether humans have instincts.
4. Do animals have emotions and intelligence? Give illustrations to defend your opinion.
5. Compare and contrast human and animal behavior.
6. Discuss different forms of learning and how they relate to acquired behavior patterns.

investigating

PURPOSE:
To examine the influence of male and female sex roles on behavior

MATERIALS NEEDED:
Pink and blue index cards, pens.

PROCEDURE:
A.   On a pink card write "female advantages" on one side and "female disadvantages" on the other side. On a blue card write "male advantages" and "male disadvantages."
B.   List as many advantages and disadvantages of being male or female as you can think of on the appropriate cards.
C.   Put the cards from male students in one pile and the cards from female students in another. Make up master lists of the advantages and disadvantages of each sex. You may wish to categorize your lists into specific areas, such as work, home, money, and responsibilities. Write the lists on the blackboard or poster paper.
   1.   Do the male and female students agree on the disadvantages and advantages of each sex?
   2.   Which items on these lists represent biological differences between the sexes and which items represent ideas that are not based on biological differences between the sexes.?
   3.   How do our ideas of being male or female affect our behavior with members of the opposite sex? How do these ideas affect our expectations?
   4.   How are sex roles changing in this country?

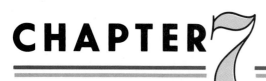

CHAPTER 7
Emotions and Human Relations

OBJECTIVES

- DESCRIBE the development of emotions through the life cycle
- IDENTIFY good and bad effects of emotions on behavior
- DESCRIBE the concept of family and its importance in society
- DESCRIBE the role of human relations in life
- STATE ways to improve communication

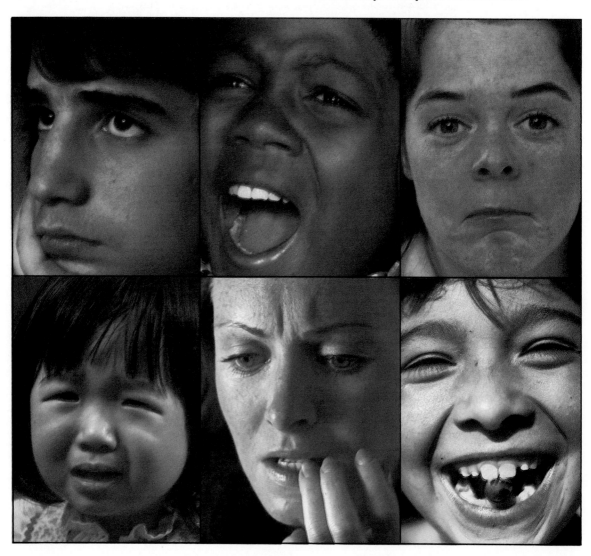

Mr. Schwartz's health class was having a guest speaker. Miss Stevens was a young psychologist who dealt with teenage problems. "Before I start talking," she said, "I'd like to hear from you. What are some things that are on your minds?" she asked. At first there was dead silence in the room. "Well, would you like to know how to be more popular, or how to control your temper?" asked Miss Stevens. Several students nodded silently. Then Roger asked shyly, "How can I get along better with my family? It seems I am always arguing with someone." Questions from other students soon followed. "How do you know when you're really in love?" "What do you think about going steady?"

Miss Stevens listened closely. "These are all good questions," she said. "Let's talk about how you really feel...your emotions. Then let's talk about getting along with others."

EMOTIONS AND YOUR PERSONALITY

Imagine what your life would be like without *emotions*. Picture yourself at a party with friends, on a date, or watching your favorite TV program. How would you act in these situations if you could not feel any emotion? Emotions are a basic part of human life.

Can you describe emotions? Emotions are feelings that add color and fullness to life. They spark mental *and* physical changes inside us. Emotions are also a unique aspect of personality. When faced with the same situation, two people may experience different emotions. Or they may each experience the same emotions but in different degrees.

Emotions themselves are neither good nor bad. It is how they affect you that is important. For example, anger can be a positive force when it is a reaction to social injustice. Then, anger can be the spark that motivates people to work for needed social change. Anger can be a negative force if expressed in ways that hurt others.

Living with your emotions is not very easy. Even the best-balanced people have to work at it all the time. You can develop a healthier personality if you understand your emotions and learn how to control them. But controlling emotions does not mean eliminating them. That would be undesirable. Wouldn't life be dull and drab without emotions?

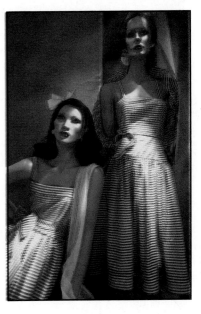

7–1. What would people be like without emotions?

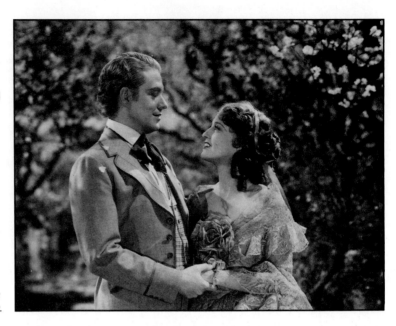

7–2. Romantic movies are often not very true to life.

LOVE: THE BASIS OF HAPPINESS

What does the word **love** mean to you? You may say that you love your parents. You may also say that you love to dance, or that you have fallen in love. Let's consider the meaning of "love" in the statement "I love you." How do you know if you love someone or if someone loves you? Love of another person is often equated with "romance" as played out in countless movies and books: boy meets girl, boy loses girl, boy gets girl, and they live happily ever after. . . . The boy and girl are almost always young and beautiful, but not very true to life. Real love does not depend on physical beauty as these stories suggest. Yet many of us tend to reject those who do not fit this ideal.

To better understand what love is, we must separate the real roots of love from the notion of romance. Real love is a deep concern for another person's welfare. When you love someone, you communicate this love not just in words but in your actions. This kind of love is not something you "fall into." It is something you work on that grows each day.

TYPES OF LOVE. Love exists in many forms. In real friendship, you love your friends and help them in any way you can in times of need. Parents and children feel a special kind of love for each other. In marital love, husbands and wives are deeply committed to each other in all aspects of their lives. People may love their country. They appreciate what their country has done for them and feel a commitment to serve in some way. The broadest type of love is love of humanity. People who truly "love their neighbors as themselves" demonstrate this kind of love.

THE NEED FOR LOVE. We are born with the capacity to love, but it must be nurtured. When babies receive love, they feel secure. In this way, self-acceptance grows. Self-love is necessary before you can love others. Do not confuse self-love with selfishness. Selfishness is seeing only oneself, not others. Self-love is seeing yourself as a worthy person in relation to other people.

Do you think that love is an important emotion? Love gives special meaning and purpose to life. How has love enriched your life?

FEAR: THE SAFETY-ALARM EMOTION

How is **fear** like a safety alarm? When you sense danger, fear sets off an inner alarm that prepares the body for a fight or flight reaction. During this reaction the muscles tense. The heart beats faster, pumping an increased energy supply to the muscles. The body is ready for action.

When the threat of danger is real, fear acts as a natural protective device. Were you ever told not to ride with strangers? Were you warned never to play with matches, or always to look both ways before crossing a street? These fears are instilled in children to protect them from harm. Fears that safeguard personal safety are a necessary part of life.

When fear stems from imagined danger, it can easily become an emotion that serves no useful purpose. For example, prejudice causes dislike and distrust of people without reason. Prejudiced people see differences in others as a threat. Why do you think this reaction occurs? Children recognize differences among people. Yet to them these differences are not a cause for alarm. Prejudice is learned like other fears.

ANXIETY: INNER FEAR. Do you feel tense before taking a test? Would you feel nervous during a job or college interview? Everyone feels some inner fear or **anxiety** (ang-**zi**-et-tee) at times even though no threat of physical harm exists. All stressful events produce the same fight or flight reaction. Fear of external dangers can be identified. The cause of anxiety can be harder to pinpoint.

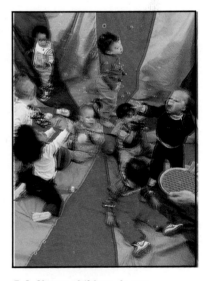

7–3. Young children do not see their race differences as cause for alarm. How do people become prejudiced?

Anxiety can be helpful if channeled in the right direction. The athlete's tenseness before a race can charge the nervous system and improve performance. Your own worry over the possibility of not passing a subject can make you study harder. Anxiety is only harmful when it interferes with health or satisfied living. How can you cope with anxiety? When you become anxious and tense, stop a minute. Try to discover the reason behind your fear. Try to think of constructive ways to reduce your tension. For example, before going on an interview, think about what questions you might be asked and prepare your answers. Practice your interviewing skills. Have a mock interview to build your self-confidence.

ANGER: AN EMOTIONAL FIRE

Anger is like an emotional fire. Within people it can rage or flare up quickly and soon burn out; or it can constantly smoulder. When you get angry does your heart pound? Does your face get red? Like fear, anger produces strong physical reactions that prepare the body for action.

Anger itself is not a good or bad emotion. It is a basic emotion that everyone feels throughout life. What situations make you feel angry? Anger usually stems from frustration because things are not the way you would like them to be. Often anger is triggered by events over which you have no control. A friend may disappoint you, or you may have a day on which everything seems to go wrong.

How can you handle anger? You can *suppress* anger or you can *express* it. Keeping anger inside you may seem easier for you or those around you. But it can be hard on you

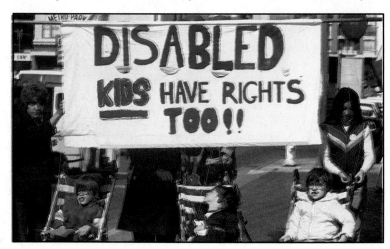

7–4. Anger can be the spark that motivates people to work for needed changes.

UNIT 2   YOUR PERSONALITY

emotionally. It may even make you sick. If you don't express anger, its tension builds inside you for a long time. Your body stays in a constant state of tenseness without release. The better solution is to express your anger, but to do so constructively.

EXPRESSING ANGER. When children become angry they may fly into a temper tantrum and scream, hit, kick, or break things. You may also feel like acting this way, but are such outbursts helpful? Once the tantrum is over, the situation that caused the anger is left unchanged. Sometimes people express anger in ways that hurt others and themselves. They may tease, pick fights, break rules, damage property, or perform other hostile or antisocial acts.

Todd and his girl friend had a bad argument. Seething with anger, Todd jumped into the car. He raced down the street ignoring the speed limit and stop signs. Within minutes he had collided with another car. Several people, including Todd, were injured.

Anger expressed without control shows emotional immaturity. Before expressing your anger, try the count-to-ten rule. Give yourself time to stop and think about the situation and why you feel angry. Decide first if the event is really important enough to rate your anger. If a person steps ahead of you in a line or a store clerk ignores you, is it worth your energy to become angry? Such events are often best overlooked or looked at in a different way. Instead of becoming angry, you might think about why people would act so rudely. It may be that they are unhappy or having a bad day.

If the situation rates your anger, decide what you can do to improve it. When others make you angry, you could discuss your feelings with them. This can ease anger but risks causing more anger, too. Have you ever felt angry all over again, just thinking about events that upset you? This can happen when you try to discuss your anger with the person involved. Without meaning to, your hoped-for discussion can quickly turn into an argument or an exchange of ugly remarks. What can you do to prevent this from happening? Before talking, give yourself enough time to get your feelings under control. Then direct your discussion *to* the *problem* not *at* the *person* involved.

When you can't discuss your feelings directly to the person who made you angry, you can use other healthy outlets for anger. You can share your feelings with a friend, a parent, or another good listener. Again, center your discussion

Discovering who you are is not an easy process. One sign of self is what a person likes and dislikes. Think about what you do and do not enjoy. Prepare two ten-item lists: *I like, I do not like.* What do your lists tell you about yourself?

around the problem, not the person involved. Do not exaggerate your side of the story. Or, reduce your anger by using up its energy through work or play. Physical exercise often helps to ease anger and allow relaxation. How did you cope with anger the last time you were upset?

JEALOUSY AND ENVY.   **Jealousy** and **envy** are considered related emotions. Both emotions stem from feelings of fear and insecurity. Jealousy makes you feel insecure because you fear losing something you already have. Envy comes from feeling insecure because you do not have possessions or advantages that others have. Envy and jealousy often lead to anger, since they are feelings of frustration.

Tom was enjoying the party with his date, Jean, who was very popular at school. When Tom left to get refreshments and returned, Jean was gone. Across the room he saw Jean laughing and dancing with Ralph. Tom rushed over and made some angry remarks to Ralph. Tom felt jealous because he thought he was losing Jean's attention.

On Valentine's Day Sally found a card from her boyfriend Mark, inside her locker. She was delighted. Later she saw her friend Karen wearing gold heart-shaped earrings. "How do you like the new earrings Bob gave me?" asked Karen. "Did you get anything from Mark?" Sally blurted a quick reply and ran off. In this case, Sally was envious.

When jealousy and envy are not controlled, they can damage personal relationships leading to unhappiness and harmful actions. Could Tom and Sally have acted differently?

RESENTMENT.   When jealousy and envy take hold of you, **resentment** often builds. Resentment is the angry feeling that life has cheated you. Self-pity keeps resentment locked inside of you. How can you free yourself from this emotion? Honest self-appraisal can help remove self-pity. It can also help you develop a worthwhile plan to improve life instead of just wishing it were better. Discussion with someone you trust may ease resentment.

GRIEF.   Everyone feels moments of sadness during life. This is a normal reaction. **Grief** and despair are similar to sadness, except they are much stronger emotions. Grief is caused by events that can never be changed or corrected such as the death of a loved person or a personal defeat. In these kinds of situations, you feel helpless and very unhappy. If grief lasts for a long time, it interferes with normal life. Though grief is a painful emotion, allowing yourself to

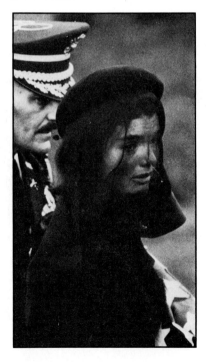

7–5. *Allowing yourself to feel grief and expressing it openly can help heal the pain of loss.*

feel grief and express it can help heal the pain of loss. If feelings of despair come over you, try to remember that few situations are hopeless. Given time, things have a way of changing. Try to talk about your feelings. Look at your situation from a distance. Try to get involved in activities, and seek help from someone you trust.

GUILT. Do you think **guilt** is as strong an emotion as love, anger, or fear? You may feel guilty when you think or act in ways that conflict with your conscience, values, or standards set by your parents and society. This helps you recognize when you have done something wrong. It lets you know when you are failing in your personal responsibilities at home, at school, or in your relationships with others.

But guilt can create unnecessary inner conflict. When a person feels guilty about minor mistakes, guilt becomes unreasonable. Sometimes the reasons for guilt feelings may lie buried in the past. For example, some parents always try to control their children's behavior by making them feel guilty. These children may grow up feeling that they are shameful, worthless people.

How can you cope with guilt? You may not be able to correct all situations that make you feel guilty, but correct those you can. Be reasonable about what you expect of yourself; no one is perfect. Try to do better the next time; you can learn from your mistakes. Let go of your guilt feelings. Punishing yourself through guilt will not change the situation or help you grow emotionally.

EMOTIONS AND THE LIFE CYCLE

INFANCY AND CHILDHOOD. From birth, infants display emotions that come from feelings of pain or pleasure. They become frightened when startled by loud, unexpected noises. When they are hungry, they show their pain by crying. When their needs are met, pleasure is felt. They start to relate feelings of pleasure with people who care. This association is the beginning of love for another.

As children mature physically, emotional growth occurs too. As they discover more about the world, their range of emotional feelings expands. Other emotions like jealousy, envy, and grief are felt. Early in life children learn that to receive affection, they must be considerate of others. They begin to give and take in their relationships. With emotional growth comes greater self-awareness.

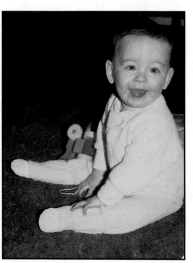

7–6. When their needs are met, babies display feelings of pleasure.

ADOLESCENCE TO ADULTHOOD. Do you ever feel as if you are on an emotional roller coaster? One day you may feel happy, and the next day you may feel sad. You can even go through many emotional changes in a single day. With adolescence comes the painful process called growing up. During these years confusion and changing feelings are natural. Adolescence *is* a time of change. You build new friendships. Old relationships often change. You grow more independent, and you learn to make decisions on your own.

As you move toward adulthood, you search to establish your identity. You enjoy new experiences. Through a process of trial and error, and then evaluation, you develop new patterns of behavior. You establish your own goals and values. As you begin thinking about what you want to achieve in life, you must look at yourself honestly. You must discover what your talents and abilities are and what you enjoy doing. Although this process begins during the teenage years, growth and development continues throughout adult life.

How do you view your future as a male or female in work, home, or social roles? Because of the changing roles of men and women in society there are many choices open to you that you may want to consider.

7–7. How do you view your future role as a male or female adult?

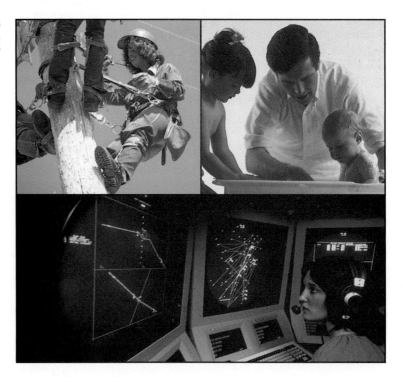

EMOTIONAL MATURITY. Physical growth is easily charted as a person grows from infancy to adulthood. Emotional growth is harder to measure. You probably know adults who act childish or children who act grown up. No two people grow at the same emotional rate. Your level of maturity depends on your experiences and how well you adjusted to them. Emotional maturity is measured by attitudes and the ability to direct emotions toward constructive behavior. It enables you to live at peace with yourself and to interact successfully with others. Table 7-1 summarizes some of the traits of the emotionally mature and immature.

EMOTIONAL GROWTH	
The Emotionally Mature	The Emotionally Immature
Are considerate of others	Are selfish and self-centered, with little consideration for others
Accept pleasures gracefully and enjoy sharing them with others	Constantly seek pleasures without regard for others
Channel emotional drives into constructive activity	Yield quickly to emotions in such explosive behavior as crying spells, depression, pouting, and temper tantrums
Accept disappointments and accept them with courage and composure	Become angry or depressed in the face of disappointments
Are confident of success and are willing to work for it and to wait	Are impatient for success and often unwilling to work for it
Adjust to other people and create a relaxed and pleasant social atmosphere	Fail to adjust to other people and create a tense and unpleasant social atmosphere

Table 7–1

FAMILY, FRIENDS, AND HUMAN RELATIONS

The most powerful influence on your emotions are the people in your life. Think about the many different people you come into contact with daily: parents, brothers, sisters, friends, teachers, neighbors. The term *human relations* is the interaction between people. Getting along with others isn't easy. It takes effort to have good relationships that add pleasure and satisfaction to your life. Learning to build good relations with others now will help you throughout life. Human relations begin with the first people in your life, your family. These relations then extend to your friends.

THE FAMILY TODAY

THE IMPORTANCE OF FAMILY. The family is the foundation of our society. It protects and cares for society's youngest members, its children. Can you list the important needs the family fulfills? A child's basic physical and emotional needs are met here. With your family, you learn your first lessons in how to communicate and share your feelings with others. You acquire attitudes, beliefs, and values from your family. Love, friendship, and acceptance are important human needs that the family provides. When these needs are met, trust grows. Then you can reach out to others outside the family circle. In these ways your family can help you grow into a happy and productive member of society.

TYPES OF FAMILIES. What does the word family mean to you? The concept of family has been changed. The *extended* family may include parents, children, grandparents, aunts, uncles, and cousins. At one time the extended family was common. Members of the extended family shared responsibilities such as financial support, household chores, and

7–8. One-hundred years ago the extended family was common. How has the family changed?

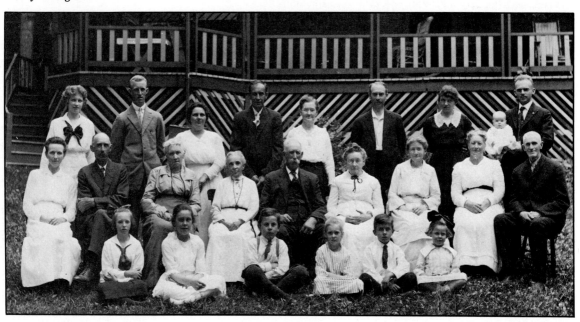

raising children. As society changed, the *nuclear* family became more common. The term "nuclear" does not refer to the nuclear age. Here, it means the "core" of the family unit. The nuclear family is composed of a mother, a father, and children. The nuclear family is still the major type of family in our country. However, the number of single-parent families is growing. The number of *blended* families, which are made up of members of two or more families, is also growing.

FAMILY TENSIONS

"I hope I get that raise," Mrs. Brown thought as she hurried to get ready for work. When she reached the bathroom, she heard the shower running. She banged on the door and shouted, "Don, hurry up! You know we agreed that I should shower first. I've got to get to work on time." "Well I've got early football practice today," Don yelled back, "that's important too." When Don finally opened the door, he and his mother just glared at each other.

Do you have disagreements in your family? Family tensions exist in even the closest families. Learning to recognize and understand the pressures of family life can help ease some of the tensions between you and your family.

FINANCIAL PRESSURES. Why was Mrs. Brown so upset? Her real concern might have been her financial responsibilities, not Don's rule-breaking. What are some costs of running a household? Rent or mortgage payments, food, and utilities are just a few expenses. Can you identify others? It is not easy for the average family to meet these expenses. Household costs may increase faster than family income. This puts added strain on family life.

Have you ever thought about cost when your request for something was denied? Families must meet their basic expenses first. Sometimes this means cutting down on less essential items such as entertainment. Many teens help out with family finances through part-time jobs. A job brings extra income and can have other benefits, too. Those who do not work can help out at home by pitching in.

PRIVACY PRESSURES. "I could have just screamed last night," Jane told her friend. "All I wanted was a few minutes to myself but everyone kept barging in on me." "It's worse in my house," said Darryl. "Whenever I come home my parents want to know every little thing that has happened. I feel I can't even keep my thoughts to myself."

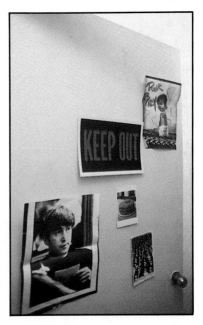

7–9. The need for privacy is a normal part of growing up.

Have you ever felt similar frustrations? The need for privacy is a normal part of growing up. Sometimes the size of your living space can make it hard to be alone. At times, a concerned parent may not realize that your need for privacy grows as you become more independent.

How can you deal with the issue of privacy at home? Talk with your family members. Calmly explain how you feel. Try to work out solutions together. In situations where this will not work, try to satisfy your need for privacy in other ways. For example, take a quiet walk so you can spend time with just your thoughts.

SIBLINGS.   Are you an only child? If you are not, then you have a **sibling.** This term means *brother* or *sister.* Siblings can be close friends. But they can also cause conflict as seen in this class discussion:

Chuck: "My older sister acts like my mother. She's always telling me what to do."

Lynn: "My little brother is driving me crazy. He either clings to me constantly or tries to annoy me in little ways. He's worse when my friends come over."

Dave: "My brothers and sisters are all so talented. I feel that I'm always being compared with them."

Pat: "My sister is the family favorite. She always gets everything she wants."

You can probably think of other problems with siblings. There are no easy answers to these situations. One key to better human relations is to look at things from another's viewpoint. In Chuck's case, his sister's actions may come from her own desire to be seen as an adult. Or she may be concerned that Chuck is actually doing something that could harm himself. Lynn would probably get along better with her little brother if she realized that he just wants her attention. Knowing this, what could she do? Pat and Dave might try to see from their parents' viewpoint. Most parents love all their children and do not deliberately compare them or play favorites. But because each child's personality is unique, parents cannot treat each child the same way. Good communication between parents and children can often help improve these situations.

PARENTS.   Do you ever feel caught between two worlds? On the one hand you may be expected to act grown up. Yet when you want adult privileges, you may be told that you are still too young. This struggle for independence is a natural part of adolescence. As a child you depended on your parents and they directed much of your behavior. Yet as you approach adulthood, the parent-child relationship changes. For both you and your parents, it can be hard to break the old behavior patterns. Parents may find it hard to accept the viewpoints of the young adult. The young adult may want more freedom but find it hard to handle new roles and independence responsibly.

Phil was ready to leave for a party when his father announced, "Be home by midnight." "I can't," protested Phil. "No one *ever* has to be home before one o'clock." "I don't care about anyone else," his father replied. "Midnight is your deadline." "Why are you always trying to run my life?" Phil shouted.

Joyce was almost ready for the party when her mother asked, "Who are you going out with tonight?" "I'm going with David," Joyce replied. "I thought we discussed that. I don't like you seeing him. He has a poor reputation." "*We* didn't discuss anything," Joyce said hotly. "*You* told *me* you didn't like him. What right do you have to choose my friends?"

Personal freedom and choice of friends are two areas in which parents and children often disagree. Here are a few others.

- Appearance
- Attendance at religious services
- Dating
- Discipline
- Grades
- Neatness
- Personal responsibilities (homework, chores, etc.)
- Spending time at home with family
- Telling the truth
- Use of leisure time
- Use of alcohol and drugs

Often conflicts stem from disagreements over rules set by those in authority. You may not like living with rules, but aren't they a necessary part of life? Schools, cities, and states all need rules so that they can operate properly. Rules provide guidelines so that people know what is expected of them.

Families have rules for the same reasons. Do you think most parents make rules just to be strict? Or do they set rules out of love and concern? Could you support a home of your own? Could you pay for clothing, food, shelter, or other necessary expenses? Are you ready to assume total responsibility for all decisions that will affect your life? Most teenagers, if these questions are answered honestly, will have to admit that the answers are no.

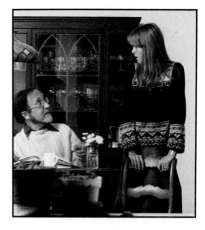

7–10. Improved communication can help resolve conflicts between parents and children.

Improved communication can help resolve conflicts between parents and children. When disagreements arise, try to avoid making demands. Instead, discuss your different points of view. In this way, you may discover what the real issues are. Then compromise is often possible. For example, Phil might learn through a good discussion that his father does not really care about an hour's time difference. Mr. Michael's real concern is Phil's driving inexperience and the greater chance of car accidents during early morning weekend hours. Knowing this, how might they reach a compromise? An open discussion does not always lead to agreement. But it can build mutual respect and understanding.

WHEN FAMILIES BREAK UP.   Essie reacted to the news of her parents' divorce with mixed emotions. At first she felt guilty and afraid. "Maybe," she thought, "this wouldn't have happened if I hadn't acted up so much. What will happen to my life now?" Then she realized divorce would mean an end to the constant fighting at home. That would be a relief.

When families break up, each family member goes through many emotions. You may feel angry that your parents could not work out their problems. You may feel hurt, confused, or resentful about the changes in your life. Anger, jealousy, and other emotions may arise when a divorced parent starts dating and you must adjust to other people entering your life.

Family experts agree that coping with divorce and your emotions takes time. You may go through several emotional stages before you really adjust. Accepting the situation, though you wish it were not so, is an important first step in dealing with divorce. It is also helpful to realize that, though children may cause pressures for parents, they do not cause divorce. Divorce is the result of problems between the two parents.

YOUR PEER GROUP

Peers are people who are considered your equals. A peer group can be defined in different ways: by age, social position, job title, or other factors. Peer groups, no matter how they are defined, are composed of people who share something in common.

How do you define your peer group? Most teenagers consider their friends and others their age as their peer group. What do you have in common with your peer group? Do you have differences, too?

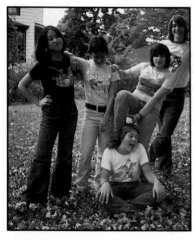

7–11. Peers can influence how you choose to look and act.

PEERS AND PERSONAL DECISIONS. How do your peers affect your life? Do they influence how you choose to look and act? Peers can have a strong effect on your behavior and how you feel about yourself. It is not unusual to feel unsure about yourself, especially during adolescence. Belonging to and being accepted by a peer group brings a sense of security and boosts self-esteem. It may seem simpler to follow the crowd than to think and act on your own. If you go against the group, you also run the risk of feeling or being alone.

Decision making involves testing your values. The decisions you make during the teen years are very important. They are the basis for the adult you will become. Think back to the last important decision that you made. Did you make that decision alone or were you influenced by peer pressure?

FRIENDSHIP AND DATING

Friendship grows from shared feelings, interests, and experiences. Making friends can be easy; keeping friends takes work. You have to be willing to give as well as receive in a friendship. When you learn to build lasting friendships, you also develop your skills in relating to others.

Dating can be an adventure in personal relationships and a source of anxiety as well. Many teenagers start dating before they are ready because of their friends. They do not want to feel left out. When the choice to date is really yours, dating can be fun. But behind its satisfaction is a more serious purpose. Dating helps you improve your social skills and can help you learn more about yourself.

DATING DILEMMAS. "I wish I knew how to be more popular," said Ellen. "I didn't have a Saturday date and I feel awful." "I had a date, but I didn't know what to say or how to act," complained Ralph. Mark joined in, "I had a first date, but when I asked about a second time, she wouldn't say yes."

These dating problems are not unusual. There is no magic formula for being popular and at ease while dating. What do people look for in a date? Appearance may attract, but it is not the most important quality in a date. People are naturally drawn to those who are easy to be with and who show a real interest in them.

Not taking yourself and dating so seriously can help you relax while on a date. If you feel tense, think about your date. He or she probably feels as awkward and shy as you

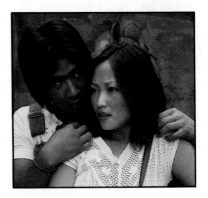

7–12. Dating can help you learn more about yourself and others.

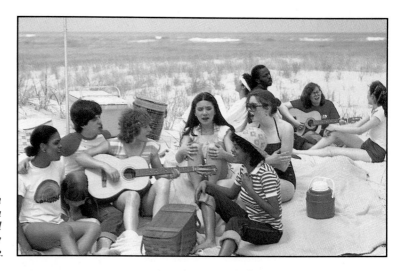

7–13. Participating in group activities gives you a chance to practice social skills and to meet a variety of people.

do. If you try to make your date feel at ease, you will probably feel more relaxed too. Then you can both have more fun on your date.

You may wonder whether you should be yourself while on a date. Changing your feelings to match what you think your date wants is seldom a good idea. You cannot feel natural and enjoy a date if you spend your time pretending to be someone you are not. After all, your date should get to know and enjoy the real you. Consider double dating or group dating activities such as parties, school dances, or sports events. Being with other couples may make you feel more at ease.

STEADY DATING. Steve felt shy around girls and seldom dated. When he met Ann, she seemed friendly and easy to talk to. Soon they were dating often, then going steady. Ann's parents thought that Steve was so "well mannered." Steve's parents were delighted to see that he was "getting out of his social shell." At school everyone thought they made a nice couple. Steve and Ann had a built-in date for every social event.

After several months, they began arguing over little things. "I just can't understand what is happening," Ann told a friend. "Since we started going steady Steve has become so possessive. Lately we just don't have much to say to each other." When Ann said she no longer wanted to go steady, Steve appeared angry. But inside he was relieved. "I thought going steady would be great," he told his best friend. "But after a while I found myself just doing things out of habit. I

162

liked Ann, but I wanted to go out with other girls, too. I felt guilty for wanting to and resentful because I couldn't."

What factors led to this couple's break up? What do you see as the plus and minus sides of dating? Dating only one person (going steady) can be convenient and can ease dating pressures. But it can also limit your chances of interacting with others and finding out exactly what personality traits are most important and best suited to you.

MATURE LOVE AND MARRIAGE

When is love a lasting emotion? When is it only a passing feeling? During dating, love and sharing with another person become mixed with feelings of physical attraction, excitement, and romance. These different aspects of love may blend so closely that it can be difficult to separate one aspect from another. These feelings can be so strong that they can temporarily blind a person to the faults and shortcomings of another.

Mature love is lasting. This is possible when two people accept responsibility for themselves and for those they love. A couple builds a satisfying life together. Yet they each maintain their identity as two unique persons. Physical attraction is a part of their relationship. It is not the guiding force. Mutual respect and trust increase the pleasure of their special friendship. Mature love forms a firm foundation for a happy marriage and a wholesome family life.

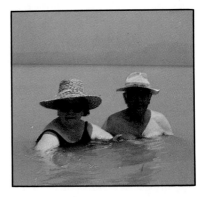

7-14. How can two people create a lasting, loving relationship?

DECIDING TO MARRY. The decision to marry is one of the most important decisions anyone makes. Yet, surprisingly, this decision often occurs without careful thought. People may become swept up in romance and being "in love" and not think beyond the wedding ceremony. They may just assume that they will live "happily ever after." A good marriage depends on *who* you marry and *when* you marry. Before making this decision ask yourself:

• Are we both emotionally mature? Are we ready to cope with the many adjustments that marriage requires? Are we each secure in who we are?

• Can we support ourselves financially? Do we have a plan that provides for all our needs, education, household, and any children?

• Do we share the same basic values and goals? Do we agree on male and female roles for household chores, money, jobs, and children?

What other questions do you think are important?

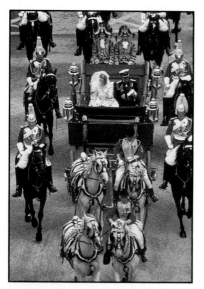

7–15. The romantic wedding of Prince Charles and Lady Diana was awe-inspiring. Yet, even they face the many challenges that marriage brings.

When two people decide to marry an **engagement** or waiting period often takes place first. It gives couples a last chance to decide whether or not they are really suited to each other and marriage. Engagement also provides time to discuss husband and wife roles and to work out concrete plans for married life. How long do you think an engagement should last?

THE CHALLENGE OF MARRIAGE

When two people exchange wedding vows, their dating relationship ends. A new relationship begins. Marriage brings special joys as well as responsibilities. It is a legal contract between two people that has certain obligations. It is also a couple's public statement of mutual commitment.

Often, when people marry they think they have reached their goal. But the challenge of marriage has just begun. A happy marriage requires constant work and attention if it is to grow and last.

At first, marriage can be as hard as it is satisfying. It may not be easy to adjust to each other's personal habits. *Living* up to new roles is tougher than just talking about them. As a marriage continues, financial worries, troubles with children, or health or family crises can arise. A couple may also fall into a routine of living together and start to take each other for granted.

Every marriage has its ups and downs. But it is the way that problems and daily conflicts are handled that is important. Regular, open communication is the key to a sound marriage.

TEEN MARRIAGES

Don and Carol were high school seniors when they decided to marry. Both their parents disapproved, but gave in when they saw that the couple was determined. After their wedding they lived with Carol's family. They couldn't afford a place of their own. They both dropped their outside school activities so they could take part-time jobs. They started saving for their own apartment. Soon, friction built between Carol and her mother. "As long as you are in my house," her mother said, "you have to respect my rules." Carol argued, "I am a married woman now. You have no right to make any demands on me." Don felt caught in between. He decided to drop out of school so he could work full time and bring in extra money. Without a high school diploma, he could only find a job that paid the minimum wage. When Don and Carol finally moved into their own apartment, things got worse instead of better. Don missed school and spent his evenings with his friends, leaving Carol at home. Carol reacted by ignoring him. Soon they divorced.

Each year over two million marriages take place. Half of these fail. Fewer teen marriages succeed. Why do you think Don's and Carol's marriage dissolved? Conflicts over money, husband and wife roles, and children are the most common reasons for broken marriages.

HUMAN RELATIONS SKILLS

We have examined many different human relationships. A common thread runs through all of those that are successful. It is good communication. You communicate in many different ways. You can tell someone directly what you think or feel. Or you can communicate through your actions. For example, you could say the words "I love you," but you could also convey this message by doing something to please someone you love. It is easy to understand a person whose words and behavior give the same message. Doubt begins when a person says one thing and acts another way.

COMMUNICATION BASICS

Good communication takes two people. You may want to talk, but the other person must be free to really listen. If the person you want to talk to is busy doing something else, politely interrupt. Arrange a specific time for a later talk. When that time arrives,

1. Learn to listen to what people say. Also read the messages in their behavior.
2. Keep your emotions under control. Do not suppress feelings, but remember to express them properly.
3. Avoid statements such as, "You can't be serious," or "You are really silly." Try to begin your statements by saying how you feel: "I was hurt when. . . ."
4. Try to see the situation from the other person's point of view. The purpose of communication is to share ideas, feelings, and information.
5. Determine the real issues before making judgments.
6. Attempt to compromise when appropriate. Your efforts to give up something will be appreciated. Others may respond in the same way.

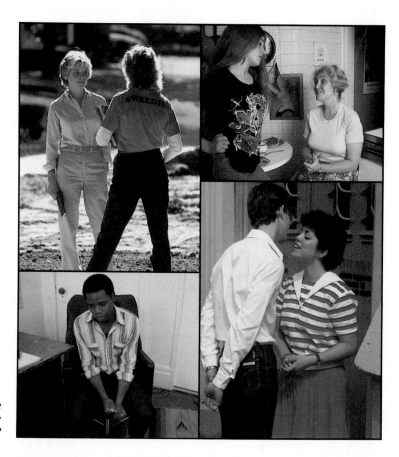

7–16. What are these people saying with body language?

SUMMARY: Emotions can have a good or harmful effect on behavior. The ability to channel emotions constructively shows emotional maturity. Love, fear, and anger are powerful basic emotions involved in human relations. Jealousy, envy, resentment, grief, and guilt are a few other complex emotions.

Human relations is the interaction between people. Establishing your personal identity and your relationships with others often causes emotional turmoil during adolescence. The family is the foundation of society. In the home you first learn human relations skills. Family tensions may stem from pressures over finances, privacy, or problems with siblings or parents. Peers can have a strong effect on personal decisions and behavior. Through friendship and dating you learn social skills. Good communication is necessary for good human relations. Marriages may fail when people are immature and fail to communicate with each other.

CHAPTER REVIEW

words at work

Which category on the right best describes the phrase on the left? DO NOT WRITE IN THIS BOOK.

1. fear anxiety anger love
2. considerate responsible confident forgiving
3. phobia apprehension prejudice anxiety
4. frustration tantrum tension resentment
5. comfort pleasure self-love mother
6. listen share compromise

a. Indications of an emotionally mature person
b. Results of anger
c. Examples of fear
d. Related to resentment
e. Related to first love
f. Communication basics
g. Influence human relationships
h. Basic emotions

review questions

1. How does love develop? What different forms may it take?
2. Explain how fear serves as a safety reaction.
3. Tell how anxiety can sometimes serve a useful purpose.
4. How can anger be a useful and a harmful emotion?
5. Explain how to deal constructively with anger.
6. Is grief a harmful emotion? Explain your answer.
7. Contrast jealousy and envy.
8. Trace emotional development from infancy to adulthood.
9. Contrast the actions of an emotionally mature and immature person.
10. Define the three types of families.
11. Explain the role of the family in society.
12. What is a sibling?
13. Identify reasons why parents and children have problems with each other.
14. Discuss how peers can influence your behavior.
15. Why is friendship important in life?
16. How does dating improve social skills?
17. Name three factors needed for a successful marriage.
18. Why do most teen marriages end in divorce?
19. Define good communication.
20. Give three suggestions for improved communication.

discussion questions

1. People seem to differ in their capacity to feel basic emotions and in how they react to basic emotions. Explain.
2. What are some common problems experienced in family life? How can these problems be solved?
3. What is the difference between real love and mere infatuation?
4. A friend is undecided about going steady and asks you for advice. What would you say?
5. Discuss common problems in dating and marriage. Identify possible solutions.

investigating

PURPOSE:

To develop listening skills that are an essential component of good communication.

MATERIALS NEEDED:

Paper and pen.

PROCEDURE:

A.   Divide the class into groups of three: (1) speakers; (2) listeners; (3) observers.

B.   Speakers may then select a topic to talk about from the list below or may choose to talk about themselves.

1. patriotism	5. friendship	9. peer pressure
2. equal opportunity	6. television	10. politics
3. school life	7. dating	11. employment
4. parenthood	8. fashion	12. sports

C.   The "speaker" talks for an uninterrupted five-minute period on the selected topic. During this time the "listener" listens carefully while the "observer" takes notes on what is being said and acts as timekeeper. (The observer should signal the speaker at the four-minute mark.) After the five-minute period, the listener repeats back to the group, as exactly as possible, what the speaker has just said. Any inaccuracies should be noted and corrected either by the speaker or the observer. After the listener has completed the recitation, any omissions should also be noted. Repeat this exercise until each person in the group has acted in each role.

D.   Discuss the exercise in class.

1.   Was it more difficult to act as a speaker or a listener? Why?

2.   Did listeners omit, add, or change the emphasis of what was said? Did speakers sometimes recall inaccurately what they had said?

3.   How important is listening in the communications process? Why? What factors affect how well someone listens? Give everyday examples of how listening might affect communications and relationships between people.

HEALTH
CAREERS

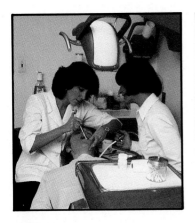

DENTIST

Today dentistry has expanded beyond tooth care. It is concerned with the entire oral area: the lips, the tongue, the gums, the jaws, and all other tissues of the mouth. In a heavy smoker, for example, the dentist can be the first health professional to spot signs of either oral cancer or precancerous conditions. In fact, bleeding gums and other oral problems may be the first signs of a more serious health problem. Most of us have had the opportunity to see what dentists do during their average workday. But have you ever thought about the manual skill and precision that this profession requires, or the extent of training necessary?

Most dentists complete a four-year college degree, then enter a three- to four-year dental school. Advanced training to become a dental specialist requires two or more years after dental school. The orthodontist, a dentist who straightens teeth, is perhaps the best-known specialist.

Whether a person works as a specialist or as a regular family dentist, dentistry is both demanding and rewarding. To learn more about dentistry, write to the American Dental Association, 211 East Chicago Avenue, Chicago, Illinois 60611.

DENTAL HYGIENIST

"An ounce of prevention is worth a pound of cure" might well be the dental hygienist's motto.

Dental hygienists provide many health services that help fight dental disease. Prophylaxis, or teeth cleaning, is one of these services. However, a hygienist's job is by no means limited to this. The hygienist also does counseling and teaching. Dental hygienists help patients understand how diet affects dental health. They also teach patients how to use toothbrushes, dental floss, and dental aids.

The training program for dental hygienists lasts for two to four years after high school. It is a college program that requires a good background in high school biology, chemistry, and math. A hygienist must like working with people and have good hand-eye coordination.

After training, dental hygienists must pass a state exam to work. Work opportunities are rapidly growing. In many states hygienists are now permitted to perform certain tasks that used to be done by dentists. Most hygienists are employed in private dental offices. However, jobs are now opening up in other places such as community health programs, schools, and dental clinics.

Information can be obtained by writing to the American Dental Hygienists Association, 444 North Michigan Avenue, Suite 3400, Chicago, Illinois 60611.

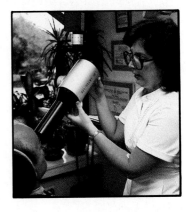

UNIT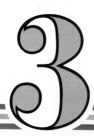

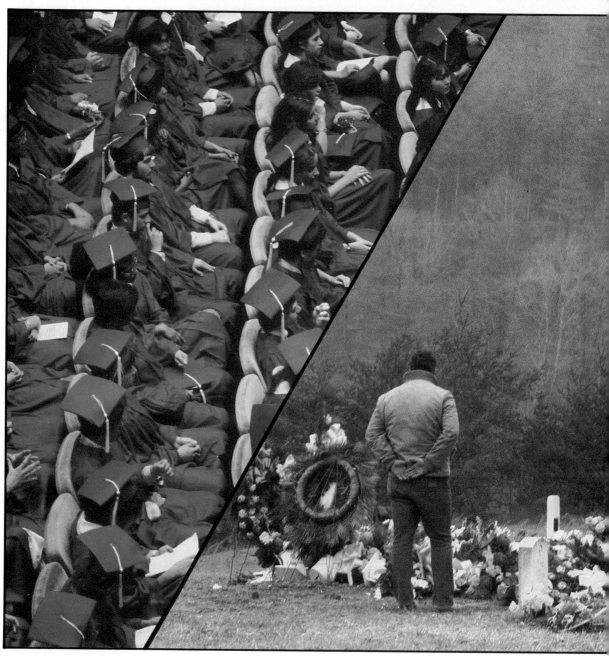

Personality Under Stress

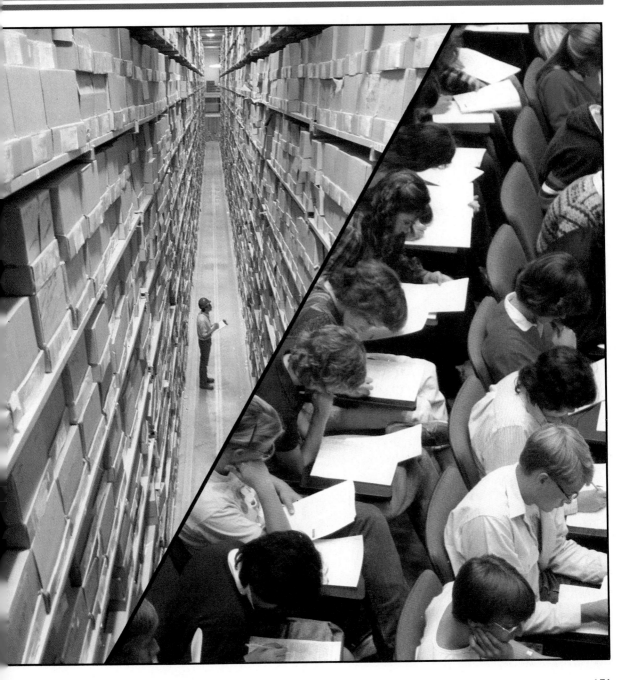

CHAPTER 8

Stress and Your Health

OBJECTIVES

- EXPLAIN the body's responses to stress
- DISCUSS the interaction of the mind and body
- IDENTIFY sources of stress
- DEFINE psychosomatic illness and OUTLINE the effects of stress on the body
- DISCUSS strategies for coping with stress

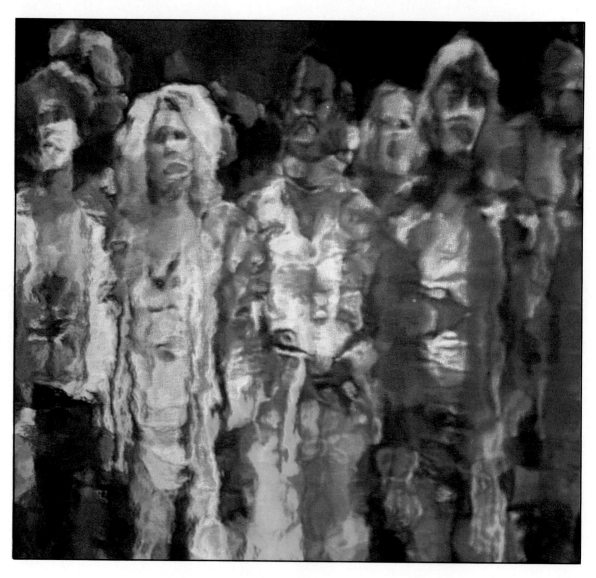

Hal could hardly believe the letter! He had gotten a full football scholarship at one of the top-ranked colleges in the country.

Within months, his life dramatically changed. He graduated from high school and moved to a college out of state. College life was different but Hal liked it. He worked hard at his studies and made the Dean's list. He starred at the football games during his first season. During Christmas vacation, he and his steady girl friend, Ann, became engaged. In April they married and moved to a small campus apartment. They were delighted when Ann became pregnant, though they had not planned on a baby so soon. Hal got a part-time job to bring in extra money.

Hal's life was hectic but happy. His only problems were his constant headaches and sleeplessness. A sedative before bedtime was the only way he got some relief. His wife told him, "Don't worry. You just had a physical. You're as healthy as a horse." Yet Hal wondered, "What's wrong with me?"

Was Hal suffering from a mysterious undetected disease? No, his real problem was stress.

THE STRESS RESPONSE

DEFINING STRESS

Whenever Dexter became angry, his heart started to pound. When Rose thought about her date for Saturday night, she felt butterflies in her stomach. As the teacher passed out the midterm exams, everyone in class felt nervous anticipation. Have you ever experienced reactions like these?

These reactions are all **stress responses.** Whenever you experience strong emotions, physical exertion, illness, or injury, you undergo stress. Even while you are asleep, you can experience emotions and stress while dreaming.

Stress is the body's way of adapting to the physical and mental demands of daily life. The stress response prepares your body for action. The heart beats faster. Blood flow increases. Breathing becomes faster.

Stress is a normal and unavoidable part of life. Without some stress, life would be dull. Stress provides the challenge we need to improve physically, mentally, and emotionally. The stress caused by a close game can help a football player run that extra yard for a touchdown. The stress you experience while working on a school project can motivate you to do your best. Physical stress such as jogging is usually helpful.

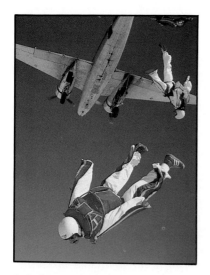

8–1. *Some people enjoy sports that contain an element of stress.*

However, prolonged or severe stress can cause physical or mental problems. In this chapter we will explore how stress affects our bodies. Chapter 10 covers the effects of stress on our minds.

YOU: MIND AND BODY

Have you heard any of these expressions: "It gives me a pain in the neck;" "It makes me sick to my stomach;" "It makes my skin crawl." These expressions point to the close relationship between the mind and body. We often think of the mind and body as separate. Yet, they actually work together as a single unit. Whenever our bodies undergo stress, our minds and personalities are affected; whenever we feel strong emotions, our bodies are affected. For example, if you get sick or physically tired, you may become irritable. When you feel strong emotions your body reacts.

NATURAL BODY BALANCE. Within your body countless physical and chemical changes occur each moment that are necessary to sustain life. When the body functions properly these changes are kept in natural balance. Your brain directs this natural system of balance. It adjusts this balance, as need be, without your conscious control. For example, when you walk briskly your body needs and uses more oxygen. As the natural oxygen level in the blood drops, and the carbon dioxide level rises, the brain signals the appropriate body systems. Breathing, blood pressure, and heart rate adjust automatically so proper balance is restored.

HOW STRESS ACTS ON YOU

THE STAGES OF STRESS. When you experience stress, a three-stage response is triggered within the body, which disrupts the body's natural system of balance. In the *alarm* stage the body prepares for action. A complex interaction of the brain, nerves, and endocrine glands (particularly the pituitary gland and adrenal glands) takes place. The hormones secreted by the endocrine glands greatly increase the heartbeat, blood flow, respiration, and sugar supply going to the muscles. These changes ready the body for "fight or flight." Stage 2 is called *resistance*. During resistance the body tries to adapt to stress and restore its natural balance. If stress continues, Stage 3, called *exhaustion*, sets in. During this stage, the body and mind become susceptible to illness unless the stress is removed.

UNIT 3 PERSONALITY UNDER STRESS

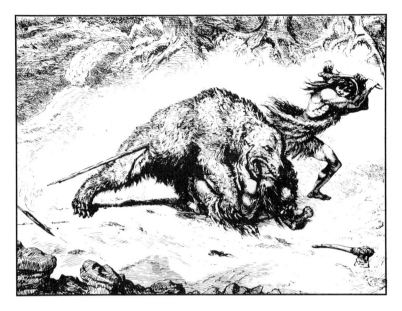

8–2. Primitive cave dwellers had to be ready for "fight or flight" reactions in order to survive.

THE EFFECTS OF STRESS.   For primitive cave dwellers, the stress response was very useful. They lived in a world full of real dangers. They constantly had to be ready for flight or fight in order to survive. In our world, it is helpful to have your body charged for action at certain times. But afterward, you need relief. When you experience repeated stress without relief, or stress that is severe or long-lasting, health problems can develop.

Do you know how a steam engine works? You can understand better how stress affects you if you think about a steam engine.

If you build a fire under the boiler of a steam engine, steam pressure in the boiler builds so that the engine runs. Without careful control too much steam pressure can build up. The boiler may then crack or even explode, causing the engine to break down. Normally this doesn't occur since steam pressure is released through the engine's cylinders and pistons as it performs useful work. Or steam escapes through the engine whistle and safety valves.

Let's say that the engine is a person: you, for instance. The boiler is your natural system of body balance. The fire is your environment with all its sources of stress; the steam pressure is stress. The cylinders and pistons represent your body and mind. The whistle is your voice. The safety valves are the activities and skills you use to cope with stress.

8–3. Like your body, the steam engine functions properly if steam pressure (stress) is carefully controlled.

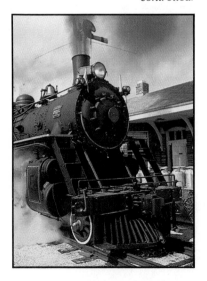

Event Rank	Life Event	Event Value
1	Death of spouse	100
2	Divorce	73
3	Marital separation	65
4	Jail term	63
5	Death of close family member	63
6	Personal injury or illness	53
7	Marriage	50
8	Fired from job	47
9	Marital reconciliation	45
10	Retirement	45
11	Change in health of family member	44
12	Pregnancy	40
13	Sex difficulties	39
14	Gain of new family member	39
15	Business readjustment	39
16	Change in financial state	38
17	Death of close friend	37
18	Change to a different line of work	36
19	Change in number of arguments with spouse	35
20	Mortgage over $10,000	31
21	Foreclosure of mortgage or loan	30
22	Change in responsibilities at work	29
23	Son or daughter leaving home	29
24	Trouble with in-laws	29
25	Outstanding personal achievement	28
26	Wife begins or stops work	26
27	Begin or end school	26
28	Change in living conditions	25
29	Revision of personal habits	24
30	Trouble with boss	23

Like an engine you need some stress to operate normally. But when the fire (source of stress) becomes too hot under the boiler, steam (stress) can build up suddenly in your boiler. If this pressure buildup lasts too long, what happens? Your blood pressure may rise, and your digestion may be affected. If stress is not relieved your boiler may explode. For example, you may suffer a heart attack. How can you prevent stress from damaging your boiler? You can use your cylinders and pistons: your mind to think stress out, and your body to work it out. You may choose to blow off steam through your whistle: talk it out. Or you can use one of your safety valves, such as a relaxation skill, to handle stress.

SOURCES OF STRESS

Factors in life that produce stress are called **stressors.** Almost any event can act as a stressor depending upon its effect on you. For example, a traffic jam might be a stressor if you were caught while rushing to an appointment. But that same situation might be a relaxing break if you were not feeling rushed. Can you identify some sources of stress in your life? The Life Stress Scale (Table 8-1) lists some of the common sources of stress. This numbered table can help you predict the likelihood of your becoming ill within the next two years because of stress.

YOUR ENVIRONMENT

PHYSICAL STRESSORS. Many elements within your physical environment can cause stress. These include elements of interior design such as color, space, and lighting. Which would you find more relaxing and conducive to recovery: a spacious, soft-green room or a hot-red, cluttered room?

There is a common expression, "Music soothes the savage beast." Noise can produce the opposite effect. Have you ever found it hard to concentrate or relax when sirens were blowing? Sometimes even the quiet hum of a motor or ticking of a clock can be disturbing. Researchers have found that people living in noisier areas see their doctors more often than people living in quieter settings. An equally upsetting environmental stressor is confinement. You have probably experienced this stressor while riding in a crowded bus or while waiting in a long line. Improper ventilation or temperature and poor air quality are just a few other environmental stressors.

SOCIAL STRESSORS.

Our social environment mainly revolves around family, friends, and school and work relationships. Social stressors, such as an argument with a friend or the anticipation of a date, produce strong emotions. Hence, these stressors are often regarded as the single, major source of daily stress in our lives.

The stress scale shown in Table 8-1 is based on events within our social environment. If you look at the scale, you will notice that it includes positive events like marriage, negative events like death, and even neutral events like eating habits. What do these events have in common? In some way they all require individuals to change familiar behavior patterns. Any change in our normal life-style produces stress. High scorers on the stress scale generally are at highest risk for health problems of some kind.

While this scale is a useful tool for measuring stress, it does not cover all sources of stress within our social environment. In our larger social world, national concerns such as the threats of nuclear disasters or wars can be sources of stress. Community concerns such as crime, personal safety, lack of recreational facilities, or employment opportunities also contribute to social stress. What concerns are foremost in your community?

OCCUPATIONAL STRESSORS.

Do you think school life is stressful? The frequent tests, competition among classmates, and the daily grind of homework put pressure on many students. In a sense, your school life is your occupation now. Later you will face certain stresses on the job.

31	Change in work hours or conditions	20
32	Change in residence	20
33	Change in schools	20
34	Change in recreation	19
35	Change in church activities	19
36	Change in social activities	18
37	Mortgage or loan less than $10,000	17
38	Change in sleeping habits	16
39	Change in number of family get-togethers	15
40	Change in eating habits	15
41	Vacation	13
42	Christmas	12
43	Minor violations of the law	11

Table 8-1 *The Life Stress Scale. Find the events that have applied to you within the last year, and then total the event value listed in the right column. If you score below 150, you have a 1 in 3 chance of becoming ill within two years. If you score between 150 and 300, you have a 50 percent chance of becoming ill. If you score over 300, you have a 90 percent chance of becoming ill.*

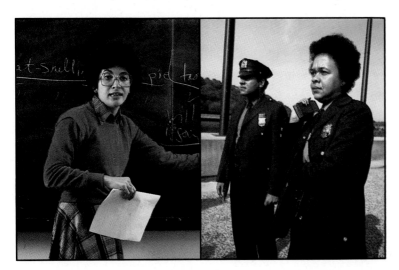

8–4. Some occupations are more stressful than others.

To better control the stress response, try to change the way you view a situation. In your mind picture the same situation in a different way. Imagine other feelings you could experience or other ways you could handle the situation. The object is to change a negative feeling into a positive or at least a neutral one. For example, a negative response to a first date could be, "He/she may not like me. What should I say or do?" A neutral response could be, "I'll be dating for a long time. This is just one night." A positive response could be, "I want him/her to have fun so I will."

8–5. Crying in times of stress helps to relieve tension.

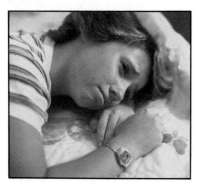

Some occupations are more stressful than others. Air traffic control, for example, is considered a highly stressful occupation. This job demands that the controller constantly be alert to avoid airplane accidents. Would you consider on-the-job stress when making career decisions?

YOUR PERSONALITY

When Tom was asked in class to give his oral report, he suddenly felt tongue-tied. Yet he had practiced it and was well prepared. His classmate Julie, on the other hand, easily gave her presentation, though she had rehearsed it only once. Why wasn't this situation stressful to both students?

No two people perceive and react to the same situation in the same way. Our personalities shape how we view a situation and how we react to it. Personality is largely determined by what we have experienced and learned in the past. Tom might have experienced past failures when he gave oral reports. Therefore, when similar situations come up in his life, he experiences stress. Julie, on the other hand, may have received positive feedback in the past when she gave oral reports. Therefore, this situation is not stressful to her.

BIOLOGICAL CHANGES. Some normal biological changes that occur during life are also sources of stress. The teen years are a time of transition from childhood to adulthood. During these years your body undergoes rapid and dramatic changes. There is a profound increase in the production of hormones, which can affect your mood and emotions. Because these normal biological changes are taking place, adolescence is often an emotional and stressful period of life.

Hormonal levels also change during the female hormonal cycle. For example, hormone levels change during the menstrual cycle, pregnancy, and childbirth. These hormonal changes can be physically and emotionally stressful. For example, following childbirth, many women experience some depression. At one time, doctors believed this feeling was only psychological. Now research has shown that the natural hormone changes following birth can explain some cases of depression.

YOUR BEHAVIOR AND LIFE-STYLE.   Have you ever delayed doing a report until just before it had to be turned in? You may have lost sleep trying to get your assignment done on time. In many ways personal behavior and life-style can become sources of physical and emotional stress. Failing to plan your time properly can create needless problems. Likewise, lack of regular exercise or sleep puts extra strain on your body. When you skip or eat meals irregularly, your energy cycle is constantly interrupted. Then your body doesn't function at its best. How often do you contribute to your own stress?

STRESS AND ILLNESS

For centuries native and folk healers have recognized the relationship between mind and body. When these healers use magic power and rituals to try to cure sickness, people often recover. Can these healers really perform magic? The body has a natural ability to fight disease and repair itself. So without magic or modern medicine, some people *will* recover from many ailments given enough time. Medicine, of course, can usually aid and speed the healing process. However, healers can actually cure many health problems. Their rituals may relieve a patient's stress, thereby producing sometimes dramatic changes in health.

At first modern medicine did not recognize the relationship between the mind, body, and illness. Doctors looked only for defects in the body or the presence of microorganisms that cause disease. If they found none, many doctors thought patients had no illness. Some doctors, however, were not convinced that physical causes were the only causes of illness. Medical research had shown that severe stress damaged the internal organs of animals. Further, research confirmed the links between mind, body, and illness in humans.

This knowledge forms the basis for two special areas of medicine. **Psychosomatic** (si-ko-so-**mat-**ick) medicine, named for the Latin roots *psyche* (mind) and *soma* (body), applies psychology and medicine to treat stress disorders. **Behavioral** medicine combines behavioral learning principles with medicine to prevent stress disorders.

WHAT IS PSYCHOSOMATIC ILLNESS?

Lately, Jim's life seemed nothing more than a series of problems. He received a failing grade in a required course. He was laid off from his after-school job. His girl friend was not speaking to him because of an argument. He was also having terrible stomach pains that worried him.

HEALTH IN HISTORY

In the early 1920's stress research began in earnest. Walter B. Connor observed that animals had an internal environment which, in the presence of physical stress such as cold, lack of oxygen or sleep, constantly adjusted to adapt to these demands. In 1929 he coined the term *homeostasis* to describe this natural system of balance and referred to it as the "wisdom of the body." Connor discovered that various hormones controlled this adaption response. He also discovered that psychological stress produced this response. For example, when cats were exposed to dogs, the cat's hormonal levels changed.

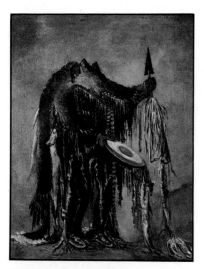

8–6. *Sometimes witch doctors actually healed sick people by relieving their stress.*

When he finally saw his family doctor he was surprised to learn that his problem was diagnosed as a **psychosomatic illness.** When Jim told his father the diagnosis, his father said, "Jim, let's go to a movie. You will forget about your pain and come back feeling like a new person." Jim's dad was wrong. Trying to forget about stress and the pain of psychosomatic illness doesn't make the problem go away. When Jim told his mother the diagnosis, she sighed with relief. "I was so worried. Thank goodness your pains are just imaginary and you are not ill." Jim's mother was wrong, too. Psychosomatic illness is often misunderstood. The pains of psychosomatic illness caused by stress are very real, and they can be harmful.

A defect in a body organ is called an **organic disease.** But when an organ has no defect in its structure, but acts up due to emotional stress, the condition is called a *psychosomatic disease* or *disorder*. These disorders disturb normal body functions. Both organic and psychosomatic diseases cause distressing symptoms. Neither is imaginary.

Have you ever tried to eat when you were really angry? Your stomach muscles tighten and you can become nauseated. An X ray would show no stomach defect. However, an X ray would also show increased or irregular churning action. This condition is a *psychosomatic disorder*. If your stomach were kept in a state of upset by continued emotional distress, an *ulcer* (an open sore in the stomach wall) could develop. In such cases, psychosomatic disease becomes organic.

Organic and psychosomatic diseases can exist together in the same organ. For example, a person with heart leakage may become alarmed about this condition. Worrying then causes the heart to beat faster. The burden of psychosomatic heart trouble is added to an already diseased heart.

STRESS AND BODY SYSTEMS

How does stress affect specific organs and body systems? Figure 8-7 illustrates the known effects of stress on the body. However, each day more is learned about the stress response and how the brain, nervous system, and endocrine system interact to affect health. So the list of stress-related problems keeps growing. Scientists believe that stress may cause a breakdown in the **immune** system. This is the body's inborn defense system against disease. The role of stress is now under serious study for diseases such as cancer and arthritis, whose causes are unknown.

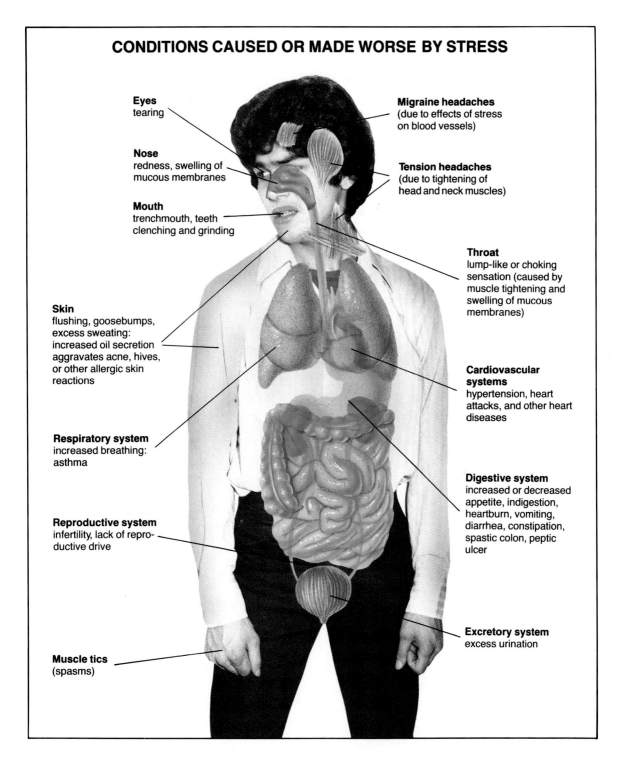

CONDITIONS CAUSED OR MADE WORSE BY STRESS

Eyes
tearing

Nose
redness, swelling of
mucous membranes

Mouth
trenchmouth, teeth
clenching and grinding

Skin
flushing, goosebumps,
excess sweating:
increased oil secretion
aggravates acne, hives,
or other allergic skin
reactions

Respiratory system
increased breathing:
asthma

Reproductive system
infertility, lack of reproductive drive

Muscle tics
(spasms)

Migraine headaches
(due to effects of stress
on blood vessels)

Tension headaches
(due to tightening of
head and neck muscles)

Throat
lump-like or choking
sensation (caused by
muscle tightening and
swelling of mucous
membranes)

**Cardiovascular
systems**
hypertension, heart
attacks, and other heart
diseases

Digestive system
increased or decreased
appetite, indigestion,
heartburn, vomiting,
diarrhea, constipation,
spastic colon, peptic
ulcer

Excretory system
excess urination

STRESS AND HEALTH RISK

Can the specific effects of stress on health be predicted for any given person? It is hard to make any good predictions. Stress may cause a headache in one person and indigestion in another. The effects of stress depend in part on a person's inherited strengths and weaknesses and present physical condition. For example, if a person has inherited a sensitive digestive system, stress is more likely to cause indigestion. A person's personality counts, too. Would you describe yourself as hard-driving or easygoing? Researchers have found that a hard-driving personality, referred to as Type A, is more prone to stress disorders than the easygoing Type B personality. Are you sensitive to stress? The questions below will help you decide whether you are a Type A or a Type B personality.

ARE YOU TYPE A OR B PERSONALITY?

Pick the number that best characterizes your behavior for each item. (In question 1, for example, pick "1" if you're always casual about appointments or pick "8" if you're never late.) Write your scores on a separate piece of paper.

| 1 | 2 | 3 | 4 | 5 | 6 | 7 | 8 |

Type B Extreme	Type A Extreme
1. Casual about appointments	Never late
2. Not competitive	Very competitive
3. Never feel rushed, even under pressure	Always rushed
4. Take things one at a time	Try to do many things at once; think about what I'm going to do next
5. Slow doing things	Fast (eating, walking, etc.)
6. "Sit" on my feelings	Express my feelings
7. Many interests	Few interests outside work

Total your score and multiply by 3. Use this scale to interpret your score.

More than 120	Very strongly Type A
106-119	Definitely Type A
100-105	Type A, but the Type B in you may save your life
90-99	Type B, but with some Type A tendencies
Less than 90	Type B

Table 8-2

MANAGING STRESS: SKILLS AND STRATEGIES

How do you cope with stress? Some people rely on alcohol, drugs, or tobacco to release tension. These strategies mask the symptoms of stress without really dealing with the root causes of problems. Dependence on such strategies can quickly become another problem that increases rather than reduces stress in life. There are many positive skills and strategies that can be used to cope with stress effectively.

Those who develop positive ways for handling stress run the smallest risk of developing stress-related health problems. For those who do not develop coping skills, stress eventually takes its toll on health.

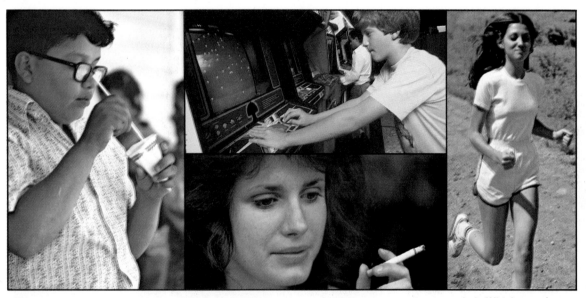

8–8. Which of these people is dealing with stress best?

BEHAVIOR STRATEGIES

You can reduce stress in your life by learning to manage your time properly. This requires planning activities before you begin them. Allow enough time to carry out activities so you can avoid a last-minute rush. When you have many things to do at once, set priorities. Decide which tasks or activities are most important and tackle those activities first. Do not put off doing things until they pile up. Then good planning becomes impossible.

Second, plan a stress-reducing life-style. Try to look ahead and anticipate major changes in life and plan for them. When possible, limit the number of changes you make in your life at any one time. Balance work and play. Make daily relaxation a priority. Then, plan relaxation time *each* day no matter how busy you may be. Practice positive life-style habits. Get regular exercise, establish regular meal times, and do not skip meals. Avoid the use of alcohol, tobacco, and other drugs.

Finally, adopt a positive attitude. Learn to change the things you can, but accept the things you cannot change. Why build up tension needlessly?

YOUR SOCIAL SUPPORT SYSTEM

Whom do you turn to in times of distress? You have a social support system made up of your family members, friends, and others you can talk to. Researchers have found that people with a good social support system enjoy better health and live longer than those people who have few personal ties. Scientists believe that social support provides a personal buffer against the harmful effects of stress. Are you in the habit of sharing your feelings with someone else? It is important to use your support system regularly and share your experiences, good and bad, with those whom you can talk to and trust.

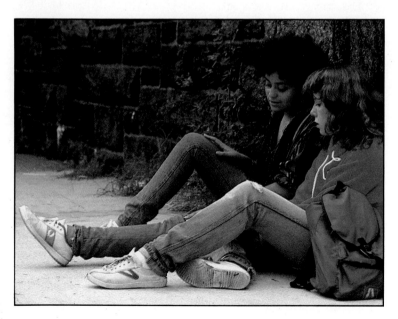

8–9. People who have good social support systems enjoy better health and live longer.

RELAXATION SKILLS

What activities help you relax? Friendly conversation, sports, and hobbies can help relax your body and mind. Even a quick nap or a few minutes of quiet each day can provide a refreshing break from daily stress. Stress experts have developed some other methods that you can use for relaxation.

RELAXED BREATHING. Have you ever noticed how babies breathe? They breathe naturally, taking deep breaths that allow their stomach and ribs to fully contract and expand. As they breathe, their stomachs rise and fall while their chests hardly move at all.

Stress alters natural breathing patterns. In stressful situations, only the chest muscles are used to breathe, and breathing becomes shallow and rapid. For those who repeatedly experience stress, shallow chest breathing can become a poor but regular breathing habit. Most teenagers and adults unconsciously breathe this way. Learning how to breathe properly can help you relax and stop the stress response when it begins. The following exercise will help you improve your breath control.

Inhale slowly and deeply with your mouth closed. Expand your *stomach* so that your lungs can fill completely with air. Imagine you are trying to bring the air all the way down to your stomach. Your stomach should rise and your chest should hardly move at all. Then slowly exhale through the mouth making an "aaah" sound. Your stomach muscles should contract as you empty your lungs completely. Practice this exercise for 5 to 10 minutes at a time until you can breathe this way without concentration. Try using this exercise to calm yourself whenever stress begins to make you feel anxious. You will be surprised to see how this simple skill can make you feel better.

PROGRESSIVE RELAXATION. **Progressive relaxation** is a simple method that reduces body tension from head to toe. First, sit or lie down in a comfortable position and use relaxed breathing. As you slowly inhale, tightly tense the muscles in one part of your body. As you slowly exhale, completely relax the tensed muscles so they feel limp. Tense and relax the muscles in each part of your body, progressing from head to toe or from toe to head. For example, first tense and relax the muscles of your face, then the neck, then the shoulders, and so on, until all muscles of the body, even fingers and toes, have been tensed and then relaxed.

BIOFEEDBACK

Can we change our heartbeat at will? Can we regulate our own blood pressure? Can we raise and lower our body temperature through conscious thought? Years ago medical scientists said that these controls were impossible. Yet even these scientists had to admit that for centuries yogis have been able to control these body functions. Today scientists are taking a second look as thousands of Americans are gaining mastery over their own bodies through a technique called biofeedback.

What does "biofeedback" mean? When you take a test in school, your grade provides you with feedback, or a measure of what you have learned. In biofeedback a mechanical apparatus provides feedback about the internal state of the body. This becomes the basis for learning. For example, the electromyograph (EMG) machine records muscle activity. By carefully listening to changes in sound, a person attached to the EMG can learn to recognize and control muscle tension. By using other machines, patients have been able to observe and eventually control changes in body temperature, blood pressure, the actions of the heart, and even the patterns of brain waves.

It is not completely understood how patients learn to control body functions through biofeedback. Some researchers compare it to learning to ride a bicycle by using training wheels. When the training wheels are no longer needed, they are discarded. In the same way, when the biofeedback machines are no longer needed, they are discarded. Patients can still maintain control over their body functions, unassisted by these devices.

What is the future of biofeedback in medicine? It is already making exciting strides in stress control and in psychosomatic medicine. It is helping patients control their bod-

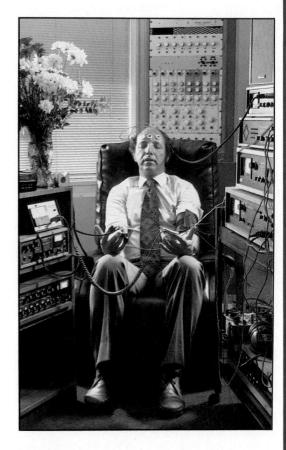

ies' negative reactions to stress. For example, patients have been able to overcome migraines, reduce high blood pressure, and control asthma attacks. Some researchers think that someday biofeedback will help prevent heart attacks by teaching people to control irregular heart rhythms.

Will biofeedback clinics become a part of traditional hospitals? Already these clinics are increasing in numbers as the interest in behavioral medicine grows. There may even be a biofeedback clinic in your own community now.

STRUGGLING WITH STRESS

Stress, properly controlled, helps you handle everyday challenges. Uncontrolled stress may cause emotional and physical problems. Are you successfully coping with stress? Table 8-3 lists some basic signs of effective stress management as well as stress warning signals.

STRESS MANAGEMENT	
Successful Coping	Warning Signs
Ability to adapt to changes	Inability to concentrate
Ability to work under authority, rules, limits, problems	Inability to slow down and relax
Ability to carry out tasks efficiently	Strong anger over minor irritations
Ability to show warmth, friendliness, love	Feeling that things often go wrong
Self-direction	Frequent prolonged feelings of boredom
Sense of humor and fulfillment	
Tolerance of others and frustration	Frequent unexplained fatigue
	Sleep problems
	Psychosomatic symptoms or disorders
	Reliance on alcohol, tobacco or drugs for relaxation
	Frequent accidents

Table 8–3

If these warning symptoms persist, consult a doctor. Your problem cannot be diagnosed before a medical examination is made. If the problem is related to stress, life-style changes may be recommended. The doctor can help, but the success of treatment depends largely on you.

SUMMARY: Stress is a normal part of life. Stressors are factors that produce stress. Stress causes many physical changes that prepare the body for action. When stress occurs often without relief, or is severe or prolonged, psychosomatic problems may develop. All systems of the body may be affected by stress. It is important to learn how to cope with stress on a daily basis in order to prevent stress-related diseases. Sports, hobbies, relaxations skills, behavioral strategies and social support can help you cope with stress.

CHAPTER REVIEW

words at work

Unscramble each word that identifies the statement next to it. DO NOT WRITE IN THIS BOOK.

1. SRESTROS: a factor that produces stress
2. SMHYPCTCAOSIO: the interdependence of the mind and body
3. NGIAORC SESEIDA: illness resulting from a structural disorder of an organ
4. ARAOVILEBH: a new branch of medicine that uses learning principles
5. MEINUM TSSYME: the body's inborn defense against disease
6. SORIPEVEGRS OXTRALEANI: a stress-reducing method

review questions

1. Define stress and give examples of stress responses.
2. Is stress helpful or harmful? Explain your answer.
3. Explain natural body balance. Why is this mechanism necessary?
4. Outline the stages of stress.
5. Give examples that show the effect of the mind on the body and the body on the mind.
6. Why is it important to understand the interaction of the mind and body?
7. What are stressors?
8. Identify three physical stressors and three social stressors.
9. Why are positive changes in life considered stressful?
10. Why is adolescence a stressful time of life?
11. Name and define two special areas of medicine concerned with stress.
12. Contrast organic and psychosomatic disorders.
13. Name an effect of stress on the stomach.
14. Give a reason why people may be more susceptible to colds during stressful times.
15. Why does stress cause different physical disorders in people?
16. Why should you avoid the use of alcohol, tobacco, or drugs to release tension?
17. Outline three behavior strategies for coping with stress.

discussion questions

1. What is the role of personality, life-style, and behavior in psychosomatic illness? Include specific examples in your discussion.
2. As it relates to stress, discuss the expression, "Failure to plan is planning to fail."
3. What occupations do you think would be very stressful? Explain the reasons for your choices. Can you suggest any ways to reduce on-the-job stress in these occupations?
4. Do you think adolescence is more stressful than adulthood? Do you think one sex experiences more stress in life than the other? Give reasons to support your positions.
5. Is it wise to block an emotional outlet, such as crying at a time of grief? Explain your answer.
6. The headline story for a weekly newspaper magazine reads, "WITCH DOCTOR CURES CANCER." Discuss group reactions to this headline. Could there be any truth to this story? Why are such headlines misleading and dangerous?

investigating

PURPOSE:
To demonstrate the sources of stress in an individual's life and ways that stress can be managed.

MATERIALS NEEDED:
Paper; pencils; index cards.

PROCEDURE:
A.   Working in groups, reread Hal's story at the beginning of the chapter on page 173.
B.   Use the Life Stress Scale on pages 176-177 to identify the stressors in Hal's life. Add any stressors not specifically mentioned in the story that you expect might also occur as a result of Hal's new life-style.
C.   Write each stressor on a separate index card with its corresponding numerical value.
   1.   What is Hal's stress score?
D.   Separate your stress cards into two groups: (a) avoidable stressors (those that can be changed; for example, stressors created by personal behavior), and (b) unavoidable stressors.
   2.   What were the unavoidable stressors in Hal's life? Discuss ways that might be used to cope with each stressor.
   3.   What were the avoidable stressors in Hal's life? How could Hal have avoided these stressors?

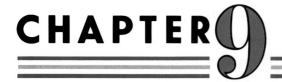

CHAPTER 9

Defense Mechanisms

OBJECTIVES

- DEFINE the mind's levels of awareness
- EXPLAIN how defense mechanisms relieve conflicts and anxiety
- IDENTIFY different defense mechanisms
- CITE examples of helpful and harmful uses of defense mechanisms

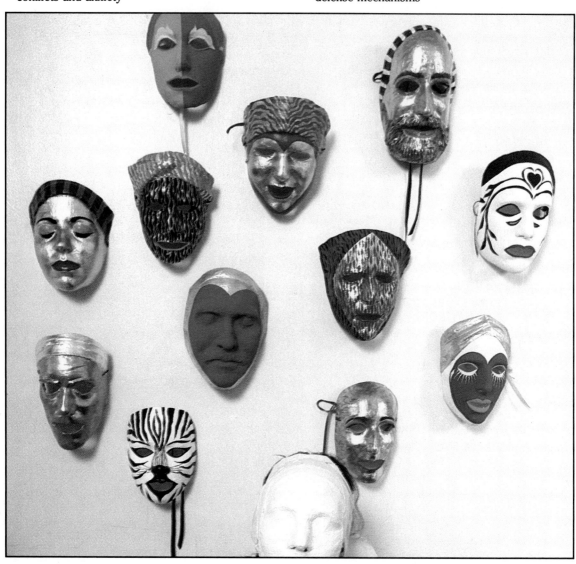

The big dance was just two weeks away. Secretly Betty hoped that Sam would ask her to go. He was very popular in the class and they had already been out together twice.

As the night of the dance grew closer, Betty still did not have a date. Sam was friendly as always but they had not gone out together again. Betty said to herself that she really didn't want to go to the dance with Sam anyway. So

when a casual friend Dan asked her to the dance, Betty said yes. Much to her surprise, Betty had a wonderful time at the dance with Dan. As they said goodnight, Betty said enthusiastically, "I had a great time, thank you, Sam, er, I mean Dan." Betty felt her face turning red with embarrassment. "How could I make such a stupid mistake?" Betty wondered.

MECHANISMS OF DEFENSIVE BEHAVIOR

LEVELS OF THE MIND

When you are aware of your thoughts, activities, and the world around you, your mind is operating on the **conscious** (**kon**-shuss) level. But beneath this conscious level, other states of awareness exist.

What did you do on your last birthday? With just a little thought, you can probably recall how you celebrated. Memories, which you are not consciously aware of but which can be tapped when necessary, are stored in the **preconscious** level of the mind. Now try to remember how you celebrated each birthday for the last ten years. This is impossible for most people to remember. Yet if you were hypnotized, you could relate EVERY detail of EVERY birthday you ever had. Events and feelings in life are never really forgotten. They are stored deep within the **unconscious** mind. Like a tape recorder, your mind records every event in the slightest detail. It also records the emotions you felt during each event. These records form impressions, which are fixed in your unconscious mind. At a later time, certain events can unlock the unconscious mind and replay these impressions. Often some small detail, such as a certain food, smell, or sound may bring back hidden memories. Have you ever suddenly remembered a long forgotten event? What triggered this memory?

Sigmund Freud M.D. (1856-1939) was a pioneer in the field of modern psychiatry. In 1894 he proposed the concept of mental defense mechanisms. In 1900 he introduced dream analysis as a method of reaching memories and conflicts hidden in the unconscious mind. Though critics disclaimed his theories at first, by 1910 Freud had gained international renown for his work.

A more dramatic example of this is when people have a sudden, close brush with death. They often report seeing their entire lives flash before them in seconds like a high-speed film. Your unconscious mind also serves as the center for your values and conscience. Whenever you want to do something that conflicts with your conscience or values, you may feel anxious or guilty.

THE NATURE OF DEFENSE MECHANISMS

We all encounter stressful events. Often these events produce feelings of guilt, fear, and insecurity. When this happens, we usually try to act as quickly as possible to relieve our discomfort. When we function at the conscious level of the mind, we can recognize the causes for our discomfort and deal with them directly. Often, however, the unconscious mind shortcuts conscious reason and effort. Instead it uses a behavior trick called a **defense mechanism.**

Have you ever been disappointed because you were not invited to a party? Did you convince yourself "I didn't really want to go anyway"? If so, you used a common mental mechanism called **rationalization.** Something you can't have becomes something you don't want.

Different defense mechanisms work in different ways. But all are mental mechanisms that operate without our conscious control. They protect us against uncomfortable feelings of anxiety. They do not ease anxiety by dealing directly with the real problem. For this reason, all defense mechanisms involve self-deception to some degree. They distort the way we see and think about a particular event. However, the situation itself remains unchanged.

9–1. The cartoon character, Dennis the Menace, often resorts to denial.

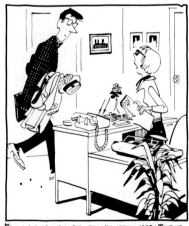

"DENNIS PHONED AND SAID TO TELL YOU NOT TO WORRY, THAT NO MATTER WHAT EVERYONE ELSE SAYS, HE DIDN'T DO IT."

MENTAL DEFENSES AT WORK
DENIAL: REJECTING REALITY

Jean had just started her senior year when her father got a new job out of state. Within weeks the whole family would have to move. Jean was very upset at the thought of leaving her friends and school life. Although she knew she would be moving, she tried out for the class play and she joined the yearbook staff.

What defense mechanism did Jean use? She resorted to **denial.** The thought of moving was too painful to accept. So she denied reality by becoming more involved in school.

Denial is used in many different situations. People who constantly fail to recognize when others are angry at them are also using denial, but to a lesser degree. People who are dependent on alcohol or other drugs often use denial. They refuse to admit they have problems and will not seek help.

REPRESSION: UNINTENTIONAL FORGETTING

"Sorry, Doctor, I forgot my appointment." Anthony had always been proud of his excellent memory. However, he had forgotten two of his last four dental appointments despite his sincere efforts to remember them. Was he losing his memory? Actually, Anthony was using **repression.** He was afraid of the grinding and drilling. Unintentional forgetting became a means of blocking out the unpleasant experience. With repression, the reality of a situation is rejected, but only briefly. Reality is soon recalled either in conscious thought or in dreams.

Did you ever make plans to do something and then forget to do it? Perhaps you *forgot* to do the task because it was associated with unpleasant feelings. This is an example of repression.

RATIONALIZATION: MAKING EXCUSES

The night before the big math exam, Juan was studying hard. Mark, on the other hand, decided to shortcut studying. He wanted to get together with a few friends instead. The day after the test Juan received a top grade. Mark received a poor grade. "Oh well, Juan's a brain. We can't all be that smart. Anyway, I would rather be popular," said Mark.

To justify his low grade, Mark used rationalization. Rationalization does not mean "rational" behavior. It is an effort to avoid a loss of self-esteem or prevent guilt feelings. When you use this defense mechanism, you make excuses for your behavior. In your own mind your actions make sense and seem right.

PROJECTION: SHIFTING PERSONAL TRAITS TO OTHERS

Sharon was not doing well in school. During her final English test, she felt a strong desire to cheat. Her conscience, however, wouldn't let her. Suddenly she began glancing around the room at the other students. After the exam she told another classmate, "Over half the class cheated."

9–2. Are you familiar with the expression "sour grapes"? It comes from an Aesop's fable about the fox and the grapes. The sweet, lush grapes were hanging on a vine high above a hungry fox's grasp. Try as he might, the fox couldn't reach a single grape. "Oh, well," said the fox as he gave up trying, "who wants sour grapes anyway." The fox was using rationalization.

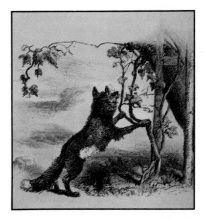

Sharon used **projection** (pro-**jek**-shun). Often people cannot accept certain faults or feelings in themselves. Unconsciously they may shift these personal traits to others. Then they see themselves in a more favorable way. In Sharon's case, she couldn't admit to herself that she had a desire to cheat. So she relieved her guilt feelings by projecting this desire onto her classmates. Projection is a common defense mechanism. For example individuals who do not like people in general may shift this trait to others and believe that "nobody likes me."

COMPENSATION: SUBSTITUTING GOALS

Ernie loved to swim, jog, play paddleball, and ski. His goal was to be good at every sport. One day Ernie went swimming in an unfamiliar lake. He ran to the water's edge and quickly dived in, before testing water depth. Tragically, he dived into shallow water. The accident left him paralyzed in both legs. At first he was angry and miserable. He felt he could never be good at anything again. However, his parents bought him a guitar. He soon discovered an interest in music. With practice, he became a very good guitar player.

Ernie used **compensation** (kom-pen-**say**-shun). When one goal cannot be reached, we turn our energies and drives toward another goal. Compensation can be a valuable device when used this way.

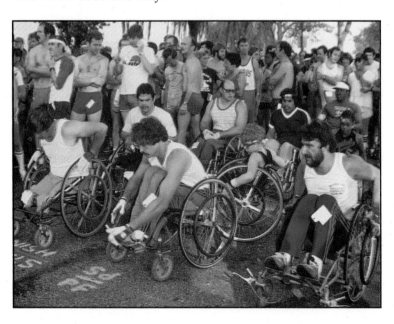

9–3. Handicapped people must find many positive ways to compensate for their disabilities.

UNIT 3 PERSONALITY UNDER STRESS

Compensation can also have a negative side. Mike felt that he was unattractive and would never be popular with girls. So, to attract female attention, he became the class clown. He often disrupted classes by cracking jokes and showing off. Mike used attention-getting to compensate for his insecurity with girls. However, his actions did not make him any more popular. Instead, he was placed on probation in school. How could Mike have used this defense mechanism in a positive way?

SUBLIMATION: REDIRECTING ENERGY

All his life Duane remembered feeling hostile toward other people. "You must have been born with a chip on your shoulder," his mother told him. At school he constantly picked fights. No one really liked him.

Finally, a helpful teacher persuaded Duane to try out for football. He made the team and became an outstanding tackle. He no longer felt the need to pick fights. He also found other rewards. His family was proud of him and he enjoyed the admiration of his classmates.

Redirecting natural energy to socially acceptable behavior is called **sublimation** (sub-lih-**may**-shun). Engaging in sports was Duane's way of redirecting his aggressive energy. Other people may choose different outlets for their feelings, such as art or public service. How do you use sublimation in your daily life?

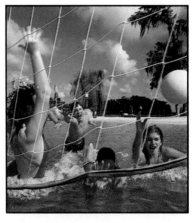

9–4. Engaging in active sports is an example of sublimation.

DISPLACEMENT: TRANSFERRING FEELINGS

Colleen angrily slammed down the telephone receiver. A girl friend had called to tell her that she had seen Colleen's steady boyfriend with another girl.

Minutes later, Colleen's mother asked, "Why are you so quiet tonight?" Colleen shouted, "Why can't you ever leave me alone? You are always picking on me." Then she stormed into her bedroom and slammed the door. What was the real reason for Colleen's behavior?

Colleen used **displacement.** She transferred her angry feelings from her boyfriend to her mother. Colleen's mother became the victim of this displacement of aggression.

Did you ever meet a stranger you instantly disliked without knowing why? It may be that this stranger unconsciously reminded you of someone else whom you didn't like. In this instance your feelings were transferred from that person to your new acquaintance.

IDENTIFICATION: FEELING CONNECTED WITH OTHERS

Lisa was tennis crazy. Her idol was the number-one player in the country. Lisa never missed a chance to see her idol play. She spent hours imitating her heroine. She talked, walked, and dressed like her. Lisa identified so closely with her idol that in her unconscious mind she *was* the great player.

In the process of **identification** you seek to connect yourself with others. You may adopt their feelings, attitudes, behavior or other personality traits. Children often use their parents as role models after whom they can pattern themselves. Do you think it is a good idea to pattern yourself after someone else? It may be helpful. However, if identification is carried to extremes, it can prevent you from fully developing your own personality.

There is a lot of truth in the saying "Misery loves company." This is another example of how identification is used. When you suffer an emotional shock, you may find it comforting to identify with someone who has had the same experience. This makes you feel that you are not alone. Identification can bring families and relatives closer together in times of grief.

Closely related to identification is the defense mechanism called **idealization** (eye-de-al-leh-**zay**-shun).

Clair was Luke's idea of the perfect girl friend. He put Clair up on a pedestal and did not believe that she had any faults.

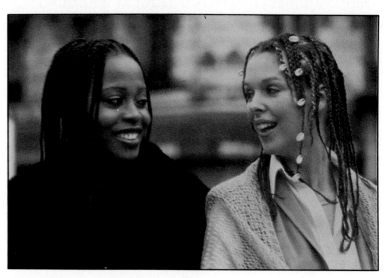

9–5. It is sometimes said that "Imitation is the highest form of praise." With whom do you identify?

He knew that she would understand completely when he had to cancel their date because of a family outing. Instead Clair became very angry. "That's fine," she said. "I'll go out with someone else." Luke was crushed. "How could I have ever thought she was so wonderful?" he asked himself.

When you use idealization, you misjudge the abilities and attributes of others. You see people you love, admire, or respect as people who are without fault. So, you expect too much from them. When they can't measure up to your ideal, what happens? You lose respect for them. Sometimes idealization is directed at oneself. You become blind to your own faults and shortcomings. This can prevent you from recognizing your mistakes and correcting them.

DAYDREAMING: FANTASY

What do you like to daydream about? Both daydreams and night dreams are expressions of our unconscious minds. In a daydream your unconscious mind creates a world as you would like it to be, not as it is. *Daydreaming* can ease the frustrations you feel when goals and desires are blocked. But waking from a dream can be more distressing when you realize that you still have not reached your goal and success is not real.

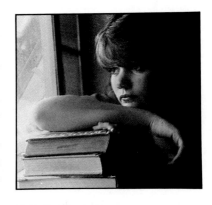

9–6. Daydreaming can sometimes ease the frustrations you feel but can be harmful if used constantly as a way to escape from reality.

George wished that he was better at sports. In his daydreams, he saw himself scoring the winning touchdown against the rival school. He was lifted to the shoulders of his teammates and carried off the field as everyone cheered. George, however, did not really apply himself during practice. So, he seldom made it off the bench during a game.

Daydreaming kept George from working toward his goal. But fantasy can be helpful at times. It can be fun to dream about the future and the possibility of success. Dreams can serve as goals to strive for. Daydreams become harmful only if they are used constantly to escape reality and if they block real accomplishment.

REACTION FORMATION: REVERSING FEELINGS

When her son Arthur was born, Nancy was just seventeen. She was still in school and unprepared to become a parent. Although her mother helped her, Nancy suddenly found herself devoting all her spare time just caring for her baby. She couldn't see her friends or join in any school activities. Nancy's family and friends all admired her dedication as a mother. Yet in Nancy's unconscious mind, she resented the loss of her freedom. She hated Arthur for being so totally dependent upon her for his every need. Whenever these feelings arose Nancy would become overprotective of Arthur. In this way, she could convince herself that she loved him with complete devotion.

Nancy used the defense mechanism called **reaction formation.** This mental defense protects a person from painful conflicts that might arise if one's true feelings were expressed. In Nancy's value system, it was unacceptable to hate one's own innocent child. As a reaction against these unconscious feelings, Nancy formed conscious feelings that were the total reverse of what she unconsciously felt.

REGRESSION: ACTING CHILDISH

Bill was a basketball star. During one game he missed some easy basket shots, and his passing was sloppy. The coach pulled him out of the game. Instead of handing the basketball over to the referee, Bill threw it up into the stands. "That was a childish thing to do, Bill," said the coach. "Why did you have to pull me out of the game just because I missed a few shots?" demanded Bill. Bill then walked off to the end of the bench, where he sulked for the rest of the game.

Bill used a defense mechanism called **regression** (re-**greh**-shun). Acting childish by throwing temper tantrums and sulking are common examples of regression.

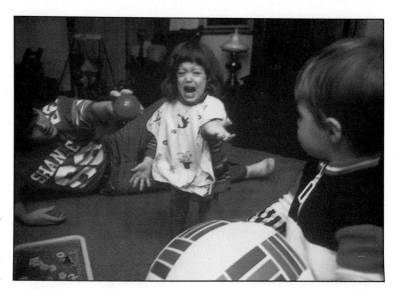

9–7. This kind of behavior is expected from young children. But in adults it is considered regressive behavior.

EVALUATING DEFENSE MECHANISMS

Are defense mechanisms helpful or harmful? Think back to the defense mechanisms you have just studied. You will find that some defense mechanisms, like *sublimation* and *compensation*, can often be helpful. Other mechanisms, such as *regression* and *denial*, are usually harmful. Other mechanisms, like *projection*, can be good or bad, depending on how they are used. For example, you may be unsure of others. You can either project a feeling of suspicion and feel that others are suspicious of you, or you can trust others and feel that others trust you.

When defense mechanisms are relied upon only from time to time, they help us feel more secure and better about ourselves. They reduce tension that can interfere with productive activity. But when they are overused or carried to extremes, troubles begin. Remember, mental mechanisms do not solve the underlying problems. They only relieve the stress that these problems cause. If the underlying problems are not eventually faced directly, they can lead to personality troubles and unhappiness.

One simple way of looking at defense mechanisms is to think of your normal rational behavior as a main highway. Then think of any problem in your environment as a roadblock. When you come to a roadblock you cannot remove, you take a mental detour, in the form of a mental mechanism. Most of these detours are short, and you have no problem returning to the main highway. Problems begin when a person STAYS on the detour and away from the main highway. This can lead to mental and emotional problems.

SUMMARY: The conscious mind is aware of thoughts and events in the environment. The preconscious level holds memories, which can be easily tapped. The unconscious mind is the center of all memories, values, and conscience. When stressful events cause conflict and anxiety, this discomfort can be relieved through conscious or unconscious action. The unconscious mind uses behavior tricks, or defense mechanisms. These mechanisms operate without conscious control to defend a person against feelings of guilt, fear, or insecurity. Defense mechanisms can be constructive or destructive forces in human behavior.

HEALTH TIP

Exercise or other vigorous physical activity is an excellent way to displace anger harmlessly. Expressing your feelings in writing can also prove effective. However, keep in mind that your written statements are meant for *you* alone not the person who has angered you. Once you have vented your anger on paper, read over your statements, then destroy the contents.

CHAPTER REVIEW

words at work

Find the word in the left column that fits one of the definitions in the right column. DO NOT WRITE IN THIS BOOK.

a. compensation
b. denial
c. unconscious mind
d. repression
e. regression
f. sublimation
g. rationalization
h. projection
i. displacement

1. The level of the mind that operates without conscious control
2. The redirection of energy
3. Unintentional forgetting
4. Substitution of one goal for another
5. The rejection of reality
6. The transference of feelings
7. Making excuses for behavior
8. Shifting personal traits to others
9. A return to childhood

review questions

1. Define the mind's levels of awareness.
2. Explain how the unconscious mind functions as a tape recorder.
3. Give an example that illustrates the different levels of the mind.
4. What is a defense mechanism? Give an example that explains your definition.
5. Name at least two characteristics of mental mechanisms.
6. Contrast the defense mechanism of repression with the mental process of denial.
7. Under what conditions might a person use rationalization?
8. Is compensation a helpful defense mechanism? Give reasons to support your answer.
9. In what respect is sublimation similar to compensation?
10. Define displacement. Describe a situation that demonstrates this mechanism.
11. Explain how the mechanisms of identification and idealization are related.
12. What is a reaction formation?
13. Give an example of attention-getting that you have observed.
14. Give an example of a helpful and harmful use of a mental mechanism.
15. When are defense mechanisms harmful?

discussion questions

1. Discuss how the use of mental mechanisms can affect relationships with others.
2. Which defense mechanisms do you think are most commonly used? Explain your answer.
3. A good friend starts to use defense mechanisms constantly. Would you be concerned about this behavior pattern? Why or why not?
4. Discuss how the unconscious and conscious minds come into play when defense mechanisms are used.
5. How can defense mechanisms be used in positive ways? How can they be used in negative ways?
6. A student auditions for a part in a school play but does not get the role. Describe how he or she might use these mechanisms: rationalization; projection; compensation; displacement; reaction formation; regression.

investigating

PURPOSE:
To demonstrate that defense mechanisms can be used to describe behavior.

MATERIALS NEEDED:
Several picture magazines; comic sections of newspapers; plain paper (poster, regular size); colored pens and/or crayons, scissors; tape; glue or paste.

PROCEDURE:
A.   Working in groups, review and identify pictures or cartoons that suggest various defense mechanisms. If no appropriate pictures can be found, draw your own.
B.   Cut out and label each picture with the correct defense mechanism. Then write a caption or a brief story to illustrate the mechanism identified.
C.   Assemble your defense mechanisms on a poster and present to the class.
   1.   What did you learn from this activity?
   2.   Are some defense mechanisms more widely observed than others?
   3.   Do posters display defense mechanisms as harmful or helpful patterns of behavior?

CHAPTER 10

Mental and Emotional Disorders

OBJECTIVES

- DESCRIBE the concepts of normal and abnormal behavior, mental health, and mental disorders
- CITE possible causes of mental health problems
- IDENTIFY common behavior patterns of major

mental disorders
- DISCUSS life crises in relationship to mental health
- STATE some signs of a troubled personality and ways to cope with crises

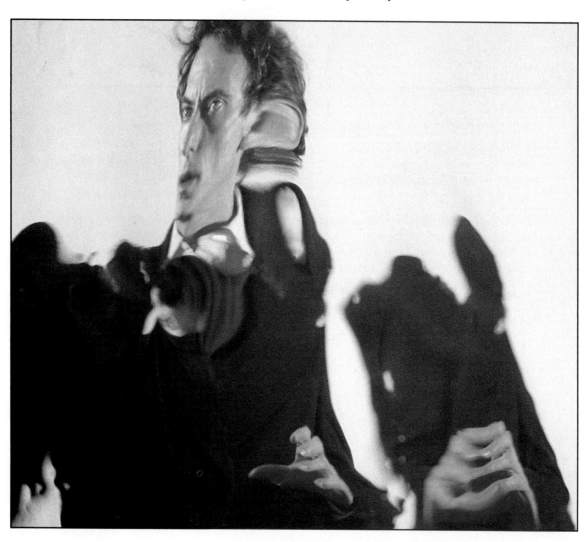

Larry was thrilled to be in New York City with his classmates. They were on their way to the World Trade Center, and he couldn't wait to see the view. Larry went up to the 110th story and walked out to the observation deck. As he looked over the city, he started to perspire. His heart raced. He suddenly felt panicky and sick to his stomach. "Why do I feel this way?" he thought. "Was it something that I ate?" He knew that heights sometimes made him feel uncomfortable, but he had never had a reaction like this. Finally Larry felt so bad that he had to leave the deck and wait for his classmates in the first-floor lobby.

What was Larry's problem? You will discover what bothered Larry as you read this chapter. You will also learn more about human behavior and mental and emotional problems.

NORMAL AND ABNORMAL PERSONALITIES

It was a bright beautiful day and John felt happy. He felt so happy that he began singing at the top of his lungs. Would you describe John's behavior as normal or abnormal? This cannot be judged without looking at other factors. For example, where and when did he begin singing?

If you overheard John singing in the shower, chances are you would not find his behavior strange. But what if his outburst occurred in the middle of English class? Normally a person's actions suit the occasion. But if they do not, his or her behavior is considered abnormal.

How often certain behavior patterns occur is another factor that must be considered when judging whether or not behavior is normal. For example, it is normal to daydream at times. But a person who daydreams constantly may start living in a fantasy world. This would not be normal behavior.

Not only outward behavior, but also inward emotions and thoughts must be considered when judging whether or not a person is normal. On the outside, a person may look and act normally, yet on the inside feel anxious, angry, or depressed all the time. Emotions and thinking can become so disturbed that people can no longer live at ease with themselves or others.

There are no sharp dividing lines between normal and abnormal personalities. Personality can be viewed as a continuous line with "normal" and "abnormal" at opposite ends.

In between there is a wide range of behavior and emotions. In general, the term *normal* describes people who view themselves and their world in a realistic way. This viewpoint helps them understand and respond properly to the people and events within their environment. Normal personalities can adapt to the stresses of life. Sometimes, behavior, emotions or thought processes break down. People are no longer able to function in their environment. In these cases, the term *abnormal* can be applied. Most people with mental and emotional problems fall somewhere on the line between normal and abnormal personalities. They are able to function at home, school, or work, but they have trouble coping with daily stresses. This robs them of a full and satisfying life.

THE NATURE OF MENTAL HEALTH

What is mental health? The term *mental health* means more than the absence of abnormal emotions, thoughts and behavior patterns. It refers to how you feel about yourself and about other people. It also refers to how well you deal with the demands of daily living. Mentally healthy people are not constantly overcome by emotions, such as anger, fear, guilt, or worry. They have self-respect as well as a tolerant attitude toward others. They are able to give love and consider the interests of others. This helps them develop satisfying and lasting personal relationships. They accept responsibilities, welcome new experiences, and use their natural talents. When problems arise, mentally healthy people react by putting their best efforts into solving the problems or adapting to situations.

THE NATURE OF MENTAL DISORDERS

At times, everyone has problems coping with their environment. There may be periods when a person has difficulty adjusting to change or in trying to get along with others. However, when these problems occur frequently or become severe and prolonged, then mental health is in trouble. Mental health workers use the term **mental disorder** to describe this condition. The term *mental illness* may also be used to describe this state. But the word *illness* may be misleading. The term *illness* suggests that a mental disorder is a disease. Many people think of a disease as a condition that may be incurable or even contagious. This is not true of mental disorders. How might this false notion affect attitudes toward mental health problems?

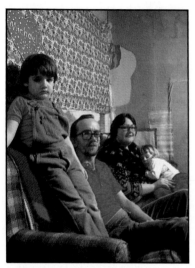

10–1. Do you think poverty adds stress to family life? What extra stresses might the family in the photo above face?

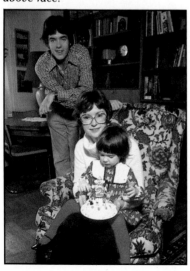

THE CAUSES OF MENTAL DISORDERS

Is stress a factor in mental and emotional problems? Are mental disorders related to heredity? Are there physical causes for mental disorders? The answer to all of these questions is yes. However the causes of all mental disorders are not fully understood.

ENVIRONMENTAL STRESS.   Throughout life we are exposed to many pressures in our environment. These produce a state of physical and mental tension that we call stress. Table 10-1 lists many common sources of stress. We cannot avoid stress entirely in our lives. In fact, some stress can be helpful. However, too much stress can lead to mental disorders.

Most experts regard the family as a major force affecting mental health. The home may be a source of stress or a source of personal satisfaction. During childhood and the teen years, an individual's patterns of behavior develop. Attitudes and outlook toward life are formed through family interaction. Growing up in an atmosphere of tension, frustration, constant criticism, fear, and insecurity can affect mental health. A person's self-image, and the ability to cope with the stress in life, can be impaired.

HEREDITY.   It is difficult to determine the role of heredity in mental disorders. Studies show that some mental disorders such as **schizophrenia** (skit-zoe-**free**-nee-ah) and **depression** occur more often in certain families. However this does not prove that the disorder itself is inherited. Family members not only share similar heredity, but they share the same environment. One generation after another may grow up under similar stressful conditions that can contribute to mental disorders. For example, families may live with the stress of poverty for generations. So it is not clear whether heredity or environment may cause the disorder. Some scientists think that a person may inherit a basic tendency toward a mental disorder. But the disorder only develops when other factors, such as family stress, are present.

PHYSICAL FACTORS.   The brain is the body's master control unit. It controls behavior, thoughts, and emotions. It is known that certain physical illnesses or injuries can affect the brain. Alcohol and some drugs also affect the brain. When the brain is affected, temporary or permanent changes in the personality can occur. When personality problems can be clearly traced to physical causes, the condition is

SOURCES OF STRESS
Physical Stressors
Noise
Confinement
Poor lighting
Improper temperature
Poor ventilation
Air pollution
Social Stressors
Conflicts with family or friends
Financial pressures
Major life events
Worry over world events
Boredom
Occupational Stressors
Constant deadlines
Heavy workload
Behavior and Life-style
Poor planning
Procrastination
Irregular meals or sleep
Inadequate exercise

Table 10-1

called an **organic mental disorder.** Syphilis, strokes, brain tumors, brain injury, and infections can cause organic mental disorders. Thus far, most cases of mental disorders cannot be linked to known physical causes. However, many researchers are now looking more closely at how the mind and body interact. They think that chemicals in the brain may play a role in the development of some mental disorders. However, the nature and the importance of this relationship are not well understood. It may be that factors such as stress affect the production of these chemicals.

CLASSIFYING MENTAL DISORDERS

Have you ever heard the terms **neurosis** (new-**row**-sis) and **psychosis** (sigh-**ko**-sis)? These terms were once used to classify most mental disorders into two major groups. These groups were based on how severe the disorders were. The term *neurosis* was used to describe the most common and milder mental disorders. People were said to be neurotic if they had frequent feelings of anxiety. The term *psychosis* applied only to certain severe disorders. People were said to be psychotic if they completely lost touch with reality.

Now, mental health specialists have devised a new classification system. This new system does not divide disorders into these two separate groups. Instead, it divides disorders according to common patterns of behavior. As a result, the term *neurosis* has been removed from the official language of mental disorders. The term *psychosis* is still used. But now it refers to any disorder that becomes so severe that the ordinary demands of life cannot be met.

Why are mental disorders classified at all? By placing mental disorders into groups, problems can be more accurately diagnosed. More precise research can be conducted. This can help determine the most successful treatment for a given mental disorder. In this way, the most helpful treatment can be prescribed for any individual patient.

We will examine some of these groups and some of the major behavior disorders within each. The major disorders that will be discussed in this chapter are summarized in Table 10-2. After reading about these disorders, you will have a better understanding of mental health problems. But do not try to diagnose yourself or others. Keep in mind that this is only a brief introduction to mental disorders. It takes mental health specialists several years of training before they can diagnose their patients.

Table 10-2

MENTAL DISORDERS
Anxiety Disorders
Phobias
Obsessions and compulsions
Generalized anxiety disorder
Dissociative Disorders
Amnesia
Multiple personality
Somatoform Disorders
Hypochondria
Conversion disorder
Personality Disorders
Schizoid personality
Avoidant personality
Dependent personality
Passive-aggressive personality
Histrionic personality
Narcissistic personality
Antisocial personality
Schizophrenia
Paranoid schizophrenia
Mood Disorders
Depression
Bipolar disorder

FOCUS ON
MENTAL DISORDERS

ANXIETY DISORDER

We've all experienced times when we feel fearful or anxious. In an **anxiety disorder,** these feelings become so strong and occur so often that they prevent a person from enjoying life. In certain situations, people troubled by anxiety disorders feel very tense. They are jumpy and are unable to relax. They may perspire a lot. Their hearts may race. They may feel dizzy or faint. Larry's problem discussed at this chapter's opening is an example of one type of anxiety disorder. This anxiety disorder is called a **phobia** (**foe**-bee-ah).

PHOBIAS: ANXIETY RELATED TO CERTAIN OBJECTS OR SITUATIONS.   To some degree, almost everyone has fears that can be termed *phobias*. Phobias are intense irrational fears of certain objects or situations. These fears can interfere with a person's normal functioning. Some common phobias are listed and defined in Table 10-3.

How do phobias develop? Phobias stem from past experiences that are no longer remembered. As a child Larry hiked into the woods all alone. He climbed a tall tree and then found he could not get back down. It was several hours

COMMON PHOBIAS	
death	*necrophobia*
doctors	*latrophobia*
heights	*acrophobia*
pain	*alcophobia*
sickness	*pathophobia*
snakes	*ophidiophobia*
storms	*astrophobia*

Table 10–3

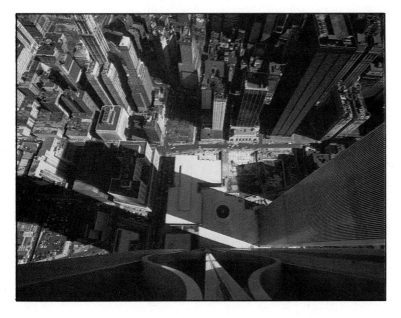

10–2. Fear of height is a common phobia.

before he was rescued. Larry no longer consciously remembers this event. Yet his mind has transferred this experience to another related situation. Sometimes phobias develop by watching the experiences of others. A child who observes a parent's fright over something may grow up with the same fear. Most people with phobias can function normally as long as they can avoid the situation that causes anxiety.

OBSESSIONS AND COMPULSIONS.   Have you ever had a silly or unpleasant thought you couldn't push out of your mind? If so, you have experienced a mild **obsession.** Obsessions are senseless or unpleasant thoughts, images, or ideas that persist against the will. **Compulsions** are repeated actions that must be performed in a very set way. Not stepping on cracks on a sidewalk is an example of a compulsion. In some way, obsessions and compulsions are defensive acts against feelings of anxiety. Often obsessions and compulsions occur together. For example, people obsessed with the idea of dirt or germs may have a compulsion to wash their hands constantly. When obsessions and compulsions are carried to extremes, they disrupt life.

Marcy usually arose at 5:00 A.M. She had to get up early because it took her three hours to get ready for school. She brushed her teeth for exactly one minute. She gave her hair twenty-five brush strokes. She chewed each mouthful of breakfast exactly twelve times. She counted every step on the way to school. She ate lunch alone so conversation wouldn't interfere with her chewing count. The step counting continued on her lonely way home. What caused Marcy to follow this abnormal routine? Marcy's problem is called an *obsessive-compulsive disorder.* As a child she only gained her parent's approval when her behavior was perfect. Her toys had to be kept in order. If her appearance, table manners, or conduct were less than perfect, she was harshly criticized. Her constant efforts to win her parents love made her feel anxious and insecure. To avoid these feelings, Marcy made an extreme effort to be perfect at home and in school. Of course, this was impossible. Her anxiety grew. Marcy's obsession with perfection led her to invent silly tasks. She did them faithfully. In her own mind, this proved she could be perfect. This eased her intense anxiety.

In moderation some obsessions and compulsions can help you achieve a worthy goal. For example, a new discovery may be made because a good idea persists. However, when carried to excess, they can be very destructive.

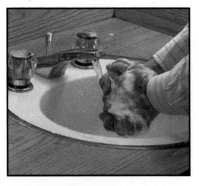

10–3. Good hygiene calls for washing hands often. However, excessive hand washing is a sign of compulsive behavior.

GENERALIZED ANXIETY DISORDER. Sometimes a person feels caught in a general state of anxiety. This feeling is not related to a specific object or situation that the person can readily identify. This feeling may be constant, or it may come as a sudden attack, lasting from several hours to several days. When this state persists for over a month, it is called a **general anxiety disorder.**

Amy entered college with mixed feelings. Her father was a highly respected judge who had graduated with honors from the same college. Partly to please her father, Amy enrolled in a pre-law course. At midsemester in college she was getting average grades. But then she couldn't concentrate on her studies. Each time she took an examination, she became tense. As a result, she started to fail. As time went on, her condition became more serious. She would wake suddenly in the middle of the night feeling frightened and she started having nightmares. She lost weight and started chain-smoking. The more she tried in school, the more frustrated she became. By the end of the semester, she was unable to continue. She decided to go home and admit her failure. Amy's condition was a generalized anxiety disorder. For several months her intense and unconscious anxiety over doing well in school had filled her life with a fear of failure.

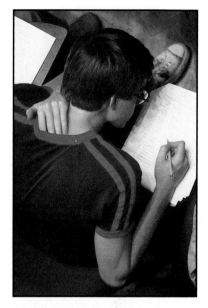

10–4. It is normal to feel anxious when taking a test. But when such feelings extend to most aspects of life and persist, a generalized anxiety disorder may be the problem.

SOMATOFORM DISORDERS

The term **somatoform** comes from the Greek word *soma* meaning body. This group of mental disorders is marked by symptoms in the body that mimic real physical illnesses. However, a person's health is not really impaired.

HYPOCHONDRIA: ANXIETY ABOUT ILLNESS. Scott was always sick. At least he always thought he was. Every time he caught a cold he worried about pneumonia. Each little ache worried him. He lived in constant fear of heart disease, cancer, or some other serious medical problem. He read every article he could find on diseases. Then he imagined he had the symptoms described in all of them. When one doctor told him nothing was wrong, he went to another. His medicine cabinet resembled a drugstore counter. He lived in a world of panic, pills, and prescriptions.

Was there anything wrong with Scott? There was nothing physically wrong with him, but he had problems just the same. Scott suffered from a disorder known as **hypochondria** (hi-poh-**kon**-dree-ah). Scott's problem could be traced

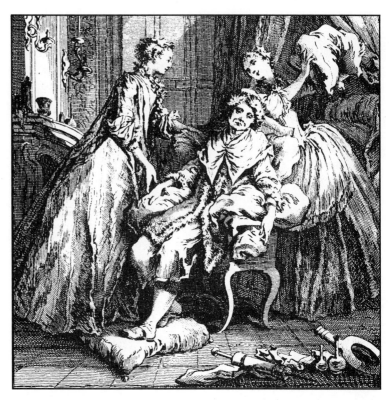

10–5. This French lithograph entitled "Le Malade Imaginaire" depicts a man with hypochondria.

HEALTH IN HISTORY

In the 1860's Jean-Marten Charcot, a renowned French neurologist, demonstrated that conversion disorder, then referred to as "hysteria," was a mental rather than a physical condition. During treatment sessions, Charcot hypnotized his patients and was able to relieve their physical symptoms. His work made a profound impression on one of his pupils, a young physician named Sigmund Freud.

to his childhood. From infancy on, Scott's mother worried about his health. Each illness was feared as if it were a fatal disease. He was constantly reminded of the danger of catching something from another person. Illness was a favorite topic of conversation in his home. Is it any wonder that Scott became a hypochondriac? Scott is not alone in his problem. Many people worry unreasonably about possible illness.

CONVERSION DISORDER. Following a minor car accident, Margaret was unable to move both legs. After a careful examination, the doctors concluded that there was no physical cause for her paralysis, yet Margaret could not walk.

Before the accident, Margaret was caught in a severe conflict. She loved a young man her parents strongly disliked. Margaret wanted to marry George, but her parents threatened to disown her if she did. Margaret loved her parents and was afraid of losing their affection. But she loved George, too, and deeply resented her parents' intrusion into her life.

How did she solve her problem? Through a **conversion disorder,** she was able to avoid resolving her problem. Margaret transferred her emotional conflict to a part of her body.

This conversion of unconscious conflict into a physical disability relieved her almost unbearable emotional state. It was also a way of getting sympathy from people involved in the conflict. As long as she was "ill," Margaret did not have to make a choice between marriage or family.

A conversion disorder may occur suddenly. In other cases the disorder may be a slow reaction to dissatisfaction with life in general. Conversion disorders can produce symptoms not only in the muscles but in the senses. A partial or complete loss of speech, hearing, or sight can result. In some cases an area of the skin may become numb and insensitive to touch, pain, heat, or cold. Dramatic reactions, such as blindness and paralysis, are rare. Most frequently, conversion disorders take the form of vague aches or pains.

SCHIZOPHRENIA

The word **schizophrenia** itself means "split mind." The split refers to a breakdown in logical thought processes. Behavior becomes strange. Words, gestures, and actions seem confused. This breakdown produces other behavior patterns:

1. *Abnormal emotional responses*. Events that normally produce joy, fear, and anger produce little or no response. Emotions expressed do not fit the occasion.
2. *Withdrawal*. The person *withdraws* into an inner fantasy life. The sense of time and space are lost.
3. *Hallucinations*. Imaginary sights or sounds, or *delusions* (false beliefs based entirely on imagination) are experienced. People that are not there are seen, heard, or talked to. People may believe they are being watched or that attempts will be made on their lives. They may also believe they receive messages from others by direct broadcasts into their minds.
4. *Severe personal distress*. People may appear desperate, or in great anguish or despair.

Not everyone who has schizophrenia shows all of these other behavior patterns. These behavior patterns may also vary in degrees of severity from case to case. However, in all cases, a person experiences a break with reality. It is the most common disorder associated with psychosis.

Schizophrenia appears most often between the ages of 15 and 35. Proper professional treatment is always required for recovery. Most people are hospitalized at some point during treatment. Some patients fully regain their mental health. However, relapses are common.

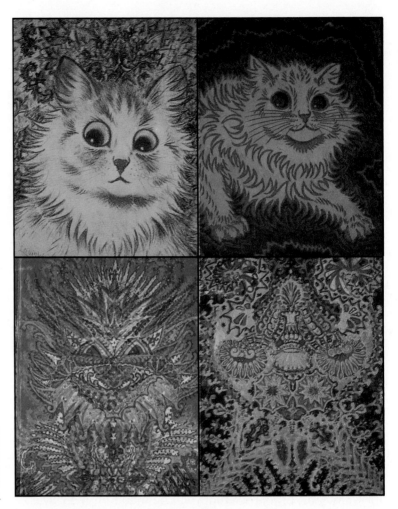

10–6. The progressive breakdown in mental processes can be seen in these paintings by artist Louis Wain, who suffered from schizophrenia.

PARANOID SCHIZOPHRENIA. The next two patients display different behavior. However, they have the same diagnosis: **paranoid schizophrenia.** This form of schizophrenia is marked by delusions either of persecution or of grandeur. Hallucinations are often present as well.

Paul, a business man, age 40, glances around the room uneasily. Since he has been in the hospital, he has been constantly on guard. He believes that his business was stolen by his partner. He is convinced that his partner has hired an assassin to kill him. Paul's delusions of persecution are terrifying and real to him. Any person around him may, in his mind, be the assassin. At times a schizophrenic patient with persecution delusions can be dangerous to others.

Mr. Higgins is neatly dressed, pleasant, and polite. At first glance, he shows no apparent behavior problem. He was hospitalized because of delusions of grandeur. The nurse begins to question him about his sleep last night. Before replying, he tells his imaginary secretary to "hold all his phone calls." He then answers all questions politely but shows his impatience with the whole conversation. He actually believes he is the president of a steamship line and makes $50,000 a month. He thinks he has important business to attend to and shouldn't be wasting his time this way. Although he gets along well with the other patients, and is no problem to the hospital staff, his delusions and hallucinations prevent him from functioning in everyday life.

MOOD DISORDERS

The normal personality has many moods, such as joy, sadness, cheerfulness, gloom, and sorrow. However, people with mood disorders have moods that are extreme and overwhelming.

DEPRESSION.   Peter had been watching the mail anxiously for weeks. When the letters he had been waiting for arrived, he was bitterly disappointed. Neither college of his choice had accepted him. For days afterward Peter moped around the house. With each week he became more withdrawn from people. He lost the desire to accomplish anything, and every movement required effort. In school he was unable to concentrate. He lost his appetite, and his sleeping habits changed. Peter was suffering from depression, a prolonged state of sadness and dejection.

Depression is one of the biggest mental health problems today. One out of every four people will suffer serious depression like Peter's sometime during life. Depression is different from normal sadness or grief. We all experience disappointments and loss that bring feelings of unhappiness. Normally these feelings ease after a reasonable time. However, people suffering from depression may have these feelings for months or even years without improvement. Suicide is a real danger for anyone suffering from depression.

Depression is a complex problem. In some cases it may be linked to unpleasant events. It may also occur for no apparent reason. As you can see in Table 10-4, depression has many different symptoms. These can range from mild to severe. In severe cases, a depressed person may lie in bed or sit in a chair staring at the floor day by day. Treatment for

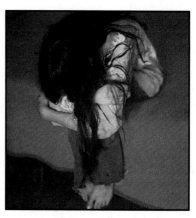

10–7. Not all signs of depression are as obvious as this one.

Table 10-4

SOME SIGNS OF DEPRESSION
Sadness
Lack of interest in friends or activities
Feelings of inferiority
Listlessness
Inability to think
Irritability
Brooding
Feeling tired, washed out
Poor appetite or overeating
Sleeplessness or excess sleep

depression often combines the use of special mood-changing drugs with other therapy discussed in the next chapter. Proper treatment can lead to a complete recovery from depression.

BIPOLAR DISORDER. Have you noticed that on certain days you feel very happy and on others you are depressed for no particular reason? This is actually normal. However, if the swing from joy to sadness occurs often and overwhelms a person, the condition is referred to as a bipolar disorder sometimes called *manic-depressive disorder*. **Bipolar disorders** have two separate phases.

The manic phase of the disorder is characterized by overactivity and restlessness. The person talks extremely fast but cannot stay on one subject. Often the manic phase brings a person great joy without any particular reason. There is delight with life and a desire to talk and laugh and sing. However, the manic phase may also center around anger. Physical activity increases to the point of violence. In the manic state people may become dangerous to themselves as well as to others.

During the depressive phase people show very little initiative, self-confidence, and physical activity. There is constant danger of suicide. They must be watched at all times, until treatment changes their attitudes and behavior.

The behavior of people suffering from a bipolar disorder is like a pendulum. The pendulum swings from great excitement to great depression. This swing may occur within a few hours. As improvement occurs during treatment, the swings into the manic or depressive stages are less severe and last a shorter time. Between these stages, behavior may be normal. With proper treatment the chance of recovery is good.

DISSOCIATIVE DISORDERS: SEPARATING MEMORY AND BEHAVIOR

Dissociate means to separate from. In **dissociative disorders,** people act as if their memories have been separated from their behavior. Their states of consciousness or identity become altered.

AMNESIA. Harvey had disappeared. Finally he was discovered by a friend of his father's in a gas station that was 100 miles from home. Even though Harvey had known his father's friend for several years, he treated him like a total stranger. When his parents arrived, he didn't know them either. He couldn't remember where or when he was born. When asked what his name was, he said it was Frank Green. Harvey was referred to a psychiatrist for treatment. His problem was **amnesia** (am-**nee**-zha).

In amnesia a person retreats from an unpleasant situation. Memory areas of the brain are blocked, and both memory and identity are lost. Harvey's memories of his life, before his new identity, were still in his unconscious mind. Through the doctor's skillful questioning and treatment, Harvey was able to recall his memories and become himself again. Why had he retreated? The doctor learned that Harvey's parents had interfered with his life in almost every detail. Harvey's unconscious drive to lead his own life had taken over completely, turning him into Frank Green.

MULTIPLE PERSONALITY.   In this disorder, emotional conflict triggers a personality split. The person withdraws from the stressful situation he or she is unable to cope with. Another personality surfaces that can cope with the situation. Sometimes more than two personalities coexist within the same person. Adults with this disorder have usually suffered extreme child abuse. Multiple personality is a very rare but fascinating disorder. It is the subject of many books and movies.

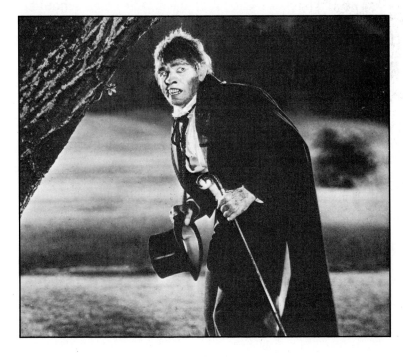

10–8. The tale of Dr. Jekyll and Mr. Hyde is perhaps the most famous case of a split personality.

PERSONALITY DISORDERS

How you think, feel, and act within your environment are all traits that form your personality. In children and teenagers, the personality undergoes many changes during the normal process of growing up. By adulthood, personality is formed and, in general, remains constant.

Certain adult personalities are classified as personality disorders. Adults with these disorders do not suffer from any severe symptoms such as hallucinations or intense anxiety. However, their peculiar personalities make them unhappy or dissatisfied with life. They usually cannot get along with others. They have trouble adapting to normal events in social or job settings. Once these abnormal personality patterns are established, they are very difficult to change. Even long-term therapy may not help unless a person is highly motivated to change.

Let's look briefly at seven common personality disorders. This will help you get a better understanding of personality disorders and how they create problems for the individual and others.

SCHIZOID PERSONALITY. If you asked people to describe Henry, they would say that he is cold and aloof. Henry always prefers to be by himself. After high school he found a job as a night watchman, so he could work alone. He prefers social isolation because he is not interested in others. Henry doesn't experience deep pleasure or discomfort from anything that happens. Understandably, he has never had a lasting friendship with anyone.

AVOIDANT PERSONALITY. Candice also prefers to be alone in social situations, but for different reasons. She has low self-esteem and is extremely sensitive to the attitudes that others might have toward her. Rather than suffer imagined rejection and humiliation, she withdraws from others as a protective device. Because of earlier and painful life experiences, Candice has learned to expect rejection and humiliation from most people. Though Candice desires friendship, withdrawal protects her from any hurt caused by attempts to relate to others.

DEPENDENT PERSONALITY. Marvin is a very dependent, yielding kind of person. He can never make up his mind about anything and constantly turns to others for advice. Leaning on others gives him a sense of security. He is very passive in social situations. He avoids any conflict that might alienate him from other people. Marvin always submits to the desires of others in order to be accepted.

PASSIVE-AGGRESSIVE PERSONALITY. Whenever his boss gives Ralph an assignment, he accepts it. Then, he handles his work in a passive, inefficient way. He dawdles over his work and forgets to complete important details. He never approaches his assignments in a positive and forceful way. He and his boss have discussed his poor performance. Yet he stubbornly resists changing his attitude.

HISTRIONIC PERSONALITY. The term *histrionic* comes from the Etruscan word *histrio*, meaning actor. Louise craves excitement and constantly draws attention to herself. She often has wild emotional outbursts. As soon as she jumps into one activity she becomes bored and her enthusiam quickly fades. She then jumps into another activity. Some people would describe Louise as popular. However, her friendships are not usually meaningful, and they are usually short-lived.

NARCISSISTIC PERSONALITY. A narcissistic personality is best described as conceited. Richard is vain and inconsiderate of others. He expects others to cater to his wishes and needs. No one enjoys talking to Richard, since he is usually so full of boast and arrogance. He needs the admiration of others. He believes that he has special talents, which others should simply recognize as obvious, without his ever having to prove them.

HEALTH ACTION

Take on of the mental disorders discussed in this chapter and explore it in greater detail. Present and discuss in class a case study representative of the disorder.

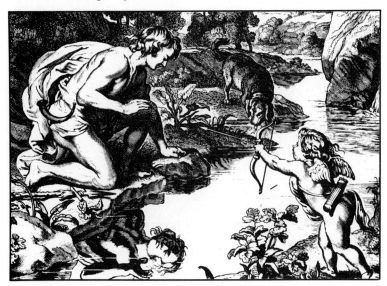

10–9. The term narcissistic *comes from the Greek legend about Narcissis, who fell in love with his own image.*

ANTISOCIAL PERSONALITY. Alvin angers quickly and seems to enjoy bullying those around him. He is suspicious of the motives of others, and he is frequently cruel and resentful. Gentleness, warmth, and consideration never seem to be a part of his behavior. He enjoys situations that allow him to display his toughness. He feels justified in getting back at others for whatever wrongs he may have experienced in life.

Behavior patterns such as these often first appear during adolescence. Teenagers with antisocial personalities behave irresponsibly and impulsively. Their antisocial acts are repeated often, despite their effects on other people. Adults with this disorder often acquire criminal records.

LIFE CRISIS

During the usual course of life, people experience many traumatic events that cause a high level of stress and emotional turmoil. These events are referred to as **crises.** Crises severely disrupt or alter normal life and often require people to make major adjustments in life-style.

A major flood forced the Ames family to leave their home. When they returned, they found that their home and their belongings had been almost completely destroyed by the flood. The entire family felt depressed and overwhelmed.

A natural disaster is just one example of a life crisis. Many other events place unusual emotional strain on families and

10–10. What changes in normal life-style do victims of natural disasters face? How might these changes affect them?

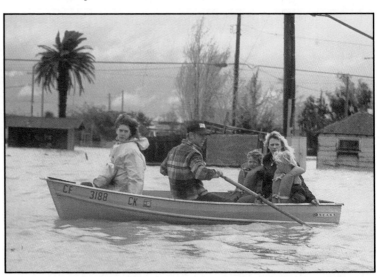

individuals. These include deaths of loved ones, becoming a victim of violent crime, major illness or injury, divorce or separation, and job loss. Often these events are unexpected. The individual often has no control over the situation. Feelings of panic, anger, depression, or helplessness are common in crisis situations.

COPING WITH CRISIS

In the case of the Ames family, they cried together over their terrible loss. Then they started to work out a plan to restore their home. Their feelings of shock lessened as they took concrete action to control their lives once again. Relatives, friends, and neighbors pitched in to help them rebuild their home.

People vary in their ability to cope with crises. The Ames family was lucky to have strong social support to ease the burden of their situation. They were able to express their emotions and share the pain of the experience together. For many reasons, people often feel alone in a crisis situation. In these cases, emotional strain can seriously affect mental health unless outside help is obtained.

SUICIDE: A SPECIAL CRISIS

Do you know the third leading cause of death among youth today? It is not cancer or any other disease. It is **suicide.** In the last 20 years suicide has increased 300 percent in young people between the ages of 15 and 24.

Depression is common in people who attempt suicide. However, attempted suicide is not always an expression of the wish to die. Often it is an expression of anger or a desperate cry for help. Among youth, suicide may be linked to a personal failure, rejection, or loss. Problems seem overwhelming and impossible to live with.

John was an average student in school. He had many friends and had never gotten into trouble of any kind. His parents were proud of him. They had high hopes that he would become a doctor. In his senior year, he began having trouble with his science courses. John felt anxious and depressed. He told his best friend, "I don't have much to live for if I can't get into college." Just before report cards came out, his mood changed. He seemed light-hearted once again. He even gave his best friend his favorite recording tapes. The next day, when his mother went to wake him for school, she found John unconscious. He had taken an overdose of pills. Fortunately, John's life was saved. With professional help he was able to learn how to cope with his feelings. He and his family learned how to communicate with each other. Eventually John returned to high school and then went on to college.

WARNING SIGNS OF SUICIDE. Many suicides and suicide attempts can be prevented if the warning signs are spotted. Most suicide victims make several pleas for help either through words or actions. Statements such as "I wish I were dead" should always be taken seriously. These statements indicate a very real problem. Prolonged depression, isolation, and withdrawal from family and friends are other warning signs. Be alert to sudden positive changes in attitude following depression. This mood shift may mean that a person has made a conscious decision to commit suicide. Giving away prized possessions also signals suicidal intentions.

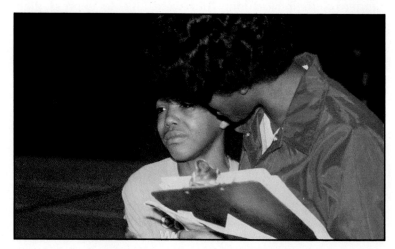

10–11. To whom can you turn in times of trouble?

POSITIVE PREVENTION. How can you help someone caught in this crisis? Mental health experts suggest the following:

1. Learn to recognize the symptoms of suicide.
2. Don't try to solve the problem alone. Tell a parent, teacher, or other adult who can help. Many cities have telephone "hotlines" staffed by trained personnel who can give assistance. Remember that a person who talks about suicide is asking for help. Do not feel that you are betraying a confidence.
3. Don't leave the suicidal person alone. Stay with the person until help arrives.

4. Listen carefully. People intent on suicide need to get real thoughts and feelings into the open. Be sympathetic and understanding, but don't try to give false reassurances and solutions. People intent on suicide need professional help. Just letting the person know that you care is the best thing you can do.

SIGNS OF PERSONALITY TROUBLE. While reading about mental and emotional problems, did you recognize any of your own feelings or behavior patterns? This is not surprising. Even the best-adjusted personalities change from day to day. When do emotional or behavior changes signal that trouble may lie ahead? Here are a few warning signs to alert you.

1. Feelings of persistent, severe anxiety without apparent cause.
2. Depression that leads to withdrawal from family, friends, or usual activities.
3. Sudden and lasting changes in moods or behavior, especially those that are not desirable or consistent with usual behavior.
4. Frequent psychosomatic complaints.
5. Placing unrealistically high standards and demands on oneself or others.
6. Performing poorly and repeatedly falling below potential.
7. Inability to cope with life's stresses.

If you or a loved one experience any of these symptoms, professional help may be needed. In the chapter ahead you will learn about the different kinds of help that are available and how help can be obtained.

SUMMARY: There are no sharp dividing lines between normal and abnormal personalities. When people feel good about themselves and about others, and they are able to meet the demands of life, they are considered mentally healthy. When people cannot adjust to situations and to other people, they may have a mental disorder. Although the causes are not fully understood, stress, heredity, and physical factors may contribute to mental disorders.

Professionals divide mental disorders into groups based on common behavior patterns. Life crises may also cause mental health problems. Whenever any mental health problem becomes severe, prolonged, or overwhelming, professional help should be sought.

CHAPTER REVIEW

words at work

Find the word in the left column that fits one of the definitions in the right column. DO NOT WRITE IN THIS BOOK.

a. phobia
b. hypochondria
c. histrionic
d. psychosis
e. narcissistic
f. depression
g. schizophrenia
h. bipolar disorder
i. amnesia
j. organic mental disorder

1. out of touch with reality
2. split mind
3. mood swings from sadness to excitement
4. physical damage to the brain
5. intense irrational fear of something
6. conceited personality
7. abnormal worry over illness
8. loss of memory and identity
9. extreme or prolonged sadness
10. attention-craving personality

review questions

1. Cite two factors that indicate abnormal behavior.
2. Distinguish between mental health and mental disorders.
3. Explain why the term "mental disorder" is preferable to mental illness.
4. Are mental disorders inherited? Explain your answer.
5. List three physical factors that can change personality and behavior.
6. Define organic mental disorder.
7. What is psychosis?
8. Why are mental disorders classified?
9. Define phobia. Give an example of a common phobia.
10. Contrast obsessions and compulsions.
11. How do conversion disorders affect behavior?
12. What are dissociative disorders? Give two examples.
13. Outline the behavior patterns related to schizophrenia.
14. Name five symptoms of depression.
15. Describe bipolar disorder.
16. Why are personality disorders classified as mental disorders?
17. Distinguish between hallucinations and delusions.
18. Name three major crises in life.
19. List six warnings of suicide.
20. When should someone seek help for mental health problems?

discussion questions

1. Discuss personality as a continuum and explain how this relates to our understanding of mental health and mental disorders.
2. A friend who is troubled by personal problems confides in you that "My situation is hopeless. Life is no longer worth living." What would you do?
3. Discuss the role of the family in the development of mental health problems. In your opinion what can be done to strengthen family life so that mental disorders are prevented and mental health is improved?
4. Why do life crises sometimes cause mental disorders? Discuss individual family and community action in times of life crisis. Use examples from experience or the media to expand your discussion.
5. Discuss your observations about impulsive and delinquent behavior in adolescence. Do you think that youths who display this behavior will develop antisocial personalities as adults?

investigating

PURPOSE:
To learn how to deal more effectively with crisis situations.

PROCEDURE:
A. Break up into groups of six or eight students.
B. Choose two people in your group to role-play a crisis situation. One student should be the person in a crisis. The other student should be a concerned friend.
C. Role-play one of these crisis situations: (a) Your best friend tells you that his parents are getting divorced and that he or she feels responsible. (b) Your neighbor's house burns down. (c) Your friend who is a freshman in college tells you he or she does not like college, but is afraid to quit. (d) Your best friend is depressed. He tells you that he has just broken up with his steady girl friend.
D. During the role-playing, other group members should observe and take notes. Record any interaction that seems effective or ineffective. After role-playing the situation for about five minutes, change students and select another situation. Repeat until each person in the group has had a chance to participate.
E. As a class, discuss what happened during the various group interactions.
    1. How did you feel as a person in crisis? As a concerned friend? What emotions did you experience?
    2. Discuss the role of communication in the interaction. Did one partner talk more than another? Was there nonverbal communication? If so, what?
    3. What seemed effective in helping the troubled friend? Ineffective? Why?
    4. In your opinion, are all these situations equally stressful? Why or why not?
    5. Do you feel this activity has helped you? Why or why not? When helping in a crisis situation, what warning signs of behavior should you be alert to?

CHAPTER 11

Therapy for the Troubled Personality

OBJECTIVES

- DESCRIBE the scope of the mental health problem
- EXPLAIN the purpose of therapy
- COMPARE different types of therapy

- OUTLINE various mental health services
- SUGGEST ways to prevent mental health problems

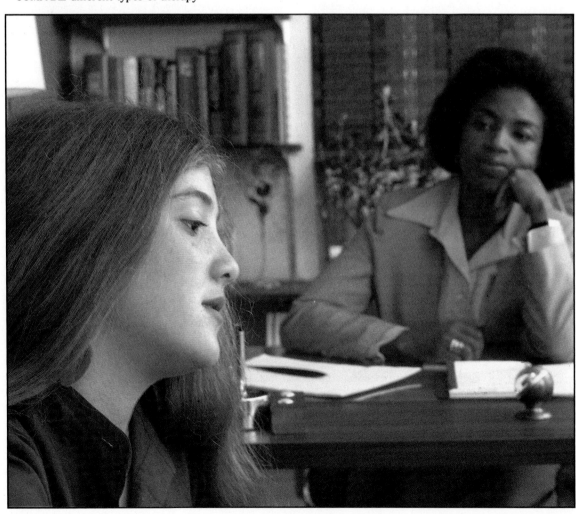

Beth:	Since Mom and Dad divorced I feel unhappy and out of sorts all the time. I'm just not interested in much of anything. I've even lost my appetite.
Steven:	That's not an unusual reaction. Have you talked to anyone about your feelings, Beth?
Beth:	Well, I tried talking to my mother. But she's pretty worried right now, too. My best friend is tired of hearing me talk about the divorce. She doesn't understand. Her family is together.
Steven:	How has your life changed since the divorce?
Beth:	Well. . . .

Who are Beth and Steven? They are not friends but they do have a special relationship. Beth is receiving psychotherapy. Steven is her therapist. Most people whom mental health services can help never show abnormal behavior. Like Beth, they carry on their lives but are not able to do or be their best. Does this fact surprise you? In the chapter ahead we will explore how therapy can help people who are troubled.

MENTAL HEALTH: TODAY AND YESTERDAY

THE PRESENT

How serious is the mental health problem in the United States today? The President's Commission on Mental Health has estimated that, at any given time, as many as one out of every four people may suffer from mental or emotional problems. At least 15 percent of the population, or 25 million people, need professional help for their problems. It is estimated that, among children, 5 to 15 percent have mental health problems. These include emotional problems, behavioral problems, and delays in psychological development.

To understand the scope of the mental health problem, you must be aware of some key facts. First, it is often hard to distinguish mental disorders from physical disorders. Often a physical illness is a result of emotional problems. Second, mental health problems cover a wide area of mental, emotional, and behavioral problems. They range from milder problems, such as mild anxiety, to severe disorders, such as schizophrenia, that require hospitalization. Third, all too often people do not receive help when early warning signs of mental health problems appear. These facts point out that more work must still be done in the field of mental health. However, a great deal has already been achieved. This becomes evident when you look at the history of mental health problems.

THE PAST

At one time, people with mental disorders were thought to be possessed by evil spirits that took over their minds. Fossil skulls from the Stone Age have been found with holes bored through them. These people believed that drilling holes in the skull would release evil spirits, thereby curing the illness. During the Middle Ages the superstition persisted. The mentally ill were thought to be in league with the devil and to have supernatural powers that caused great harm. The remedy was to drive the demons out of the body by burning, beating, starving, or other methods of torture. During the eighteenth century, mental illness was considered a mark of weakness and a family disgrace. The mentally ill were put into asylums as a solution to the problem. Instead of receiving care and treatment, the patients were treated as prisoners. They were chained in cells and hidden from public view. Recovery, or even improvement of patients, was thought to be almost impossible.

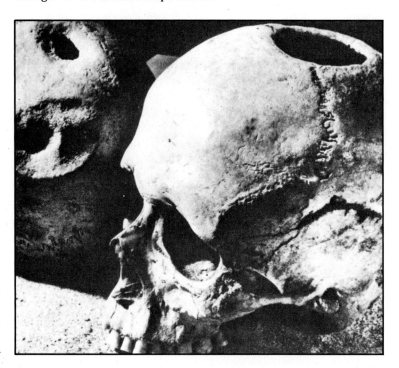

11–1. During the Stone Age, it was believed that drilling holes in the skulls of the mentally ill would release the evil spirits within.

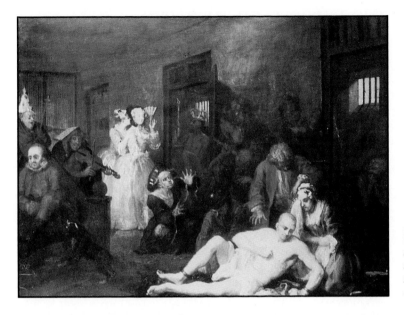

11–2. A painting by William Hogarth depicting the inhuman treatment of the mentally ill in a nineteenth century insane asylum.

Just before the start of the nineteenth century, movements began in England and France to break the chains that confined the mentally ill. In America in 1812 the great social reformer Dr. Benjamin Rush wrote a book entitled *Medical Inquiry and Observations Upon the Disease of the Mind*. He was one of the first to advocate humane treatment for the insane. He believed that mental diseases were as subject to healing as physical diseases. Dr. Rush's work on mental disorders brought about a new specialty in medicine that became known as **psychiatry** (sigh-**ki**-at-tree). Psychiatry is the study and treatment of disorders of the mind. The rise of psychiatry brought new hope to patients.

In the 1840's a young American schoolteacher, Dorothea Dix, became a crusader for founding mental hospitals. She helped found the first public hospitals for humane treatment of the insane. But change came slowly. Most mental hospitals only provided custodial care. Almost a hundred years went by before patients began to receive any effective treatments.

In 1908 Clifford Beers, a former patient in a mental hospital, published *A Mind That Found Itself*. This book brought to light the terrible truth about mental hospitals. Public opinion was so aroused that a national citizens' group was formed to fight the problems of poor mental health. The group still continues its work today under the name Mental Health Association.

THE PURPOSE OF THERAPY

Many people do not understand what therapy is and what it is supposed to do. The word *therapy* means *treatment*. In treating mental health problems, two major approaches are used. One approach is medical treatment. The other approach is called **psychotherapy** (sigh-ko-**ther**-ap-pee). It involves communication between a trained therapist and a patient. Sometimes both approaches are used in therapy. Regardless of the type of therapy used, they all have a single goal. It is to help people change their behavior so that they may live fuller, more satisfying lives. Therapy is used to treat all kinds of personal problems in which emotional factors play a part. Many people are seeking help to overcome a variety of emotional problems, including mental disorders, reactions to crisis situations, addictions, and psychosomatic disorders. Increasing numbers of people are seeking therapy for personal growth rather than for personal problems.

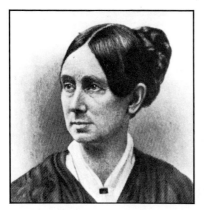

11–3. Dorothea Dix helped found the first public mental hospital for humane treatment of the insane.

TYPES OF THERAPY

PSYCHOANALYSIS: UNLOCKING THE UNCONSCIOUS MIND

Psychoanalysis (sigh-ko-ah-**nal**-eh-sis) is the best-known type of psychotherapy. It dates back to the work of Sigmund Freud at the turn of the century. Freud was the founder of psychoanalysis. He was the first to recognize the role of the unconscious mind in personality and behavior. Even today Freud's techniques are used in psychoanalysis and other therapies.

Freud believed that mental disorders resulted from painful memories stored in the unconscious. He believed that these disorders could be cured by psychoanalysis. Psychoanalysis brings these memories to consciousness. It is an in-depth study of a person's past from birth to the present. It concentrates on the person's unconscious mind and any repressed conflicts. To solve the patient's problems, these hidden feelings and experiences must be explored. As a result the patient gains an understanding of how past experiences have affected present actions and emotions. How is the unconscious mind reached? During the therapy sessions the patient is encouraged to say *everything* that comes to mind. No thought is considered too minor. Dreams, expressions of the unconscious, are discussed and analyzed.

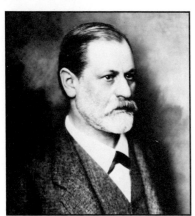

11–4. Sigmund Freud was the founder of psychoanalysis. Today, his techniques, as well as others, are used in psychotherapy.

Unfortunately, psychoanalysis is both costly and time consuming. Patients visit therapists several times a week for about two to six years. Supporters of psychoanalysis, however, believe that in many cases it is the only way to bring about a lasting cure. Others argue that alternate methods are just as good, less costly, and help the patient change behavior more rapidly.

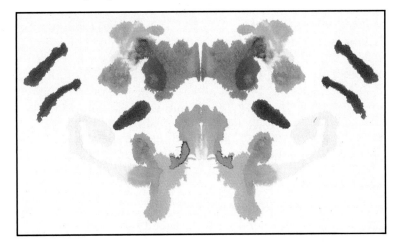

11–5. What do you see in this inkblot? The inkblot test was devised by Hermann Rorschach. It allows the projection of one's feelings onto an ambiguous picture. Reaction to this test can help a therapist gain some insight into a person's personality structure.

CLIENT-CENTERED THERAPY: A NONDIRECTIVE APPROACH

Client-centered therapy was developed by the psychologist Carl Rogers. Rogers uses the term *client* since the term *patient* implies sickness. This therapy differs from psychoanalysis in one major way. Psychoanalysis focuses on a person's past. Client-centered therapy focuses on the client's *present* attitudes and behavior. The therapist assists the client in this process by studying and clarifying the client's attitudes. Emotions are identified and discussed with the client. For example, if the client has just discussed an upsetting event, the therapist might respond by saying "You feel angry about that, don't you?" It is then up to the client to understand the problem and change behavior. Client-centered therapy is also called **nondirective.** The client decides the goals of the treatment. The therapist does not tell the client how to act in any situation. The therapist helps a client see choices but the client must make the decisions.

At the crux of client-centered therapy is the comfortable, accepting environment that the therapist creates. This atmosphere is free from pressure and criticism. The therapist conveys to the client a total belief in the individual's self-worth. As a result, the client learns to speak freely about problems. He or she develops a stronger sense of self-esteem and is able to cope better with problems.

BEHAVIOR MODIFICATION: CHANGING ACTIONS THROUGH LEARNING

Behavior modification is based on the belief that most behavior is learned. There is one basic difference between behavior modification and other psychotherapies. In behavior modification, there is little or no concern for gaining insight into the unconscious or in making major personality changes. The therapist focuses only on specific behaviors that need to be changed. The therapist helps to change specific behavior patterns by teaching the patient new responses to old situations. Many different methods are used. These include controlling reinforcements, desensitization, and modeling.

CONTROLLING REINFORCEMENTS. A child's tantrums are staged to get attention. If parents try to soothe the child or react by becoming upset, the child receives the desired attention. This reinforces the child's behavior. The next time attention is desired the child will have another tantrum. The tantrums could be stopped by "controlling the reinforcement" given to the child. For example the parents could ignore the tantrums and/or reward proper behavior. Then the tantrums would soon disappear.

11–6. Token economics *is a form of behavior modification used in mental hospitals. The staff reinforces "healthy" behaviors and ignores "others." Patients decide what rewards they want to work for and are given tokens as visible evidence that they are making progress.*

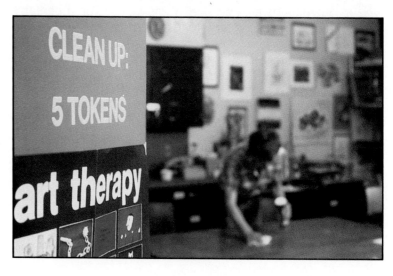

Therapists have sometimes achieved dramatic results by **controlling reinforcement.** In one such case a male schizophrenic patient had not spoken for nineteen years. The therapist's goal was to make him talk again. A stick of chewing gum became the reinforcement. At first, when the patient just moved his lips, he was rewarded with a piece of gum. Later, if he made a sound of any kind, he received another stick of gum. Gradually, he began to say the word "gum," and only then was he rewarded. The reinforcement of the gum was eventually replaced by other rewards. Soon the patient was speaking again.

DESENSITIZATION.   Have you ever watched a parent help a child overcome a fear of water? The parent introduces the child to the water by degrees. First, only the feet touch the water, then the legs, and so on. Soon this step-by-step process helps the child get over the fear.

Behavior therapists use a similar method called **desensitization** (dee-sen-sit-tih-**zay**-shun) to help patients overcome their fears and anxieties. First, the therapist and patient identify all events that produce anxiety. These events are ranked from least to most disturbing. Then relaxation techniques are taught to the patient. Once these techniques are mastered, the patient is then told to imagine the least stressful event. The patient learns to remain relaxed when thinking about this event. The same procedures are followed as more stressful events are introduced. When a patient then confronts the same events in real life, he or she no longer experiences anxiety.

MODELING.   **Modeling** is based on the principle that people learn by example to form a new behavior. Bill's fear of snakes prevented him from gardening or even hiking in the woods. During a group behavior therapy session, Bill watched another person, called a model, handle a live but harmless king snake. The model showed no fear. The therapist then encouraged each patient to imitate the model in handling the snake. Finally they were persuaded to hold the snake and let it coil around them. The treatment helped almost everyone in the group, including Bill, to overcome their fear of snakes.

GROUP SESSIONS

Traditional therapy involves just two people: the therapist and the person seeking help. Group sessions are based on the premise that people have similar problems and can learn from one another. Today, a variety of group sessions are available, including family therapy, group therapy, encounter groups, and self-improvement and self-help groups.

FAMILY THERAPY. There was a great deal of tension in the Ferris household. Mr. Ferris had just been laid off from his job. Lately, it seemed the couple quarreled a lot. Often their arguments concerned their son, Adam. He stayed out late at night against their wishes. At school he was a constant discipline problem. When Adam was threatened with suspension, his parents decided to seek professional help. A therapist interviewed Adam. The therapist saw that, while Adam's problems were serious, they were only part of a more complex problem affecting the whole family. In this case the therapist recommended family therapy for each of the Ferrises.

What is the basis for family therapy? The family is a close knit unit where human-relation skills are learned. Therefore, a person's problem can sometimes reflect conflicts and communication breakdown within the family. In these situations, the problems of the person seeking help are seen as symptoms of the troubles that weigh down the entire family.

The therapist observes the entire family, since what is needed is *family therapy*, not individual treatment. The therapist observes how each family member responds to the others and contributes to the problems that they all share in common.

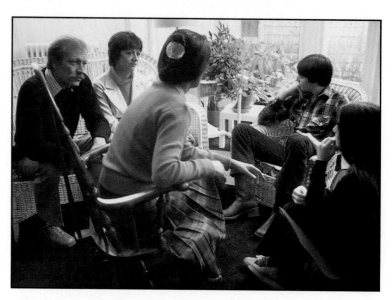

11–7. The family therapist helps to promote new and more wholesome attitudes and behaviors among family members.

UNIT 3 PERSONALITY UNDER STRESS

The therapist works with several or all members of the family, sometimes together, sometimes apart. The major areas of conflict are examined. The therapist points out the harmful ways the family members are relating to each other. The therapist also helps to establish good communication. Areas of anger and fear are rooted out. In time, the therapist breaks down the attitudes and behaviors that caused the family's problem. As a result family members learn to express their feelings toward each other in helpful ways. The therapist promotes new, more wholesome attitudes and behaviors.

GROUP THERAPY. In group therapy, a therapist guides several people. Usually the therapist takes a passive role and does not try to lead the conversation. Instead the patients discuss their problems, share experiences, and interpret each other's behavior. Patients realize that they are not alone in their problems and learn from each other. For example, teenagers with drug abuse problems may gain insight into their actions and motives by participating in group therapy with other drug abusers.

SELF-IMPROVEMENT GROUPS. The purpose of self-improvement and encounter groups is to help people learn to relate more openly and honestly with each other. These are *not* therapy sessions. They are not intended for people who seek help with emotional problems. They are designed to help people better understand how they interact with others.

HEALTH ACTION

Research a type of psychotherapy (not already discussed) and report your findings to the class. When studying the therapy, be sure to note its basic theory of mental disorders and specific methods used in treatment. Does the therapy claim a success rate? What evidence does it offer for its claims?

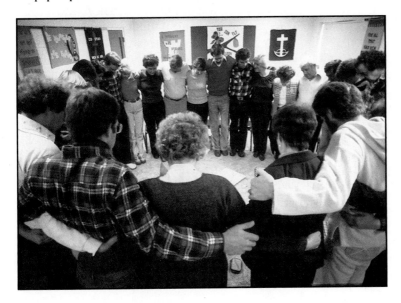

11–8. Self-improvement groups help people relate to one another openly and honestly.

A group leader, sometimes called a trainer or facilitator, encourages the group to experience and express emotions. These groups have become popular in recent years. Before deciding to join one, it is wise to learn as much as possible about the group, its methods, and the leader.

SELF-HELP GROUPS. Are you familiar with the names "Alcoholics Anonymous" and "Weight Watchers"? These groups are just two examples of self-help groups. Self-help groups are formed by people with a common problem. Those who join help one another overcome the problem they all have in common. These groups are not, as a rule, run by professional therapists or group leaders. They are self-directed by the group members. These groups are proving to be a powerful force in helping people overcome many problems related to mental health. For example, there are groups for single parents, for the divorced, and for children of alcoholics. Recovery, Inc. is one self-help group for people with emotional problems.

MEDICAL THERAPY: CHEMOTHERAPY

Any discussion about the treatment of mental and emotional problems would be incomplete without learning about **chemotherapy.** Chemotherapy is treatment that involves the use of drugs. It is often used in combination with other therapy. Three major classes of drugs are used today:

1. **Antianxiety drugs.** *Tranquilizers* are the most widely used drugs. They reduce emotional tension and anxiety. They also help calm patients, making psychotherapy more effective. In psychotic patients tranquilizers can reduce hallucinations and delusions. They are also used to treat physical symptoms caused by emotional problems.
2. **Antidepressant drugs.** These drugs are also called **psychic energizers** because of their mood-elevating effects. They are used to combat severe depression by creating an emotional uplift.
3. **Antimanic drugs.** These drugs help reduce the severely excited manic state. Drugs, such as *lithium*, have made it possible for many patients to resume normal activity.

The use of chemotherapy has sometimes been criticized. Some argue that drugs may change a patient's moods but do not change the basic underlying problems. Some of these drugs, such as lithium and a certain class of antidepressants called MAO inhibitors, also have dangerous and unpleasant side effects. And with drug use, there is always the potential for abuse. Although these statements are true, chemotherapy is still considered valuable. Chemotherapy can help patients reach a state of mind that makes other therapy possible. Also, patients who would have remained hospitalized years ago can today live in their own homes with the help of drugs.

THE EFFECTIVENESS OF THERAPY

With over 200 therapies available, you might well ask, "Which therapy works best?" This question cannot be easily answered. Almost all therapies will work, but for certain people, and not for others. No two people have the same personalities, problems, or life experiences. Also, no two therapists, even when trained in the same therapy methods, have the exact same methods.

In some cases people with mental and emotional problems get well without any therapy at all. It may be that, given enough time, many people learn to cope with their problems in their own way. Social support or other factors could also improve, which might help to correct some people's mental and emotional problems.

However, it has been found that most people with emotional problems can be helped with therapy. Researchers have found that more people with emotional problems who received therapy improved their mental health than those who did not receive therapy. The effective methods have the following traits in common:

1. The patient respects the therapist as a model of a mentally healthy person. Patients usually open up and talk about their problems when they trust their therapist.
2. The therapy provides a warm, supportive environment. Sincere expressions of warmth and acceptance of "abnormalities" can provide an atmosphere in which change can occur.
3. The therapy provides feedback to patients about their behavior and how their environment affects their thoughts and feelings.
4. The therapy builds on strengths rather than weaknesses. Criticism seldom changes thoughts or behavior patterns. The therapist motivates the patient to grow and change.

MODERN MENTAL HEALTH SERVICES

Until 1955, 75 percent of all mental patients were treated in large state hospitals. These hospitals were overcrowded and understaffed. They were isolated from the community. Patients were often locked into wards. Physical restraints, such as straightjackets, were frequently used. Good professional treatment was seldom available.

The mental health picture has changed greatly. Today 75 percent of all mental patients receive help as outpatients in public or private settings. This means that they may remain at home while receiving treatment. Inpatient care, when necessary, is more generally available within the community. State hospitals still continue to provide most inpatient care for those with long-term problems. General hospitals with mental health units, or community mental health centers, now provide most short-term inpatient care.

INPATIENT HOSPITAL CARE

When someone's problems become very severe, he or she may no longer be able to function at home. Inpatient care in a hospital may be required. Psychotic patients, for example, usually need inpatient care. Most patients improve after two to six weeks of intensive treatment in a hospital. After this treatment, most patients only require partial inpatient care or outpatient care.

Soon after admission to a hospital the patient meets with doctors and other specialists. They study the condition, diagnose the problem, and recommend treatment. A full life history is prepared, including information about the patient's home, social, and educational background. This is necessary in order to understand the patient's problems thoroughly. The patient also receives a thorough physical examination. Most hospital treatment focuses on psychotherapy and chemotherapy. This treatment is supplemented by **milieu** (meel-**you**), or environment, therapy. In milieu therapy, the patient's environment is changed in order to encourage changes in attitudes and behavior. Recreation and occupational therapies help patients gain touch with reality so that they can function again in their homes and communities. In recreation therapy, games, crafts, or other enjoyable activities are used to motivate patients and to help them express their feelings. Special art, music, or dance

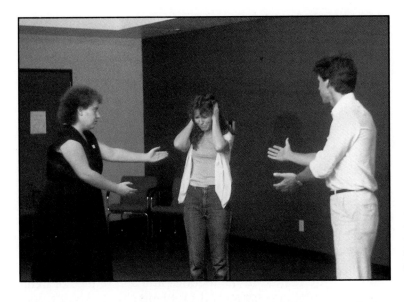

11-9. In this drama-therapy session, the girl in the middle is playing herself. The other two people are playing her divorced parents.

therapists help patients express their feelings creatively. Occupational therapists help patients learn the skills of daily living, such as basic home management, social, and job skills.

COMMUNITY MENTAL HEALTH CENTERS

Community mental health centers were set up to help bring mental health care directly to the community. People who have mental or emotional problems already have a lot to cope with. If they are moved away from their families and communities, they must cope with yet another problem: adjusting to new surroundings. Treating patients near their homes, especially if their illnesses are treated early enough, can be more effective. Also, research has shown that patients treated near their homes do not need to be treated for as long a time, and their return to society is less difficult. Mental health centers provide a range of services. Among the services provided are outpatient and short-term inpatient care, emergency services, and partial hospitalization. Partial hospitalization means that patients work by day and return to the center at night. Or they may receive treatment at the center during the day and return to their homes at night.

CRISIS INTERVENTION SERVICES. Many communities have set up 24-hour services for people in need of immediate help. These services exist for crises such as suicide, child abuse, drug abuse, or other pressing problems. Sometimes these services may be part of existing programs at hospitals or community mental health centers. Or they may be run by other community groups. They may be staffed by professionals and/or trained volunteers. Some operate as drop-in centers while others function as telephone hotlines. These services have proven to be very effective in helping people cope with life crises.

PRIVATE THERAPISTS

Almost every community has therapists in private practice, including:

- *psychiatrists*, who are doctors that specialize in mental and emotional disorders. They may use drugs as well as psychotherapy to treat problems. Some psychiatrists specialize in working with children or the aged.
- *psychologists*, who are specialists in human behavior. They are trained in the theories and techniques of treating mental and emotional problems. They are not doctors and cannot prescribe drugs. Psychologists hold a master's or Ph.D. degree.
- *psychiatric social workers and nurses*, who are trained to perform a wide range of jobs related to mental health. They often work in mental hospitals, clinics, mental health centers, or community agencies. Some do private counseling and therapy. They generally hold a master's degree in social work or nursing and have extra training in mental health.

Before starting therapy as a private patient, always check the background of the therapist. In many states, there are no laws that state the training required to practice therapy. Hence, some people call themselves "therapists" even though they do not have the proper training.

FINDING HELP

If you or a friend or a relative ever needed help, where would you turn? You could start by asking your family doctor, clergyman, or a school nurse or guidance counselor. You could also contact your local hospital or mental health center. Groups such as family service agencies or chapters of the Mental Health Association can help too. Self-help groups, hotlines, and other mental health services are listed in the phone book. So, too, are family service agencies. Many communities have information and referral services to link consumers with needed services. Check the phone book for listings such as "Information Referral Service" (or system,) "Community Service," "Action Line," "Hotline," "HELP," and "CONTACT." Also, look in the Yellow Pages under "Mental Health" or "Social Services." The telephone operator can often be of great help in locating mental health services.

In a crisis, do not hesitate to go to a hospital emergency room or call the police. Most police are trained to handle crises. They can help put you in touch with crisis intervention services. Most people only need short-term therapy. This is particularly true when problems are brought on by a personal crisis.

PREVENTING MENTAL PROBLEMS

COMMUNITY ACTION

Mental health is a community concern. By working together community groups and local citizens can help improve mental health in their area. Sources of stress within a community can be reduced by improving housing and recreation, reducing unemployment, and cutting down on crime. Day-care and after-school programs can help reduce stress for parents who work. Volunteer programs such as Big Brothers, Big Sisters, and Foster Grandparents provide youth with added social support. Self-help groups provide social support while helping people learn new ways to cope with problems. The community mental health movement is growing. Find out what is happening in your community.

PERSONAL ACTION

What can you do to contribute to the prevention of mental disorders? One important way is to develop and maintain your own mental health. The following are some helpful suggestions:

1. Learn to handle stress and tension.
2. Develop a positive self-image. Self-respect is the foundation for good mental health.
3. Accept your shortcomings and failures.
4. Deal with problems as they occur. Solve problems or learn to adjust to them.
5. Set realistic goals and strive to achieve them. Doing

your best will help you accomplish positive goals. It will also help you build a positive self-image.

6. Participate in activities at school and your community. Helping others will make your own problems seem less significant.

7. Seek help early if a problem develops.

You can contribute to the prevention of mental disorders in other ways. Learn more about mental health problems. Examine your own attitudes toward mental health problems. Experts believe that if we were all more tolerant toward behavior we don't understand, the social stigma of mental health problems would be reduced. What effect might this have on community mental health?

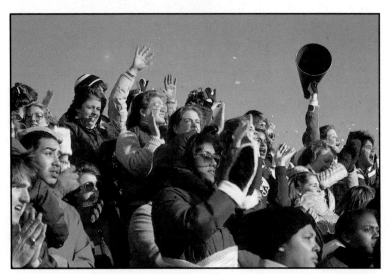

11–10. Participation in school and community activities helps you develop and maintain your own mental health.

SUMMARY: Until the twentieth century, mental problems were rarely understood. Treatment was almost nonexistent. Today people with mental health problems receive psychotherapy, chemotherapy, or both. Psychotherapists use insight or behavior methods to change behavior. Psychoanalysis, client-centered therapy, and behavior modification are examples of different psychotherapies. Therapy may be provided on an individual or group basis. Community mental health centers provide many mental health services. When problems are severe, inpatient hospital care is available. Crisis intervention services can help in emergency situations. Improving mental health is everyone's responsibility. Communities and individuals must work together to achieve this.

CHAPTER REVIEW

words at work

Match the category on the right that best describes the words in the series on the left.
DO NOT WRITE IN THIS BOOK.

a. desensitization, modeling
b. dreams, unconscious memories
c. psychoanalysis, behavior modification
d. antimanic, antidepressive, and antianxiety drugs
e. recreation and occupational therapy, psychodrama
f. outpatient clinics, crisis centers

1. chemotherapy
2. psychoanalysis
3. milieu therapy
4. mental health services
5. behavior modification
6. psychotherapy

review questions

1. Describe the relationship among physical disorders, mental disorders, and the mental health problem.
2. Name three facts that affect the scope of the mental health problem.
3. How does the put-them-away approach to mental disorders contrast with the modern concept of mental illness?
4. Define therapy.
5. Describe the two major approaches used in the treatment of mental health problems.
6. List five reasons why people might seek therapy.
7. Describe two methods into which all psychotherapies can be divided.
8. Who founded psychoanalysis? Describe the theory of this therapy.
9. How does psychoanalysis reach the unconscious mind?
10. Outline some drawbacks of psychoanalysis.
11. Describe client-centered therapy. How does it differ from psychoanalysis?
12. Describe a behavior modification technique.
13. Why is family therapy valuable for some patients?
14. Name three classes of drugs used to treat mental disorders. What does each do?
15. Contrast group therapy and encounter groups.
16. What are self-help groups? How do they work?
17. Why are community mental health centers vital to the mental health program?
18. What services are available for mentally troubled people?
19. Name four health professionals who provide mental health services.
20. How can communities help prevent mental disorders?
21. Describe six ways in which mental disorders can be prevented.

discussion questions

1. Discuss the stigma of mental disorders and psychotherapy. How can it be reduced?
2. Do you think drug therapy should be used in treating mental disorders? Defend your answer.
3. A friend's behavior changes drastically. What would you do?
4. A friend seeks help in obtaining mental health services and asks you how to find services, which method is most effective, and advice about therapists. How would you reply?
5. Outline a program of personal and community action that would help prevent mental disorders.
6. In your opinion, how serious is the mental health problem? Use your own observations, not statistical facts to support your answer.

investigating

PURPOSE:
To develop a "mini-directory" of mental health services in your community.

MATERIALS:
Phone book and index cards.

PROCEDURE:
A.   Find as many listings as you can in your local phone book for mental health services. Look under Action Line, Alcoholics Anonymous, Child Abuse, Community Service, CONTACT, Hotline, Help, Information Referral Service or System, Parent Helpline, Social Service Hotline, and Victims Services. Also look in the Yellow Pages under Mental Health or Social Services.

B.   Assign different members of the class to ask your school nurse, guidance counselor, members of the clergy, and family doctors for other listings.

C.   As a class, write each listing on an index card. Alphabetize the cards.

D.   Assign different class members to find out either by calling or by visiting about the mental health services that have been identified in your community. Answer these questions on the cards:

1.   What services are offered?
2.   What are the hours?
3.   What are the fees?
4.   If therapy is offered, what kind is it?
5.   What is the background of the staff?
6.   Do volunteers work in the organization? In what capacity?

E.   Collect all the cards. Make a mini-directory with the information that has been gathered.

HEALTH
CAREERS

PSYCHOLOGIST

Psychiatrists and psychologists basically perform the same job: true or false? The answer is both true and false. It is true because psychiatrists and clinical psychologists treat patients with emotional, or mental, disorders. However, since psychiatrists are specialized physicians, their treatment may include drug therapy. Psychologists are nonmedical specialists and may not prescribe or administer drugs. What, then, is a psychologist? A psychologist is a specialist who studies human behavior. To become a psychologist you must earn at least a

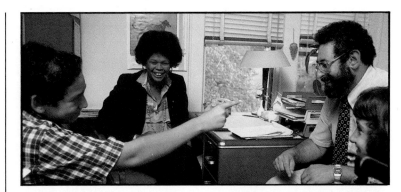

master's degree. Most often, however, a Ph.D. is required. Many states also have other requirements for certification. Hospitals, schools, private practice, industry, and research are just some areas in which psychologists are needed.

If human behavior interests you, perhaps you should consider a career as a psychologist. To find out more about this field, write to the American Psychological Association, 1200 Seventeenth Street, N.W., Washington, D.C. 20036.

OCCUPATIONAL THERAPIST

A teenager with emotional problems prepares to enter the working world; a young

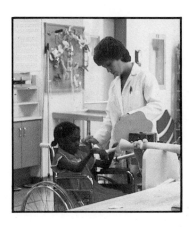

child has learning difficulties in school; a skilled laborer loses a limb and can no longer perform his job. Each person, each problem, is different, but all can be helped by an occupational therapist. Occupational therapists are life specialists. They work with any person whose life is upset by physical injury or accident, birth defects, aging, or emotional or developmental problems. Therapists first evaluate the patient and problem, and then plan and direct a therapy program. You can begin a career as an occupational therapist by

completing a four-year college program and then passing a national examination. There is also a one- to two-year program that prepares you to work as an occupational therapy assistant. Assistants help with patient evaluation and treatment. Therapists and assistants may work in hospitals, clinics, nursing homes, schools, day-care centers, and psychiatric centers. Learn more by writing to the American Occupational Therapy Association, 1383 Piccard Drive, Suite 301, Rockville, Maryland 20850.

UNIT 4

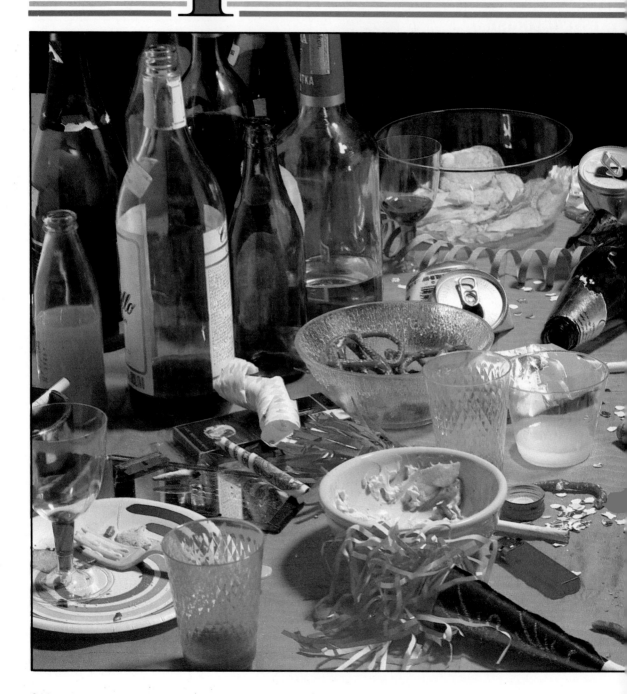

Substance Use and Abuse

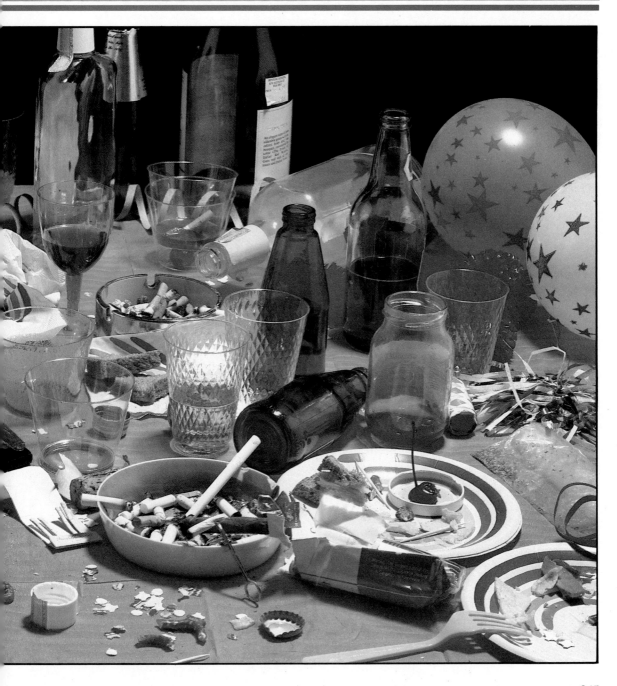

CHAPTER 12

Drugs

OBJECTIVES

- DEFINE the term "drug" and DISTINGUISH between over-the-counter and prescription drugs
- EXPLAIN the basic guidelines for proper drug use

- IDENTIFY the problems of drug abuse
- COMPARE and DESCRIBE how different drug groups affect the mind and body
- FIND resources for drug treatment in your community

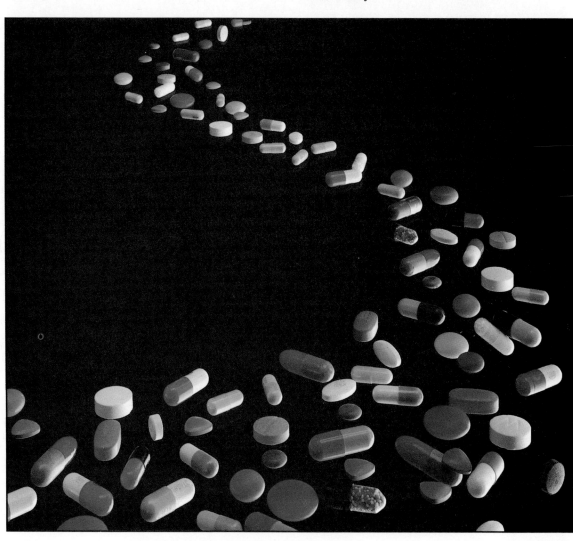

When Gene met his two best friends after school he could see that they both looked excited. "Have I got a surprise for you," said Floyd. Floyd looked around carefully and then pulled out a cigarette. He lit it and took a long puff. Gene recognized the smell of marijuana. Floyd then passed the cigarette to Mark, who also inhaled deeply. "Your turn," said Mark as he offered the cigarette to Gene. Gene hesitated.

He was curious about drugs, but had never used them. He had read about their harmful effects. "Go on," urged Floyd, "this stuff is terrific. It never *hurt* anyone." "That's right," Mark chimed in, "take it."

Gene, Floyd, and Mark are not real people, but their situation is. Do you think marijuana is harmless? What decision do you think Gene made? What would your decision have been?

DRUGS: PROPER USE VS. ABUSE

Modern drugs can indeed do wonderful things. The so-called "wonder drugs" have essentially wiped out disease epidemics such as smallpox and polio. Antibiotics such as penicillin can fight many different kinds of infectious diseases. People with diabetes can take insulin to control the sugar levels of their blood. Many people are alive today because of these modern drugs.

Modern drugs serve many other functions as well. Drugs such as aspirin can relieve pain. Anesthetics such as novocaine can cause numbness to pain. There are drugs that affect blood pressure, fertility, and appetite. But have we become a drug-dependent country? We have drugs to give us energy, drugs to put us to sleep, and drugs to relieve our anxiety. When used under medical supervision these drugs serve a useful purpose. When used without medical supervision, they can cause serious problems. A healthy body and mind do not depend on drugs to achieve a sense of well-being.

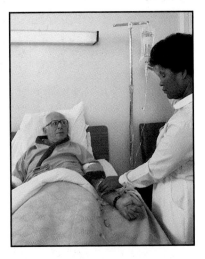

12–1. Modern drugs serve very useful purposes when used under medical supervision.

WHAT IS A DRUG?

A **drug** is *any* chemical substance that alters either the mind or the body. In fact, many substances thought to be harmless are actually drugs that can be harmful if misused. Vitamin A, for example, is essential for healthy eyes. However,

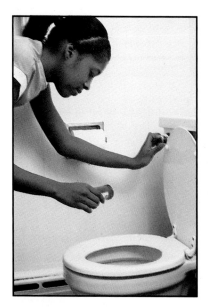

12–2. Flushing away leftover prescription drugs is a safe way to dispose of them.

it can produce blurred vision, headaches, or other problems when used in excess. Aspirin, which is used to relieve headaches, is also a drug. Vitamins, aspirin, antacids, and cold remedies are just a few of the drugs many people take without thinking twice. Since they are classified as *over-the-counter (OTC) drugs,* a prescription is not needed to buy them. How many other OTC drugs can you name?

Prescription drugs cannot be legally purchased without a doctor's written permission. These drugs are controlled substances. This means that the federal government regulates the manufacture, import, export, distribution, and use of these drugs. Stiff penalties are imposed for illegally making, selling, or using these drugs. This is because they are powerful and can be dangerous when improperly used.

Before using any drug, whether prescription or OTC, think about it seriously. Remember, *no* drug is absolutely safe. Aspirin, for example, can irritate the stomach. The first rule of proper drug use is to use them with caution.

YOUR DRUG PRESCRIPTION.   Have you ever received a drug prescription? If so, the prescription was written expressly for you. Before writing the prescription, your doctor considered more than your medical problem. Your medical history, your weight, and your general health were also considered. All these factors can affect how a drug acts in your body. For example, your size and weight determine the drug's dosage. As a rule, the larger you are, the greater the dosage.

This is why your prescription should be used only by you and for the specific purpose for which your doctor prescribed it. Follow the exact directions carefully. If in doubt about how to use the drug, always ask your doctor or pharmacist for more advice.

DRUG REACTIONS

TOLERANCE.   Drug **tolerance** is the body's ability to become used to a drug's effects. As tolerance grows, the body requires larger and larger doses to produce many of the same effects. Do all drugs produce tolerance? No, but many drugs that can be abused do produce tolerance.

DEPENDENCE.   Many drugs produce a state of **dependency,** either physical, psychological, or both. If users are physically dependent on a drug, their bodies require a constant supply of the drug to function normally. This is also

HEALTH IN HISTORY

What is the origin of the symbol "Rₓ," meaning prescription? In ancient Greece, physicians asked the blessing of the gods before writing a prescription. Eventually, to save time, the prayer was reduced to a mere written sign. Rₓ is the symbol for the god Zeus. This symbol also may have come from an abbreviation for the Latin word *recipe* meaning "you take."

called **addiction.** When dependent users do not get the drug, they undergo *withdrawal* sickness. They may experience severe nervousness, nausea, trembling, stomach pains, and muscle cramps. If the drug is taken again, these symptoms disappear at once, indicating that a state of addiction exists.

People who are psychologically dependent on drugs lead a life-style that is focused on drugs. Dependent users cannot mentally resist drug use whether or not they have an actual physical need for drugs. Since the mind and body are interrelated, it is hard to distinguish between physical and psychological drug dependency. A person's mental craving for a drug may be so strong that it seems like a physical need for the drug. There may be a wish to experience the feelings, emotions, and sensations that the drug produces. Of course, these needs are only satisfied for a short time. The user's basic problems remain. In fact, as psychological dependency grows, the user's problems almost always get worse.

Dependence-producing drugs are not limited to prescription drugs. Some OTC drugs such as certain cough medicines can also cause dependence. Usually their labels carry this warning: "Caution: this product may be habit-forming."

INTERACTIONS.   Though people may react differently to the same drug, some general effects can be expected for a given drug. However, when two or more drugs are in the body at the same time, the effects cannot be simply added. Often, they multiply and are much greater than and very different from those of any single drug. This is called a **synergistic effect** (sin-ner-**jis**-tick). For example, taking alcohol and depressant drugs *separately* and in small doses is not usually dangerous. However, when these drugs are used together in certain doses, they can cause lung failure and even death. But not all drugs produce such effects. When some drugs are used together, they cancel or limit each other's effects.

Drugs can also interact with other things, such as food. Some drugs can make the skin more prone to sunburn. This is another precaution to take when using prescribed drugs: *always* ask your physician or pharmacist about possible interactions and precautions you should take.

DRUG ABUSE

Why do people abuse drugs? Easy access to drugs is an invitation to drug abuse. Why do some people, especially

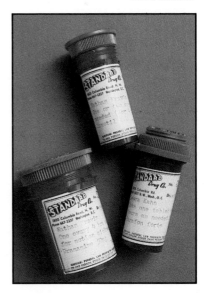

12–3. Carefully read and follow the directions of your prescriptions. If in doubt, always ask the pharmacist or doctor for more advise.

teenagers, accept the invitation? Below is a list of reasons sometimes given. What other reasons have you heard?

1. To ease peer pressure
2. To satisfy curiosity
3. To relieve boredom
4. To express dissatisfaction
5. To hurt self or others
6. To expand the mind
7. To relax
8. To be more alert
9. To have fun
10. To be social
11. To escape
12. To cope with stress

Look at all the reasons. Do they have something in common? People who abuse drugs depend on them to change the way they feel, instead of learning to change themselves through constructive action. Abusers generally do not understand the risks that drugs pose to physical, mental, and emotional well-being. Drug abuse, especially among the young, can disrupt the lives of users. Drugs often lead to problems at home, at school, or at work. A student may lose interest in school. Grades may slip and a student may even drop out. At home, an abuser may withdraw from family and friends as he or she becomes more dependent on drugs. At work, the influence of drugs may cause a lack of motivation. Poor work habits, such as lateness or carelessness on the job, may develop. What effect would this have? This could lead to the loss of a job.

PATTERNS OF ABUSE. Studies have revealed that there are four general patterns of drug abuse. Every pattern of abuse poses a physical and psychological risk. All drugs have the potential for harmful reactions, even if taken only once. Also, those who use drugs infrequently never expect that their use may lead to dependency.

- *Experimental users* try different drugs once or twice. They are more curious about a drug's effects than the drug's dangers. They feel that they can try a drug a few times and then stop. Sometimes they do. However, their experiments often lead to recreational use.
- *Occasional users* take drugs to have a good time with friends. They think that drugs make them more sociable and more acceptable to their peers. Without their realizing it, occasional use may turn into a regular habit.
- *Regular users* take drugs often to maintain a drugged feeling. Though they would deny it, regular users become psychologically dependent on drugs. Although these users try to carry out their daily activities at home, school, or work, their actions are usually ineffective.

250

- *Dependent users* rely on drugs physically and psychologically and will go to great lengths to get them. Without drugs they become severely distressed, mentally and physically.

Do you know someone who fits into one of these patterns? Dependent users all started with experimental use of drugs. Can you see how drug abuse can progress from one pattern to another? What kind of physical, emotional, and legal risks might result from even a one-time drug experiment? Think about these important questions as you read about different types of drugs.

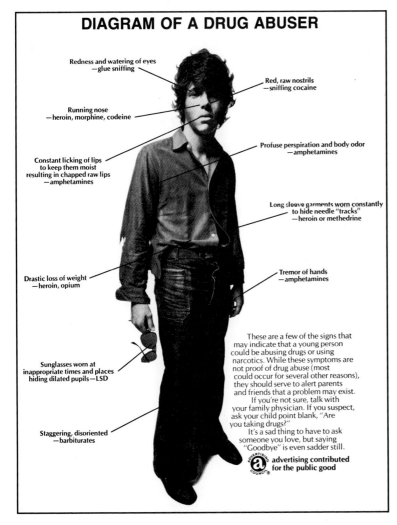

DIAGRAM OF A DRUG ABUSER

Redness and watering of eyes
—glue sniffing

Red, raw nostrils
—sniffing cocaine

Running nose
—heroin, morphine, codeine

Profuse perspiration and body odor
—amphetamines

Constant licking of lips
to keep them moist
resulting in chapped raw lips
—amphetamines

Long sleeve garments worn constantly
to hide needle "tracks"
—heroin or methedrine

Drastic loss of weight
—heroin, opium

Tremor of hands
—amphetamines

Sunglasses worn at
inappropriate times and places
hiding dilated pupils—LSD

These are a few of the signs that may indicate that a young person could be abusing drugs or using narcotics. While these symptoms are not proof of drug abuse (most could occur for several other reasons), they should serve to alert parents and friends that a problem may exist.
If you're not sure, talk with your family physician. If you suspect, ask your child point blank, "Are you taking drugs?"
It's a sad thing to have to ask someone you love, but saying "Goodbye" is even sadder still.

Staggering, disoriented
—barbiturates

ⓐ advertising contributed
for the public good

12–4. *Do you know someone who has these symptoms?*

TYPES OF ABUSED DRUGS

INHALANTS

What do room deodorizers, nail polish, model airplane glue, household cement, paint thinner, varnish, and shellac all have in common? Besides being household products, they all contain chemicals that evaporate and can be inhaled. Any substance that is inhaled may be called an **inhalant.** Many inhalants are used in medicine to relieve symptoms such as those of asthma. But inhalants that are abused contain dangerous drugs that can cause serious health damage. Inhalants such as nitrous oxide, aerosol propellants, amyl nitrite (snappers, poppers), and butyl nitrite (Rush, Bullet, Jac Aroma, Locker Room) are also dangerous.

The effects of inhalants on behavior are similar to those of alcohol. They cause dizziness, loss of muscle coordination, slurred speech, blurred vision, nausea, and depression. They can also cause imaginary sights and sounds, loss of color perception, ringing in the ears, and sometimes violent behavior.

The initial effects last for 15 to 45 minutes. However, in the second stage, which may last for an hour or more, drowsiness and sometimes unconsciousness occur. Sniffers almost always receive more than they expect. The poisonous fumes they sniff can cause brain and nerve damage, as well as liver, kidney, and bone damage. Low blood pressure and weight loss have also been reported. Inhalants can cause sudden death in one of several ways. Sniffing highly concentrated aerosols can cause heart failure. Some inhalants depress breathing until it stops. The toxic fumes can displace oxygen in the lungs causing suffocation.

Some inhalants produce tolerance quickly. At first a user may need only a few whiffs to feel high. But, as the person becomes a regular user, increased amounts of the chemical are needed for the same effects.

Who are inhalant abusers? Because inhalants can be obtained easily, children as young as age 7 use these drugs. But teenagers, particularly boys, are the most frequent users.

STIMULANTS

Stimulants are drugs that increase certain functions of the central nervous system. When taken, the user becomes more active, alert, and nervous. If you have ever drunk coffee, tea, or cola, then you have taken caffeine, one of the most com-

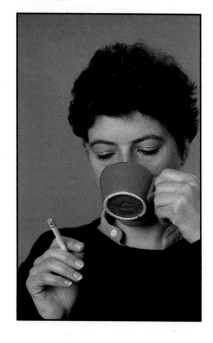

12–5. Nicotine and caffeine are commonly used stimulants.

monly used stimulants. Caffeine is also found in many OTC products. When used in excess, caffeine can produce a jittery feeling or nausea. Another familiar stimulant is nicotine, found in tobacco products.

There are stronger and more dangerous stimulants, such as *amphetamines* and *cocaine*. They give the user a quick elevation of mood and a false sense of well-being, self-confidence, power, and energy. Psychological dependence grows quickly. Heart action increases and blood pressure rises. These effects are heightened if stimulants are injected.

When a stimulant's effect wears off, the user feels tired and depressed. This is sometimes called the down phase, or crashing. Tolerance to stimulants builds with repeated use. Withdrawal from stimulants after heavy use can cause mental breakdowns and suicidal depression.

AMPHETAMINES (peaches, uppers, bennies, speed).

In medicine, **amphetamines** are sometimes used to combat fatigue, prevent drowsiness, reduce appetite, and treat nervous system disorders. When prescribed, the doses are small. They are given only for short periods of time. The medical names for some amphetamines are Benzedrine, Dexedrine and Methedrine.

All amphetamines stimulate the nervous system. Sometimes they cause dilation of the pupils, a dry mouth, sweating, headaches, and diarrhea. Regular use of these drugs can damage physical and mental health. Heavy users may become fearful and mistrustful of others. This mental state can lead to violent behavior. An overdose can cause collapse of the circulatory system, convulsions, coma, and

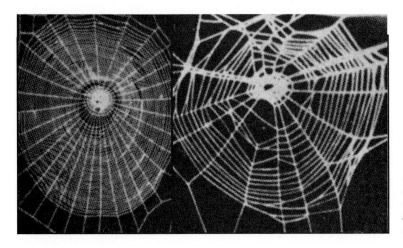

12–6. On the left is a normal symmetrical spider web. On the right is an abnormal web spun by a spider that was subjected to amphetamines.

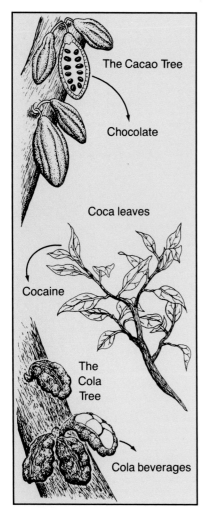

The Cacao Tree

Chocolate

Coca leaves

Cocaine

The Cola Tree

Cola beverages

12–7. Cocaine is made from coca leaves. Cola beverages are made from decocainized leaves of the coca plant and cola nuts. Chocolate is made from the cacao plant.

death. An injection produces a much greater effect than that of a pill. In the drug culture, *speeding* refers to the repeated use of amphetamines, often Methedrine, in high doses over a short period of time. Speeding is extremely dangerous and can even be fatal.

Many people do not realize that amphetamines have dangerous side effects. Therefore, they are widely abused. Some students may use them to stay awake while cramming for exams. Long-distance truck drivers have used them to stay alert on trips, thereby causing traffic accidents.

COCAINE (snow, big C, coke, nose candy). What did the Incas and Sigmund Freud have in common? They were all users of *cocaine*. The history of cocaine goes back to the Incas, who first discovered the powers of coca leaves, from which cocaine is made. The Incas chewed the leaves for energy and strength, and believed that they were gifts from the gods. For a short time, Freud used cocaine in psychiatry. He first tried it himself, and then prescribed it to patients as a cure for depression. Later he realized that cocaine had harmful effects, so he no longer used it himself or prescribed it to his patients.

Today doctors still use cocaine as a local anesthetic during ear, nose, or throat operations. When applied, it numbs the skin or mucous membranes. For the most part, new anesthetics have now replaced cocaine.

When abused, the drug is usually sniffed or snorted in powdered form. It is then absorbed by the mucous membranes of the nose and throat. Sometimes cocaine is eaten or injected into a vein. When cocaine is smoked in its pure base form, called "freebase," it produces a much stronger and more dangerous effect.

What is a cocaine high? It is similar to a strong amphetamine high. It is a temporary feeling of pleasure. Fatigue seems to vanish and appetite is reduced. A regular user often experiences hallucinations of touch, taste, sound, or smell. When the effects of the cocaine wear off, the user experiences a feeling of depression and sometimes a paranoid fear.

Cocaine can be physically damaging as well. Sniffing cocaine can severely damage the nasal membranes. It can also increase the heart rate by 50 percent and speed respiration. Such dramatic changes in the body have caused deaths by heart attack or lung failure. Cocaine deaths are most common when the drug is injected or smoked.

Can you become addicted to cocaine? While there is still some debate about whether cocaine is physically addictive, there is no doubt that users quickly become psychologically dependent on it. This dependence is so strong that users are unable to quit even when cocaine use severely damages their personal lives. Despite the illegal drug's high cost, the abuse of cocaine is unfortunately becoming more common.

DEPRESSANTS

How do **depressant** drugs affect the body? We do know that they reduce the action of the nerves, heart, and skeletal muscles. They also slow down breathing and lower blood pressure. Depressants have legitimate medical uses and may be prescribed to treat emotional disorders.

Alcohol, a depressant, is the drug most often abused in this country. When used with another depressant, the combination is very dangerous. The body systems can be slowed down to the point of coma or death.

BARBITURATES (barbs, bluebirds, blue devils, reds, downers, goofballs, rainbows, yellow jackets). Barbiturates are often classified according to how long their effects last. Phenobarbital (Luminal) is the best-known long acting barbiturate. Short to intermediate-acting barbiturates include amobarbital (Amytal), pentobarbital (Nembutal), and secobarbital (Seconal). Ultrashort-acting barbiturates are used primarily as anesthetics. An example of one is thiopental (Pentothal). All of the barbiturates are derived from barbituric acid. Usually barbiturates can be recognized by their names. If you look at the drugs listed, you will notice that they all have names that end with the letters "al."

When used without medical supervision, barbiturates have unpredictable effects. Their effects not only vary from person to person but they also vary within the same person from one time to the next. The effects are often similar to those of excess alcohol. Users experience mental confusion, slurred speech, staggering, and deep sleep. Barbiturates may also bring on extreme depression, causing users to feel tired and hopeless. When in this depressed state, users may reach for the rest of a bottle and "end it all" on purpose. They may also become confused and forget how many tablets they have already taken. Then they may take an overdose by accident. This explains why barbiturates are a leading cause of drug-related deaths. Because barbiturates can distort vision and slow reaction time, they can cause accidents of all kinds.

Barbiturates are strongly addicting, both physically and mentally. The body also develops a tolerance to these drugs. Users must take more and more of them to ward off withdrawal sickness. Sudden withdrawal causes nausea, severe cramps, convulsions, delirium, and coma. A person undergoing withdrawal must be hospitalized for several weeks.

TRANQUILIZERS. Tranquilizers are known for their quieting effects. You may be familiar with tranquilizers by the trade names Equanil, Miltown, Thorazine, Librium, and Valium. These drugs are prescribed for anxiety and for certain psychological problems.

Ordinarily, tranquilizers do not produce mind-altering effects. Since they were once considered to be relatively harmless, they were widely prescribed. Now, however, both the National Institute on Drug Abuse and the National Institute for Mental Health urge that physicians and patients use these drugs more cautiously. Misusing tranquilizers can cause physical and psychological dependence. Taking tranquilizers and alcohol together can cause death.

METHAQUALONE (ludes, quads, sopor, sopes, 714's). Methaqualones are known by the trade names Quaalude, Parest, Optimil, Somnafac, and Sopor. These drugs were once thought to be safe, but today we know that this is untrue.

Small doses produce feelings of calm and well-being. Large doses produce feelings of elation. Methaqualone has many harmful side effects, including headaches, nosebleeds, dizziness, diarrhea, loss of coordination, skin numbness, and arm and leg pain. Tolerance and psychological and physical dependence develops with continued use. Withdrawal can produce symptoms similar to barbiturate withdrawal. The practice of "luding out," combining this drug with alcohol, can cause death.

MARIJUANA (Acapulco gold, ganga, grass, Mary Jane, pot, weed). Marijuana's botanical name is *Cannabis sativa*, but most people simply refer to it as marijuana. This plant has been grown for centuries. The stems are used for rope, and its oil is used in paint. However, today it is most widely used for its mind-altering effects.

How is marijuana used as a drug? The dried leaves and flowers of the plant are crushed.Then it is put into pipes or

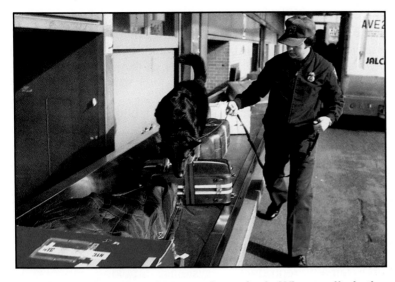

12–8. At airports, police dogs are trained to sniff out drugs hidden in luggage.

rolled into cigarette papers and smoked. When rolled, the cigarettes are known as reefer, joints, sticks, and smoke. The smoke from the drug has a distinctively sweet odor, like that of burning dried grass or rope. In powdered form marijuana is sometimes sniffed or taken with food. *Hashish*, also known as hash, is a concentrated form of marijuana. "Hash oil" is a concentrated liquid extract made from marijuana.

The mind-altering effects of marijuana vary from person to person. The effects also vary depending on the amount taken in and the amount of **tetrahydrocannabinol** (te-tra-hi-dro-ka-**na**-be-nul), or THC, the marijuana contains. THC is the main psychoactive substance in marijuana. Since 1975, THC levels of marijuana available in the United States have greatly increased. Therefore, marijuana today may pose greater risks to users than ever before.

After alcohol and nicotine, marijuana is the most widely abused drug in our country. Its widespread use has led many people to believe that it is harmless. In low doses marijuana produces feelings of drunkenness. The user may feel light-headed, giddy, relaxed, or peaceful. Some users have reported that marijuana distorts the senses of taste, touch, sound, and smell. Marijuana increases heart rate, lowers body temperature, and reduces blood sugar levels. This latter effect causes a craving for food. The eyes become red and the mouth and throat become dry.

Marijuana also distorts a sense of time and space, causes memory loss, and impairs judgment. Some users become unsteady and have trouble with coordination. In this state

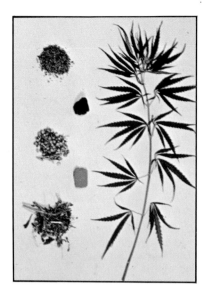

12–9. The marijuana plant and its derivatives

they cannot respond quickly. These effects last several hours after the drug is taken. Like alcohol, driving after or during marijuana use is hazardous. Marijuana impairs learning ability and sports performance. Because of its effect on memory, users are unable to concentrate and comprehend in the classroom.

Sometimes marijuana can produce feelings of depression and moodiness. Marijuana can cause feelings of intense fear and anxiety, often called a "pot panic." Larger doses of the drug can cause hallucinations. This is why marijuana is sometimes classified as a hallucinogenic drug.

How dangerous is marijuana? Its long term effects are still being studied. Evidence suggests that marijuana is more harmful than was once thought. After using marijuana, the chemicals in it remain in the body for up to a month. Studies indicate that marijuana disrupts the functioning of the male and female reproductive systems. Smoking tobacco is known to cause lung diseases. What about smoking marijuana? Marijuana smoke contains some of the same chemicals that are found in tobacco smoke. One of these chemicals is a known cancer-causing agent. Marijuana smoke contains 70 percent more of this chemical than tobacco smoke contains. Marijuana smokers inhale more deeply, and hold the smoke in their lungs for longer periods. Also, marijuana cigarettes lack filters to cut down on the harmful chemicals inhaled. Scientists believe that ongoing research will prove that marijuana smoking increases a user's risks of getting lung diseases as much as, or even more than, cigarette smoking.

Do you know what the term "burn out" means? It has been used to describe the effects often observed in heavy, long-term marijuana users. Burned-out users may believe they are fine, but to others their thinking seems slow and confused. In most cases, a user's mental state improves after several weeks of not using marijuana. It is not known whether or not prolonged use causes irreversible damage.

Although marijuana may not be physically addictive, strong psychological dependence often develops. Tolerance may develop with regular users. Because of its effects on the mind, body, and learning, doctors are especially concerned about marijuana use during adolescence. Young people are still maturing sexually, physically, and mentally. They are learning skills and gaining knowledge needed for a lifetime. Any of the effects just discussed may prevent a teenager from becoming a healthy, normal adult.

HALLUCINOGENS

Hallucinogens, sometimes called *psychedelics*, are drugs that produce hallucinations. They have been proclaimed as quick trips to bliss or shortcuts to discovering the inner self. Often what they produce are quick rides to the hospital. After taking these drugs, the physical senses and the feelings of time and space are altered. Although some think that such effects can expand the mind, users know that they can be terrifying, and do not lead to inner discovery. Under the influence of hallucinogens, fact and fantasy are so confused that violent acts and accidental death can result.

Users develop a tolerance to hallucinogens, but not physical dependence. The chances of developing psychological dependence on these drugs is great.

LSD (acid). If you asked most people to name a hallucinogenic drug, they would probably say LSD. LSD is the abbreviation for lysergic acid diethylamide. It is a very potent hallucinogen, and tolerance builds quickly. An average dose, no bigger than a speck of dust, can produce effects that last eight to ten hours. A dose can be taken on a sugar cube, a cracker, or a cookie. LSD can also be taken in the form of a pill. LSD has no current medical use.

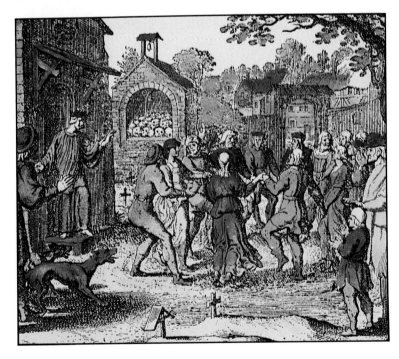

12–10. A phenomenon called the St. Vitus Dance *occurred in fourteenth century Europe. For unknown reasons, people danced convulsively on the streets. Today, drug researchers theorize that the St. Vitus Dance was caused by a mold on grain that produced a substance similar to LSD.*

What happens on an LSD trip? The effect of LSD cannot be predicted. LSD users experience physical changes, such as an increase in heart rate or a rise in blood pressure. Chills, fever, trembling, loss of appetite, and nausea can also occur. Some users see strange visual images and brighter, more intense colors. Sometimes LSD seems to cause confusion in the brain's sensory areas. Music may appear as colors or colors as flavors or odors. Some users experience panic when they realize that these effects cannot be stopped. Others become terrified because they think that their lives are being threatened. These symptoms are the same as those of paranoid schizophrenia. In this state of mind users are dangerous to themselves and to others.

Anxiety, depression, and loss of a sense of reality may last from days to months. Flashbacks of an LSD trip may occur days, weeks, and even months after use.

PCP (angel dust, crystal, peace pills, superjoint, busy bee, green tea leaves, elephant tranquilizer, DOA or dead on arrival, hog). In the 1950's and the 1960's, this potent drug was used as an anesthetic on humans. However, its use was banned because of its unpleasant side effects. In 1967, PCP surfaced from underground laboratories and could be bought on the streets. Although its common slang name is "angel dust," this synthetic drug is no heavenly experience. It has been related to many murders, suicides, and accidental deaths.

Why does PCP claim so many lives? Its effects are wildly unpredictable. In one user a dose of PCP can produce a state of drunkenness. In others, the same dose can produce depression, paranoia, hallucinations, and thoughts of death. In large doses the drug can cause violent rages, psychosis, stupor, coma, and death.

Usually, PCP is sprinkled on parsley, mint leaves, or marijuana. Then it is smoked. It can also be snorted like cocaine, swallowed as a pill, or injected. Once taken, PCP stays in the system for a long time. Behavioral and psychological changes can persist even after the PCP is no longer in the system. If overdoses of PCP are taken, treatment is difficult. Those who overdose must be hospitalized.

Why would anyone take such a dangerous drug? Since more people are learning the real facts about PCP, its use is on the decline. But there are still many people who are unaware of its dangers. Some drug users take PCP as a new high. Others may think they are actually buying LSD, THC, or cocaine.

12–11. PCP rock crystal. PCP is one of the most dangerous drugs to surface in many years.

Control of this drug is difficult. There are many home-made PCP labs across the country. Today narcotics agents are working to uncover and get rid of these makeshift operations. Many past users of PCP are helping the authorities to stop illegal traffic of the drug. What does that tell you about the effects of PCP?

PEYOTE AND MESCALINE (beans, buttons, cactus, mesc, mescal, moon). The Aztecs discovered that the peyote cactus could produce strange visions. The substance in peyote that causes hallucinations is mescaline, and it can be made synthetically.

In its natural form peyote is chewed or brewed in tea. In its synthetic form it is injected or swallowed.

The effects of peyote can be severe. It is common to experience nausea, cramps in the stomach, sweating, and vomiting for several hours. Following this, the user experiences hallucinations for a period of four to twelve hours.

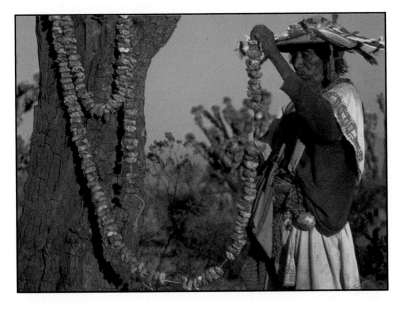

12–12. The Huichol Indians in Oaxaca, Mexico use peyote in sacred rituals.

PSILOCYBIN AND PSILOCYN (sacred mushroom, magic mushroom). Have you heard of mushrooms that cause hallucinations? There are such mushrooms, from which psilocybin, a psychoactive drug, is made. They have been used for centuries in ceremonies of the Mexican and Central American Indians. Usually they are swallowed, and the effects, similar to those of mescaline, last for about six hours.

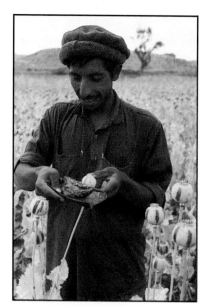

12–13. Opium is harvested from the unripened pods of poppies.

12–14. During the Civil War, morphine was used to relieve pain. As a result, many soldiers became morphine addicts.

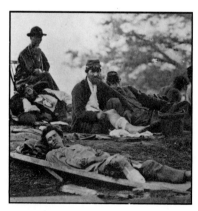

NARCOTICS

Narcotic drugs, sometimes called *opiates*, are a product of the opium poppy. Legally, narcotics are used in medicine as pain relievers or cough suppressors and as remedies for diarrhea or other intestinal problems. These drugs depress the central nervous system and create a short-term sense of elation. They also induce drowsiness or sleep. Decreased physical activity and visual ability are also common. Physicians prescribe narcotics for patients carefully. Tolerance grows quickly with narcotic use. These drugs cause strong physical and pyschological dependence. Which drugs belong to the narcotics family? Opium, morphine, codeine, heroin, and methadone are the best-known narcotics.

OPIUM. Opium is made from unripened pods of poppies. All other narcotics are made from opium. Afghanistan, Iran, Pakistan, Laos, Thailand, and Mexico are the countries in which opium is produced for illegal sale.

In the early 1900's, opium was often smoked in a pipe. Today it is no longer widely abused in the United States. Opium brings on a dreamy stupor or unconsciousness that lasts for several hours.

Paregoric, a mild narcotic made from opium, is used in medicine. Since it slows the contractions of the smooth muscle in the digestive tract, paregoric relieves abdominal and digestive pain and diarrhea.

MORPHINE (cube, first line, hocus, Miss Emma, mud). Have you ever heard the saying "the arms of Morpheus"? Morpheus was the Greek god of dreams and the namesake for the drug *morphine*. In its pure form, morphine is a fine, white powder with a bitter taste. It is also a very effective pain-killer. During the Civil War morphine was widely used as a pain-killer for injured soldiers. Many of these soldiers became postwar morphine addicts. Today morphine is often used after surgery or for cancer cases. Small doses relieve pain, and larger doses induce sleep.

CODEINE. If you have ever had a severe cough or toothache, you may have been given a prescription for a codeine preparation. Aspirin plus codeine tablets (APC) are prescribed for pain relief. When used in cough medicines, codeine quiets the cough reflex.

Codeine is the least addicting drug of the narcotics. Nonetheless, anyone using codeine products should follow his or her physician's directions carefully.

HEROIN (big H, horse, junk, scag, smack).   When heroin was first made from morphine in 1874, it was thought to be a cure for morphine addiction. Several years later physicians realized that heroin also produces dependency. Today its medical use is illegal in the United States.

Addicts often begin using heroin by sniffing or smoking the drug in powdered form. Since tolerance develops quickly, addicts resort to injecting a heroin solution into their veins to heighten its effects. This practice is called *mainlining*. As the senses become dull, the user's tensions, fears, and worries ease. This stage is followed by a stupor that can last several hours. In this stupor, hunger and thirst are reduced.

What happens when heroin use stops? Within 12 to 16 hours, addicts experience severe withdrawal symptoms, including sweating, shaking, chills, nausea, diarrhea, abdominal pain, and cramps in the legs. Severe mental and emotional anguish are also experienced. The only way to stop these symptoms is to take another dose of the drug.

What other health hazards do heroin addicts face? Death at an early age is not unusual. Some addicts die from overdoses because they buy drugs of unknown strength and purity. As tolerance grows, it becomes more difficult to distinguish between safe and dangerous drug doses. Another common problem is due to using dirty needles, which can cause severe infections such as blood poisoning and liver disease. Severe malnutrition and self-neglect are other common problems of the addict.

Because of heroin's high cost, getting money to pay for a daily supply becomes a bigger and bigger problem for an addict. Heroin can be purchased only from pushers, who are usually part of a drug ring. To get the money for drugs, the addict often resorts to stealing or other crimes.

METHADONE.   When World War II created a morphine shortage, chemists made *methadone*. Its effects are similar to morphine and heroin. Medically it can be used to relieve pain or to treat heroin addiction. Methadone blocks the addict's need for heroin and prevents the onset of withdrawal symptoms. Careful medical supervision is required to control the dosage. When used illegally by those who are not dependent on heroin, it produces a narcotic effect. A methadone overdose can cause death. Methadone, like other narcotics, can become addictive. Addicts go through withdrawal sypmtoms when they stop taking the drug abruptly.

CONTROLLED SUBSTANCES: USES AND EFFECTS

	Drugs	Often Prescribed Brand Names	Medical Uses	Physical Dependence Potential	Psychological Dependence Potential
NARCOTICS	Opium	Dover's Powder, Paregoric	Analgesic, antidiarrheal	High	High
	Morphine	Morphine	Analgesic	High	High
	Codeine	Codeine	Analgesic	Moderate	Moderate
	Heroin	None	None	High	High
	Meperidine (Pethidine)	Demerol, Pethadol	Analgesic	High	High
	Methadone	Dolophine, Methadone, Methadose	Analgesic, heroin substitute	High	High
	Other Narcotics	Dilaudid, Leritine, Numorphan, Percodan	Analgesic, antidiarrheal	High	High
DEPRESSANTS	Chloral Hydrate	Noctec, Somnos	Hypnotic	Moderate	Moderate
	Barbiturates	Amytal, Butisal, Nembutal, Phenobarbital, Seconal	Anesthetic, anticonvulsant, sedation, sleep	High	High
	Glutethimide	Doriden	Sedation, sleep	High	High
	Methaqualone	Optimil, Parest, Quaalude, Somnafac, Sopor	Sedation, sleep	High	High
	Tranquilizers	Equanil, Librium, Miltown, Serax, Tranxene, Valium	Antianxiety, muscle relaxant, sedation	Moderate	Moderate
	Other Depressants	Clonopin, Dalmane, Dormate, Noludar, Placydill, Valmid	Antianxiety, sedation, sleep	Possible	Possible
STIMULANTS	Cocaine	Cocaine	Local anesthetic	Probable	High
	Amphetamines	Benzedrine, Biphetamine, Desoxyn, Dexedrine	Hyperkinesis, narcolepsy, weight control	Possible	High
	Phenmatrazine	Preludin	Weight control	Possible	High
	Methylphenidate	Ritalin, Bacarate, Cylert, Didrex	Hyperkinesis	Possible	High
	Other Stimulants	Ionamin, Plegine, Pondimin, Pre-Sate, Sanorex, Voranil	Weight control	Possible	Possible
HALLUCINOGENS	LSD	None	None	None	Degree Unknown
	Mescaline	None	None	None	Degree Unknown
	Psilocybin-Psilocyn	None	None	None	Degree Unknown
	PCP	Sernylan	Veterinary anesthetic	None	Degree Unknown
	Other Hallucinogens	None	None	None	Degree Unknown
CANNABIS	Marijuana, Hashish	None	None	Probable	Moderate

Tolerance	Duration of Effects (in hours)	Usual Methods of Administration	Possible Effects	Effects of Long Term Use or Overdose	Withdrawal Syndrome
Yes	3 to 6	Oral, smoked	Euphoria, drowsiness, respiratory depression, constricted pupils, nausea	Slow and shallow breathing, clammy skin, convulsions, coma, possible death	Watery eyes, runny nose, yawning, loss of appetite, irritability, tremors, panic, chills and sweating, cramps, nausea
Yes	3 to 6	Injected, smoked			
Yes	3 to 6	Oral, injected			
Yes	3 to 6	Injected, sniffed			
Yes	3 to 6	Oral, injected			
Yes	12 to 24	Oral, injected			
Yes	3 to 6	Oral, injected			
Probable	5 to 8	Oral	Slurred speech, disorientation, drunken behavior without odor of alcohol	Shallow respiration, cold and clammy skin, dilated pupils, weak and rapid pulse, coma, possible death	Anxiety, insomnia, tremors, delirium, convulsions, possible death
Yes	1 to 16	Oral, injected			
Yes	4 to 8	Oral			
Yes	4 to 8	Oral			
Yes	4 to 8	Oral			
Yes	4 to 8	Oral			
Yes	2	Injected, sniffed	Increased alertness, excitation, euphoria, dilated pupils, increased pulse rate and blood pressure, insomnia, loss of appetite	Agitation, increase in body temperature, hallucinations, convulsions, possible death	Apathy, long periods of sleep, irritability, depression, disorientation
Yes	2 to 4	Oral, injected			
Yes	2 to 4	Oral			
Yes	2 to 4	Oral			
Yes	2 to 4	Oral			
Yes	Variable	Oral	Illusions and hallucinations, poor perception of time and distance	Longer, more intense trip episodes, psychosis, possible death	Withdrawal syndrome not reported
Yes	Variable	Oral, injected			
Yes	Variable	Oral			
Yes	Variable	Oral, injected, smoked			
Yes	Variable	Oral, injected, sniffed			
Yes	2 to 4	Oral, smoked	Euphoria, increased appetite, disoriented behavior, short term memory loss	Lung damage, possible reproductive damage, loss of motivation	Insomnia, hyperactivity, and decreased appetite reported in a limited number of individuals

TREATMENT AND PREVENTION

How widespread is the drug problem? According to estimates, since the mid-1970's the number of heroin addicts has remained at about half a million. Accurate statistics on the overall number of drug abusers are almost impossible to obtain. This is because drug abuse by teenagers and adults often goes unnoticed until a crisis occurs. However, a national survey on drug abuse, conducted yearly on behalf of the National Institute on Drug Abuse, provides information on trends in drug use. It reported a dramatic increase among teenagers and adults in marijuana and cocaine use since 1972. This fact has alarmed public health officials. They realize that more must be done to prevent drug abuse.

AID FOR ABUSERS

EMERGENCY AID. Do you know when emergency treatment is needed for drug abuse? Signs of a drug overdose or other serious reactions needing urgent care include unconsciousness, semiconsciousness, or confused mental state. The person may not be alert enough to answer questions. He or she may have severe difficulty in breathing. Bizarre or violent behavior and threats of suicide are other signs of an overdose.

When a person is unconscious, apply first aid as outlined in Chapter 27. In all cases, call for help or seek immediate medical care at a hospital emergency room or community mental health center. Both deal with mental and physical emergencies caused by drug abuse. Once the crisis is past, the person is directed to other sources of help.

DETOXIFICATION. When users are physically dependent on drugs, chemical **detoxification** is the first step in treatment. During detoxification, the drug is excreted from the body. The abuser receives medical treatment, either as a hospital inpatient or as an outpatient. In cases of heroin addiction, methadone is often prescribed to reduce withdrawal symptoms. Once detoxification is complete, ongoing help must be provided. This is because strong psychological dependence on drugs still remains. Without ongoing help, the ex-addict usually starts taking drugs again.

MAINTENANCE PROGRAMS. For the heroin addict, ongoing treatment often includes methadone maintenance. Regular, medically supervised doses of methadone are given

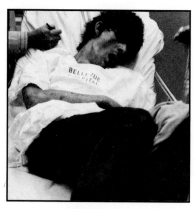

12–15. Detoxification may produce acute withdrawal symptoms.

as a drug substitute to block the physical effects of heroin. Usually this treatment lasts for a year or longer. During this time counseling and other services are provided. When rehabilitation is completed, the addict is gradually weaned from methadone.

DRUG-FREE PROGRAMS. Therapeutic communities are for drug abusers who are drug-free. Their purpose is to help abusers overcome their psychological cravings for a drug life-style. Members of these communities live together, either full time or part time. They support one another in overcoming their mental dependencies. Besides peer support, counseling or therapy is provided. Members learn how to handle their problems without drugs. They may also participate in job training programs.

Other types of drug-free programs may provide services such as individual or group therapy, conversational (rap) sessions, recreational activities, remediation, and job counseling and training. Most programs encourage parents to participate in their activities. Some programs operate independently or as part of drug-free clinics sponsored by hospitals or community mental health centers. Are you familiar with the programs available in your community?

FINDING HELP. Could you find help if you or a friend had a problem? Your parents, doctor, clergy member, school nurse, teacher, or other adults may be able to assist you in finding the help you need. Also, check the yellow pages of the telephone book under listings such as drugs, drug abuse, counseling, youth, family, mental health, or social services. In many communities there are drug abuse or crisis hotlines. Their numbers can be obtained from your local telephone operator. Many drug programs are entirely free, and they are confidential.

DOES TREATMENT WORK? The answer to this question is yes, if there is a desire on the part of the individual user to change. Studies show that detoxification alone seldom brings lasting results. However, for those who want to free themselves from drugs and who participate fully in ongoing treatment, the success rate is high. Yet, many abusers don't truly recognize that they have a problem. They simply go through the motions of attending a treatment program, denying that they need help. These abusers usually drop out of treatment programs and go back to using drugs. Before drug abusers can be helped, they must want to help themselves.

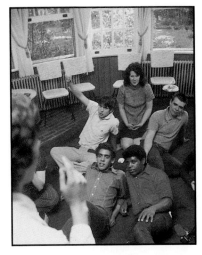

12–16. Rap sessions are often a part of drug-free programs.

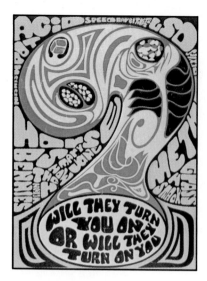

12–17. How do you interpret this message?

PREVENTION: THE ANSWER TO ABUSE

How can drug abuse be prevented? Under state and federal law, stiff penalties are imposed for the illegal sale and possession of drugs. Under international agreements, strict control measures have been designed to stop illegal drug traffic. Strict law enforcement together with effective treatments for drug abuse must continue.

However, the only real answer to drug abuse is prevention. First of all, people must learn the facts about drug abuse so that they can make better decisions. But this is only a first step. Learning to make decisions that help you avoid drug abuse is what prevention is really all about. Decision-making is not always easy. It can be very hard when it means taking a stand that differs from that of your peers. But each time you make a decision on your own, you exercise your most important right as an individual. This is the right to choose what is best for you and for others. Prevention also extends to your friends. When your friends need advice or just someone to listen, you can show by your presence that you care. In this way, you can help prevent others from turning to drugs as an escape from problems.

DECISIONS AND DRUGS

Throughout life, you will need to make decisions about the proper medical use or abuse of drugs. However, during the teenage years, the pressure to abuse drugs can be especially strong. You want to be accepted by your peers. Your problems may seem too large to solve. Or you may feel that you have no one to whom you can talk. Instead of trying to escape from your problems by taking drugs, consider the positive ways to cope with your emotions. To some teenagers, trying drugs seems no different than experimenting with other new ways of doing things. As you have learned, drug abuse *is* different from other activities. There are serious risks that should be considered before making a decision about drugs. What do you have to lose by your actions? Is there anything that you really gain? You owe it to yourself and others to consider these questions carefully. Every time you get involved in a worthwhile activity, you are choosing an alternative to drugs. Activities that help you relax, make you feel good about yourself, or teach you something new are all healthful and promote well-being. Using drugs can never be a substitute for these healthful activities. Figure 12-18 shows some of these activities. What others can you add?

HEALTH TIP

Always turn on the bathroom light when you take drugs at night. Never take drugs in the dark. Many pills and bottles look alike. Each year people needlessly experience harmful drug reactions when the wrong drug is taken.

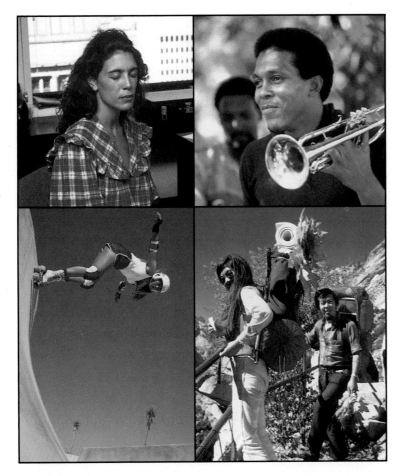

12–18. Here are some alternatives to drug abuse. Can you think of others?

SUMMARY: A drug is any chemical substance that alters the mind or body. Drugs can produce tolerance, and psychological and physical dependence. All abused drugs affect the nervous system, distort the senses, cause emotional upsets, and change behavior. Inhalants are volatile chemicals that cause intoxication when inhaled. Stimulants excite the central nervous system and make users feel tense and alert. Depressants slow the action of the nervous system. Hallucinogens produce sensory distortions and emotional instability.

Treatment varies for drug abusers. Chemical detoxification is necessary when a user is physically addicted to a drug. Ongoing help is needed for abusers to break psychological drug dependence.

Prevention is the best answer to drug abuse. This involves learning not only the facts about drugs, but how to make decisions about drug use.

CHAPTER REVIEW

words at work

Find the word in the left column that fits one of the definitions in the right column. DO NOT WRITE IN THIS BOOK.

a. synergistic
b. detoxification
c. addiction
d. butyl nitrite
e. tolerance
f. opium
g. methadone
h. PCP
i. marijuana
j. cocaine

1. a stimulant
2. larger drug doses producing the same effect
3. a depressant
4. increased drug effects through drug interaction
5. a synthetic narcotic
6. a hallucinogen
7. an inhalant
8. a natural narcotic
9. physical and psychological dependence
10. removal of drugs from the body

review questions

1. Is vitamin C a drug? Explain your answer.
2. Define the term *over-the-counter* (OTC) drug. Give an example of an OTC drug.
3. What is a prescription drug? Give an example of a prescription drug.
4. List several medical uses of drugs.
5. Why are many drugs limited to prescription use?
6. Name three factors that are considered by physicians when prescribing drugs.
7. Why should a drug prescription only be used for whom it was written?
8. Describe the synergistic effect of drugs.
9. What is psychological drug dependence?
10. Name four types of drug users and describe their patterns of drug abuse.
11. Explain the cause of withdrawal sickness.
12. Name four types of drugs that are abused and their effects.
13. Describe the action of barbiturates on the nervous system.
14. To what extent are barbiturates addicting?
15. Why is cocaine use harmful?
16. Describe the harmful side effects of methaqualone.
17. Why is it dangerous to drive after marijuana use?
18. Name the possible long-term effects of marijuana use.
19. Define the term *narcotic*. Give an example of natural and synthetic narcotics.

20. Name four symptoms of a drug overdose.
21. Outline the steps that should be taken when emergency aid for drug abuse is needed.
22. How does "detoxification" aid in the treatment of drug abusers?
23. Describe three services of drug-free treatment programs.

discussion questions

1. Do you think drug abuse among young people is rising or declining? State evidence to support your views.
2. Discuss why and how people get "hooked" on drugs. Describe any differences between adults and teenagers in this addictive process.
3. Compare physical and psychological dependence. In most cases, do you think these problems coexist in the addicted person? If so, why?
4. How does addiction affect a person's life and behavior? Is drug use among young people more damaging than adult abuse? Why or why not?
5. In your opinion, what actions might help prevent drug abuse among young people? Discuss the role of parents, peers, and the school.

investigating

PURPOSE:
To apply the decision-making process to real-life situations.

MATERIALS NEEDED:
Paper and pen.

PROCEDURE:
A. Study the decision-making tree in the Appendix.
B. Reread the opening story of Gene found on page 247.
C. Draw a decision-making tree for Gene based on the assumption that he chose not to use drugs. Refer to the information in the chapter as necessary. Consider and include all possible positive and negative effects that might affect his choices such as health, family, friends, and legal considerations.
D. Write an ending to the story describing how Gene later assesses his decision.
E. Compare and discuss each step of your tree and your story endings in class.
    1. What three effects would you rank as most influential in Gene's decision-making process? Why? (Rank the top three.)
    2. Look at Step 4 on your decision-making tree, the positive and the negative effects of each choice.
    3. Which three effects would you rank as least influential? Why?
    4. If Gene had chosen to smoke the marijuana, which factor do you think would have most influenced his decision? Why?

CHAPTER 13

Alcohol

OBJECTIVES

- IDENTIFY patterns of alcohol use and some reasons for this behavior
- EXPLAIN why alcohol is a drug and OUTLINE its effect on the mind and body
- DISCUSS the effects of alcohol on society
- DEFINE alcoholism and CITE its signs and stages and effects on life
- DESCRIBE programs that help alcoholics and their families

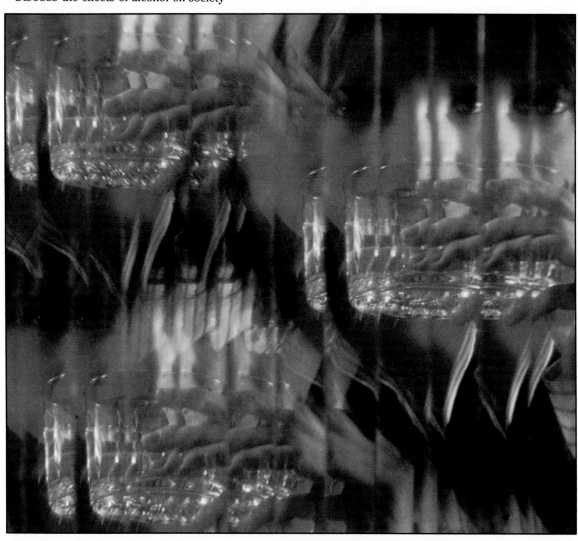

Vanessa was excited about her first date with Wade and the New Year's party. "What would you like to drink?" Wade asked Vanessa. "Is there any soda?" she said. "Sure," Wade replied. "But you don't want that. It's New Year's Eve." "That's right," added his friends, Sue and John. "This is a party, remember?" Vanessa refused. "OK," said Wade grudgingly, as he continued to sip his wine.

By the party's end, there had been lots of celebrating. "C'mon, everyone, let's grow, I mean go." Wade announced. "Are you sure you can drive, Wade?" Vanessa asked nervously. "Don't worry," Wade said, "I know I've had too much wine tonight, so I just drank a couple of cups of strong, black coffee to fix me up." "Why don't I drive?" John suggested, "I feel high but I know I can't be drunk. After all, I've just been drinking beer." "Hey, everyone!" Sue giggled, "I'll drive. Before the party I drank a big glass of milk to coat my stomach, so I'm sober." Vanessa looked at her friends and wished she were old enough to drive. "Was anyone sober?" she wondered. "What should I do?"

AN OVERVIEW OF ALCOHOL DRINKING PATTERNS

Just how much do Americans drink? Each year they consume about 9 billion liters (2 1/3 billion gallons) of alcoholic beverages. About two-thirds of the adult population drinks. Many teenagers drink, too, even though it is illegal for minors to do so. In 1982 the National Institute on Drug Abuse sponsored a survey of high school students. Although each school and community is different, the survey showed that 93 percent of high school seniors have had a drink.

For many people alcohol is a traditional part of life. It is commonly used at celebrations. If you attend a wedding, the newlyweds may be toasted with champagne. Can you think of any other occasions when alcohol is usually served? But alcohol's popularity causes many problems. Drinking and driving is a leading cause of traffic deaths and injuries. Alcohol is the cause of many other problems that range from disrupting personal relationships to causing birth defects.

REASONS WHY PEOPLE DRINK

Many adults drink because it is a social custom that they enjoy. Some people believe that alcohol in small amounts can be relaxing and can add pleasure to a meal or a

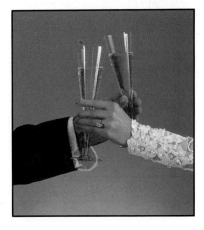

13–1. Alcohol is commonly used at celebrations, such as weddings.

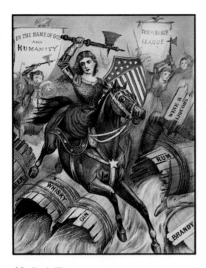

13–2. A Temperance League poster from the 1800s.

get-together. However, some people drink alcohol to escape from problems. For these people, alcohol use can slip into dangerous alcohol misuse. Some of the reasons for alcohol misuse are:

- To escape pressures or problems, or to relieve stress.
- To change bad feelings about oneself, to forget loneliness, or to boost self-confidence.
- To replace unsatisfying personal relationships.

Why do teenagers drink? They may drink for the same reasons that adults drink, and for other reasons as well. Some drink to appear more adult or to be accepted by their friends. Others drink as an experiment or an act of rebellion. These reasons for drinking can also lead to the misuse of alcohol. Regular use can cause psychological and physical dependence.

MANY PEOPLE DON'T DRINK

About one-third of all adults choose not to drink. Some people may not like the taste of alcohol. Many people do not drink because of religious beliefs or different social traditions. In some cases, the nondrinking person may have been a previous drinker who is fighting *alcoholism*. Can you think of other possible reasons for this decision? To use or not use alcohol is a personal decision that a mature person makes responsibly.

WHAT IS ALCOHOL?

What is found in dynamite, perfume, and food wrap? What do people pour into their cars as antifreeze? What is used in disinfectants and in tinctures? The answer to all these questions is alcohol. There are different kinds of alcohol. *Isopropyl alcohol* is rubbing alcohol. **Methanol** (**meth**-a-nahl) is a form of alcohol used in paint thinners, varnishes, and shellac. It is highly poisonous. Have you ever noticed this label on a methanol product: "Caution: Do Not Use in Closed Places?" Just breathing methanol's powerful fumes can be harmful. *Ethyl alcohol*, or **ethanol** (**eth**-a-nahl), is another form of alcohol. This is the alcohol that is found in beverages. *Denatured alcohol* is a mixture of methanol and ethanol. This mixture is highly poisonous and is widely used for industrial purposes.

Ethyl alcohol is not just a drink. It is a drug that is classified as a depressant. It decreases the activity of the body

HEALTH IN HISTORY

The temperence movement began in the United States in the early 1800's. It reached its peak in 1919 with the passage of the 18th Constitutional Amendment. The amendment, which became law in January 1920, remained in effect until December 1933. During this time, the export, import, manufacture, sale, and transport of beverages containing one-half of 1 percent or more alcohol by volume was prohibited.

functions and acts like a tranquilizer. This is why some people rely on it as a relaxant in social situations. For centuries ethyl alcohol was used as an anesthetic to induce unconsciousness.

Like most drugs, alcohol is neither good nor bad. It depends on how alcohol is used. If used wisely, it can be harmless. In fact, recent research suggests that adults who drink small amounts of alcohol daily, no more than one or two drinks, may have a lower risk of heart disease. If misused on a regular basis, alcohol can become an addictive drug. It can cause strong physical and psychological dependence. Alcohol is powerful enough to cause coma and even death. About 95,000 deaths from alcoholism or alcohol-related problems occur annually. This makes the abuse of alcohol a major drug problem.

ALCOHOL PRODUCTION

Have you ever tasted fresh, unprocessed cider and then sipped the same cider a week later? The difference in taste is caused by the formation of alcohol. Alcohol is formed by a process known as **fermentation.** Through the action of yeast, the sugar in the cider is chemically broken down into alcohol and other by-products. All alcoholic beverages are made by this process. The fermentation of sugar in grapes, berries, or fruits produces wine. Beer is made from fermented malted barley. Rum comes from fermented molasses. Corn, wheat, and potatoes are also used to produce alcoholic beverages. The alcohol contents of drinks vary. To know the alcohol content of a beverage, you must check the label. The alcohol content of beer and wine is expressed as a percentage. Beers produced in the United States contain 3.2 to 6.4 percent alcohol. The alcohol content of wines varies from about 10 to 20 percent. The alcohol content of

13–3. Some alcoholic beverages are made by fermenting the sugar in these plant products.

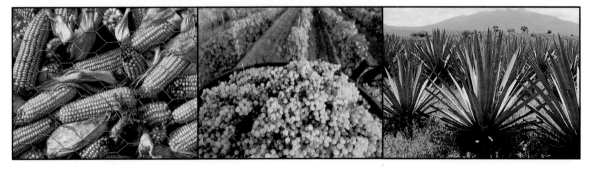

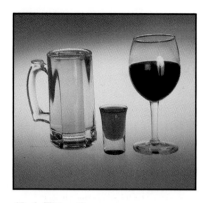

13–4. These three beverages contain the same amount of alcohol.

distilled or hard liquors, such as whiskey, rye, vodka, and gin, is expressed on the label as "proof." The *proof* is twice the alcohol percentage. For example, 80 proof whiskey contains 40 percent alcohol.

Look at Figure 13-4. All of these alcoholic beverages contain equal amounts of alcohol. A 355.2-milliliter (12-oz) can of beer or a 147.9-milliliter (5-oz) glass of wine contains as much alcohol as a 44.4-milliliter (1.5-oz) shot of 86 proof hard liquor. Each contains 14.8 milliliters (.5-oz) of alcohol. Alcohol, whether consumed in beer, wine, or liquor, affects the nervous system in the same way.

WHAT HAPPENS WHEN A PERSON DRINKS?

MIND-BODY INTERACTION. Because the mind and the body interact, even one alcoholic drink can affect a person's behavior and body functions. With each additional drink, a person loses more control of his or her coordination and speech. Drinking alcohol also causes changes in personality and mental functions. Normal inhibitions loosen and emotions such as anger or sadness may be heightened. Clear thinking and judgment are impaired.

Teenagers are often more susceptible to the ill effects of alcohol. This is because teenagers have less experience with alcohol than adults. They may overestimate their ability to handle alcohol and then drink beyond responsible, safe limits. Also, teenagers are still learning social relations skills and emotional control. For this reason, they are often unable to cope with the social problems that drinking may create.

BLOOD ALCOHOL CONTENT. Blood alcohol content, **BAC,** is a measure of the alcohol content in the bloodstream per 100 milliliters of blood. It is expressed as a percentage. The higher the BAC, the more powerful the effect of alcohol on the mind and body. Body weight is an important but often overlooked factor in drinking. A single beer for a person weighing 52 kilograms (120 lb) results in a higher BAC than it does for a person weighing 82 kilograms (180 lb). Most medical and traffic safety authorities consider a BAC of .10 percent as the intoxication level. A 63-kilogram (140-lb) person would reach this level after drinking four beers in a single hour. How can an understanding of BAC help you? It can show you the relationship between how much a person drinks and alcohol's effects. Using Table 13-1, find the BAC of a 63-kilogram (140-lb) person who has drunk two beers in a single hour.

APPROXIMATE BLOOD ALCOHOL CONTENT (BAC) AND DRIVING RISK									Table 13-1
	Body Weight–Kilogram (Pound)								
Number of Drinks in One Hour	45 (100)	54 (120)	63 (140)	72 (160)	81 (180)	90 (200)	99 (220)	108 (240)	
1	.04	.03	.03	.02	.02	.02	.02	.02	Drive with caution
2	.08	.06	.05	.05	.04	.04	.03	.03	
3	.11	.09	.08	.07	.06	.06	.05	.05	
4	.15	.12	.11	.09	.08	.08	.07	.06	Driving impaired; very risky
5	.19	.16	.13	.12	.11	.09	.09	.08	
6	.23	.19	.16	.14	.13	.11	.10	.09	
7	.26	.22	.19	.16	.15	.13	.12	.11	
8	.30	.25	.21	.19	.17	.15	.14	.13	Illegal: do not drive
9	.34	.28	.24	.21	.19	.17	.15	.14	
10	.38	.31	.27	.23	.21	.19	.17	.16	
	Percent Number of Alcohol in the Blood								

One drink = 44.4 milliliters (1½ oz) of 86 proof liquor or 355.2 milliliters (12 oz) beer or 147.9 milliliters (5 oz) wine.

THE MULTIPLIER EFFECT. When alcohol is taken in combination with other drugs, such as tranquilizers, the effects are immediately and often dramatically increased. Tranquilizers and alcohol are both depressants. Many accidental deaths have occurred from mixing these two drugs. Even over-the-counter drugs, such as aspirin or antihistamines, can change the way alcohol acts on people. Unfortunately the effects cannot be predicted in advance. To be safe, never mix alcohol with other drugs. Table 13-2 summarizes some of the effects of mixing alcohol with drugs.

INDIVIDUAL DIFFERENCES. Both Pete and Paul weigh the same amount, yet Pete feels high while Paul seems unaffected after one beer. Each person's body has a different chemistry and reacts differently to alcohol. Some people find that, regardless of how little they drink, their bodies do not tolerate alcohol. The circumstances under which a person drinks can make an important difference, too. When people have not eaten, are especially tired, are emotionally upset, or are recovering from a recent illness, alcohol can have a stronger effect. The effects of alcohol also depend on the social situation. For example, when drinking with friends, a teenager's behavior may become loud and rowdy. When drinking in the presence of parents, that same person may be quite subdued.

Table 13-2

THE EFFECTS OF MIXING ALCOHOL WITH DRUGS

Alcohol mixed with:

antibiotics = flushing, drowsiness, vomiting

antihistamines = drowsiness

aspirin = stomach and intestine bleeding

high blood pressure medicine = increased effect, blood pressure can be lowered to dangerous levels

narcotics = depression of central nervous system, can arrest respiratory system

non-narcotic pain killers = stomach and intestine irritation and possible bleeding

oral antidiabetic drugs = flushing, vomiting, drowsiness

sedatives and tranquilizers = depression of central nervous system

Tolerance level is another individual difference. Like many addictive drugs, tolerance develops with repeated alcohol use. As tolerance grows, a person must drink more to feel the same effects. Tolerance is not a sign that you've learned to control alcohol. As you'll see later, it is a sign that *alcohol* is beginning to control *you.*

HOW DOES ALCOHOL AFFECT THE BODY?

What happens when someone swallows an alcoholic beverage? Let's follow the route alcohol takes through the body and find out.

THE INTAKE

Alcohol first passes over the sensitive membranes of the mouth and esophagus. If the alcohol content of the drink is high enough, these delicate membranes become irritated. A warm or burning sensation is felt. In heavy drinkers these membranes are constantly inflamed. Heavy drinkers run a much higher risk of developing cancer of the mouth and throat. Combining heavy drinking with heavy smoking increases the risk of mouth and throat cancer even more.

THE STOMACH

Have you ever heard the warning, "Don't drink on an empty stomach"? Once alcohol reaches the stomach, it does not have to be digested. The alcohol molecule is very small and can easily pass through the stomach lining. In an empty stomach alcohol is rapidly absorbed into the bloodstream. Food in the stomach, particularly high-protein food, slows the rate of alcohol absorption. Carbonation in beverages speeds alcohol absorption.

Alcohol in small amounts increases the flow of gastric juices from the stomach lining. This is why small amounts of alcohol can stimulate the appetite. Greater amounts of alcohol dull the appetite. Heavy drinkers often suffer from malnutrition, since they fill up on the empty calories in alcohol. Excessive alcohol use also stimulates an excessive flow of gastric juices, whose acid content is high. This irritates the stomach lining. Repeated irritation can cause an open sore in the stomach called an *ulcer.*

THE CIRCULATORY ROUTE

About 20 percent of the alcohol is absorbed into the bloodstream through the stomach. The remaining 80 percent passes to the small intestine where it is quickly absorbed into the bloodstream. Once in the bloodstream, the alcohol is evenly distributed throughout the circulatory system and all body tissues.

Should you ever rely on alcohol for extra warmth during a camping trip? Don't. As alcohol enters the bloodstream, it dilates (widens) the blood vessels. This causes a greater flow of blood to the skin (blushing) and a temporary feeling of warmth. When blood is carried to the skin, there is increased heat loss from the body surface. Therefore, body temperature decreases rapidly.

THE BRAIN

When alcohol reaches the brain, it immediately begins to affect the brain's ability to control behavior and body functions. As BAC increases, the drinker loses more control.

BAC .1 PERCENT. Alcohol first starts to affect the centers of the brain that control intelligence, perception, and motor ability. Next, alcohol affects the centers for emotions. People tend to become more talkative. Their emotions and inhibitions are relaxed. Good judgment and self-control decrease. Some feel powerful and attempt dangerous acts, such as driving on the wrong side of the road. Studies have shown that even a single drink affects perception and reaction time.

BAC .2 PERCENT. Can you guess what happens as BAC rises? The brain centers for intelligence, emotions, and sensory and motor abilities are affected even more. It becomes difficult to think clearly. Memory is impaired. Emotional behavior cannot be predicted. Some people become easily excited or angered. Even simple movements, such as walking a straight line or buttoning a coat, become difficult or even impossible tasks.

BAC .3 PERCENT. During this phase alcohol throws the body into a state of complete confusion. The sense organs are seriously affected. Speech becomes slurred and a person may experience double vision. Hearing can also be impaired. Distances are difficult or impossible to judge. A person can no longer walk normally. Moods can change suddenly or become exaggerated.

BAC .4 PERCENT. Are you familiar with the expressions "getting stiff" or "I was paralyzed?" This is literally what happens at the .4 percent BAC level. At this stage the brain can barely function. The entire nervous system is ineffective. The person becomes almost unconscious. The body seems frozen and unable to move. The drinker is no longer able to walk or to stand. Vomiting or uncontrolled urination may occur.

BAC .5 PERCENT. At .5 percent a person slips into a deep coma with little or no reflexes. The rates of breathing, heart action, and blood pressure are decreased. The brain loses its ability to control body temperature. If the breathing centers of the brain become paralyzed, death can and often does result.

THE KIDNEYS

The intake of alcohol has a *diuretic* effect on the kidneys. This means that it increases the formation of urine. Alcohol does this by acting on the *pituitary gland* which lies beneath the brain. This gland secretes a hormone that controls urine production. Alcohol suppresses the secretion of this hormone, causing more urine to be produced by the kidneys. This is why a person is dehydrated and thirsty after drinking.

THE LUNGS

Did you ever sniff a strong liquor and suddenly feel lightheaded? When you inhale alcohol fumes, the alcohol is rapidly absorbed through the lungs. It then quickly reaches the brain. While breathing out, alcohol leaves the body in small amounts through the lungs. Even after a single drink, the odor of alcohol can be smelled on the breath.

About 5 percent of the alcohol taken into the body leaves through the kidneys, lungs, and skin. The rest is removed by the liver.

THE LIVER

Drinkers are advised to sip, never gulp, drinks. There is a good reason for this. When alcohol reaches the liver, the process of removing it begins. **Oxidation** converts alcohol into water and carbon dioxide. This occurs at a rate of 14.8 milliliters (.5 oz) of alcohol or .01 to .02 percent BAC per hour. Gulping alcohol at a faster rate causes a rapid build-up of alcohol in the bloodstream.

LIVER DAMAGE. Alcohol can interfere with the liver's ability to break down fats. Fats then collect in the liver and cause a condition known as fatty liver. More than 75 percent of all alcoholics have a fatty liver. It has also been found in moderate drinkers. When drinking stops, the condition is usually reversed.

Cirrhosis means scarring. Heavy alcohol use destroys normal tissues of the liver and replaces them with scar tissue. This decreases blood flow and the functioning of the liver. Progressive cirrhosis can cause death. Other conditions can cause cirrhosis, but it is usually caused by alcoholism.

AFTER EFFECTS: THE SOBERING PROCESS

Until alcohol is completely oxidized, it continues to circulate through the bloodstream. As alcohol is oxidized, the BAC level drops and the sobering process occurs. Can anything speed up the sobering process? So-called cures, such as black coffee, cold showers, and walks in the fresh air, may make a drinker feel more awake. But nothing can speed the sobering up process. A person's reaction time and reasoning ability improves only when enough time has gone by for oxidation to reduce the BAC level.

A hangover is the body's way of saying, "I have had too much alcohol to drink." Although hangovers may be joked about, they are really no laughing matter. Hangover symptoms include headaches, extreme fatigue, and nausea. People can also experience psychological symptoms, such as anxiety, guilt, and depression, especially if they cannot remember or regret their behavior during and after their drinking. What is the cure for a hangover? Home remedies do not work. Only time, rest, and solid food can help.

ALCOHOL AND SOCIETY
ALCOHOL AND ACCIDENTS

"Drinking and driving don't mix." The facts speak for themselves. Studies show that at a BAC of .05 percent the risk of highway accidents doubles. At a BAC of .10 percent the chances are seven times greater. At a BAC of .15 percent the accident risk increases twenty-five times. Would you like to play those odds? Many people do. Alcohol is involved in 50 percent of the highway accidents each year. About 30 thousand people die, and half a million are injured in these

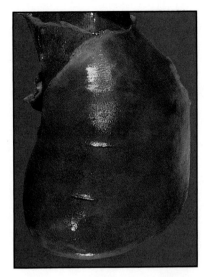

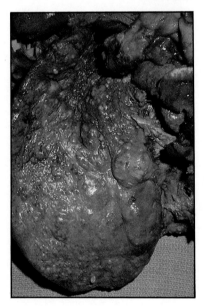

13–5. A normal liver compared to a liver with cirrhosis, caused by alcoholism.

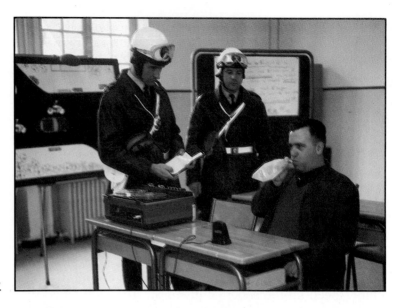

13–6. Police officers use a breathalyzer to measure the alcohol content of the blood.

accidents. Alcohol-related car accidents are the leading cause of death of young people. Many states have increasd the legal drinking age in an effort to reduce these traffic deaths.

Drunk driving, also called DWI (driving while intoxicated), is against the law in every state. In most states, drunkenness is defined as .10 percent BAC. Most police officers use breath analysis to measure BAC. The person exhales into a *breathalyzer*. This machine quickly measures BAC (see Figure 13-6). BAC can help drinkers determine if they have reached the drinking danger zone (.05 percent BAC) or the drunken zone (.1 percent BAC). But since even one drink can reduce judgment and reaction time, the safest course is not to drink and drive at all.

Alcohol-related deaths do not stop on the highway: 80 percent of fire deaths, 65 percent of drownings, 70 percent of fatal falls, and about 40 percent of deaths while on the job are linked to alcohol use. Alcohol is a factor in an estimated 80 percent of all suicides.

ALCOHOL AND CRIME

Alcohol is a factor in 34 percent of the rapes, 41 percent of the assaults, and 64 percent of the murders in this country. Of all arrests in the United States, 55 percent involve alcohol misuse. Why is alcohol related to crime? It clouds judgment and reduces self-control. A simple argument can turn into a fistfight or lead to a more serious crime.

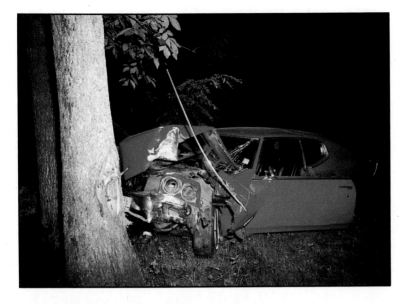

13–7. Alcohol-related car accidents are the leading cause of death among young people.

ALCOHOL AND FAMILY LIFE

It is estimated that about one out of every four families has been seriously affected by alcohol. Alcohol misuse hits at the core of family life. When one or both parents abuse alcohol, the chances of child abuse and neglect increase. Experts may not agree on the cause of child abuse, but 60 percent of all reported child abuse cases involve alcohol misuse. Recent studies show that alcohol is often a factor in cases of spouse abuse.

ALCOHOLISM: THE DISEASE

At one time most people looked down on alcoholics. People saw this problem as a sign of personal weakness. But, through public education, the attitudes of society are changing as more people understand what alcoholism is.

WHAT IS ALCOHOLISM?

Alcoholism is not just a social and behavioral problem. The American Medical Association considers alcoholism a chronic, progressive, and sometimes fatal disease that requires professional treatment. It is marked by drug tolerance, physical dependency, and disease-like changes in body organs. All these factors are the direct or indirect result of drinking. Alcoholism shortens life by 10 to 15 years. Since about 10 million Americans suffer from alcoholism, it is one of the most serious public health problems today.

WHO IS AN ALCOHOLIC?

How would you describe a typical alcoholic? Do you think of a person in torn or ragged clothes, sleeping in public places? Less than 3 percent of alcoholics fit this picture. Alcoholics can be mothers, fathers, business people, doctors, laborers, secretaries, teachers, and students. Anyone who drinks runs the risk of becoming an alcoholic, regardless of age, intelligence, profession, or wealth.

WHAT CAUSES ALCOHOLISM?

Alcoholism is puzzling. There are several theories about why people become alcoholics. Some theories point to personality problems. Social theories focus on the way alcohol is treated in a particular society or culture. Biological theories focus on heredity and body chemistry.

Not everyone who drinks becomes an alcoholic. Most people are social drinkers. They enjoy drinking small amounts at home or on social occasions. Life is not that simple for *problem drinkers*, who are mentally dependent on alcohol. Their drinking creates problems for themselves and other people. In certain situations these people drink too much and then drive, or they drink despite their doctors' orders. But problem drinkers are not always alcoholics. They can control their drinking *if* the situation demands. For example, a teen may drink too much with friends but stop drinking if he or she is trying to impress a date. The third category of drinkers, alcoholics, cannot control drinking. Alcoholics drink beyond responsible limits no matter how this behavior hurts themselves or others.

HIGH-RISK GROUPS. Anyone who drinks runs a risk of developing alcoholism. One out of every ten drinkers becomes an alcoholic. Studies suggest that drinking during the teen years may increase the risks of developing this disease. Children of alcoholics are also at higher risk. They develop the problem more often than children of non-alcoholics. This suggests that biological factors, such as inherited body chemistry, may affect the onset of this disease. Older people are also more likely to develop this disease. Increased leisure time, the stress of losing loved ones, and health problems have been posed as possible reasons. Also, alcohol may have a stronger effect on older people because of changes in their nervous systems.

ALCOHOL AND PERSONAL LIFE. The alcoholic has trouble carrying out duties at home, school, and work. If an alcoholic is a wage earner, money problems usually result. Work output decreases, and lateness or absence from work increases. Alcoholics often lose their jobs. Alcoholism creates other money problems, too. Since alcoholics have more health problems and accidents, they have extra medical bills or repair bills to pay. Also, more money is taken from the household budget to purchase alcohol.

Alcoholism is considered a family disease since it disrupts family life. As an alcoholic's life centers on drinking, there is little time for anything else. Families often feel bitter and lose respect for the alcoholic member. Children may feel helpless in the situation. They may develop behavior problems in school or do poorly at their schoolwork. Some families feel guilty and think they caused the problems. Others feel ashamed. They begin to shy away from friends to hide the problem. As pressures mount, separation or divorce may occur.

WHAT ARE THE SIGNS AND STAGES OF ALCOHOLISM?

Where does problem drinking stop and alcoholism begin? Since alcoholism usually develops slowly, it is hard to tell. But as the disease progresses, signs of the disease begin to appear. As a drinker slips into the first stage of alcoholism, he or she develops an increased tolerance to alcohol. Even large doses have little effect. The drinker makes promises to quit but can't keep them. Personality change is noticeable. The person becomes more and more cross or forgetful. There are periods called blackouts, when the drinker cannot remember actions or thoughts. The alcoholic drinks more alcohol to escape from problems.

As the disease progresses, the alcoholic is caught in a vicious cycle of drinking, isolation, guilt, and more drinking. The following signs become more noticeable in the middle stage:

1. Drinking starts in the morning or when the drinker is alone.
2. Tolerance builds even further.

3. Drinking becomes an important daily event.
4. Performance on the job, at school, or at home decreases.
5. The drinker denies or hides the addiction.

When the alcoholic reaches the final stage of the disease, denial is no longer possible. The alcoholic's drinking is clearly visible and uncontrolled. Work is no longer possible. Family life falls apart. Other signs are apparent, as follows:

1. The alcoholic becomes isolated from family and friends.
2. The changes in personality are severe. The alcoholic is tense, cross, and distrustful of people who want to help.
3. The alcoholic lives on an alcohol diet and does not eat properly. Liver diseases often develop. When drinking stops, the alcoholic may have severe withdrawal symptoms called **delirium tremens** (de-**leer**-ee-um **tree**-menz) (DT's). Trembling of the body and hallucinations occur. In rare cases, convulsions and death occur.

WHAT ARE THE SIGNS OF PROBLEM DRINKING?

Young people can develop problems with alcohol just as adults do. Today, about 3.3 million teenagers are problem drinkers. Would you be able to spot signs of problem drinking in yourself or your friends? This checklist can be used to determine whether you or someone you know has a drinking problem. If you answer yes to any of these questions, you should carefully evaluate your behavior and perhaps seek help.

1. Can you enjoy parties, sports events, or other social activities without drinking?
2. Does drinking greatly change your personality?
3. Do you take, or do you want to take, a drink after a disappointment, an argument with your parents or friends, or a disagreement with a teacher?
4. Do you try to drink more than your friends?
5. Do you find that you have to keep drinking more to get the same effect?
6. Have you ever gotten into trouble at school, on the highway, or at home because of drinking?
7. Has a friend or a date ever complained about your drinking habits?

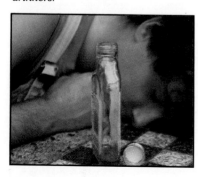

13–8. About 3.3 million teenagers are problem drinkers.

8. Do you ever drink alone?
9. Do you make promises to drink more responsibly that you cannot keep?
10. Have you ever missed school because of drinking?
11. Does drinking make you feel more confident?
12. Do you often drink to become intoxicated?

THE TREATMENT OF ALCOHOLISM

Many different sources of help exist for alcoholics. A physician or counselor can help the alcoholic find treatment, so can the National Council on Alcoholism. This is the only national voluntary group founded to combat the disease of alcoholism. Through its networks of local councils on alcoholism, it helps direct alcoholics and their families to treatment centers. Alcoholism cannot be cured, but it definitely can be arrested. With proper treatment as many as two-thirds of all alcoholics recover. If an alcoholic is physically addicted or has other health problems, he or she may need to spend some time in the hospital first. Under medical care the alcoholic is detoxified, meaning the body is rid of alcohol. Medical treatment helps restore the body's normal functioning as much as possible. Sometimes drugs, such as *Antabuse* (disulfiram), are given to prevent drinking. When alcoholics take Antabuse, even the smallest amount of alcohol makes them violently ill. Other treatment focuses on helping the alcoholic overcome psychological addiction to alcohol. The alcoholic can also be aided in readjusting to life without the drug.

Alcoholics Anonymous, simply known as AA, is perhaps the best-known source of help. AA is an organization of men and women working together to help each other arrest their disease. The alcoholic attends meetings with recovered alcoholics and people in the process of recovering. Discussions at the meetings allow the alcoholic to share experiences with the group. How does someone join AA? Simply by attending an AA meeting. AA is listed in the telephone directory of most cities. There are no rules or members' dues to pay. AA is completely supported through contributions. The only requirement for membership is a desire to stop drinking. Once alcoholics recover, can they ever drink again? Most authorities agree that alcoholics can never return to social drinking. The disease is arrested, but it is never cured. Not drinking alcohol must become a way of life for the recovered alcoholic.

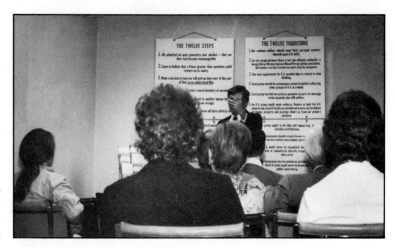

13–9. Members of Alcoholics Anonymous work together to help each other arrest their disease.

ALANON AND ALATEEN: THE FAMILY LIFELINE

Whether or not alcoholics decide to seek help, there is help for their families. Alanon and Alateen are two groups that can be a family's lifeline. They help prevent an alcoholic's family from being destroyed by alcoholism. Alanon is for anyone affected by close contact with an alcoholic. Members include relatives, employers, and many alcoholics.

Young people in the 12 to 20 age group can join Alateen. Alateen members learn to cope with the problems caused by the alcoholics around them. Neither group is linked with AA, but they are the same in many ways. There are regular meetings where members share their experiences and encourage and support one another. They learn facts about the disease that affects their lives. Both groups are supported entirely by voluntary contributions.

DECISIONS ABOUT DRINKING

Have you made a decision about drinking? Many teenagers choose not to drink alcohol. If this is your decision, be firm. Don't apologize. After all, it is your body, your life, and your right. Do you respect the decision of others not to drink? Or do you debate the issue or otherwise try to exert pressure on others? Can any reason justify such actions?

If you drink to escape problems and pressures, you may be headed for trouble. Preventing alcohol abuse means knowing how to use alcohol wisely. Will alcohol be a problem in your life? It's your choice.

FOCUS ON HEALTH

SADD, Students Against Drunk Driving, is giving growing numbers of parents, teachers, law officers, and teenagers a reason to be glad. SADD is a prime example of how young people can turn peer pressure into positive peer power.

SADD's goal is simple: to help teenagers save their own lives and the lives of others by waging an all out war against drunk driving. SADD members use education to bring their message home to other students. They also plan and provide activities such as "Day High," an alcohol-drug free class party for graduating seniors.

SADD is unique among alcohol abuse prevention programs. It was student organized in the Boston area in 1981. Today it is in all states, is still growing and is still student run. Members freely pledge "not to drink and drive, or let a friend drink and drive." "Friends don't let friends drive drunk" is one

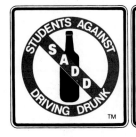

of SADD's slogans. The programs's success has come from the fact that members realize that teenage drunk driving is *their* problem. Teenagers must accept responsibility for it and solve this problem themselves through education and positive peer pressure. Members are making SADD's motto true: "If we can dream it, it can be done." For more information on SADD write: SADD, 66 Diana Drive, Marlboro, MA 01752.

SUMMARY: Alcoholic beverages are widely used. It is a depressant drug that acts on the brain and affects behavior. As BAC rises, physical, emotional, and mental activities are impaired. Proper functioning can be restored through the oxidation of alcohol. Body weight, tolerance, and the presence of other drugs in the body or food in the stomach are some factors influencing alcohol's effects. Alcohol misuse is a major social and health problem. Traffic and home accidents, fire, child abuse, and crime are all linked with alcohol misuse. People who cannot control their drinking suffer from a complex disease called alcoholism. This disease affects not only alcoholics, but also their families, friends, and employers. Alcoholism cannot be cured, but it can be arrested. Therefore, it is important to recognize the signs of this disease, particularly in its early stages. Many sources of help exist for the alcoholic, including the National Council on Alcoholism, Alcoholics Anonymous, Alateen, and Alanon. Those who choose to drink should drink responsibly. They should drink within reasonable limits and never endanger themselves or the lives of others.

CHAPTER REVIEW

words at work

Find the word in the left column that fits one of the definitions in the right column. DO NOT WRITE IN THIS BOOK.

a. alcoholic
b. cirrhosis
c. delirium tremens
d. depressant
e. ethanol
f. methanol
g. Antabuse
h. BAC
i. oxidation

1. a dangerous liver condition
2. beverage alcohol
3. a substance that slows up body processes
4. poisonous alcohol
5. visual hallucinations
6. blood alcohol content
7. psychologically dependent on alcohol
8. alcohol becomes water and carbon dioxide
9. prescribed to prevent drinking

review questions

1. How many adults drink alcoholic beverages? Cite 3 reasons for their social use.
2. List three reasons why some adults choose not to drink.
3. Identify four reasons for drinking that can lead to alcohol misuse.
4. Teens may drink for different reasons than adults. Cite at least 3 such reasons.
5. Distinguish between ethanol and methanol.
6. Explain alcohol's classification as a drug.
7. Compare the proof and alcohol content of beer, wine, and hard liquors.
8. Describe the general affects of alcohol on the mind and body.
9. Define BAC. What is the relationship between BAC and the effects of alcohol?
10. Trace the effects of alcohol at different percentages of BAC.
11. Cite five factors that can alter the effects of alcohol on an individual.
12. Trace the path of alcohol through the body.
13. Discuss alcohol misuse as a safety problem.
14. Why is alcohol use associated with crime?
15. Name two effects of alcohol misuse on family life.
16. Define alcoholism. Why is it considered a family disease?
17. Compare social drinkers, problem drinkers, and alcoholics.
18. What three groups are at a higher risk of becoming alcoholics?
19. Name three effects of alcoholism on personal life.
20. Trace the progression of alcoholism.
21. Outline treatment that is available to help people recover from alcoholism.

discussion questions

1. Compare and contrast drinking patterns among adolescents and adults. Are teenagers more vulnerable to alcohol misuse?
2. In your opinion, what should be our attitude toward alcoholics?
3. Is it your business if other people drink? Discuss your answer.
4. What action(s) can help reduce alcohol-related traffic deaths? Do you think increasing the legal drinking age is an effective method?
5. What does responsible alcohol use mean to you?
6. Discuss behavior that may indicate alcoholism. What would you do if you observed these signs in yourself or others?

investigating

PURPOSE:
To develop self-assertion skills that can be applied to prevention of alcohol abuse.

PROCEDURE:
A.   On a sheet of paper, give an example of an assertive, nonassertive, and aggressive response to these situations:
   1.   You loan a friend your best sweater and it is returned soiled.
   2.   Your best friend telephones you to discuss something that happened at school. You are studying for an important test and do not want to talk.
   3.   You are eating out. When your food arrives, the order is wrong.
B.   Compare and discuss your responses in class.
   1.   Was it difficult to think of assertive responses? Why or why not?
   2.   How do you think most people would respond to these situations? Give examples of other situations in which self-assertion skills would be helpful.
C.   On the reverse side of the paper, now write an assertive response to counter alcohol misuse in these situations:
   1.   You have promised your parents that you will not drink at a party. Once you are there, your best friend insists that you take a drink.
   2.   You are on a date and your date begins to drink excessively.
   3.   You are a passenger in a car. The driver pulls out a beer and begins drinking.
D.   Divide the class into groups of three to six students. Select two students to role-play one of the situations in Exercise C. In the role-play, one student must act out his or her assertive response while the other student responds accordingly. Non-acting students should observe and take notes. Repeat and alternate situations until each student has practiced an assertive response.
E.   Discuss the role-play situations in class.
   4.   Was it difficult to act assertively in the role-play situation? If so, how?
   5.   What kinds of pressure was the "assertive" student subjected to? What risks did the "assertive" student take by maintaining his or her position?
   6.   Discuss other situations where self-assertion skills would be helpful.

CHAPTER 14

Tobacco

OBJECTIVES

- DISCUSS the motivation for smoking and why tobacco use is addictive
- OUTLINE the effect of mainstream and sidestream smoke on the body
- DESCRIBE the health risks of smoking
- EXPLAIN why tobacco is harmful to health
- DEVELOP strategies for action to combat the tobacco problem

join the great american smokeout

Carlos was meeting his new friend Jake after baseball practice. Carlos took one look at his friend and exclaimed, "Hey, what's wrong with you? You've got a lump in your cheek just like I did when I had a bad toothache." "I'm fine," Jake laughed, "haven't you ever seen a man chew tobacco? I decided to try chewing when I saw my favorite pro player in a chewing tobacco ad. He says he can enjoy tobacco by us-ing 'moist smokeless tobacco.' I figure if he's doing it, it must be safe. After I've used up the plug of tobacco I just bought, I'm going to try dipping." "Dipping?" Carlos said quizzically. "That's when you put a pinch of snuff between your cheek and gum. It gets your mouth juices flowing. And then you spit." "What a disgusting habit," thought Carlos silently.

THE SMOKING HABIT
PAST TO PRESENT

In the early 1900's, when automobiles and telephones were becoming a part of American life, cigarette smoking was almost unknown. Most tobacco users chewed their tobacco, smoked it in pipes or cigars, or inhaled it as snuff. Only a few mastered the art of rolling shredded tobacco in papers to make cigarettes.

The production of cigarettes started with the development of cigarette-manufacturing machines, convenient packaging, and advertising. Cigarettes quickly grew in popularity. They were inexpensive, mild enough to be easily inhaled, and more socially acceptable than other forms of tobacco use. Consequently, in the 1920's cigarette smoking became a habit among the majority of adults. This is no longer true today. Since 1965 there has been a steady annual decline in the percentage of adults who smoke. Currently only one-third of the adult population smokes. Over a half million adults quit smoking for good each year. Yet more cigarettes are being produced and smoked than ever before. Who is doing the smoking today?

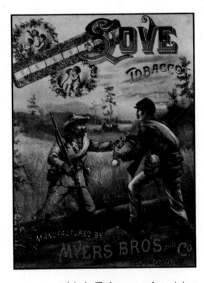

14–1. Tobacco advertising has been around since the beginning of the tobacco industry.

THE SMOKING POPULATION TODAY

Although the percentage of people who smoke has decreased significantly, our population has grown. So the absolute number of smokers is larger today than in 1965.

HEALTH IN HISTORY

When the first English settlers arrived in America, they found that native American Indians used tobacco. The basic techniques used by the native Americans to grow and cure tobacco were remarkably similar to modern production methods. In 1610 John Rolfe introduced tobacco as a cash crop in the Jamestown colony. Thus, tobacco production is considered America's oldest industry.

Research also suggests that the average smoker today consumes more cigarettes than a smoker of twenty years ago.

An estimated fifty-five million people smoke. Of these smokers, sixty percent claim that they have tried to quit the smoking habit but so far have failed. The smoking habit among youth may begin as early as ages twelve to fourteen. However, the average age when young people become regular smokers is sixteen. As age increases, so does the percentage of young people who smoke. Look at Figure 14-2, which shows the percentage of high school students who smoke frequently. Notice that in 1974, males smoked more than females. Today, though the percentage of both male and female smokers in this age group has declined, girls smoke more than boys.

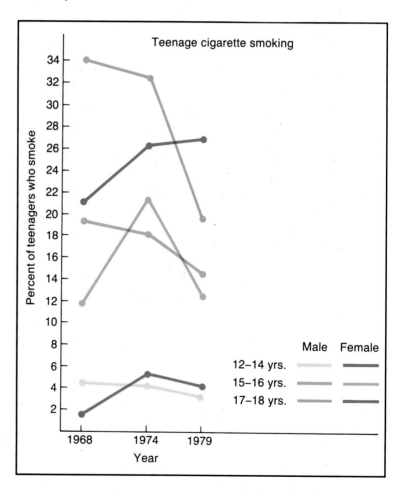

14–2. The percentage of girls who smoke regularly has increased steadily.

WHY DO PEOPLE SMOKE?   Most smokers agree that their first experience with cigarette smoking was unpleasant. They had to learn the smoking habit. Why do young people willingly acquire an unhealthy habit that they might not be able to break for the rest of their lives? Is it the attraction of cigarette advertising? Do they follow the example of older siblings, parents, or adult role models who smoke? Undoubtedly, these factors have some effect. But surveys among high school students indicate that most young people learn the smoking habit from friends who smoke. The approval of peers provides initial social reinforcement. Eventually the smoking habit is carried over to other situations, such as becoming a way to handle boredom. A person then smokes whether or not peers are present. Handling the cigarette is a part of the ritual that helps fix the smoking habit.

The declining smoking rates for youth show that most young people prefer a more positive, smoke-free life-style. For health, appearance, and social reasons they choose not to smoke. Although some may experiment with smoking, they soon quit. They can then enjoy life that is not regulated by a smoking habit. Unfortunately, others continue smoking at least until middle age.

If you ask a group of smokers why they continue to smoke, you'll receive several different answers. What arguments against smoking could you give in reply to each of the following statements?

1. I enjoy it.
2. It gives me something to do when I'm relaxing.
3. It gives me a lift.
4. It helps me feel better when I'm depressed or upset.
5. It creates a sociable atmosphere.

You will not often hear smokers admit that they simply can't stop. But smoking quickly becomes a habit, and most smokers find the habit hard to break.

TOBACCO ADDICTION

What is tobacco? The answer depends on who you ask. A botanist might describe tobacco as a plant whose leaves are used for cigarettes, cigars, pipe blends, snuff, and chewing products. A tobacco farmer might call it a profitable crop. A doctor might call it an addictive substance and a cause of cancer. A chemist might refer to the 2,000 chemical compounds that are produced when tobacco is burned. These include **tar** and the drug **nicotine** (**nik**-a-teen).

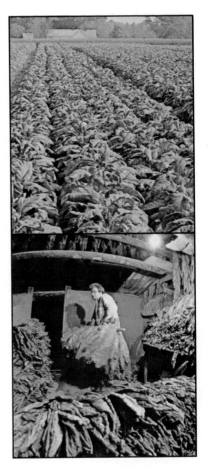

14–3. Tobacco production involves growing, harvesting, drying, curing, and shredding tobacco leaves.

Tar is the residue formed when tobacco smoke condenses. Certain chemicals found in tar may be the principal cancer-causing agents in tobacco smoke. Medical scientists have done extensive research on the effects of smoking. In tests, they found that tar applied to the skin of mice causes both cancerous and noncancerous tumors.

The nicotine present in tobacco acts primarily as a stimulant drug. Nicotine raises blood pressure, increases heart rate, and decreases body temperature. It also dulls the appetite. Like other stimulants, the aftereffect of nicotine is a depression of body functions. Some people find that nicotine has a calming effect in stressful situations.

Nicotine is an addictive drug that can have strong effects. If the *pure* nicotine content of two cigars were injected into a person's bloodstream, death would result. When tobacco is smoked, the nicotine in it reaches the brain in just seven seconds. That is twice as fast as another addictive drug, such as heroin, reaches the brain by injection.

Nicotine, like many other drugs, causes both psychological and physical dependence. A pack-a-day smoker takes more than 70,000 puffs of nicotine a year. Because nicotine is the only drug that is used constantly each day, throughout the day, strong dependence builds with cigarette use.

As tolerance to nicotine grows, the initially unpleasant side effects that most new smokers experience subside. Once a person becomes a frequent tobacco user, irritability, nervousness, and other withdrawal symptoms may occur when the smoker stops smoking.

People who are dependent on smoking fall into common daily behavior patterns. For example, they usually begin their day with a morning cigarette. This sends a burst of nicotine to the brain that stimulates the smoker and may produce a sense of well-being. Throughout the day, the smoker tries to maintain this feeling by smoking off and on. If too many cigarettes are smoked, nicotine levels build in the bloodstream. Then overdose symptoms such as nausea may be experienced. If too few cigarettes are smoked, blood nicotine levels drop. A person then feels he or she needs a cigarette just to feel normal again.

MAINSTREAM AND SIDESTREAM SMOKE

Smoke directly inhaled from a cigarette is called **mainstream smoke.** It carries all the tar, nicotine, and other dangerous chemicals directly into the body. When a smoker

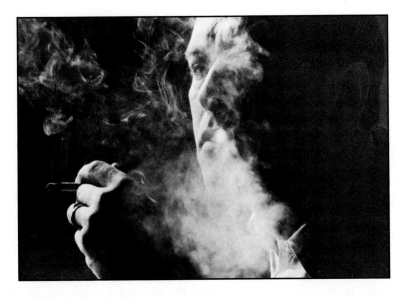

14–4. Sidestream smoke is inhaled by everyone nearby.

exhales, some mainstream smoke is returned to the air. Mainstream smoke enters and leaves the lungs about eight or nine times per cigarette.

A cigarette burns almost a full twelve minutes, continuously polluting the air. The smoke-polluted air, called **sidestream smoke,** is inhaled by everyone nearby. As a result, nonsmokers unwillingly become passive smokers. Figure 14-4 is a typical example of sidestream smoke.

What does sidestream smoke contain? It has the same substances as mainstream smoke, but in greater concentration. It has about twice as much tar and nicotine, three times as much benzopyrene (a known cancer-causing agent), three times as much carbon monoxide, and seventy times as much ammonia as mainstream smoke. Whether you smoke yourself or are forced to be a passive smoker, you should understand the major effects of smoking.

HEALTH IN HISTORY

Dr. Benjamin Rush, a signer of the Declaration of Independence, issued one of the earliest warnings about tobacco's effects on health. In 1798 Dr. Rush declared that tobacco had ill effects on the stomach, nerves, and oral cavity.

HOW DOES SMOKING AFFECT THE BODY?
THE CARDIOVASCULAR SYSTEM

Do you consider auto-exhaust fumes a health hazard? **Carbon monoxide** (**kar**-bon muh-**nock**-side) fumes from car exhaust are indeed deadly. Carbon monoxide fumes are released into the air when tobacco is burned also.

When oxygen from the air enters the bloodstream, it easily combines with the hemoglobin in the red blood cells. The oxygen is then transported to all the cells in the body. When oxygen and carbon monoxide enter the bloodstream together, they compete for **hemoglobin** (**hee**-mow-glow-bin). The power of carbon monoxide to combine with hemoglobin is about 230 times greater than that of oxygen. When carbon monoxide combines with hemoglobin, a new product called **carboxyhemoglobin** (kar-box-ee-**hee**-mow-glow-bin) is formed. As blood levels of this product increase, the oxygen supply in the blood decreases. Vital body tissues are robbed of needed oxygen. In time, this causes damage to the heart, blood vessels, and other organs. Exposure to carbon monoxide is especially harmful to those already suffering from heart or lung disease.

Studies have shown that even short-term exposure to the carbon monoxide in tobacco smoke can be harmful. One study revealed that smoking ten cigarettes in a nonventilated car produced high levels of carbon monoxide in the air. This doubled the carboxyhemoglobin level in the blood of both smokers and nonsmokers in the car. It also slowed the driver's reaction time. Another research study with animals showed that exposure to the carbon monoxide in sidestream smoke over four or five weeks also caused heart and brain damage in the animals.

When smoke enters the lungs, nicotine is also absorbed into the bloodstream. Nicotine causes the blood vessels to narrow, which increases blood pressure. As a result, the heart's workload can increase by as much as twenty-eight beats per minute.

THE RESPIRATORY SYSTEM

The respiratory system is equipped with a natural cleaning brush. Delicate, hairlike **cilia** (**sih**-lee-ah) project from the mucous membranes of the air passages (see Figure 14-5). The cilia act like bristles on a broom. They "sweep" dust, mucous, and other foreign particles out of the air passages, toward the throat.

The nicotine and carbon monoxide in tobacco smoke paralyze the cilia. Therefore, they cannot expel all of the particles in tobacco smoke. These particles irritate the mucous membranes lining the air passages. This causes them to swell and secrete more mucous. As the membrane swells, cilia can no longer function. These foreign particles must be

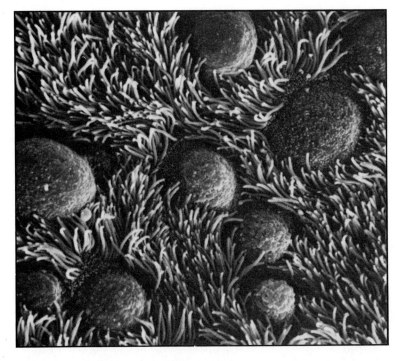

14–5. The cilia, magnified 3840 times, act like bristles on a broom to sweep foreign particles out of the lungs.

coughed out. This is called a smoker's "hack." Improper function of the cilia also sets the stage for more frequent respiratory infections. This is one reason why respiratory illnesses are more frequent not only in smokers but in young children whose parents smoke.

Do you know why athletes should never smoke? Tobacco smoke swells the air passages, and thus diminishes the flow of air to and from the lungs. So smokers experience shortness of breath during physical activity.

INTERACTION OF TOBACCO WITH DRUGS AND FOOD

Would it surprise you to learn that smokers require larger doses of certain painkillers than nonsmokers? This is just one example of how drug effects can go up in smoke with tobacco use. The action of nicotine and other tobacco chemicals speeds the body's use of many drugs. To get the same benefit from certain drugs as nonsmokers, smokers may need larger doses of these drugs and may need doses more often.

Therefore, before medications are prescribed, smokers should alert the doctor to their tobacco habit. This is important for another reason. Smoking can change a smoker's response to certain routine medical laboratory tests. Unless the patient's smoking habit is known, proper diagnosis becomes more difficult. The doctor may subject the smoker to additional testing procedures to confirm or rule out certain diseases. How might this affect the patient?

Tobacco smoke interferes with the digestion and use of food as well. Smoking affects the way the body uses vitamin C and certain B vitamins. Research also indicates that smoking changes the body's ability to break down proteins, carbohydrates, and fats. This may be one reason why mothers who smoke tend to give birth to smaller, lighter babies. Low birth weight puts these babies at higher risk of infant death and illness.

WHAT ARE THE HEALTH RISKS OF SMOKING?

Have you ever looked at the end of a filter cigarette after it was smoked? The dark film in the filter was caused by trapped tar and nicotine. But filters do not catch all the harmful products in tobacco smoke. Look at Figure 14-6. It shows a smoker's lung and the cigarette residue collected from it. Compare this with the picture of the nonsmoker's clean lung. Continued smoking causes abnormal changes not only in the lungs, but in the mouth, throat, and cardiovascular system as well.

14–6. A smoker's lung compared to a nonsmokers lung; gross specimens; and tissue cross-sections.

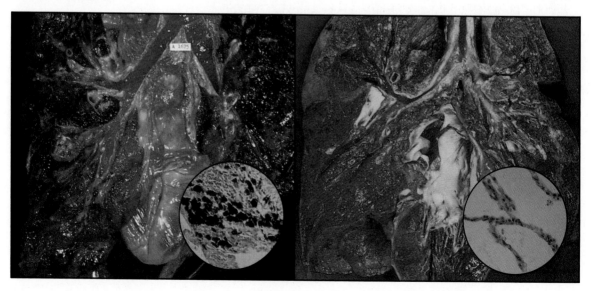

The health risks due to smoking are summarized in Table 14-1 on page 302. The risks of developing these diseases are considerably higher for smokers than for nonsmokers. This is true for both men and women. Keep in mind that the risks vary with the following factors:

- number of cigarettes smoked
- amount of each cigarette smoked (from the entire cigarette to just a few puffs)
- number of puffs during cigarette consumption
- depth and length of the inhalation
- tar and nicotine content of the cigarette smoked
- how long a person has smoked

Notice that the health risks go beyond lung cancer and heart disease. The risks of developing many other types of cancers and other health problems increase when a person smokes. When nicotine enters the digestive tract, it stimulates an increase in stomach acid. This can cause *peptic ulcers*, which are open sores in the stomach. Pregnant women who smoke increase their chance of a miscarriage or stillbirth. Smoking also poses increased risks of developing allergies and impairing the immune system.

What about the risks posed by passive smoking? Researchers are still gathering data on its harmful effects. The absolute risks have not been determined. However, studies have found a higher rate of cancer among nonsmoking wives whose husbands smoke compared to those whose husbands do not smoke. Another study suggests that the health of the unborn baby can be hurt if even only the father smokes!

ARE SOME FORMS OF TOBACCO SAFE?

LOW-TAR/NICOTINE CIGARETTES. Have you heard of a low-tar/nicotine (T/N) cigarette? It is the tobacco industry's attempt to eliminate the health hazards of cigarette smoking. Studies show that low-T/N cigarettes result in lower death rates from cancer and coronary heart diseases. However, death rates among smokers of low-T/N cigarettes are still *far higher* than for those who have never smoked. This may be due to the fact that carbon monoxide levels are not reduced with these cigarettes.

Can someone switch to low-T/N cigarettes and then smoke more, and still minimize the harmful effects of smoking? Definitely not. Death rates among those who smoke one to two packs of low-T/N cigarettes a day are much higher

SMOKING AND HEALTH

	Health Risks for Smoker Versus Nonsmoker	Benefits of Quitting
Life Span	The life expectancy of a two pack a day smoker, age 25, is 8.3 years less than for a 25 year old nonsmoker.	After 15 years, an ex-smoker's life span becomes similar to that of a non-smoker.
Lung Cancer	Heavy smokers (two packs a day or more) have 15–25 times greater risk of lung cancer: other smokers have 10 times the risk. The risk is greater for smokers in certain occupations, e.g., asbestos-related jobs.	Risk decreases gradually after quitting. After 15 years an ex-smoker's risk of lung cancer becomes similar to that of a non-smoker.
Cancer of the larynx, mouth, esophagus	Larynx: Heavy smokers have 20–30 times greater risk of death due to this cancer. Pipe and cigar smokers have at least a 5 times greater risk. Mouth: All smokers have a 3–10 times greater risk of developing mouth cancer. Esophagus: All smokers have a 4–5 times greater risk of getting cancer of the esophagus. Risk of developing these cancers greatly increases when smoking is combined with alcohol use.	Risk decreases gradually after quitting. Risk becomes similar to that of nonsmokers after 10–15 year period. Some immediate benefit from reduced or no alcohol use in combination with tobacco use.
Bladder Cancer	7–10 times greater risk for cigarette smoker. An even greater risk for smokers in certain occupations, for example dye-related jobs.	After 7 years ex-smoker's risk similar to that of non-smokers.
Cancer of the Pancreas	2–5 times greater risk for cigarette smokers.	Data not available. Risk appears related directly to cigarette consumption. Therefore reduced or no smoking should decrease risk of disease.
Coronary Heart Disease (CHD)	Tobacco is a major risk factor for this disease. There are over 120,000 deaths each year from CHD due to smoking.	Risk decreases sharply after one year of quitting. After 10 years, risk is same as for people who have never smoked.
Chronic Bronchitis and Emphysema	4–25 times the risk for smokers. Lung damage apparent even in young smokers.	Symptoms such as smoker's hack disappear within weeks. Decline in lung function slows and may improve.
Peptic Ulcer	Among smokers, peptic ulcers are more common and harder to cure.	Ex-smokers who have peptic ulcers will recover more quickly than smokers.
Pregnancy	Stillbirths and low birthweight infants are more common among smoking mothers. Low birthweight babies are more prone to birth defects and illness and death.	Risk of stillbirth and low birthweight becomes similar to that of nonsmokers, provided smoking stops before 4th month of pregnancy.
Allergy/Immune System	Evidence for increased allergies and impairment of the immune system.	Risk greatly reduced by stopping.

Table 14–1

than for those who smoke less than one pack a day of high-T/N cigarettes. There is no such thing as a safe cigarette.

PIPES AND CIGARS.   Are pipe and cigar smokers safe from smoking hazards? The health facts say no. These forms of smoking can reduce some health hazards. Usually, pipe and cigar smokers do not inhale hot, damaging smoke. Therefore, the risk of heart and lung disease is lower. However, the risks of developing cancers of the mouth, throat, larynx, and esophagus are equal among pipe, cigar, and cigarette smokers. Pipe smoking is suspected to be a direct cause of lip cancer. Overall, people who do not smoke have a greater life expectancy than pipe and cigar smokers.

Cigarette smokers who switch to smoking cigars or pipes may be exposing themselves to even greater health risks. Research indicates that this group of smokers has fixed inhaling patterns. They are likely to inhale the stronger, more irritating smoke from cigars or pipes.

SMOKELESS TOBACCO.   The use of **smokeless tobacco** is becoming more popular among young men. Many have started chewing and dipping tobacco. How come? They may be attracted by the persuasive advertising campaigns. These ads often use well-known sports personalities who imply that this habit is a safe alternative to smoking. In fact, though these products are not as yet required by law to contain warning labels, smokeless tobacco has many health risks. Like other forms of tobacco use, chewing and dipping deliver nicotine and other harmful chemicals to the body. Direct contact with tobacco irritates the lining of the mouth. The inside soft oral tissues form leathery white patches called *leukoplakia*. These patches are considered a precancerous condition. Dippers and chewers have a greatly increased risk of cancer of the mouth and esophagus. The irritating tobacco juices also damage the teeth and gums. Smokeless tobacco contains grit and sand that can wear away tooth surfaces. It also contains sugar that can lead to tooth decay and gum disease. The gums recede, and the teeth drift, loosen, and fall out.

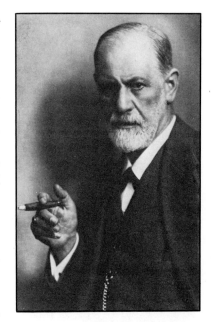

14–7. Sigmund Freud, a well-known cigar smoker, had cancer of the jaw.

WHAT ARE THE SOCIAL EFFECTS OF TOBACCO?

Before you decide to smoke, dip, or chew tobacco, consider the social effects of tobacco use. Advertising strives to promote tobacco use as being socially appealing. But what is attractive about stained fingers, discolored teeth, and bad breath? Smoking also causes increased facial wrinkling. Smoking odors cling to hair and clothes. Most nonsmokers find this tobacco "perfume" offensive. Most people find spitting, which is part of the dipping-chewing habit, extremely offensive. This habit once drew public outcries of disgust. At that time, spitting was banned for health and social reasons. Today chewing tobacco is being promoted in advertising campaigns. The ads claim that chewing tobacco is very appealing and masculine. What do you think?

Each person, of course, must weigh the social effects of using tobacco for himself or herself. Begin by asking yourself these two questions: Does the tobacco habit add real "fun" to my life? Does it honestly make me more masculine or feminine and appealing to others?

SMOKING AFFECTS EVERYONE

Who is affected by smoking? Everyone, smokers and nonsmokers alike, is affected by the smoking habit. Society pays a high price for smokers' habits. The estimated price we pay is $30 billion per year. This includes the total of all medical and hospital expenses, lost income due to cigarette-related illnesses, and property damage and injuries caused by fires started by cigarettes. This price does not include the emotional cost of accidents, premature disability, or death from causes related to smoking. What can we do, as individuals and as a nation, to eliminate this health problem?

REPORTS TO THE NATION

The first public warnings on the dangers of cigarette smoking were issued by the Surgeon General in 1957. This was followed in 1964 with the Surgeon General's report on Smoking and Health. This report made the public aware of the strong scientific evidence indicating that smoking causes lung cancer and chronic bronchitis, and is also related to deaths from heart disease.

As a result, several steps were taken at the national level to safeguard public health. All cigarette packs must be clearly labeled with the warning shown in Figure 14-8. In 1970 all cigarette ads were banned from radio and television. In 1979 the Surgeon General issued another report which confirmed that cigarette smoking is dangerous, far more dangerous than was supposed in 1964. The 1979 report reinforced the original conclusions. It also found, through years of additional scientific evidence, that (1) smoking is associated with serious and extensive atherosclerosis of the aorta and coronary arteries; (2) smoking produces a certain amount of lung damage even in young smokers (there is a greater tendency to develop a regular cough, phlegm, wheezing, or other respiratory symptoms among young people who smoke); and (3) the smoking habits of children are influenced by their family and peers.

Since 1980 the Surgeon General has issued a series of reports entitled "Health Consequences of Smoking." The 1980 report stressed the harmful effects of smoking on women's health and on unborn children and infants. The 1981 report dealt with the increased use of low-tar/nicotine cigarettes. The 1982 report emphasized that tobacco use causes many forms of cancer. About 30 percent of all cancer deaths can be attributed to tobacco use. Imagine how many lives could be saved if people would forego this habit.

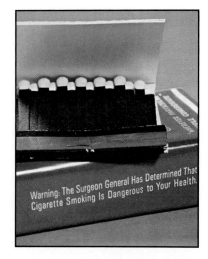

14–8. Do you think that this warning is strong enough?

A SMOKE-FREE ENVIRONMENT

Although it sometimes seems like a smokers' world, nonsmokers are in the majority. Even many smokers support nonsmoking policies. For example, in several states there are now laws that forbid smoking in many public places. Most smokers agree that smoking cigarettes should be banned in more places than it is now. Smoking and nonsmoking sections on planes, interstate buses, and trains have already been established. Many employers are establishing smoke-free work sites. Still there is much you can do to protect the air you breathe.

The National Interagency Council on Smoking and Health has adopted a nonsmokers' Bill of Rights. The Bill lists three basic rights:

1. Nonsmokers have the *right to breathe clean air*, free from harmful, irritating tobacco smoke. When this right conflicts with the smoker's rights, clean air comes first.
2. Nonsmokers have the *right to speak out*, firmly but politely, about their discomfort from tobacco smoke. When smokers light up without asking permission, nonsmokers have the right to voice their objections.
3. Nonsmokers have the *right to act* through legislation, social pressure, or any valid means to prevent or discourage smokers from polluting the atmosphere.

HEALTH TIP

Inhaling sidestream smoke can detract from the pleasure of a restaurant meal. Today more restaurants across the country are catering to nonsmokers. Select a restaurant that has a nonsmoking section or, before you are seated at one, find out if there is a nonsmoking section. If not, do not hesitate to request seating away from smokers' tables.

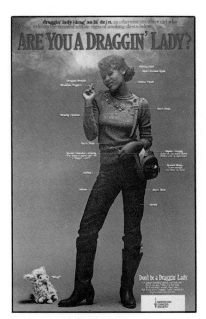

14-9. Improving your health and appearance is a good incentive to stop smoking.

THE SMOKERS' STRATEGY

If you are a smoker, now is the time to quit the habit. As you grow older quitting can be harder as the tobacco habit becomes an established behavior pattern. You will need a lot of willpower and a good reason to quit. There is no single method that works for everyone. Some people stop immediately whereas others taper off gradually. Here are some suggestions that ex-smokers recommend. Plan your strategy carefully. Make a list of the reasons you want to quit. Review your list each day. Keep a record of when you smoke and how much. Attach this record to a cigarette pack. Review progress daily. Cut down the number of cigarettes you smoke gradually. Limit the times when you smoke. Don't smoke when you first feel the nicotine craving. When you do smoke, smoke only half a cigarette. Make yourself more aware of each cigarette you smoke. You can do this by using methods such as smoking with the opposite hand. Let friends know you are quitting so they can help. Avoid your regular smoking routine. Start enjoying a smokefree lifestyle. Exercise more. Try new activities.

The first few days and weeks can be the most difficult. Real success is usually achieved in two to four months, when you can go through your regular activities without wanting to smoke. What's the reward? You will have far greater lung power for your favorite sports. Food will taste better. Your teeth and breath will improve. Your lungs will begin repairing themselves at once, as soon as smoking stops. The risks of developing cancer and heart diseases drop, and eventually become close to or the same as the risks for nonsmokers. Remember, over 30 million people have quit smoking. You can do it too!

SUMMARY: Tobacco use in any form is harmful to health. The health risks of tobacco use include certain cancers and heart and lung disease. Risks vary with the amount of chemicals consumed through tobacco and the length of time tobacco is used. Nonsmokers can be affected by tobacco smoke when they inhale sidestream smoke. Nicotine, tar, and carbon monoxide are some of the major toxic substances in tobacco smoke. Nicotine is an addictive, stimulant drug that affects the cardiovascular system. Tar contains cancer-causing agents. Carbon monoxide robs the body of oxygen so that the cardiovascular system must work harder. In the respiratory system gases and particles of smoke injure the cilia and clog the lungs.

HEALTH ACTION

Devise two or three original warning labels for cigarette packages. The wording should be brief and should clearly convey the message.

UNIT 4 SUBSTANCE USE AND ABUSE

CHAPTER REVIEW

words at work

Unscramble each word that identifies the statement next to it. DO NOT WRITE IN THIS BOOK.

1. C T I N N E O I: an addictive drug found in cigarettes
2. G M O N I O H E L B: oxygen-carrying part of the blood
3. C R O N A B O M E D I X O N: a hazardous gas present in smoke
4. L A I C I: hairlike projections in the air passages
5. C N R A H L O B M O B G E Y O X I: compound formed when hemoglobin combines with carbon monoxide
6. T M E A R E D I S S: the smoke a nonsmoker inhales
7. K S S L E S E M O C A O C B O T: chewing and dipping

review questions

1. What is the current trend in the number of smokers among youths and adults?
2. Cite three factors that may influence the decision to smoke.
3. Name three reasons why people smoke.
4. Define tar and nicotine.
5. Describe two effects that nicotine produces, proving it is an addictive substance.
6. Distinguish between sidestream and mainstream smoke.
7. What is passive smoking?
8. Is sidestream smoke harmless?
9. Define carboxyhemoglobin and describe its effects on the body.
10. How does nicotine affect the cardiovascular system?
11. What causes a smoker's "hack?"
12. Why should smokers alert physicians about their smoking habit?
13. Name five parts of the body that are damaged by tobacco use.
14. Cite three health risks that smoking poses to an unborn child.
15. Does passive smoking pose a health risk? Explain your answer.
16. Describe the health hazards of low-tar/nicotine cigarettes.
17. Compare the health hazards of cigar, pipe, and cigarette smoking.
18. Should chewing tobacco carry a warning label? Explain your answer.
19. How does tobacco use affect appearance?
20. Summarize the findings of the Surgeon General's reports.
21. List five ways to help break a smoking habit.

discussion questions

1. Does smoking concern all of us? Give evidence to support your answer.
2. To deter tobacco use among youth an advertising ban on the use of live models has been proposed. Do you think this would be effective? Why or why not?
3. Discuss smoking as a physical and psychological addiction. What common behavior patterns have you observed among addicted smokers?
4. Smoking in school among students is a problem in many areas. Discuss policies that you think would be effective in addressing this problem.
5. A friend asks for help in breaking a tobacco habit. What would you do?
6. Discuss positive ways nonsmokers can assert themselves when a smoker lights up in (a) an elevator, (b) a restaurant, and (c) a bus.

investigating

PURPOSE:
To investigate the effects of smoking on the cardiovascular system.

MATERIALS NEEDED:
An adult smoker who has *not* smoked for at least three hours prior to this activity; cigarettes; matches; a clinical thermometer; wristwatch or clock with a second hand; paper; graph paper; pencil.

PROCEDURE:
A. Have the smoker hold the sensitive end of the thermometer between the fingers. After two minutes, read the thermometer and record the temperature.
B. Place two fingers on the thumb side of the smoker's wrist and find the pulse. Use the second hand of a watch or clock and count the pulse rate for 60 seconds. Record your results. Repeat until three pulse readings have been obtained. Average the three readings to obtain a "normal" pulse rate.
C. Instruct the smoker to light and smoke a cigarette. After the smoker has taken four or five puffs of the cigarette, take and record the 60-second pulse rate and finger temperatures again. Repeat and record these ratings every 15 minutes until the pulse rate and finger temperature return to normal. (Note: for accuracy, the smoker should not increase his or her activity during this period.) Chart your findings on a graph.

   1. How did smoking affect the finger temperature and the pulse rate? What changes in the cardiovascular system produced these effects?
   2. Based on your results, determine about how many extra times the subject's heart must beat as a result of smoking one pack of cigarettes. With each heart beat, the heart pumps about 70 ml of blood. Calculate the extra blood volume that must be pumped by the heart as a result of smoking one pack of cigarettes.
   3. Discuss smoking as a risk factor in the development of heart disease.

PHARMACIST

Which member of the health team do people utilize most often? If your answer is pharmacist, you are right. Pharmacists are an important link between consumers and doctors. Pharmacists do more than dispense drugs and health products. Pharmacists also help people maintain their health by giving them needed information. They sometimes direct people to appropriate health services or help them to practice preventive medicine. Pharmacists also keep individual patient profiles. These profiles are the records of all drugs prescribed for each customer. Before filling patients' prescriptions, pharmacists check these records carefully for potential harmful reactions that might occur from taking more than one drug at a time. A pharmacist becomes a specialist in the science of drugs by completing a three- or four-year course in pharmacy and passing a state licensing examination. For more information write to the American Association of Colleges of Pharmacy, 4630 Montgomery Avenue, Bethesda, Maryland 20814.

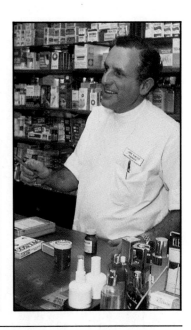

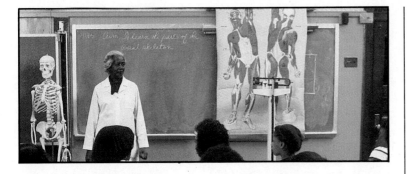

HEALTH EDUCATOR

One health professional who plays a special role in preventing health problems is the health educator. The health educator helps people improve their health by distributing health information and by motivating people to use it. If your health and the health of others interest you, you can make this interest a career. School health and community health education are two areas from which you can choose. As a school health educator, you might teach many subjects, including first aid, safety education, nutrition, personal hygiene, and community and environmental health. Through you, your students could be started on a lifetime of healthful living. To become a health educator, you must have a four-year college degree in health or community health education. Many jobs also require a master's degree.

For information about a career as a health educator, contact the American School Health Association, P.O. Box 708, 1521 S. Water Street, Kent, Ohio 44240, and the Association for the Advancement of Health Education, 1900 Association Drive, Reston, Virginia 22091.

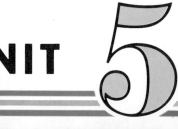

UNIT 5

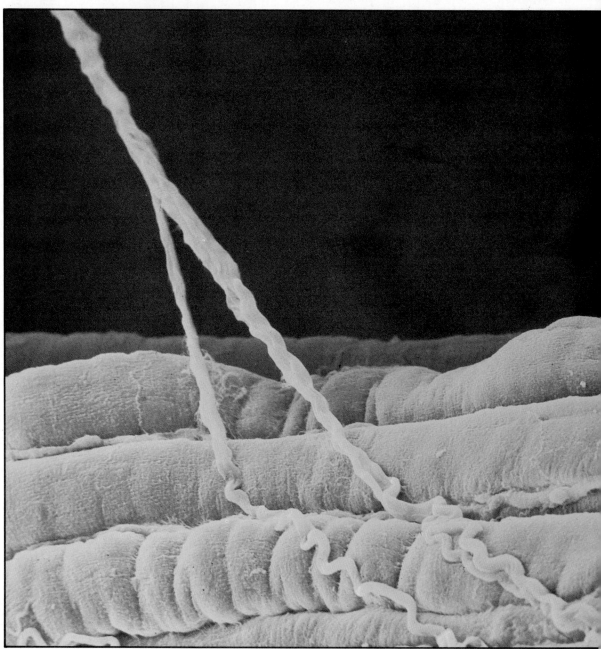

Your Control Systems

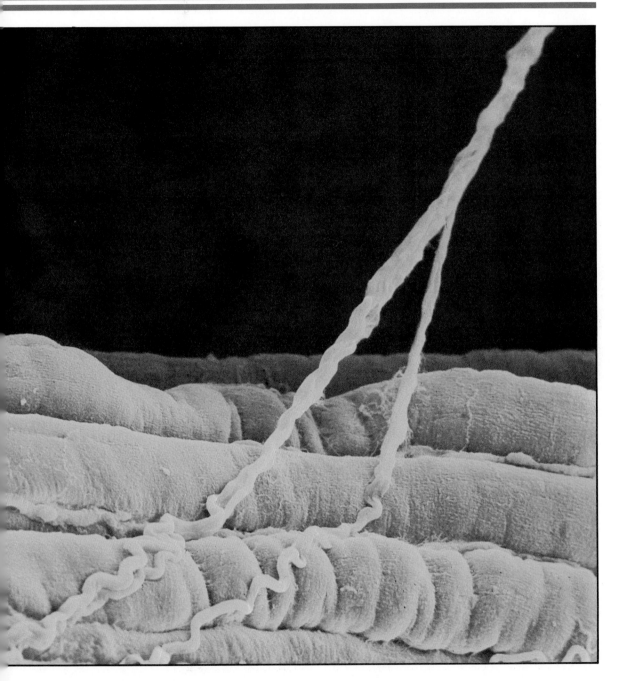

CHAPTER 15

The Nervous System

OBJECTIVES

- LOCATE and DESCRIBE the central and peripheral nervous systems
- DESCRIBE the parts of a neuron and TRACE the pathway of a nerve impulse
- DESCRIBE the parts of the brain and the function of each part
- STATE the functions of the sympathetic and parasympathetic nervous systems
- DESCRIBE the damage to the nervous system caused by skull and spine injuries and disease, and how they are diagnosed

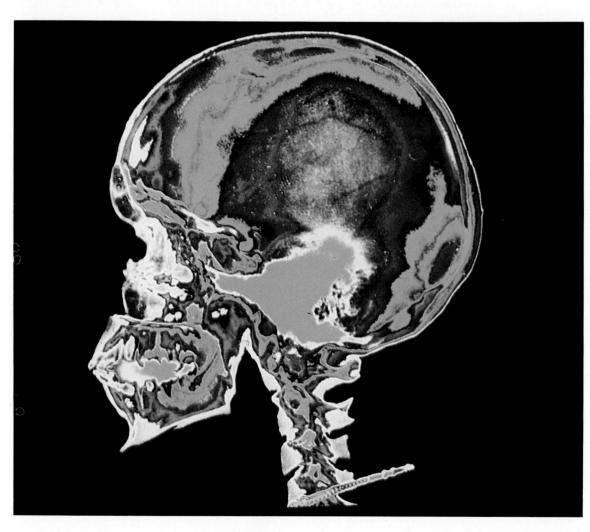

Twenty-four hundred years ago Hippocrates located the center of the intellect inside the skull. Before this it was believed that humans thought with their hearts. Today scientists suspect that all human behavior can be described in terms of a series of electrochemical impulses. However, unraveling the mystery of how these impulses determine human behavior is a complex task. There are billions of nerve cells in our bodies. The simplest response involves millions of these nerve cells. Our remarkable nervous system is vital and irreplaceable. In this chapter you will learn about how the nervous system functions and how to take care of it. You will also learn about some of the disorders of the nervous system.

STRUCTURE AND FUNCTION

The human nervous system is awesomely complex. It is made up of a network of over 25 billion nerve cells that lead from the brain and establish contact with every portion of the human body. The brain is the central control unit. Messages travel over nerve cells from every part of the body to inform the nerve cells in the brain of everything going on inside and outside the body. The nerve cells in the brain process this information and send out messages over other nerve cells. In response, people laugh, cry, sing, walk, talk, and otherwise behave as human beings.

NEURONS

Nerve cells, called **neurons** (**ner-**rons), are the building blocks of the nervous system. Neurons are capable of responding to stimuli and passing these responses to other neurons. This ability makes the neuron a transmitting unit capable of passing information from one part of the body to another.

Not all neurons are alike. There are three different types: **receptor, connecting,** and **motor neurons.** Each type performs a special job. Receptor, or input, neurons detect changes in the environment and in the body and relay this information to the brain. There are separate receptors for heat, cold, touch, and pain. There are also receptors for hearing, sight, taste, balance, and smell.

Sensory receptor neurons are unevenly distributed throughout the body. In the fingers there are many touch

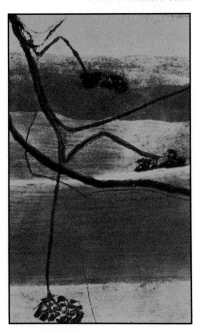

15–1. These are branches of a motor neuron, magnified 768 times, which carry impulses from the brain to muscle cells.

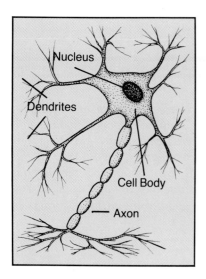

15–2. The entire nervous system is composed of individual cells called neurons.

15–3. Neuron fibers, magnified 600 times, are bound together as nerves, like cable wires.

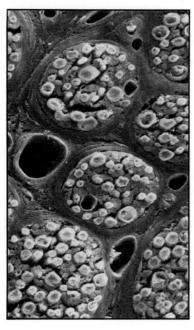

receptors but there are fewer in your back. This is why the fingers are more sensitive to touch than the back. Within the eye there are the greatest number of pain receptors. Even the entrance of a tiny speck of dust can cause pain. Hearing receptors are found only in the ears, and vision receptors are found only in the eyes.

The connecting neurons in the brain act as a message-relay center. They react to incoming sensory information, process this information, and then pass messages back to the motor neurons.

The motor neurons receive orders from the brain and carry them to the muscles, the glands, and the internal organs. They are responsible for every movement of the body, from the movement of the hand to the act of breathing.

STRUCTURE OF A NEURON.   You can begin to understand how neurons work by examining a single neuron, such as the one shown in Figure 15-2. Nerve cells are very different from other body cells in structure and function. In the diagram you can see that a neuron, like all cells, has a **cell body** and a **nucleus.** But, unlike other cells, it also has special threadlike fibers that lead to and from the cell body. These fibers have a separate mission. The **dendrites (dendrites),** fibers leading to the cell body, are receivers. They receive messages and carry them to the cell body. The **axon,** the single long fiber leading away from the cell, is a transmitter. It transmits the messages away from the cell body to the next nerve cell.

Neurons are so small that they can be seen only with a high-powered microscope. To understand the relative dimensions of the neuron parts, think of this example. If the cell body were the size of a tennis ball, its axon might extend up to a mile in length but would be only half an inch in diameter. The dendrites would branch to fill a large room.

Neuron fibers, axons and dendrites, are usually bound together into nerves. There may be thousands of neuron fibers in a single nerve. They can be compared to the wires in a telephone cable. Each is insulated from the others and acts independently (see Figure 15-3).

NEURONS IN ACTION.   It is a cloudy, cool day. You are sitting outside in a stadium, wearing a heavy sweater. You are watching your school team compete in a relay race. Suddenly the sun comes out, and the temperature rises. You soon begin to feel uncomfortable, and you remove your sweater. Although this sequence of events seems simple,

314

there were actually millions of nerve cells involved. Let's find out what happened.

The sequence of events inside your body can be compared to a relay race. As the temperature increased, the heat receptors in your skin picked up a message. The message was then transmitted into a signal called a *nerve impulse*. Nerve impulses are somewhat like an electrical current, but are different in that they depend upon the activity of living cells. Chemical changes as well as electrical changes are involved in the transmission of nerve impulses. Neurons conduct impulses at the rate of about 2 to 120 meters per second.

When the heat receptors are stimulated, the nerve impulses move along the dendrites to the cell body. Then they travel down the axon until they reach the end of the fiber. There, dendrites from the next sensory neuron are waiting to receive the message. However, before the message can be relayed, the impulses have to cross a microscopic gap known as a **synapse** (**sin**-ahps). This is made possible by chemical messengers. Tiny sacs at the end of the axon produce these chemical messengers. When a neuron impulse reaches the end of the axon, these sacs release the chemicals, which travel across the synapse, and cause the next neuron to fire. The nerve impulse travels from one neuron to the next until it reaches the spinal cord. In the spinal cord, connecting neurons join the race, relaying the impulses to the brain. In the brain the impulses are translated by other neurons into a meaning: "It is too warm." Other neurons translate these impulses into a suggestion: "Remove your sweater." The neurons in the brain then send a message back through motor neurons. The motor axons ending at the muscles receive the message and follow the orders of the brain. They instruct certain muscles to contract and others to relax in orderly patterns. Therefore, you remove your sweater and the relay race ends.

THE PARTS OF THE NERVOUS SYSTEM

Part of the nervous system is housed in the skull and spine, while part extends throughout the remainder of the body. The part that is centrally located, the brain and the spinal cord, is called the **central nervous system.** There are also nerves that are connected to the brain and spinal cord and extend to the exterior, or periphery, of the body. This is called the **peripheral nervous system.**

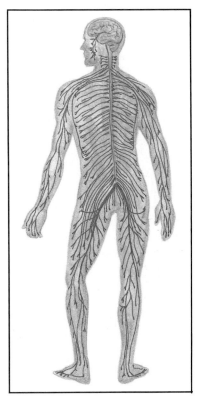

15–4. The central and peripheral nervous systems

THE BRAIN

Years ago the heart was considered the body's most important organ, the center of life. Today the brain is considered to be the master control unit. The brain is responsible for emotions, for learning, for perceptions, and for basic life functions. In fact, as understanding of the brain's importance grows, even the definition of death changes. Today most physicians pronounce a patient dead when the brain is dead, even if the heart still beats. Why is brain death used as a measure of life? Our hearts are just mechanical pumps, which can be made to work by artificial means. But when the brain stops working, its functions cannot be replaced.

What does the brain look like? Imagine a giant walnut, about 1.35 kilograms (3 lb), and you have a good picture of the brain. Like a walnut, the brain has many folds and wrinkles. These increase the surface area of the brain, thereby increasing the number of neurons. Altogether there are more than 25 billion neurons in the brain.

BRAIN PROTECTORS.   If you touched the brain, it would feel like a balloon filled with water. Since your brain is so fragile and so vital an organ, it is well protected. The brain is housed within its own protective helmet, the *cranial cavity* of the skull. The brain is also surrounded by tough membranes called **meninges** (men-**in**-jees). The outer meninx lies directly against the skull. The inner meninx covers the brain. The third one lies between the other two. Another form of protection is the clear **cerebrospinal fluid** (ser-ree-bro-**spy**-nal). This liquid fills the space between the middle and inner meninges. The fluid also fills certain inner spaces of the brain, called **ventricles** (**ven**-trick-kulz). This fluid, which acts as a shock absorber, cushions the brain against injury. It also helps to feed nerve tissues and to remove waste products from them.

PARTS OF THE BRAIN.   The brain has four main parts. The largest part of the brain is the **cerebrum.** Beneath the cerebrum are the **cerebellum,** which is the second largest part of the brain, and the **interbrain.** The **brainstem** is the elongated portion of the brain that looks like a stalk for the cerebrum.

THE CEREBRUM.   The cerebrum is divided into two halves by a deep groove, much like a walnut. These halves are then further divided by folds into areas called *lobes.*

The cerebrum is the center of intellect, memory, language, and consciousness. All nerve impulses are meaningless until they reach the cerebrum. For example, even though pain receptors respond to a cut, pain is not felt until the impulse reaches the cerebrum. There the impulse is translated into its meaning, in this case, pain. If action is necessary, the cerebrum further translates the message into muscle commands. This process is similar to that of a computer. When the brain receives a nerve impulse, it relies on its memory bank. From information stored there, the brain chooses the appropriate action. Next it instructs the body about how to carry out that action. Precisely how that occurs is unknown. What is known, however, is that each part of the cerebrum has a specific task. The cerebrum forms a higher proportion of the human brain than it does of the brain of any other animal. It is responsible for our highly developed human intelligence.

A MAP OF THE CEREBRUM.

Figure 15-5 outlines each area of the cerebrum and its job. The sensory areas receive impulses from the sense organs and relay messages through

15–5. The control areas of the cerebrum. Notice that the motor and sensory areas for different parts of the body are adjacent.

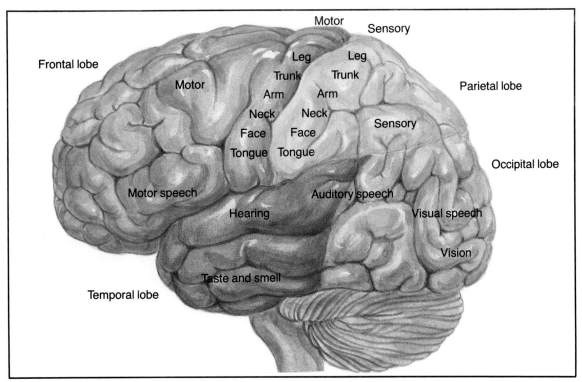

FOCUS ON HEALTH

RIGHT AND LEFT BRAINS

Although the two halves of the brain look identical, evidence indicates that they have totally different functions. The left brain controls the right side of the body, and the right brain controls the left side of the body. The two halves also have different ways of thinking. The left brain can be called the logical brain. As you read these words, your left brain is comprehending their meaning. The left brain recognizes groups of letters as words and groups of words as sentences. Your left brain is also capable of doing arithmetic. In fact, it is the left brain that has many of the same functions as a computer. It takes in information and processes it in a very logical fashion. People who study math and science use their left brains a great deal.

What does the right brain do? When you draw a picture or listen to music or recognize a face without putting a name to it, your right brain is involved. The right brain is mute, and interprets the world through patterns, meanings, and emotions. Artists and musicians use their right brains a great deal.

How were the separate functions of the right and left brains discovered? This information first emerged when doctors began to perform operations to cure epilepsy. There is a bundle of nerve fibers between the two halves of the brain called the *corpus callosum.* The corpus callosum is the main communication line between the right and left brains. Cutting this connection in epileptics reduced the number of seizures that occurred. The operation also isolated the two halves of the brain. This allowed researchers to study the separate functions of the two halves. A split-brain patient could name an object placed in his right hand by touch alone. The sensory data went to the left brain, where the verbal center lies. But the same split-brain patient could not name an object placed in his left hand. The sensation went to the right hemisphere, where the verbal center was poorly developed. Usually, this information would cross over from the right brain to the left brain.

With the use of EEG readings, more information is now being gathered about the different functions of the right and left brains. Electrodes are placed on the left and right sides of the scalp. Nerve activity at each electrode is recorded as the subject performs different tasks. When writing a letter, there is more activity in the left hemisphere. When drawing a picture, there is more activity in the right hemisphere. During any kind of activity, there is some nerve activity on both sides of the brain, although activity on one side is usually greater than on the other. The musician pictured below uses mostly his right brain. The dotted lines show the paths of nervous impulses.

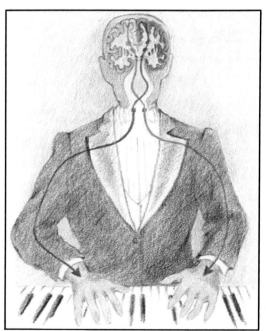

special areas of the brain. Motor areas control movements. Association areas, the least understood, are the centers of emotion and intelligence.

The speech areas, which control communication, involve several areas of the brain. For example, what happens when you SEE the word "car?" Immediately your mind pictures a four-wheeled vehicle. To get that picture, you draw information from a memory bank in the visual speech area of your brain. Then you link it to an image associated with that word. At this point the word takes on meaning. Had you HEARD the word "car" instead, you would have also connected the word to a memory picture. However, that picture would have come from a different center of the brain, the auditory speech center. When this linkage is made, sound takes on meaning. To say the word "car," you must use the muscles in your lips, tongue, larynx, and respiratory system. That requires coordination between your motor speech area, which controls muscles, and your auditory speech area, which tells you the sounds to make. But to write the word "car," the visual speech area and the motor areas of your brain must communicate and cooperate.

Since the motor area works closely with all parts of the speech areas, damage to one can upset the other. Such a situation can cause problems with reading, writing, or speech. Many children who have learning difficulties in school are now known to have a problem in one or more areas of the brain.

THE CEREBELLUM. The word "cerebellum" means "little brain," but don't let that name fool you. Even though it's small in comparison to the cerebrum, the cerebellum performs a big job. It is the control for smooth, coordinated muscle movements. Do you enjoy sports? Do you like to dance? These activities would be impossible without help from the cerebellum.

The cerebellum receives impulses from the balancing centers of the inner ear, from the muscles and joints, and from the motor areas of the cerebrum. The cerebrum initiates muscular movements. The cerebellum ensures that these movements are carried out smoothly and effectively. Like the cerebrum, each part of the cerebellum has a special function.

INTERBRAIN. The interbrain is composed of the **thalamus** and the **hypothalamus.** The thalamus is the main relay center conducting information between the spinal cord and the cerebrum. The hypothalamus is an important link between mind (the cerebrum) and body. It controls the secretion of chemicals called hormones that affect several body functions. It also helps maintain water balance and temperature in the body, and contains centers for appetite and thirst.

THE BRAINSTEM.   The brainstem is the lower portion of the brain. It has three parts. From top to bottom, they are the *midbrain*, the *pons*, and the *medulla*. The midbrain connects the brainstem with the cerebrum and parts of the cerebellum. The midbrain mediates visual and auditory reflexes, and controls certain eye movements. The word "pons" means bridge. The pons forms a bridge mainly between the medulla and other parts of the brain. The pons also helps regulate chewing, facial expressions, respiration, and certain eye movements. The medulla, a small bulb of the brain, is where the spinal cord joins the brain.

15–6. A lateral view of the human brain

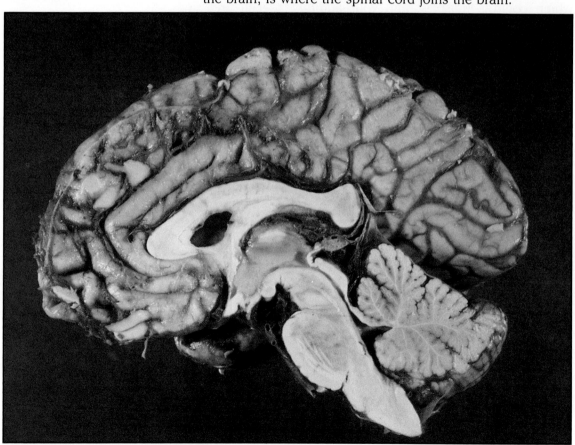

A CLOSER LOOK AT THE MEDULLA. In the medulla most nerve fibers on the right side of the brain cross over to control the left side of the body. Fibers from the left side of the brain control the right side of the body.

The medulla is also a vital control center. As you read this page, your medulla is hard at work. You never consciously have to command your lungs to breathe. The medulla controls this as well as other basic body functions, such as digestion, blood pressure, and body temperature.

Figure 15-7

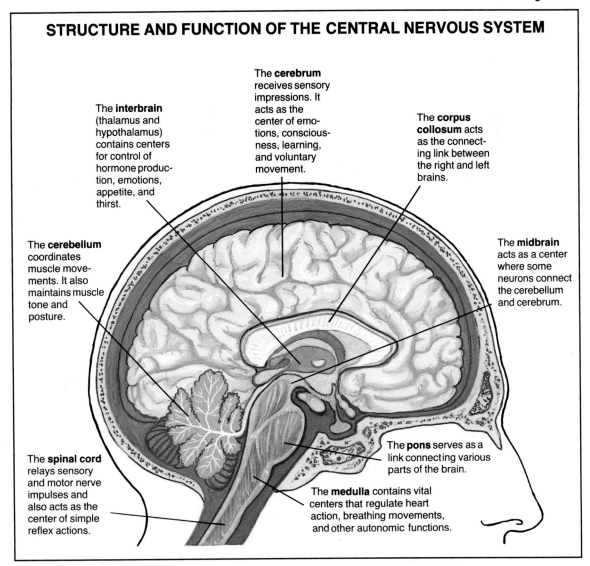

STRUCTURE AND FUNCTION OF THE CENTRAL NERVOUS SYSTEM

The **interbrain** (thalamus and hypothalamus) contains centers for control of hormone production, emotions, appetite, and thirst.

The **cerebrum** receives sensory impressions. It acts as the center of emotions, consciousness, learning, and voluntary movement.

The **corpus collosum** acts as the connecting link between the right and left brains.

The **midbrain** acts as a center where some neurons connect the cerebellum and cerebrum.

The **cerebellum** coordinates muscle movements. It also maintains muscle tone and posture.

The **spinal cord** relays sensory and motor nerve impulses and also acts as the center of simple reflex actions.

The **pons** serves as a link connecting various parts of the brain.

The **medulla** contains vital centers that regulate heart action, breathing movements, and other autonomic functions.

What happens when you become frightened? You breathe harder, and your heart beats faster. That is because the actions of the medulla can be triggered by the sense organs and the emotional centers of the brain.

The medulla sits at the base of the skull and juts out slightly. It is the body's most vulnerable spot. A single blow to the medulla can be instantly fatal. Damage to this part of the brain can cut off control of vital body functions.

THE SPINAL CORD: A CABLE FROM THE BRAIN

The **spinal cord** is a nerve cable extending down the spinal column from the medulla. The spinal cord is vital, and the neurons composing it are unable to replace themselves. If the spinal cord is severed, there is permanent paralysis from that point downward. Thus, there is a great need of protection from injury. The bones of the spine provide a great deal of protection. The meninges, or membranes surrounding the brain, continue down the spinal cord to provide it with a protective covering. Cerebrospinal fluid fills the area between the middle and inner meninges.

A cross section of the cord is shown in Figure 15-9. The dark area in the center is gray matter, and surrounding it is the white matter. The gray matter forms a shape like that of

15–8. Structure of the spinal cord

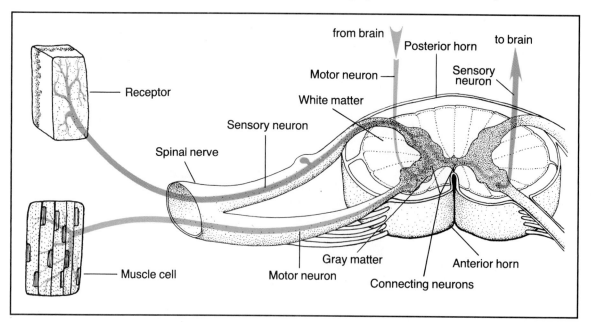

UNIT 5   YOUR CONTROL SYSTEMS

a butterfly with spread wings. The pointed tips of the wings of gray matter are called *horns*. The posterior pair points toward the back of the spinal cord. Here, sensory nerves go into the cord from the outlying areas of the body. The anterior pair points toward the front of the spinal cord. Here, motor nerves leave the cord and extend to the muscles.

White matter, surrounding the gray matter, consists of a dense mass of nerves that pass up and down from the brain. Sensory nerves carry impulses up the cord to the brain. Motor nerves carry impulses from the brain.

15–9. Cross-section of the spinal cord

THE PERIPHERAL NERVOUS SYSTEM

The *peripheral nervous system* is well named. Peripheral means "located away from the center." The peripheral nervous system sends information from the central nervous system to other parts of the body. It also sends sensory information from the body back to the central nervous system.

Part of the peripheral nervous system (the cranial nerves) extends from areas of the brain to parts of the head. There are 12 pairs of these cranial nerves. The cranial nerves transmit information to the brain from the nose, eyes, ears, and tongue. They also bring orders from the brain to the muscles that control the eyes, face, jaw, neck, tongue, and throat.

The spinal nerves form the other part of the peripheral nervous system. The spinal nerves lead away from the spinal cord. These large nerve cables begin in the neck and extend down the length of the spinal cord. There are thirty-one pairs of spinal nerves, one pair between each vertebra. One nerve of each pair goes to the right side of the body, and one goes to the left. Since the spinal nerves contain both sensory and motor fibers, they are called *mixed nerves*.

Just outside the cord, each nerve cable splits into a "Y". The branch leading to the back of the spinal cord contains fibers of sensory neurons, which carry incoming impulses. The other branch leading from the front of the spinal cord contains fibers of the motor nerves, which carry outgoing impulses. The motor branch joins the sensory branch within the gray matter of the spinal cord. Here, sensory and motor neurons synapse with each other. They also connect with neurons that lead to and from the brain. To picture this, you might think of a spinal cord as a main highway with traffic moving in two directions. Traffic entering and leaving this main highway travels on two different one-way roads.

REFLEXES. During a routine physical examination, the doctor hits your knee with a small hammer. What happens? Your leg jerks upward. The knee-jerk reflex is an example of a *simple reflex*. The stimulus is the tap of the hammer, and the jerk of your leg is the response. During this reflex response a part of the nervous system other than the brain is involved. How is the brain bypassed?

When the knee is hit, the muscle is stretched, and sensory fibers within the muscle are stimulated. They send the impulse along the sensory nerves, and the impulse enters the spinal cord through a posterior branch. The impulse then moves across a synapse to the ending of a motor neuron. Next, the impulse leaves the spinal cord, through its anterior branch, and moves along a motor nerve to the knee muscles. This sequence of events causes the knee to jerk. It happened without your control. This is called a *reflex arc*. Trace the path of a reflex arc in Figure 15-10.

15–10. The reflex arc

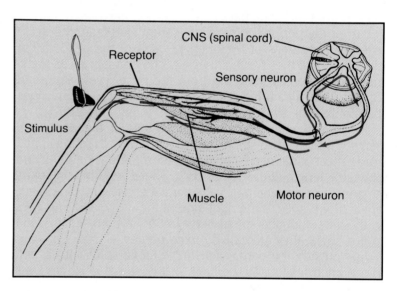

PROTECTIVE REFLEXES. If you accidentally touch a hot stove, you immediately pull your hand away. Afterward, you suddenly become aware of pain. That response is also a simple reflex, although it is more complex than a knee jerk. Before the pain impulse reaches the brain, a reflex impulse is relayed to the muscles controlling the hand. By the time the brain tells you "pain," your hand is already safe. This reflex arc acts as a natural protective device.

THE AUTONOMIC NERVOUS SYSTEM

The **autonomic nervous system** controls body functions without your conscious control. It might well be called the "automatic" nervous system. To accomplish its task, it uses its two nerve networks: the sympathetic and parasympathetic systems. The sympathetic nerves arise from the midportion of the spinal cord and lead to all vital internal organs and glands. These include the liver, the pancreas, and the salivary and sweat glands. The parasympathetic nerves arise from the brain and lower spinal cord. These nerves also innervate most of the internal organs (see Figure 15-11).

Most of the internal organs are innervated by both the parasympathetic and sympathetic systems. Like two teams in a tug-of-war, the two systems generally work in opposite directions. In this way, they act as a check and balance for each other. The function of the sympathetic system is to speed up the body and prepare it for a "fight or flight" reaction. It increases blood pressure, heartbeat rate, breathing, and blood flow to the skin and muscles. The parasympathetic system, however, acts as the brake. It slows the heart, opens the blood vessels, and lowers the blood pressure. It allows the body to rest and repair itself.

15–11. The autonomic nervous system regulates the internal organs of the body. What are the functions of its two divisions?

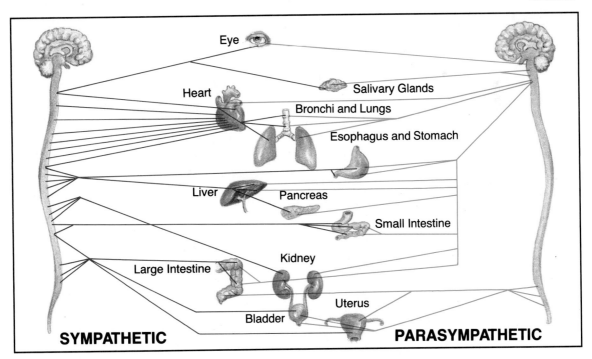

Eye Nose
Heart Salivary Glands
Bronchi and Lungs
Esophagus and Stomach
Liver Pancreas
Small Intestine
Kidney
Large Intestine
Uterus
Bladder

SYMPATHETIC **PARASYMPATHETIC**

Both of these systems are influenced by emotions and by your external and internal environments. For example, if you become frightened, your mouth becomes dry. That is because impulses, carried to the salivary glands by the sympathetic system, tell the glands to stop working. What happens when you are hungry and smell food? Does your mouth begin to water? That is because a message is carried to your salivary glands by the parasympathetic system, which prepares you to start eating.

The autonomic nervous system is not entirely without conscious control. For centuries yogis have shown that it is possible to gain control over many automatic activities. We now know that, by using biofeedback, people can be taught how to control blood pressure, heart rate, headaches, and muscle tension.

ATTACKS ON YOUR NERVOUS SYSTEM

Your nervous system can encounter health problems. Headaches are common problems, but they are usually not causes for concern. Other problems are more serious and require prompt medical attention. What makes the nervous system sometimes go haywire? How do physicians detect these problems? What can they do to treat them?

IDENTIFYING THE PROBLEM

Frequent and severe headaches, memory lapses, pain or numbness in the arms or legs, speech disturbances, trembling, weakness, and failing eyesight are just a few of the complaints that indicate nervous system disorders. A neurologist is a physician specializing in diagnosing and treating disorders of the nervous system. Although a symptom or complaint may not mean that there is something seriously wrong, it could be a warning of trouble. The neuroglogist must be an expert sleuth. No clue is overlooked during the examination.

The neurological examination begins with a detailed history of the patient's problem. A skilled neurologist can determine from the patient's answers if the nervous system is in trouble. After a history is taken, the entire nervous system is checked carefully through a series of simple but important tests. Before making an actual diagnosis, the neurologist

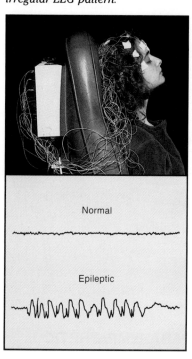

15–12. The EEG records the electrical activity of the brain. Abnormalities, such as epilepsy, produce an irregular EEG pattern.

Normal

Epileptic

may also use several laboratory tests or other techniques to discover the problem in the nervous system. Two long-standing tests are the electroencephalogram (EEG for short) and the spinal tap.

EEG.   The EEG records the electrical activity of the brain. Tiny electrical signals are produced by nerve cells in the brain. Electrodes are placed on the scalp to pick up these signals. Can the EEG read your mind? No, but it can tell when you are asleep or when you are concentrating on solving a problem. The brain patterns for each of these activities are different. EEG's can be used to diagnose abnormalities, such as epilepsy caused by a tumor, which produces a special pattern on an EEG (see Figure 15-12).

THE SPINAL TAP.   Have you ever seen a maple tree being tapped for syrup? A spinal tap works in much the same way. A doctor inserts a needle between the vertebrae of the spinal column and draws a small amount of the spinal fluid for analysis. It is only through this procedure that certain diseases can be diagnosed and treated properly.

THE CT.   Computerized tomography, CT, combines a computer with X rays. The CT can produce pictures of the human body that are impossible with ordinary X rays. On a so-called *CT scan,* images of cross sections of the head can be viewed. Different colors indicate different densities. The most dense structures, such as bone, appear white. A brain tumor can be seen on the CT scan pictured in Figure 15-13.

NUCLEAR MAGNETIC RESONANCE (NMR).   NMR is a new invention that may eventually replace the CT scan to detect body abnormalities with greater accuracy. The patient is placed inside a huge magnet, and the body's response to magnetic waves is recorded by a computer.

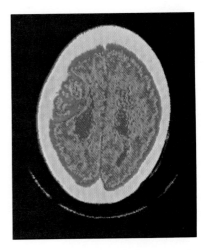

15–13. Notice the tumor in the left brain on this CT scan.

HEADACHES

Headaches are a common problem that affect approximately 90 percent of the population. Although headaches rarely involve the nervous system, people commonly fear that headaches can be due to a brain disorder.

Tension can cause a headache if the muscles in the scalp and back of the neck tighten. Headaches can last hours, days, weeks, or even years. However, most headaches can usually be relieved by aspirin, massage, or applied heat. Headaches may recur if the problem is emotional tension.

HEALTH TIP

Handling stress is one of the best ways to avoid headaches. Exercising relaxes the body, especially the muscles at the back of the neck, which tend to stiffen. Also, taking a rest in a quiet place, avoiding stuffy rooms, or getting fresh air can help.

Another kind of common headache is called the *migraine headache*. Migraines can be severe. They can begin with changes in sight, such as seeing spots or flashes of light before the eyes. The sensory changes last a short time. Then the throbbing pain of the migraine begins. The pain is usually on one side of the head, but it can occur on both sides. Vomiting sometimes occurs with migraine headaches. The exact cause of the migraine is unknown. Stress, fatigue, or an upset in body chemistry may trigger migraine headaches. Prescription medications can relieve the pain of migraine headaches and reduce their frequency. Biofeedback has also been found to be effective.

Sometimes serious brain problems can cause headaches. Infections or bleeding of the meninges, brain tumors, or abnormal cell growth in the brain can cause headaches. Therefore, if you have unusually long headaches, or if a severe headache develops suddenly, see a doctor.

BRAIN INJURIES

Although your nervous system is well protected, injury and direct damage, either temporary or permanent, can occur.

CONCUSSIONS.   A severe blow to the head may cause the soft mass of the brain to strike the hard inner surface of the skull. This causes temporary unconsciousness followed by a headache. The treatment is rest, and recovery is usually complete.

CONTUSIONS.   Do not confuse a concussion with a contusion. A contusion is much more serious. It is actually a bruising of the brain or nerves. Recovery is possible, but it takes a long time. A contusion of the brain almost always causes unconsciousness. When unconsciousness is deep and prolonged, the patient is said to be in a coma. A contusion can cause a blood clot in the brain. These clots must sometimes be removed by surgery.

FRACTURES.   A skull fracture (a break in the bone) sounds dangerous, and often it is. Given a period of absolute rest, a patient's bones will usually mend without complications. Nonetheless, the simplest of skull fractures can become serious if a blood clot forms or the cerebrospinal fluid leaks into certain parts of the skull. Then either the clots must be removed or the leak must be sealed through surgery. A fracture is also serious when there is a complete break, not just a crack, in the skull. This is because skull fragments can press on the brain and cause paralysis. Again, surgery is usually necessary, either to adjust or to remove broken bone from the brain's surface.

NERVE AND SPINAL CORD INJURIES

The nerves and the spinal cord are sometimes damaged by a partial tear or complete cut. Household, work, and car accidents are the most frequent causes of these injuries.

Sometimes an injury to the peripheral nerves can be repaired through surgery. Then each of the damaged nerve ends is cut and sewn together. Such a procedure is comparable to the splicing of torn film. Once sewn, the nerve fibers slowly begin to grow together. Since their rate of growth is very slow, the fibers take a long time to heal.

Most spinal cord damage occurs when a splinter from a fractured vertebra pinches or cuts the spinal cord. It can also occur when a vertebra slips out of place. Improperly moving a person with a spinal cord injury might move the splinter or vertebra further. This may cause permanent paralysis.

Are you familiar with the terms *paraplegia* and *quadraplegia*? *Paraplegia* means paralysis of the legs and lower body. *Quadraplegia* is paralysis of both the arms and the legs.

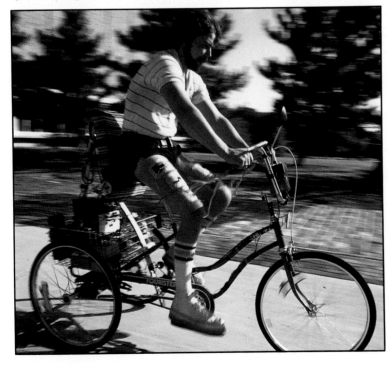

15–14. Computer-controlled electrical stimulation of muscles allows a person with paraplegia to ride a bicycle.

Many paraplegics and quadraplegics still lead productive lives, despite their paralysis. Biomedical research promises an even brighter future for them. Experiments are proving that paralyzed limbs can be made to work again when aided by electrical computerized devices.

DISORDERS OF THE NERVOUS SYSTEM

CEREBRAL PALSY. Cerebral palsy, which affects about 700,000 people in our country, is a group of disabling conditions caused by damage to the central nervous system. It is not contagious. Damage can occur either before or during birth if oxygen to the brain is decreased or temporarily cut off. During birth, pressure on a baby's delicate head can damage the motor areas of the brain. Accidental injury, lead poisoning, or certain illnesses early in life can also lead to cerebral palsy.

What are the effects of cerebral palsy? That depends on the area of the brain that is damaged and the seriousness of the injury. Most often people with cerebral palsy have spastic muscles that are tense and contracted. Although the muscles are not paralyzed, they do not move with ease and coordination. Walking and speech may also be difficult. Don't confuse a physical disability with a mental disability. Most people with cerebral palsy have average or above-average intelligence.

Even though no cure exists for cerebral palsy, exercise, speech therapy, special training of the muscles, and braces can help people with cerebral palsy lead active lives.

EPILEPSY: ELECTRICAL STORMS. Epilepsy is not a disease but a disorder of the nervous system. It is caused by a sudden electrical imbalance in the brain that triggers an electrical storm. This brain "storm" causes a **seizure.** Seizures can be very severe, lasting two to five minutes, or less severe, lasting ten to thirty seconds. During severe seizures, an epileptic may fall to the floor and completely lose consciousness. The entire body shakes violently in a **convulsion.** Once the seizure passes, the victim may feel sleepy or have a headache, but usually there is no memory of the incident.

Less severe seizures, which are most frequent in children, are so tiny they can easily go unnoticed. A person may seem out of touch with his or her surroundings or stare blankly into space. A child who has learning difficulties in school or who is labeled a daydreamer may actually have this type of undiagnosed epilepsy.

Epilepsy does not have a single cause. Brain injury before or during birth or at any other point in a person's lifetime can cause this disorder. Or there may be other causes, such as a high fever in childhood, an intake of poisons, an infection, a chemical imbalance, or a tumor in the brain. If a chemical imbalance or tumor is the problem, the epilepsy is sometimes correctable. Many children with epilepsy simply outgrow it by their teen years.

Most often epilepsy is incurable. However, epilepsy can usually be controlled by special drugs. Today these drugs are so effective that convulsions and seizures can be eliminated in 50 percent of all patients. Ultimately, drugs may even be able to control the disorder totally.

MULTIPLE SCLEROSIS. This disease affects some 300,000 people in the United States alone. Multiple sclerosis is a mysterious crippler of young adults. It disables by attacking the insulation of the nerve fibers. Because multiple sclerosis destroys the fibers in patches, nerve impulses can no longer pass easily to and from the spinal cord and brain. The complications multiple sclerosis creates are unpredictable. They depend on which nerves are attacked. One person may experience a loss of balance or coordination, and another person may be paralyzed by the disease. Speech and hearing difficulties can also develop. Sometimes the symptoms mysteriously disappear for months or years, only to suddenly reappear. Multiple sclerosis is usually a progressive disease, but it rarely causes death.

PARKINSON'S DISEASE. People usually do not contract Parkinson's disease before age 40. Most people with this disease are over 60. It usually causes trembling of the arms and legs and often produces muscle stiffness, which makes walking, and sometimes speech, difficult. A masklike unchanging facial expression may occur. To people who do not understand the problems of this disease, such an expression can be misunderstood.

Parkinson's disease requires careful diagnosis. Although no cause or cure is known, the drug L-dopa has dramatically reduced the disease's effect on many patients. Some who were once handicapped can now function again.

Until 1954, many thousands of people of all ages suffered permanent paralysis or even death from poliomyelitis, a viral infection of the spinal cord. Former President Franklin D. Roosevelt was a victim of this disease.

After many years of research, Dr. Jonas Salk perfected the first successful polio vaccine in 1953. Today, the Sabin vaccine, taken orally, is widely used. Polio has nearly been eradicated in this country.

15–15. Wild animals can carry rabies. If bitten by an animal, seek medical attention at once.

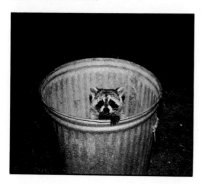

INVADERS OF THE NERVOUS SYSTEM

When bacteria or viruses enter the body, such invaders can multiply and cause trouble. Sometimes the nervous system is directly attacked by the infection. Sometimes other parts of the body are attacked first, and then the infection spreads to the nervous system.

NEURITIS AND SHINGLES. Neuritis and shingles are common nervous system disorders. In the United States alone, over 7 million people suffer from neuritis. Neuritis, which means inflammation of the nerves, can be caused by a virus, another organism, or some unknown agent. If a sensory nerve is affected, pain develops. If a motor nerve is affected, there can be weakness or paralysis. Vitamin therapy, antibiotic drugs, and rest can help fight the infection. Of course, neuritis can sometimes clear by itself, like a cold.

Shingles is caused by a virus closely related to the virus that causes chicken pox. The two viruses may be the same. When the virus attacks a sensory nerve, blisters appear on the skin along the path of that nerve. Severe pain also results. New drugs are now available to help relieve the pain and inflammation caused by shingles.

ENCEPHALITIS: "SLEEPING SICKNESS." A virus carried by the common mosquito is the cause of encephalitis. The virus destroys the gray matter of the brain. Because encephalitis often causes a coma, the common name for the disease is "sleeping sickness." Public health measures, such as eliminating stagnant pools in which mosquitoes breed, have greatly reduced encephalitis cases.

MENINGITIS (Cerebrospinal Meningitis). Meningitis is an infection of the meninges of the brain or spinal cord. The most common form of meningitis is highly contagious and is spread by a discharge from the nose, the throat, or the eyes of people carrying meningitis bacteria (meningococci). The symptoms of this disease are severe headache, rash, fever, and chills, which appear quickly after infection. Then, within 24 hours, a stiff neck and back pain develop. Meningitis affects mostly children and teenagers, and it can kill. However, now more than 90 percent of patients can survive if the disease is treated with antibiotics in its early stages.

RABIES. Rabies, or hydrophobia, is a viral disease of the central nervous system. The rabid virus enters the body by a bite from a diseased animal. Wild animals, such as foxes, skunks, raccoons, or squirrels, as well as household pets, can carry this disease. Vaccines available from a veterinarian can protect pets against rabies. If a person is bitten by an animal, seek medical attention at once.

WELLNESS WATCH

Do you take chances with your nervous system, or do you handle it with care? Take this quiz to find out whether or not you are taking proper care of your nervous system. Copy your answers on a separate sheet of paper.

If you can answer *yes* to these questions, you have started taking important steps in keeping your nervous system protected. Do you know why each of these questions is important for the health of your nervous system?

1. Do you wear seat belts in a car?
2. Are there safety reflectors on your bicycle?
3. Do you know how to operate a power mower and other power equipment safely?
4. Do you wear protective head gear when motorcycling and/or speed bicycling?
5. Do you always check for water depth before diving into the water?
6. Do you avoid the use of mind-altering drugs?
7. Do you avoid excessive drinking of alcoholic beverages?
8. Do you eat balanced meals regularly?

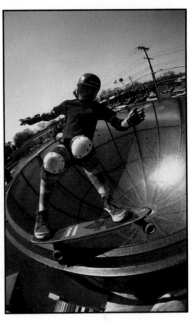

15–16. Wearing protective head gear can help prevent brain injuries.

SUMMARY: Neurons are the basic building blocks of the nervous system. They form the nerves, the brain, and the spinal cord. The nervous system is divided into two parts. The spinal cord and brain make up the central nervous system, the center of all activities of the mind and body. The peripheral nervous system, composed of the cranial and spinal nerves, is the messenger system. It carries the nerve impulses of the senses and other parts of the body to and from the brain. The autonomic system is also part of the peripheral nervous system. The sympathetic and parasympathetic systems work together to regulate the body's unconscious functions, such as breathing, heart beat, and digestion. The nervous system is delicate and irreplaceable. Although it is well protected by bones, membranes, and fluid, it can be damaged in accidents or by disease.

CHAPTER REVIEW

words at work

Complete the following sentences. DO NOT WRITE IN THIS BOOK.

The ___1___ is sometimes compared to a computer. Its cells are called ___2___. Some of these cells carry messages to the brain. They are called ___3___. The ___4___ receive messages from the brain and carry the messages to the parts of the body. In a reflex response, messages do not go to and from the brain but through the ___5___.

Your vital body functions are controlled by a part of the brain called the ___6___. Two nerve networks control the involuntary body functions. The ___7___ acts to slow down body functions. The ___8___ generally speeds up the body functions.

The largest part of the brain is the ___9___. Another part, the ___10___, is the key to smooth, coordinated muscle movements.

If a disease condition exists in the nervous system, a medical doctor, called a ___11___, can be consulted. This doctor may use an ___12___ to determine the electrical activity of the brain cells. An electrical imbalance of the brain that can be detected using this device is called ___13___.

review questions

1. Describe the parts of a neuron.
2. Describe receptor, connecting, and motor neurons.
3. Describe the action necessary for a group of neurons to respond to a simple stimulus, such as being too warm.
4. Locate and describe the central and peripheral nervous systems.
5. List the major parts of the brain.
6. Describe the control areas of the cerebrum.
7. What is the chief function of the cerebellum?
8. List and identify the three parts of the brainstem.
9. What function of the medulla makes it vital to life?
10. Describe the spinal cord.
11. Identify the peripheral nervous system.
12. How do the sympathetic and the parasympathetic systems of the autonomic nervous system act as a system of checks and balances?
13. Describe a simple reflex. How do reflexes serve as protectors of the body?
14. What tests might neurologists possibly give in making a neurological examination?

15. Distinguish between migraine and tension headaches.
16. Define a concussion and a contusion.
17. Why may a skull fracture be extremely dangerous?
18. What is the most common cause of injuries to the spinal cord?
19. Describe cerebral palsy.
20. Identify the following infections or disorders of the nervous system: (a) neuritis; (b) shingles; (c) encephalitis; (d) meningitis; (e) multiple sclerosis; (f) Parkinson's disease.

discussion questions

1. Compare the nervous pathways involved with a protective reflex, such as touching a hot object, to a conscious action, such as picking up a pencil.
2. Why is the brain considered the center of life? Outline the vital functions of the brain.
3. Do you follow good health habits to protect your nervous system? Describe ways to reduce the risk of nervous system disorders.

investigating

PURPOSE:
To do a brief "neurological examination" of reflexes.

MATERIALS:
Flashlight.

PROCEDURE:
A.   To test the reflexes needed for maintaining balance: Have a partner put both feet together and close his or her eyes. See if he or she can maintain balance, even if given a slight push. Nerve fibers in the muscles sense changes in the tensions and positions of muscles and relay this information to the spinal cord.

    1.   Why do you think this test is done with the eyes closed?

B.   To test knee-jerk reflexes: Have your partner sit so that his or her legs dangle. Then, strike the tendon just below the kneecap with your third finger or the edge of a ruler or thin book. If there is no knee jerk, have your partner clasp his or her hands and grip hard. This usually takes the attention away from the leg so that the reflex reaction can occur freely.

    2.   Draw a diagram illustrating the path of the nerve impulses that cause the knee-jerk reflex.

C.   In a darkened room, examine the pupils of your partner's eyes. Then shine a light near, but not directly into, his or her eyes.

    3.   What happens to the pupils?

    4.   What is the purpose of this reflex reaction?

CHAPTER 16

Sense Organs

OBJECTIVES

- DESCRIBE the anatomy of the eyes and ears
- EXPLAIN how the eye and ear function
- DESCRIBE common vision problems and how they are corrected

- OUTLINE the steps for eye and ear care
- DESCRIBE loss of sight and hearing
- DESCRIBE the organs of smell, taste, and touch

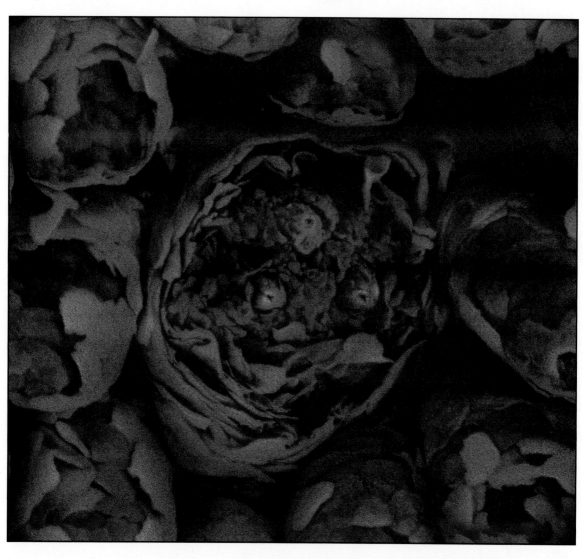

Gerry and Russ were rehearsing in the basement with their rock band, the Vultures. Gerry plays lead guitar; Russ plays bass. Gerry's sister, Kay, yelled down the stairs, "Will you pipe down! The dishes are rattling up here!"

She screamed louder. Since nothing happened, she went downstairs and turned the amplifier down. "Gerry, does it have to be so loud? My ears are ringing!"

Loud music and loud noises are very much a part of modern living. What effect do you think they have on people's hearing?

THE SENSES

The senses are highly specialized receiving stations, which are sensitive to various kinds of energy in the environment. The sense organs collect energy and translate it into nerve impulses. These impulses travel to the brain where they are interpreted. Without the senses, the brain would be imprisoned in the darkness of the skull, unable to learn or communicate with others.

We usually recognize five different senses: sight, hearing, touch, smell, and taste. Sometimes the sense of balance or position is considered a sixth sense. However, classification of the senses is not this simple. Each includes several different sensations. For example, we see form, light, color, and direction. Our ears can distinguish different properties of sound, like pitch, volume, and tone quality. Skin sensations include touch, pressure, pain, heat, and cold. The taste buds are sensitive to four chemical sensations: sweet, sour, salty, and bitter. Some researchers estimate that the smell receptors may be sensitive to as many as fifty different chemical sensations.

EYES

If you were asked to rate your sense organs in order of their importance, what would you put first? In humans, the eyes are the most highly developed sense organs. Through them we have the ability to discern events not only close by, but at great distances as well. We receive more information through our eyes than through any other sense organs.

HEALTH TIP

Some of the best sunglasses have polarized lenses. This means that light passing through the lenses is blocked when it strikes at certain angles. To test sunglasses to make sure that they are polarized, hold two lenses together and look through them. Rotate one lens and keep the other still. The amount of light passing through should change.

PROTECTION OF THE EYE

Like other organs, the eye is carefully protected. The bones in the skull protect the eyes. The eyebrows help to shade them and to catch perspiration from the forehead. Eyelids are folds of skin that protect your eyes and keep them moist by blinking. The **sclera** (**skler-**ah) is the white of your eye. It is a tough outer layer covering all but the front of the eyeball. The front of the eyeball is protected by the transparent **conjunctiva** (con-junk-**tie-**vah). The eyelashes keep small particles out of the eye by causing the lids to blink.

Where do tears come from? Tears come from glands in the upper, outer edges of the eye sockets. Tears reach the surface of the eyeball through tiny tubes, the tear ducts. Tears drain through ducts in the corner of each eye, close to the nose. These ducts empty into a larger duct, which drains into the nose. Tears are important to the eyes. They keep the eyeballs moist and wash out dirt and other foreign particles. Tears contain salt, making them slightly antiseptic. Thus, tears help reduce the danger of infection.

NERVE RECEPTORS IN THE EYE

The **optic nerve** (**op-**tik **nerv**) connects the eye to the brain. This nerve is a cable of over one million bundles of nerve fibers. The optic nerve spreads out inside the eye to form the **retina** (**ret-**in-ah), which contains millions of nerve fiber endings, or receptors. The receptors are of two kinds: **rods** and **cones.**

Rods register light and darkness. They are used in dim light to see objects in shades of black, gray, and white. Vision in the rods requires a pigment, visual purple. You don't see bright light with the rods because light breaks down visual purple. However, visual purple is restored in dim light, and the rods begin to function again. When you go from a bright room directly into darkness, you cannot see at first. Gradually, you begin to see objects in black and white. You were **night-blinded** until the rods re-formed visual purple. Some people don't have enough visual purple. They are night-blind all the time, making night driving dangerous.

Cones register color in bright light. Some people have a visual impairment called **color blindness** (see Figure 16-2). This condition is inherited and found mostly in males. Most color blindness is very mild, and affects seeing shades of red or green. A person who is completely color-blind sees only shades of gray, black, and white.

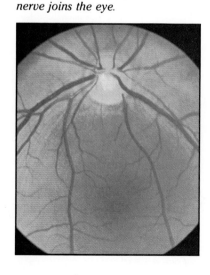

16–1. The human retina, as viewed through an ophthalmoscope. Notice the retinal blood vessels and the optic disc (light area) where the optic nerve joins the eye.

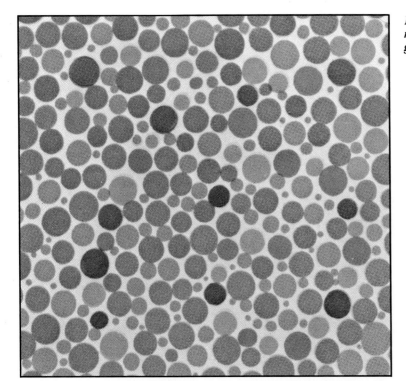

Stop reading this book for a moment. Focus your eyes on a small object in the room. You see the object and a small area around it clearly. Notice, too, that you see indistinctly a larger area surrounding what you see clearly. Vision out of the corner of your eye is called **peripheral vision.** There is a spot near the center of the retina measuring about .21 centimeter (one-twelfth of an inch) in diameter. A pit in the center of this spot, called the **fovea** (**foe**-vee-ah), contains many cones but no rods. Rays of light hitting this region are seen distinctly. Rays of light hitting the area around the fovea are seen indistinctly.

HOW IS AN IMAGE FORMED?   To some extent, an eye can be compared to a camera. Rays of light travel from objects into the eye through the pupil. The iris acts like the diaphragm of a camera, controlling the amount of light entering the eye. The iris has two sets of muscles. One set pulls away from the pupil, making it larger. This happens in dim light. The other set of muscles is arranged in a circle around the pupil. In bright light these muscles contract and the pupil becomes smaller.

STRUCTURE AND FUNCTION OF THE EYE

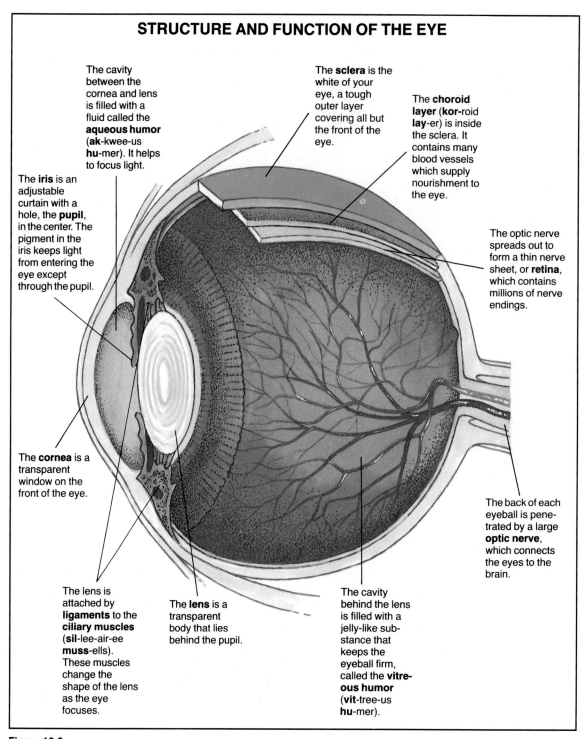

The cavity between the cornea and lens is filled with a fluid called the **aqueous humor** (**ak**-kwee-us **hu**-mer). It helps to focus light.

The **sclera** is the white of your eye, a tough outer layer covering all but the front of the eye.

The **choroid layer** (**kor**-roid **lay**-er) is inside the sclera. It contains many blood vessels which supply nourishment to the eye.

The **iris** is an adjustable curtain with a hole, the **pupil**, in the center. The pigment in the iris keeps light from entering the eye except through the pupil.

The optic nerve spreads out to form a thin nerve sheet, or **retina**, which contains millions of nerve endings.

The **cornea** is a transparent window on the front of the eye.

The back of each eyeball is penetrated by a large **optic nerve**, which connects the eyes to the brain.

The lens is attached by **ligaments** to the **ciliary muscles** (**sil**-lee-air-ee **muss**-ells). These muscles change the shape of the lens as the eye focuses.

The **lens** is a transparent body that lies behind the pupil.

The cavity behind the lens is filled with a jelly-like substance that keeps the eyeball firm, called the **vitreous humor** (**vit**-tree-us **hu**-mer).

Figure 16-3

Light rays are bent by the *cornea* and the *lens* and are focused onto the retina, just as the lens of a camera focuses light rays onto the film. In passing through the cornea and lens, light rays from different parts of the object cross, making the image of the object appear upside down, or inverted, on the retina. In a normal eye, light rays traveling from a distant point meet at the retina. When light rays come from nearby objects, the *ciliary muscles*, which control the lens, contract to thicken the lens. This causes light rays to meet on the retina. We call this process **accommodation** (see Figure 16-5).

You might think that the upside-down image on the retina would confuse the brain. However, the brain forms the image in an upright position. A camera takes upside-down pictures, too, but the image is corrected by holding the developed photographic print in an upright position.

Rays of light stimulate millions of nerve endings in the retina. Each stimulated nerve ending sends an impulse along a fiber of the optic nerve to the brain. Brain cells receive millions of impulses to form a complete picture.

STEREOSCOPIC VISION.   Unlike a camera, we can see in three dimensions. We can also change the direction of our vision by rotating our eyes. Three pairs of muscles turn each eyeball in its socket. Normally, the muscles in both eyes work together so that both eyes are directed to the same spot. This is called **binocular vision** (bye-**nok**-cue-lar **viz**-shun). When you see an object with both eyes at once, you see it from two slightly different angles. This gives you the

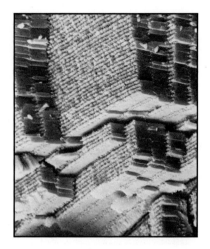

16–4. *Human lens cells magnified 490 times. Note the precise alignment of cells in rows.*

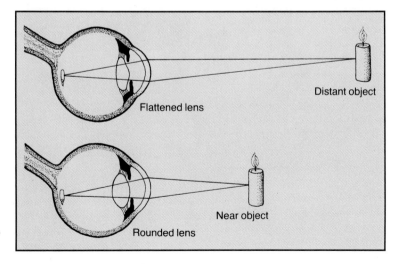

Flattened lens

Distant object

Near object

Rounded lens

16–5. *Accommodation of the eye lens*

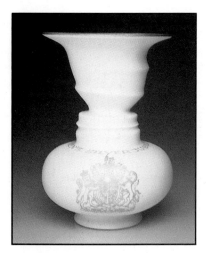

16–6. Do you see the profiles of Queen Elizabeth and her husband, Prince Philip?

depth of vision known as **stereoscopic vision** (stare-ee-oh-**scop**-ik **viz**-shun). The objects you see have depth, length, and width. If your eyes did not work together, you would see two flat images, rather than a single image in three dimensions.

PERCEPTION IN THE BRAIN

Neural impulses from the retina reach the brain, where they are perceived as three-dimensional objects. Our brains can perceive size, shape, color, brightness, motion, and direction. Certain visual clues allow the brain to perceive distance and depth. For example, objects appear smaller with increased distance. The relative positions of several objects together are indicated by how they overlap and how they cast shadows. How the brain perceives an object also depends on past experience and knowledge about the object.

Sometimes the eye and the brain are deceived. Visual cues from an object may be unclear and the brain then perceives the object in two different ways. This is called an *optical illusion*. Look at Figure 16-6. Do you see the two profiles? Look at Figure 16-7. Why do the people on the right look so much bigger than those on the left? The walls they are standing against do not meet at right angles, as in most rooms. Also, the right wall is smaller than the left.

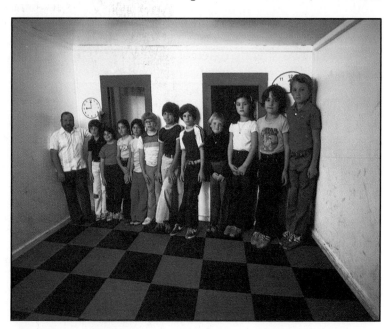

16–7. How was this optical illusion created?

THE EYE SPECIALISTS

An *ophthalmologist* is a medical doctor who specializes in the diagnosis and treatment of eye diseases and vision defects. Ophthalmologists also perform eye surgery. Sometimes examination of the eyes reveals a disorder in another part of the body. Ophthalmologists are trained to recognize those kinds of symptoms. They are the only specialists who use drugs in treating eyes.

The *optometrist* is a specialist in problems of vision. Optometrists can recognize and diagnose eye diseases and diseases of other parts of the body that affect the eyes. When they diagnose vision problems they may prescribe corrective spectacle lenses, contact lenses and/or eye exercises to improve vision. They are also specialists in the rehabilitation of the visually handicapped.

An *optician* is an expert in the grinding of lenses and fitting of glasses. Opticians fill the prescription written by ophthalmologists or optometrists.

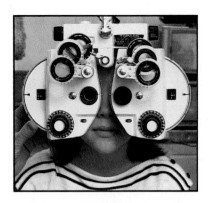

16–8. Optometrists use this instrument to fit lenses.

TESTING VISION

When was the last time you had your eyes tested? Eyesight is commonly tested with a Snellen Chart. You have probably seen Snellen Charts hanging on the wall of a doctor's office or in a school clinic. The top row of letters is printed in very large type, and each successive row is printed in smaller type. The chart is read from a distance of 6 meters (20 ft). Each eye is tested separately. You read down the chart as far as you can. Each line of letters is marked with a number that indicates the distance at which a normal eye could read the letters. If you can only read part way down the chart, to the 20/40 line for example, this means you can read letters at a distance of 20 feet that a person with perfect vision could read at 40 feet. Your vision would be 20/40, about a 50 percent reduction in the sharpness of seeing (see Figure 16-9). Legal blindness in most states is defined as vision of 20/200 even when aided by glasses.

VISUAL PROBLEMS

Visual problems result when (1) the eyeball is not shaped normally; (2) the lens cannot focus properly; (3) the transparent parts of the eye become cloudy or opaque; (4) the retina is damaged; or (5) the optic nerve is defective. Common visual problems can usually be corrected.

16–9. The Snellen eye chart. An individual with perfect vision (20/20) can read line 8 of a full-sized chart at a distance of twenty feet.

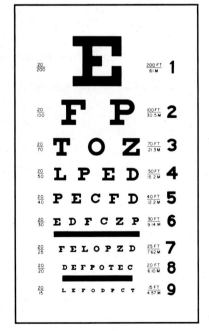

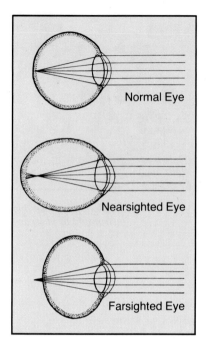

16–10. Normal vision, nearsightedness, and farsightedness

16–11. It is important to follow your doctor's instructions for the proper use and care of contact lenses.

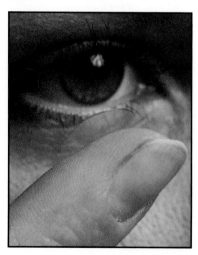

In **farsightedness,** or **hyperopia**, the rays of light focus at some point behind the retina. This condition is caused by a short eyeball. The muscles in the eye used for accomodation must work extra hard to focus images on the retina. This results in considerable eye fatigue, headaches, and in extreme cases may even cause crossing of the eyes. Farsightedness makes it difficult to maintain clear vision comfortably when reading for long periods of time.

Someone who is farsighted finds the printed page a blur. A farsighted child entering school may develop irritability, inattention, or an aversion to close eye work. It is important for young children to be examined in order to discover such visual impairments, which can be aided by corrective lenses.

As an individual grows older the lenses of the eyes become more rigid. They cannot change shape, or accommodate, to focus the eye on near objects. This condition is usually noticed by persons between ages 40 and 50. As a result, older people need reading glasses or bifocal lenses for reading and close work. This is a normal part of the aging process. Vision continues to change with advancing age.

In **nearsightedness,** or **myopia**, the rays of light focus in front of the retina. This happens when an eyeball is too long from front to back. Distant objects are always blurred. Corrective lenses throw the point of focus farther back onto the retina to restore clear vision.

Astigmatism (ah-**stig**-mah-tiz-um) is the result of an irregular cornea or lens. If either is out of shape, light rays are not bent equally from all angles. This causes a blurred image, like that seen through the corner of a curved windshield. Astigmatism is remedied with corrective lenses. The lenses are shaped so that certain areas bend the light rays, compensating for the irregular cornea or lens.

CONTACT LENSES. **Contact lenses** are plastic lenses that fit over the corneas. The hard lenses are made of a stiff, durable plastic that can easily be cleaned daily. The soft lenses are more flexible and fragile. They are not as likely to scratch the eye and can also change shape. For this reason, some wearers find them more comfortable than hard lenses. The soft lenses need to be sterilized daily and treated chemically weekly. Recently, soft plastic lenses have been developed that may be worn by some people for up to two weeks at a time, even during sleep. These lenses "breathe"; that is, they allow oxygen to pass through them. Other developments include the introduction of bifocal contact lenses.

OTHER EYE DEFECTS

EYE-MUSCLE DEFECTS. Muscles in normal eyes work together, allowing us to see *stereoscopically,* or in three dimensions. However, in some eyes the muscles do not work together. When this occurs, the eye turns toward the stronger muscle. If the pull is toward the nose, the person becomes cross-eyed. Some babies are born with eye muscles that do not work together. This defect may be corrected at an early age by special lenses, surgery, or both. By doing eye exercises, the eyes can be trained to work together.

MISMATCHED VISION. *Mismatched vision* in the two eyes is another common defect. If a child sees normally in one eye and the other eye is farsighted, nearsighted, or has astigmatism, the eyes are unable to adjust. To avoid the confusion caused by a blurred image from one eye and a clear image from the other eye, the child unconsciously learns to depend only on the normal eye. The eye that has poor vision becomes worse due to lack of use.

This condition may be remedied by corrective lenses and a patch over the normal eye. This forces the weaker eye to exercise, which makes it stronger. Early treatment improves the chances for correction.

EYE INJURIES

At least 160,000 children of school age suffer eye injuries each year. Most of these occur among junior high school students and could have been prevented if the students had worn safety glasses or protective goggles in their school shops and science labs.

You should see an eye doctor immediately if you have any eye injury. Removing a speck of dirt from a lid is the ONLY eye treatment you should perform. If a speck lodges in your eye, excess tears usually wash it to one of the lids. If you pull down the lower lid, you may find the speck in the fold. Lift it off with a cotton swab or the edge of a CLEAN handkerchief. If it is under the upper lid, pull this lid over the lower lid to dislodge it. Do not rub it under any condition. The speck may be embedded in the cornea, and rubbing could push it in even deeper.

Embedded particles should be removed by a doctor. Bits of steel, chips of glass, and grains of sand are common causes of eye injuries. If you work with these materials, wear shatterproof goggles.

EYE INFECTIONS

Pinkeye, known medically as *epidemic conjunctivitis,* is a common contagious infection of the conjunctiva. It causes reddening and swelling of the membranes of the eyes and lids and produces a milky discharge. It is easily spread by infected towels and other articles.

There are other forms of conjunctivitis that are not contagious. These include irritation by smoke, dust, bright lights, chemicals in pools, and infected sinuses. You should see your doctor if you have persistent conjunctivitis.

Styes are infections of the glands of the eyelids. They are caused by the same bacteria that cause pimples and boils. These bacteria may reach the eyes by rubbing them with dirty hands. Styes may be treated by using hot, moist compresses on the infected area.

EYE DISEASES

According to the National Society for the Prevention of Blindness, approximately half a million people in the United States are considered legally blind. Each year nearly 47,000 Americans lose their precious sight. A few eye diseases cause most of this tragic blindness. How much do you know about these diseases: **glaucoma** (glau-**ko**-mah), **cataracts** (**kat**-tar-rakts), **corneal scarring,** and **detached retina?** These diseases can damage the eyes and destroy sight.

GLAUCOMA. About 2 million Americans over the age of thirty-five have glaucoma. Studies show that half that number have early glaucoma without knowing it. There are 300,000 new cases of this dreaded disease each year.

Chronic glaucoma usually strikes older people. It progresses slowly and may destroy much of the vision in an eye before the victim realizes it. Glaucoma is characterized by a buildup of fluid pressure in the eye. Either too much aqueous humor is produced, or openings at the outer margin of the iris close, preventing drainage. As a result, fluid pressure builds up, which can permanently damage the eye. This makes the eyeball hard, rather than soft and pliable. The early stages of glaucoma can be detected with a tonometer, which measures the fluid pressure in the eyes. By the time glaucoma is noticeable to an individual, vision loss has already begun. Although lost vision cannot be restored, medicine or surgery can prevent further loss. However, if glaucoma is detected early, little or no vision is lost.

16–12. Eyeball pressure is measured with an instrument called a tonometer. Older people should have their eyes tested for glaucoma at least every two years.

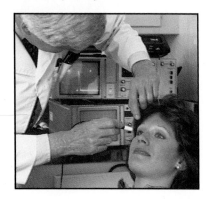

UNIT 5 YOUR CONTROL SYSTEMS

CATARACT. You may have seen cataracts in the eyes of older people. They appear as milky spots in the lens. If they cover the whole lens, they can block vision. Unlike glaucoma, the retina is not destroyed. Sight is restored by removing the natural lens and substituting convex glasses or contact lenses, which focus light rays on the retina. Cataract surgery is highly effective, restoring sight in 98 percent of the cases. In some cases, surgeons can now implant plastic lenses that do not need to be removed.

Cataracts may occur in infants or young people as a result of an eye injury, diabetes, maternal German measles (rubella) during pregnancy, or from other causes. However, two thirds of the cases of cataracts occur in people over 55 years of age. The cause of this condition in older people is not known.

CORNEAL SCARRING. An eye injury or disease may cause the cornea to become scarred or cloudy, leading to blindness. Some 400,000 Americans are victims of corneal blindness. An eye operation, called *corneal transplant,* removes the cloudy cornea and grafts a clear one onto the eye (see Figure 16-13).

These donor corneas are removed quickly from a deceased person. Permission to do so is arranged through relatives of the deceased. Individuals may also make arrangements to have their eyes donated after death. In some states you may donate your eyes and note it on your driver's license. Eye banks are maintained in many sections of the country. They arrange air shipments of donor corneas, packed in ice, to hospitals. The Eye Bank for Sight Restoration in New York City and Lions Clubs in many states supply corneas for transplantation.

DETACHED RETINA. Various conditions can cause the attached retina of one or both eyes to separate from the choroid layer of the eyeball. The choroid layer is inside the sclera. It is dark brown and contains many blood vessels that supply nourishment to the eye. When a portion of the retina detaches, fluid collects beneath it, and vision in that area is destroyed. The area of separation increases until the retina separates completely, destroying the retina and all vision.

Retinal detachment is more common in people beyond middle age. Often it is associated with an injury to the head. However, the condition may occur in younger people, especially among those who are extremely nearsighted.

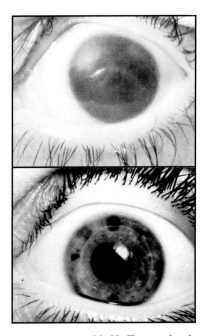

16–13. Top, a cloudy cornea. Bottom, the same eye after a corneal transplant.

Retinal detachment (see Figure 16-14) usually begins along a margin of the retina. This causes a black area in the field of vision. Another sign of a detached retina is the sensation of flashing lights. The symptom often appears suddenly and signals the need for immediate examination by an ophthalmologist. The detached portion of a retina can be reattached by a delicate operation performed by an eye surgeon. Surgery is effective in a majority of the cases. Today, laser beams can be used to repair detached retinas.

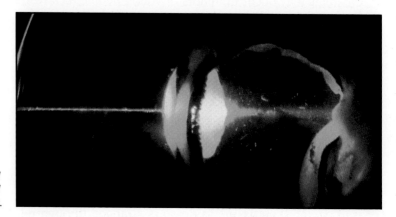

16–14. This detached retina is being repaired with a laser beam.

WELLNESS WATCH

1. Have you had your vision checked at least once since grade school?
2. If you have prescription lenses, do you use them when you are supposed to?
3. Do you always use safety glasses or goggles when doing work hazardous to your eyes?
4. When you are reading or doing close work, do you give your eyes enough light and avoid glare?
5. When you are doing close work, do you rest your eyes every half hour for a few minutes?
6. Do you protect your eyes from bright sunlight by wearing sunglasses?
7. If you get something in your eye, do you avoid rubbing?
8. Do you avoid using eyewashes?
9. If you wear contact lenses, do you follow your doctor's instructions on their proper care?
10. If your eyes itch or hurt for more than a few days or if you notice any eye defects, do you see a doctor?

HEARING

The ears are the most important part of your communication system. Hearing allows you to learn and share ideas. Hearing music gives you pleasure. Hearing horns and other signals warns you of potential danger. Most people think of the ear only as an organ of hearing. However, it is a complex organ that has other functions as well. For example, we would find it hard to even stand if our ears were damaged.

Figure 16–15

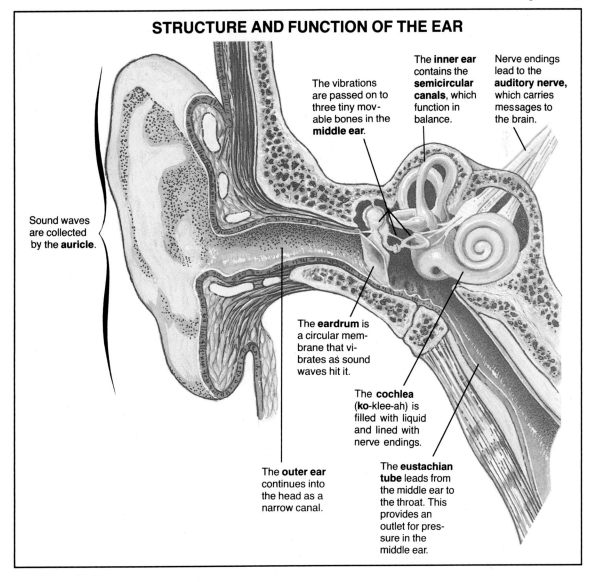

STRUCTURE AND FUNCTION OF THE EAR

The vibrations are passed on to three tiny movable bones in the **middle ear**.

The **inner ear** contains the **semicircular canals**, which function in balance.

Nerve endings lead to the **auditory nerve**, which carries messages to the brain.

Sound waves are collected by the **auricle**.

The **eardrum** is a circular membrane that vibrates as sound waves hit it.

The **chochlea** (**ko**-klee-ah) is filled with liquid and lined with nerve endings.

The **outer ear** continues into the head as a narrow canal.

The **eustachian tube** leads from the middle ear to the throat. This provides an outlet for pressure in the middle ear.

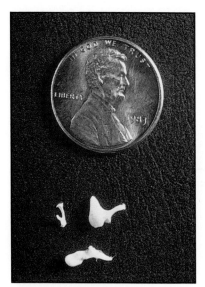

16–16. The hammer, anvil, and stirrup are the three smallest bones in the human body.

HOW WE HEAR

Sounds are the impressions the brain receives when sound waves strike the eardrum. These waves vibrate against the eardrum. The vibrations correspond to the pitch and loudness of the sound waves that strike it. High-pitched sounds make the eardrum vibrate faster. Louder sounds make the eardrum move farther in and out. The vibrating eardrum sets the hammer, anvil, and stirrup vibrating (see Figure 16-15). These bones act as a series of levers to magnify the inward and outward movements of the eardrum. The stirrup vibrates with a force more than twenty times greater than that of the eardrum. The cochlea of the inner ear is filled with a liquid and is surrounded by a membrane. This membrane stretches across the opening of the cochlea, called the oval window. The vibrating stirrup sets this membrane vibrating, which in turn causes the liquid inside the cochlea to vibrate. Waves in this liquid vibrate against a membrane that stretches the full length of the cochlea. The cochlea is widest at the opening and gets narrower as it spirals inward. High-pitched sounds start the membrane vibrating near the opening of the cochlea, which stimulates nerve endings there. Low-pitched sounds start the membrane vibrating near the narrow end of the cochlea. In this way, different-pitched sounds activate different nerve fibers, which carry the appropriate messages to the brain.

HOW WE MAINTAIN OUR BALANCE

Balance, or equilibrium, is sometimes called the sixth sense. If you are standing straight, leaning, or lying down, you are aware of it. If you spin around, you confuse this sense and become dizzy.

The semicircular canals of your inner ear are organs of balance. The canals contain fluid and are lined with nerve endings. There are three semicircular canals at right angles to each other in each ear. If you bend forward and backward, you rock the fluid in one of the canals. Leaning from side to side moves the fluid in another canal. Turning around affects the third canal. Movement of the fluid in the semicircular canals stimulates nerve endings. From these nerve endings, impulses are carried to the center for balance in the brain.

Another sense, called the **kinesthetic** (kin-ess-**thet**-tick) sense, is your feeling of position and movement. It lets you know how your body is positioned. There are nerve endings in the muscles that transmit this information to the brain.

HEALTH TIP

If you have a tendency toward motion sickness when riding in a car or bus, keep your eyes on the horizon in front of you. Do not try to read or to look out the side windows.

Ears need little care except to guard against middle-ear infections. Wax, normally present in the ear canal, may accumulate and harden over the eardrum. This interferes with hearing. *Under no conditions should it be removed with any type of instrument.* This could pierce the eardrum or introduce an infection. If you think excess wax is present, see your doctor, who can remove it easily and painlessly.

Most ear infections are caused by germs that find their way from the throat to the middle-ear through the Eustachian tube. Swimming is a common cause of middle-ear infections in teenagers. You can get water into your ears through your nose and the Eustachian tube. However, this can be avoided. If you jump into the water feet first, hold your nose. If you are underwater or are swimming with your face down, blow out through your nose gently.

Have you ever been given the advice not to blow your nose very hard when you have a cold? Blowing your nose improperly during a cold can cause the infection to travel up the Eustachian tube. To avoid this, hold a handkerchief to your nose loosely. Keep both nostrils open and blow gently.

MIDDLE-EAR INFECTIONS.   When an infection from the nose or throat travels to the middle ear, the Eustachian tube becomes filled with pus. The tube swells and closes, building up pressure. As pus pushes against the eardrum, it causes great pain. The pressure can cause the eardrum to burst. Although a tear resulting from a ruptured eardrum may heal, scar tissue forms, which can cause some permanent hearing loss. If there is too much pressure built up in the Eustachian tube, the doctor may lance the eardrum to relieve the pressure if it is absolutely necessary. The small opening caused by lancing will heal quickly and leave no scar tissue. Prompt use of antibiotics can cure the infection and prevent a rupture or the need for lancing.

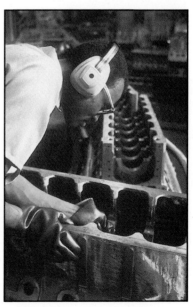

16–17. This worker wears earmuffs to protect his ears from noise.

If an infected ear is not treated properly, it may flare up again and again and become a chronic infection. The infection could enter the **mastoid bone** (**mas-**toid) behind the middle ear. This causes a serious bone infection, called *mastoiditis.* An infected mastoid bone in the middle ear can cause deafness in a short time. Not long ago mastoid operations were quite common. Today effective drugs clear up this infection without surgery.

NOISE POLLUTION.   There is an old saying, "Silence is golden." In our modern world of jet planes, motorcycles, and sirens, "golden silence" has grown increasingly scarce.

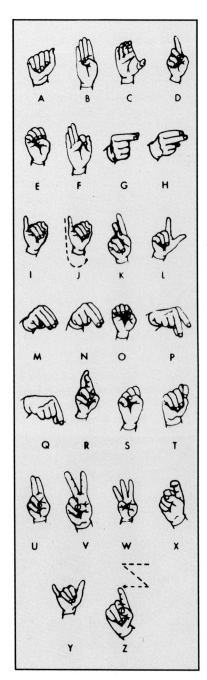

16–18. The alphabet in sign language

The loudness of sound is measured in decibels. A sound that is barely audible registers 10 decibels, whereas a jet taking off can generate as many as 130 decibels. Sounds above 100 are above the pain threshold.

It is not known exactly what intensity or duration of noise can lead to hearing loss. Most experts advise you to let your ears be your guide. If noise is loud enough to interfere with your ability to hear others near you talking, or if noises cause pain or ringing in your ears, the noise is potentially dangerous. Workers at airports, in boiler factories and foundries, and musicians or discotheque fans may develop nerve deafness. Wherever noise cannot be kept below a safe level, workers should wear earplugs, earmuffs, or helmets.

LOSS OF HEARING

About 16 1/2 million people in America, or about 8 percent of our population, have some degree of hearing loss. About 11 million of these struggle along without any form of correction for their hearing loss.

Many of the victims of hearing loss have had middle-ear infections. Middle-ear infections not only damage the eardrum, but they may cause *adhesions.* These are bands of tissue that bind the bones of the middle ear. This prevents transmission of vibrations to the inner ear. This condition is called chronic adhesive deafness.

Another important cause of deafness, which may be hereditary, is known as otosclerosis. People with this condition can have varying degrees of deafness, caused by an overgrowth of bone. This closes the oval window, fusing the stirrup bone to the window. It is estimated that 10 percent of the population has some degree of *otosclerosis.*

AID FOR THE HARD OF HEARING

Too many people try to cover up a hearing loss because of embarrassment or false pride. They struggle along, missing much that is said. They feel left out of things. Emotional problems often follow if the condition is not corrected.

HEARING AIDS. Many people with hearing loss have helped themselves through the use of hearing aids. There are two types of hearing aids. One is a miniature public address system, which amplifies sounds. The user wears a small microphone and amplifier and has a receiver in his or her ear canal.

In the other type, amplified vibrations are carried to the bones of the skull. This is done by an attachment, which fits against the bone behind the ear. Some people get discouraged when they first use a hearing aid. At first it may be difficult to distinguish conversation from all the other magnified sounds. With practice, many become used to their hearing aids. Hearing aids should be bought only if recommended by a physician, since not all types of deafness are helped by these aids.

SURGERY FOR DEAFNESS. In recent years an operation, called *stapes mobilization,* has partially restored hearing in large numbers of people. This operation is performed in cases of chronic adhesive deafness, as well as for otosclerosis. The surgeon loosens the stapes bone from the oval window. More recently surgeons have been able to build new eardrums and reconstruct or replace middle-ear bones.

Formerly there was little hope for people with severe nerve deafness. Researchers are at work on a computer program that would retune incoming sounds. A tiny device would be implanted under the skin behind the external ear. A wire would carry the current to an electrode implanted in the cochlea, restoring at least some degree of hearing.

EDUCATION FOR THE DEAF. As of the end of 1982, there were 643 schools and classes for children and adolescents with severe deafness in the U.S. The total enrollment was 46,257. Most schools teach "total communication," involving the use of sign language (using the hands to form letters and words); lip reading (also called "speech reading"); visual materials, such as movies; and hearing aids for all but the totally deaf.

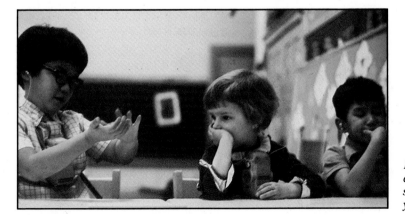

16–19. Children who are deaf learn to speak using sign language at a very young age.

HEALTH ACTION

Mix solutions of water with sugar, salt, lemon juice, and unsweetened chocolate. Using cotton-tipped swabs, test the different areas of your tongue to see which areas taste the different flavors.

16–20. The Paccinian corpuscle, magnified 120 times, is a specialized pressure receptor found in the skin.

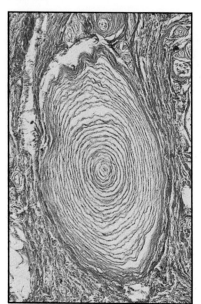

A SENSE OF TOUCH

When you think of feeling in the skin, you think of touch. This is only one of several different sensations registered in the skin. You can also sense pressure, pain, heat, and cold. Skin sensations are registered in nerve endings all over your body. The sense receptors are not evenly distributed over the surface of the body. The fingers and lips have greater concentrations of sense organs than other areas and, therefore, are more sensitive to touch. Nerve fibers carry impulses from the sense organs to your spinal cord, and then to your brain. It is here that all these feelings register.

When you place your hand lightly on an object, your first sensation is touch. As you press harder, you sense pressure. If the object has a rough surface and you press hard enough, you may feel pain. These senses are closely related, yet they are distinct from one another. There are many different types of touch, pressure, and pain receptors. Some are free nerve endings, and others have specialized structures.

Your skin has receptors for both heat and cold. If you could distinguish only heat and not cold, you would run the danger of freezing to death. If you could sense only cold, you would not know when you were being burned.

SENSES OF TASTE AND SMELL

What are your favorite foods? What do you like about them, their taste or their smell? It is difficult to distinguish between these two senses. What you interpret as taste may in fact be smell. Have you ever noticed that food seems tasteless when you have a cold? This is because your sense of smell is blocked. Food loses its taste because of this.

The senses of taste and smell are chemical senses. That is, the organs for taste and smell are stimulated when chemicals come in contact with them.

SMELL. The sense of smell is much more sensitive than the sense of taste. The receptor sites for smell are two small patches of cells in the roof of each nasal cavity, having a total area of less than one square inch. These patches consist of closely packed cells with highly specialized smell receptors between them. Unlike the taste buds, which are sensitive to only four chemical sensations, the smell receptors may be sensitive to as many as fifty. Mixtures of these sensations produce a broad range of odors that we smell.

TASTE. The tongue is covered with thousands of **papillae,** or tiny projections. There are moats around each papilla. **Taste buds,** the organs for taste, project into these moats. (See photo of papillae on page 336.) The taste buds are bathed in dissolved foods. Chemicals in the food stimulate the taste buds. The taste buds only respond to tastes of sweetness, sourness, bitterness, or saltiness. You cannot taste all four of these flavors on every part of your tongue. Figure 16-21 shows the areas on your tongue that taste the four different flavors.

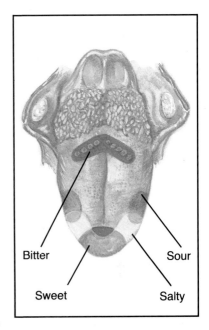

Bitter

Sour

Sweet

Salty

16–21. Different areas of your tongue taste the four different flavors.

SUMMARY: The sense organs are highly specialized. Sensory nerves carry impulses from the senses to the brain. The human eye is the most specialized of our sense organs. It receives light rays through the pupil and focuses them on the retina. Sound is the sensation that the brain receives when sound waves strike the eardrum. Skin sensations such as touch, pressure, pain, heat, and cold are registered in many different kinds of sensory receptors. The nasal cavity contains the receptor sites for smell, and the tongue contains the taste buds. Proper health care is a must to ensure the protection of your sense organs.

CHAPTER REVIEW

words at work

Find the word in the left column that fits one of the definitions in the right column. DO NOT WRITE IN THIS BOOK.

a. accommodation
b. cochlea
c. cones
d. conjunctiva
e. fovea
f. hyperopia
g. myopia
h. retina
i. semicircular canals
j. vitreous humor

1. The fluid that fills the eyeball behind the lens
2. The nerve sheet of the eye
3. Organs of balance
4. Nerve endings that function in bright light and color vision
5. The membrane that covers the sclera on the front of the eyeball
6. The focusing of light rays on the retina
7. Farsightedness
8. A small pit in the retina in which vision is most distinct in bright light
9. Nearsightedness
10. The hearing apparatus of the inner ear

review questions

1. Name the layers of the eyeball, from outside to inside.
2. Locate the crystalline lens of the eye.
3. Distinguish between the aqueous and vitreous humors of the eye.
4. How do rods and cones function in vision?
5. Explain why you can hardly see when you enter a dark theater but see much more clearly a short time later.
6. Why is peripheral vision less distinct than central vision?
7. How does the crystalline lens of the eye function in accommodation?
8. Describe the shape of the eyeball in hyperopia and in myopia.
9. Why is the visual image blurred in astigmatism?
10. Describe the work of three kinds of specialists engaged in various phases of correcting vision defects.
11. What is stye conjunctivitis?
12. Contrast the nature of vision loss in glaucoma and cataracts.
13. List several precautions necessary for proper eye care.
14. Describe the transmission of vibrations from the eardrum to the oval window.
15. Explain how the mastoid bone may become involved in an ear infection.

16. Describe the function of the Eustachian tube.
17. What are the causes of deafness?
18. List several steps for ear care.
19. What function besides hearing does the inner ear perform?
20. List five distinct skin sensations.
21. Describe the flavors that register on the taste buds of the tongue.
22. Locate the olfactory nerve endings.

discussion questions

1. Debate the statement: "Human beings are supreme among living organisms because of their highly developed sense organs."
2. Rate your sense organs according to their importance to you. Compare your list with those of other classmates.
3. Discuss the advantages and disadvantages of wearing contact lenses or regular glasses.
4. Cite examples to show how noise pollution contributes to defective hearing.

investigating

PURPOSE:
To find your blind spot and to test your eyes for dominance and peripheral vision.

PROCEDURE:
A.   There is a blind spot where the optic nerve joins the retina. Draw two large dots about 7 cm (3 in.) apart on a piece of paper. Hold the paper directly in front of your eyes. Close one eye and move the paper back and forth until one of the dots disappears. Repeat with the other eye.
    1.   How far was the paper from your eyes when one of the circles disappeared?
B.   Look directly in front of you. Have a partner hold a pencil behind you and then slowly move it in a circle around your head.
    2.   At approximately what angle could you first see the pencil out of the corner of each eye?
C.   One of your eyes is dominant. That is, one of your eyes judges the position of objects in relation to other objects. Hold a pencil, eraser end pointing up, about 8 inches in front of your eyes. Look at a distant reference point, such as the edge of a window or door. Line up the edge of the pencil with the edge of your distant reference point. Close one eye, then the other.
    3.   The dominant eye should not jump while looking at the pencil. Which is your dominant eye?

CHAPTER 17

Chemical Regulators

OBJECTIVES

- LOCATE the endocrine glands in the body
- STATE the function of each endocrine gland
- DESCRIBE how glands interact
- DESCRIBE the consequences of endocrine malfunction and treatment required

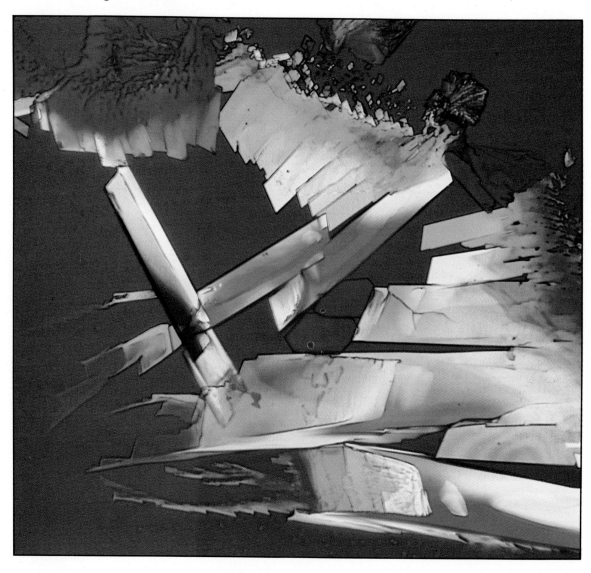

Al and Jack were lifelong friends. When they finished school, they joined the fire department. One night the alarm sounded for a raging fire in an old paint factory. The flames had not yet reached a large tank of paint solvent. If it exploded, it would blow up the whole block. Al and Jack approached it through an unburned area. After dousing it with foam, they were about to leave when the floor above caved in, pinning Jack's legs under a huge beam, which was afire at one end. Al didn't stop to think. With a great heave he lifted the beam off Jack's legs and dragged him to safety.

What gave Al the strength to do what it would have taken at least four men to do under ordinary circumstances?

WHAT ARE ENDOCRINE GLANDS?

What causes the body to change so rapidly during adolescence? Why are some people energetic while others are sluggish? What regulates the menstrual cycle in women? The answers to these questions can be found within the endocrine glands. These are organs in the body that manufacture and secrete chemicals called hormones.

There are two kinds of glands, *exocrine* and *endocrine*. "Exo" means outside. Exocrine glands secrete their products through ducts to the outside of the body or into the digestive tract. The salivary glands, mucous glands, sweat glands, and tear glands are all exocrine glands. "Endo" means inside. Endocrine glands do not have ducts. They secrete their products directly into the bloodstream, which carries them to all parts of the body. The endocrine glands (see Figure 17-1) consist of the **hypothalamus** (hi-poe-**thal**-ah-mus) and **pituitary** at the base of the brain, the **thyroid** and **parathyroids** (pear-ah-**thi**-royds) at the base of the neck, the **adrenals** (ah-**dree**-nals) above the kidneys, the **pancreas** in the abdomen, and the **ovaries** (**oh**-var-rees) in the pelvis and **testes** (**tes**-tees) in the scrotum.

ENDOCRINE SECRETIONS

The chemical messengers secreted by the endocrine glands are called **hormones,** from the Greek word *hormon*, which

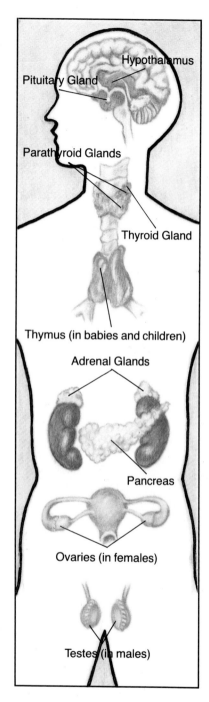

17–1. The endocrine system

means to arouse to activity. Hormones affect most body activities. Most endocrine glands secrete at least small amounts of their hormones all the time. There are at least thirty to forty different hormones in the body at any one time. Tiny amounts of hormones have powerful effects on the body. They control and monitor the chemical balance within each organ, tissue, and cell of the body. They affect growth and activity and, most important of all, they allow the body to make proper adjustments to changes in the outside world.

The activities of the endocrine glands must be carefully balanced. If they are not working properly, the entire body is affected. If a gland is too active and secretes too much hormone, illness results. Likewise, if a gland is underactive and does not secrete enough hormone, illness also results.

THE PITUITARY

How are the activities of the glands regulated? The **pituitary gland** acts as the master control unit. It secretes many hormones that affect the activity of many other glands, including the sex glands, thyroids, and adrenals. It is sometimes called the master gland, and the glands it controls are called target glands. The pituitary responds to the level of hormones in the blood secreted by the target glands. For example, if there is too little *thyroxine* in the blood, the pituitary responds by secreting a thyroid-stimulating hormone that is carried to the thyroid. The thyroid then responds by secreting more thyroxine.

MIND-BODY INTERACTION

Do you remember what the **hypothalamus** is? It is located at the base of the brain and is connected to the pituitary. What does this tell you? The hypothalamus serves as a link between the mind and the body. It is part of the nervous system, but must also be considered part of the endocrine system. It secretes hormones called releasing factors, which stimulate the release of specific hormones of the pituitary. Also, hormones from other endocrine glands act on the hypothalamus. If you will recall, the hypothalamus is the control center for the autonomic nervous system. The autonomic nervous system controls the essential body functions such as digestion, breathing, and heartbeat. The hypothalamus is the center for emotions as well. Can you see why there is a close interaction between the endocrine glands, the emotions, and the autonomic nervous system? By way of the hypothalamus, your emotions can change the activity of your glands. Likewise, your glands secrete hormones that influence your emotions and the autonomic nervous system.

Have you ever experienced superhuman strength in a time of danger, like Al in the story? Emotions of fear or anger stimulate the hypothalamus to send messages by way of nerves to the adrenal glands. In response, the adrenals secrete **adrenaline** (ah-**dren**-nal-lin), which prepares the body for fight or flight. This happens instantly. Blood pressure and pulse increase, reserve sugar is poured into the blood, and the body is thrown into a state of readiness. After the crisis is over, anxiety feelings may remain until adrenaline levels in the body return to normal. As you learned in Chapter 8, continued stress can cause the body and mind to be in a constant state of anxiety, due to this same stress response.

HOW THE PITUITARY FUNCTIONS

Let's take a closer look at how the pituitary functions. The pituitary gland, about the size of an acorn, is made up of two lobes. The **anterior lobe** is toward the front. The **posterior lobe** lies behind it. Each lobe secretes different hormones. For this reason, the pituitary is really a double gland.

THE ANTERIOR LOBE.   The anterior lobe of the pituitary gland secretes powerful hormones that affect other endocrine glands. For example, **ACTH, adrenocorticotropic hormone** (ah-**dree**-no-kort-ee-ko-**trop**-ik **hor**-moan), stimulates the cortex, or outer layer, of the adrenal glands. **Thyrotropic hormone** (thi-row-**tro**-pik) is a thyroid-stimulating hormone, often referred to as **TSH.** It regulates both the size and the activity of the thyroid gland. **Somatotropic hormone** (so-**ma**-to-trop-ik), often called growth hormone, regulates the growth of the whole body. Usually, this hormone stimulates bone growth and allows a person to grow to his or her normal size.

What happens if the pituitary is underactive, and the body does not receive sufficient somatotropic hormone? The result will be pituitary dwarfism (see Figure 17-2). This condition produces a normally proportioned person who is much smaller than average size. Another kind of dwarfism, not due to lack of somatotropic hormone, causes shortened arms and legs but a normal-sized trunk. If pituitary dwarfism is

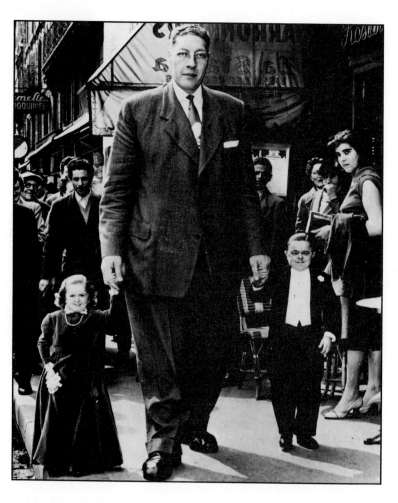

17–2. What causes giant-
size and midget-size
people?

recognized early in life, treatment with somatotropic hormone may result in growth to normal size.

If a tumor develops in the pituitary's anterior lobe the pituitary secretes too much somatotropic hormone. When this
happens during the growing years, the bones lengthen abnormally, producing a giant-sized person. If oversecretion of
the somatotropic hormone occurs after growth is completed,
the result is quite different. The bones do not lengthen. Instead, they thicken, especially the bones of the jaw, hands,
and feet. While this is happening, the soft tissues over the
bones enlarge, changing a person's appearance. The face
looks massive, and the hands and feet are large and awkward. This condition is called **acromegaly** (ak-crow-**meg**-
ah-lee) and may be treated surgically or by X-ray therapy.

What causes changes in your body during adolescence? During the years in which a child grows to an adult, the anterior pituitary gland secretes **gonadotropic hormones.** These hormones stimulate the gonads or reproductive organs (the testes in the male and the ovaries in the female) to produce sex hormones. The sex hormones cause dramatic changes in physical, mental, and emotional characteristics during the adolescent years. This is one reason why adolescence can sometimes be a period of confusion.

The gonadotropic hormones are also important in regulating the menstrual cycle and pregnancy in women of childbearing age. They interact with hormones secreted by the ovaries to control the sequence of events during the menstrual cycle and pregnancy. After childbirth, a high level of female hormones stimulates the anterior pituitary to secrete **lactogenic hormone.** This hormone causes secretion of milk in the mammary glands of the mother.

The pituitary and the gonads act as a system of checks and balances. When there are low levels of sex hormones in the blood, the pituitary starts secreting more gonadotropic hormones. This, in turn, stimulates the production of more sex hormones by the gonads. When the level of sex hormones in the blood is high again, the pituitary stops secreting gonadotropic hormone. Then the gonads stop producing sex hormones. This dynamic balance between the pituitary and the gonads is especially important in regulating the menstrual cycle, which is explained in more detail later on.

POSTERIOR PITUITARY.   The posterior lobe of the pituitary secretes the **antidiuretic hormone,** or **ADH.** This hormone regulates water balance in the body. Normally, much of the water in the blood is removed as it passes through the kidneys. ADH regulates the kidneys to give most of the water back to the blood as needed. If they did not, a person would have a serious internal water shortage. This condition is called **diabetes insipidus.** People who have it crave water constantly. They drink gallons every day and lose most of it as urine. Although these symptoms are similar to those of true diabetes, the two diseases have different causes and should not be confused.

Oxytocin is the other known hormone of the posterior pituitary lobe. This hormone stimulates smooth muscles to react. Smooth muscles are found in the walls of the internal organs, such as the digestive organs, the blood vessels, the uterus, and the mammary glands.

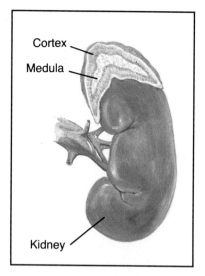

17–3. The adrenal glands are located on top of the kidneys.

17–4. The excitement of competition produces an extra surge of adrenaline that can help to break world records. Salazar has broken the world's record for the marathon.

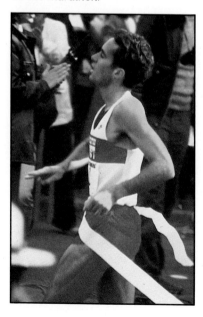

THE ADRENALS

Located above the kidneys are two vital members of the endocrine family: the adrenal glands (see Figure 17-3). The adrenals are double glands, like the pituitary. The **cortex** is the outer part of an adrenal gland, and the **medulla** is the inner part. These parts produce different hormones.

The adrenal cortex secretes a complex mixture of hormones. These hormones regulate the balance between salt and water in the body tissues. They control the metabolism of proteins, fats, and carbohydrates. They also regulate the production of certain types of white blood cells. Other hormones reduce inflammation in the joints. Probably the best-known adrenal hormones are *cortisone* and *aldosterone*.

There is also a check-and-balance system between the pituitary and the adrenal cortex. ACTH is a hormone produced by the anterior pituitary gland. ACTH stimulates the adrenal cortex to secrete its hormones. The increased hormone secretion of the adrenal cortex in turn inhibits the production of more ACTH by the pituitary. This interaction is called negative feedback.

THE EMERGENCY GLANDS. As you have already learned, the adrenal gland secretes adrenaline, the hormone responsible for the stress response. It is actually the adrenal medulla that produces this hormone. Adrenaline is important to you in times of danger. A sudden noise on a dark night can make you run a quarter of a mile like a track star. When athletes are tense with excitement, they surpass their normal performance. Coaches call this "keying up."

THE MEDICAL USES. Adrenaline is used as a heart stimulant. It can also be used to reduce allergic reactions, such as hives, because it constricts blood vessels in the skin. Adrenaline also expands tiny air passages in the lungs, relieving the discomfort of asthma.

Cortisone also has many uses in medicine. It reduces inflammation in joints and is helpful in the treatment of arthritis. It is also effective in the treatment of asthma.

THE THYROID GLAND

The thyroid gland reaches across your throat just below your voice box. There is a lobe on each side of the trachea, connected by a narrow bridge, or isthmus (Figure 17-6). One of the hormones produced by the thyroid gland is called **thyroxine.** Thyroxine controls your **metabolism.** When doctors speak of your metabolism, they are referring to the rate at which cells produce energy.

How does the thyroid gland work as a thermostat? Every cell in your body is a small power plant. Each cell oxidizes food and releases energy for all life activities. Your body depends on this supply of energy. If your thyroid gland is underactive, not enough food is burned in your cells. Therefore, not enough energy is produced. If the thyroid produces too much thyroxine, the result is a tremendous speedup, or increase of energy.

AN OVERACTIVE THYROID

If the thyroid is overactive, the body oxidizes food too rapidly. Weight loss and a ravenous appetite are symptoms of an overactive thyroid. Other abnormal changes are extreme nervousness, restlessness, dizziness, and difficulty in sleeping. Sweating when you should be cool is another symptom. In certain cases the eyes bulge, giving a staring look. The gland may become somewhat enlarged.

How can an overactive thyroid be slowed? At one time surgery was usually necessary to remove part of the gland. But now a drug is available that blocks or slows down thyroid hormone production.

A more recent treatment for an overactive thyroid consists of giving radioactive iodine orally. The radioactive iodine reaches the bloodstream and is then picked up by the thyroid. The iodine is not picked up by any other tissue except the thyroid. Here it bombards the gland with radioactive particles, destroying some of the gland tissue.

AN UNDERACTIVE THYROID

In a person with an underactive thyroid, food is not oxidized fast enough. Much of it is changed to fat, causing weight gain. The person feels sluggish. There is not even enough energy to keep warm. The hands and feet are cold all the time. A person with an underactive thyroid can be helped with thyroid hormone in the form of pills. However, this condition is not common. Most weight gain stems from poor eating habits and too little exercise.

Simple goiter is an enlargement of the thyroid gland, often accompanying iodine deficiency. Iodine is vital for the production of thyroxine. Lack of iodine decreases the output of

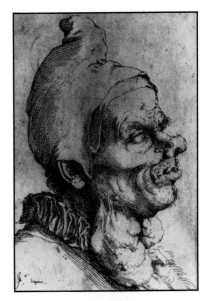

17–5. Historical drawing of a goiter condition. This condition is no longer common since most people have adequate iodine in their diets.

HEALTH IN HISTORY

At one time goiter was common in inland regions where the soil lacked iodine salts. On the other hand, simple goiter was rare along the seacoasts. The oceans contain salts of iodine, which are taken up by the marine plants and animals. People eating seafood receive abundant iodine. Today, large quantities of marine life reach inland markets to supply iodine in the diet. The addition of iodine to table salt has also eliminated large numbers of iodine-deficiency problems.

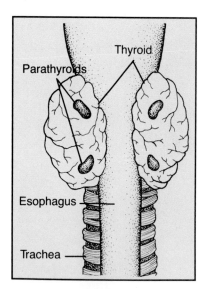

17–6. The location of the thyroid and parathyroids in relation to the trachea and esophagus

17–7. X ray of a child, showing the thymus

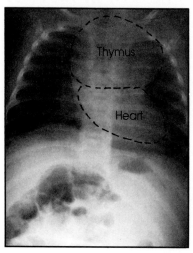

thyroxine. This condition, in turn, causes the anterior lobe of the pituitary gland to increase its secretion of thyrotropic hormone. This stimulates the thyroid gland, which must work harder to produce thyroxine when there is not enough iodine. The thyroid gland may get larger in order to do all this extra work.

A person with simple goiter can prevent further increase in the size of the thyroid gland by taking iodine prescribed by a doctor. However, this treatment seldom reduces the size of the gland. Surgery may be necessary to return the gland to normal size.

THE FOUR PARATHYROIDS

There are four parathyroids, each no larger than a small pea, that lie in back of the thyroid, two on each lobe. They secrete *parathyroid hormone.* The parathyroids regulate the balance of calcium and phosphorus. Calcium and phosphorus are minerals necessary for the growth of bone and proper muscle contraction. If the parathyroids are underactive, the level of calcium in the blood falls. This causes muscles to develop painful spasms, called *tetany.* If the parathyroids are overactive, calcium is taken out of the bones and enters into the bloodstream. Muscles over-relax and weakness results.

A new hormone called *calcitonin* has been discovered to treat people with overactive parathyroids. It directly opposes the effects of the parathyroid hormone. It reduces the calcium level of the blood and promotes calcium buildup in the bones.

THE THYMUS

The thymus lies under the breastbone, in front of the heart. It weighs about 14 grams (1/2 ounce) in the newborn and reaches its maximum size at ages 12 to 14. After that it gradually grows smaller. It is a center for the production of a type of white blood cell called a lymphocyte. Lymphocytes play an important role in protecting the body against disease. The thymus is most active early in life when infants, children, and adolescents need it most to prevent infection. Most adults have already developed immunity to many infectious diseases because of exposure to them early in their lives. Therefore, they no longer need a large thymus. You can read more about this in Chapter 23.

THE PANCREAS

The pancreas serves a double function. The bulk of its tissue secretes digestive enzymes. Scattered throughout the enzyme-secreting tissue are tiny groups of cells called the **islets of Langerhans** (**eye-**lets of **lan-**ger-hanz). These islet cells secret the hormones *insulin* and *glucagon*.

Insulin regulates the use of glucose (blood sugar) in the body in several ways. Glucose is the primary nutrient that is used by body cells to produce energy. Normally, glucose is transported in the bloodstream from the digestive organs to the liver. In the liver most glucose is changed into starch, or glycogen. Insulin enables the liver to store glucose in the form of glycogen. Insulin also stimulates cells to take up glucose. What do you think happens if the islets of Langerhans do not produce enough insulin? The liver cannot store glucose and the body cells cannot take it up. Glucose stays in the blood and cells are deprived of energy. This is one of the causes of **diabetes mellitus** (die-ah-**bee-**tees **mel-**lie-tus), also referred to as sugar diabetes, or true diabetes.

Glucagon has the opposite effect. It changes the stored glycogen back to glucose, which is then released into the blood for delivery to the tissues. This change occurs when the body needs more energy and doesn't have enough glucose.

INSULIN OVERPRODUCTION

Several conditions can cause the islet cells of the pancreas to produce excess insulin. Excess insulin results in a condition called **hypoglycemia** or low blood sugar. The

HEALTH TIP

Some athletes use steroid drugs to build muscles and increase strength and weight. However, steroids are powerful drugs with potentially dangerous side effects. They can affect the normal production of sex hormones in males and females, and can seriously damage normal reproductive development and function. Never use these powerful drugs unless under the supervision of a physician.

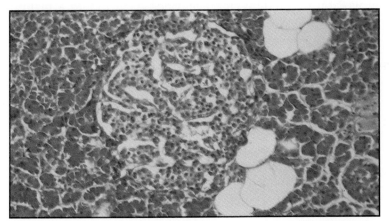

17–8. *Cross-section of the pancreas showing an islet of Langerhans (the group of cells in the center of the photo)*

presence of excess insulin causes a dramatic fall in the blood glucose level of a person. The result is weakness, headaches, and fatigue. Temporary hypoglycemia can be caused by fasting or skipping meals. True hypoglycemia is a rare condition that occurs much less often than does diabetes. Tumors in the islets of Langerhans may cause this problem. A diet high in sugar has also been linked to the condition. Diagnosis can be made after a special test that measures the sugar level of the blood over a period of hours, after ingestion of high-sugar solution.

THE OVARIES AND TESTES

The ovaries in the female and testes in the male are the reproductive organs. These organs produce the sex cells, but they also secrete hormones. Cells in the testes secrete a hormone called **testosterone** (tes-**tos-**ter-roan). The cells in the ovaries secrete the hormones **estrogen** (**ess-**trow-jen) and **progesterone** (pro-**jes-**ter-roan). (See photo of estrogen crystal on page 358.)

Sex hormones are responsible for the changes that occur during adolescence. They produce the secondary sex characteristics that bring about the deepening of the male's voice, the broadening of arms and legs, and the growth of a beard. In females they cause the hips to broaden, the waist to become more slender, the breasts to develop, and menstruation to begin. Along with these physical changes come important mental and emotional changes.

MENSTRUATION

In women of child-bearing age, once each month a mature egg, or ovum, is released by the ovaries and begins its journey to the uterus. By this time, the uterus lining has been prepared in case the egg is fertilized. The lining has grown thick with nutrients and blood that can nourish a developing embryo. If pregnancy does not occur, the lining breaks down, and the blood and nutrients that compose it are discharged during the menstrual period. Each cycle, from the beginning of one menstrual period to the next, lasts an average of about 28 days. However, there is extensive variation from one person to the next, and from one period to the next in the same person. What regulates the timing of the menstrual cycle? Why is the egg released at precisely the right time? What causes menstruation to begin?

THE FOUR HORMONES
OF THE MENSTRUAL CYCLE

The ovaries and the pituitary secrete hormones that regulate the menstrual cycle. These hormones determine when ovulation takes place, and when and how long menstruation occurs. To some extent, they also affect moods and general health. Two hormones, estrogen and progesterone, are secreted by the ovaries. The pituitary produces the other two: **follicle-stimulating hormone (FSH)** and **luteinizing hormone (LH).** As you have learned, the pituitary interacts closely with the hypothalamus. The hypothalamus reacts to emotions and hormones in your body and, in turn, signals the pituitary by means of messenger hormones. Do you see how emotions can affect the menstrual cycle, and vice versa? The hypothalamus senses stress and sends out a message to the pituitary. The pituitary then stops producing LH and FSH. A menstrual period might start later than expected, or it might be missed altogether.

PREMENSTRUAL TENSION

Look at Figure 17-10. Note the changing levels of hormones during the menstrual cycle. About one week before menstruation, hormone levels are very high and then begin to fall rapidly. It has been estimated that about one week before each menstrual period, at least 50 percent of all women of reproductive age experience emotional stress. These women also note general swelling and puffiness of their ankles and faces. Such women are advised to limit their use of salt during this time or to use diuretics to rid the body of excess salt and water. Tea is a natural diuretic. Hormone therapy may benefit some women.

DYSMENORRHEA

The term **dysmenorrhea** (dis-men-o-**re**-ah) comes from the Greek, meaning "painful menstrual flow." Most women have some cramping during menstrual periods, but some have severe pain. Hormones that are synthesized by many tissues, called prostaglandins, may be responsible. **Prostaglandin** (pros-tah-**glan**-din) secretion increases during menstruation and may cause uterine muscle spasms. However, it may be traced to other disorders. Women should consult a doctor in cases of severe dysmenorrhea.

HEALTH TIP

A warm heating pad will sometimes help relieve menstrual cramps. Exercising regularly will also reduce menstrual cramps.

THE MENSTRUAL CYCLE

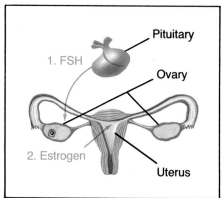

1. FSH
Pituitary
Ovary
2. Estrogen
Uterus

Preovulation. The pituitary secretes FSH, which causes an egg to mature in the ovary. FSH also causes the ovaries to secrete **estrogen**. Estrogen causes the uterus to develop a lining rich in nutrients and blood for the developing egg.

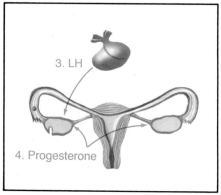

3. LH
4. Progesterone

Ovulation. At mid-cycle, the egg leaves the ovary. This is signaled by LH (lutenizing hormone) from the pituitary. LH also stimulates the ovary to secrete progesterone which prevents another egg from developing.

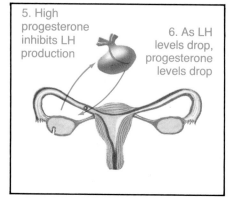

5. High progesterone inhibits LH production
6. As LH levels drop, progesterone levels drop

Postovulation. The ovary continues to secrete progesterone. If the egg is not fertilized, progesterone in the blood reaches a high concentration which inhibits the production of LH. As LH levels decrease, so does progesterone production.

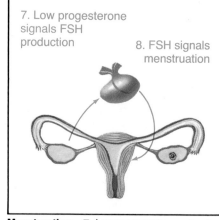

7. Low progesterone signals FSH production
8. FSH signals menstruation

Menstruation. Lower progesterone levels signal the pituitary to produce FSH, and another egg begins developing. FSH also signals the beginning of the menstrual flow.

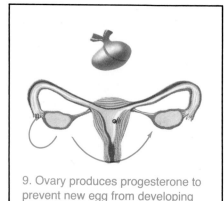

9. Ovary produces progesterone to prevent new egg from developing

Pregnancy. If the mature egg is fertilized, the ovary continues to produce progesterone throughout the pregnancy. A hormone secreted by the placenta stimulates progesterone production. Therefore, no new eggs begin to develop, and no menstrual periods occur.

Figure 17-9

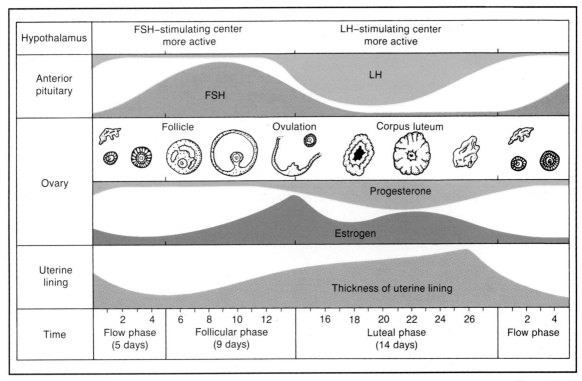

Figure 17–10

ENDOCRINE GLANDS AND THEIR SECRETIONS

Gland	Location	Hormone	Activity Stimulated by Hormone
Pituitary Anterior lobe	Base of brain	ACTH	Stimulates secretion of hormones produced by the cortex of the adrenal glands
		Thyrotropic	Stimulates activity of the thyroid
		Gonadotropic	Stimulates activity of certain cells of the reproductive glands
		Somatotropic	Regulates growth of the skeleton
		Lactogenic	Stimulates secretion of milk produced by the mammary glands
		Luteinizing	Helps regulate the menstrual cycle
		Follicle stimulating	Helps regulate the menstrual cycle
Pituitary Posterior lobe	Base of brain	Antidiuretic hormone (ADH)	Regulates water balance in the body
		Oxytocin	Stimulates smooth muscles of the uterus and mammary glands
Adrenal cortex	Above kidneys	Aldosterone	Regulates balance between salt and water in body tissues
		Cortisone	Regulates breakdown of protein foods
			Controls production of bone, ligaments, certain white blood cells, and other connective tissues
Adrenal medulla	Above kidneys	Adrenaline (epinephrine)	Increases heart action, constricts blood vessels, and stimulates the liver (to release glucogen) and nervous system
Thyroid	Neck, below voice box	Thyroxine	Regulates the rate of metabolism
Parathyroids	Back surface of thyroid lobes	Parathyroid	Regulates balance of phosphorus and calcium in tissues
Islet cells of the pancreas	Behind stomach	Insulin	Enables the liver to store and utilize sugar
		Glucagon	Changes stored glycogen into glucose
Testes	Testicles	Testosterone	Produces male secondary sex characteristics
Ovaries	Lower abdomen	Estrogen Progesterone	Produce female secondary sex characteristics

Table 17–1

SUMMARY: The endocrine glands, working as a team with the nervous system, control most of the body's activities. This includes control of the rate of growth; the maturing process from childhood through adolescence to adulthood; the ability to cope with emergencies; the body's salt, water, and sugar balance; and the rate at which we burn food. The endocrine glands also control heart rate and blood pressure and the menstrual cycle in women. They operate together as a system of checks and balances. When the balance is upset, serious diseases may result.

CHAPTER REVIEW

words at work

Find the word in the left column that fits one of the definitions in the right column. DO NOT WRITE IN THIS BOOK.

a. acromegaly
b. adrenals
c. antidiuretic hormone (ADH)
d. Islets of Langerhans
e. estrogen
f. hyperthyroidism
g. goiter
h. hypoglycemia
i. ovaries
j. parathyroids

1. Glands regulating calcium and phosphorus balance
2. Produce insulin
3. Somatotropic hormone excess in adulthood
4. Responsible for regulating water balance in the body
5. Thyroid hormone excess
6. Caused by insulin excess
7. Female sex hormone
8. Female reproductive organs
9. Superchargers of the endocrine system
10. Condition due to iodine deficiency

review questions

1. How are endocrine glands fundamentally different from glands such as the salivary glands?
2. List and locate the endocrine glands.
3. What is a hormone?
4. In what ways do hormones affect the body?
5. Why is the pituitary sometimes referred to as the master gland?
6. What is the function of the hypothalamus?
7. What causes pituitary dwarfism?
8. What causes a giant-sized person?
9. What causes the body changes that take place during adolescence?
10. Describe the adrenal glands.
11. What are some of the medical uses of adrenaline?
12. How does the thyroid gland serve as the body's thermostat?
13. What effect does an overactive thyroid gland have upon the body?
14. What are the symptoms of an underactive thyroid gland?
15. What is the function of the parathyroid glands?
16. Discuss the function of the thymus gland.
17. What hormone is produced by the male reproductive organs?
18. Describe the menstrual cycle.

discussion questions

1. Discuss the effect of emotions on the endocrine system.
2. Why do coaches give "pep talks" before the start of a big game?
3. Discuss the dynamic balance (the process of negative feedback) of the endocrine system.
4. Can you name any body function that is not affected by the endocrine system?
5. Discuss possible new horizons in the use of hormones in the medical field.

investigating

PURPOSE:

To illustrate the function of the endocrine glands in everyday life.

MATERIALS NEEDED:

Magazines; paper; pens; paste; scissors.

PROCEDURE:

A.   Review Table 17-1 on the endocrine glands and their secretions on page 372.

B.   Look through old magazines for pictures of people, keeping in mind the functions of the endocrine glands listed on the chart. Cut out pictures that illustrate endocrine function. For example, a photograph of a child and a grown person would illustrate the function of gonadotropic hormone. Find pictures to illustrate at least one function of each gland. Glue each picture to a separate piece of paper.

C.   Write captions for your pictures, explaining what gland and hormone function the picture illustrates.

D.   As a class, designate different areas of the classroom walls for each gland. Tape up your pictures where they belong.

E.   As a class, describe the functions of each gland as illustrated in the pictures.

   1.   Describe how hormones regulate your body functions during the course of a normal day.

   2.   Describe what would happen if your glands secreted too much or not enough of the following hormones: somatotropic hormone; thyroid hormone; parathyroid hormone; and insulin.

THE SKELETAL-MUSCULAR SYSTEM

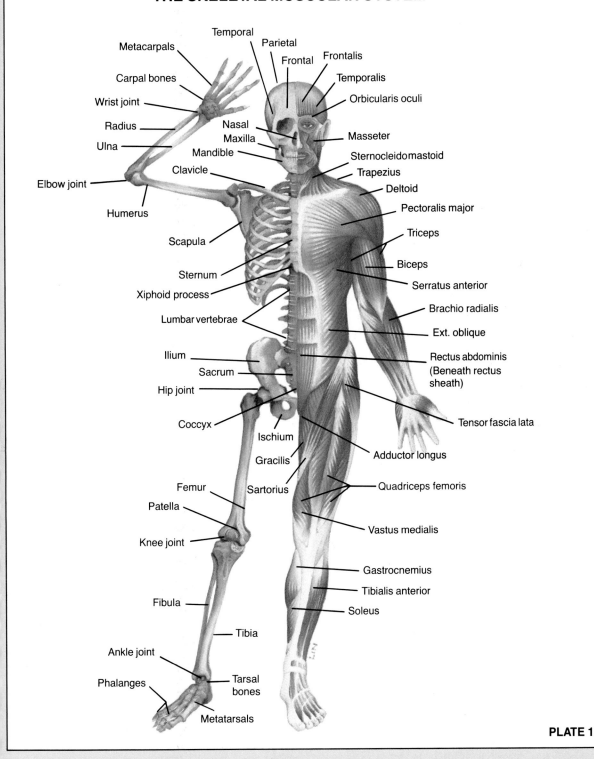

Temporal
Metacarpals
Parietal
Frontal
Frontalis
Carpal bones
Temporalis
Wrist joint
Orbicularis oculi
Radius
Nasal
Ulna
Maxilla
Masseter
Mandible
Sternocleidomastoid
Clavicle
Trapezius
Elbow joint
Deltoid
Pectoralis major
Humerus
Triceps
Scapula
Biceps
Serratus anterior
Sternum
Xiphoid process
Brachio radialis
Lumbar vertebrae
Ext. oblique
Rectus abdominis
Ilium
(Beneath rectus
Sacrum
sheath)
Hip joint
Coccyx
Tensor fascia lata
Ischium
Gracilis
Adductor longus
Femur
Sartorius
Quadriceps femoris
Patella
Vastus medialis
Knee joint
Gastrocnemius
Tibialis anterior
Fibula
Soleus
Tibia
Ankle joint
Phalanges
Tarsal
bones
Metatarsals

PLATE 1

THE NERVOUS SYSTEM

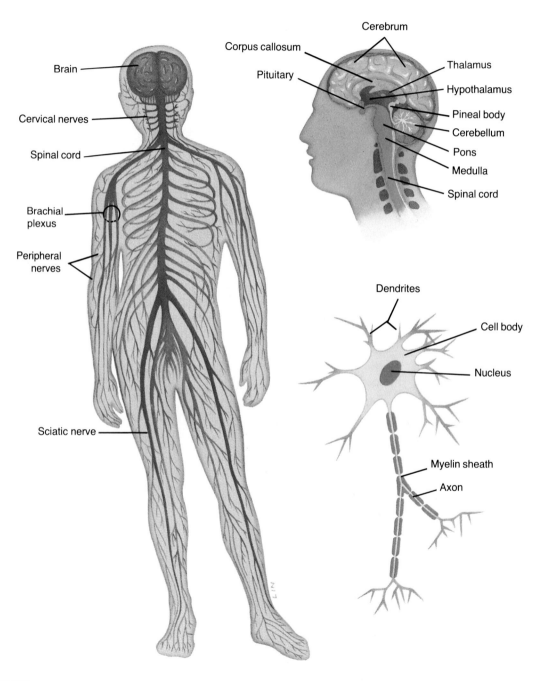

Brain

Cervical nerves

Spinal cord

Brachial plexus

Peripheral nerves

Sciatic nerve

Cerebrum

Corpus callosum

Pituitary

Thalamus

Hypothalamus

Pineal body

Cerebellum

Pons

Medulla

Spinal cord

Dendrites

Cell body

Nucleus

Myelin sheath

Axon

PLATE 2

THE FIVE SENSES

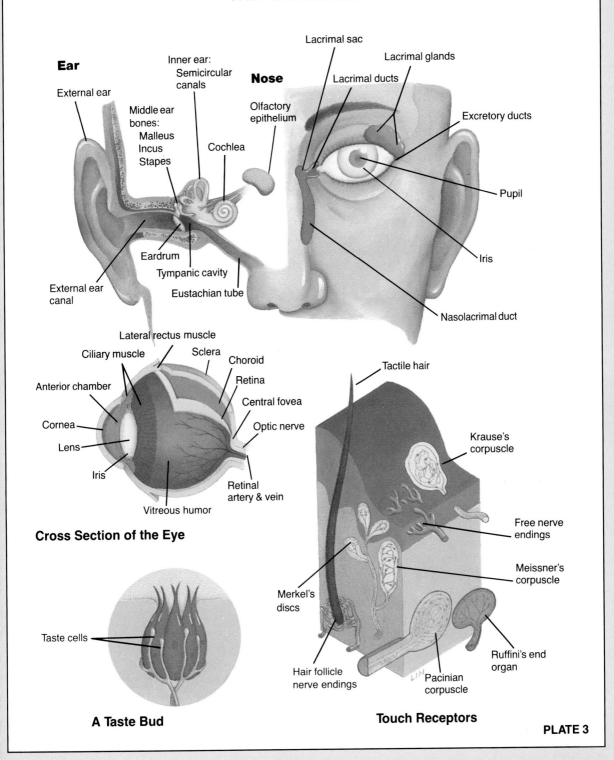

Lacrimal sac

Inner ear:
Semicircular canals

Lacrimal glands

Lacrimal ducts

External ear

Middle ear bones:
Malleus
Incus
Stapes

Olfactory epithelium

Cochlea

Excretory ducts

Pupil

Eardrum

Tympanic cavity

External ear canal

Eustachian tube

Iris

Nasolacrimal duct

Lateral rectus muscle

Ciliary muscle

Sclera

Choroid

Retina

Tactile hair

Anterior chamber

Central fovea

Krause's corpuscle

Cornea

Optic nerve

Lens

Iris

Free nerve endings

Retinal artery & vein

Meissner's corpuscle

Vitreous humor

Cross Section of the Eye

Merkel's discs

Taste cells

Hair follicle nerve endings

Pacinian corpuscle

Ruffini's end organ

A Taste Bud

Touch Receptors

PLATE 3

VEINS AND ARTERIES

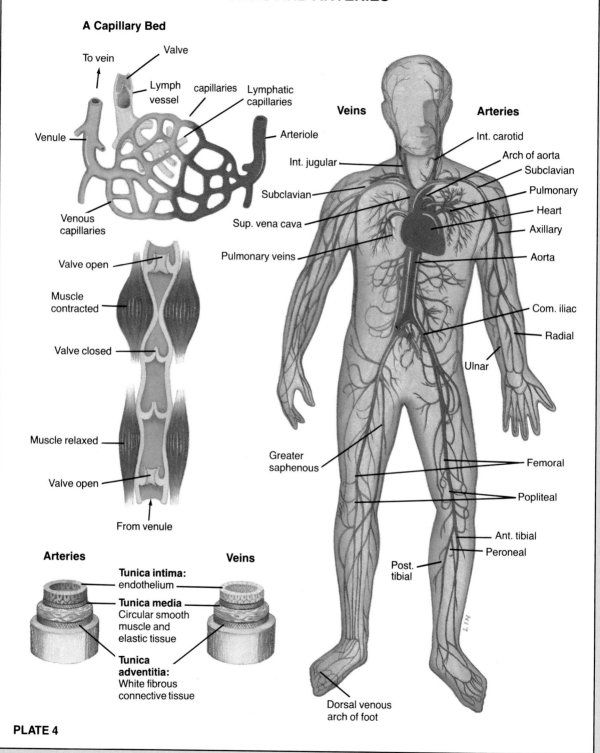

A Capillary Bed

To vein

Valve

Lymph vessel

capillaries

Lymphatic capillaries

Venule

Arteriole

Venous capillaries

Valve open

Muscle contracted

Valve closed

Muscle relaxed

Valve open

From venule

Veins

Arteries

Int. jugular

Subclavian

Sup. vena cava

Pulmonary veins

Int. carotid

Arch of aorta

Subclavian

Pulmonary

Heart

Axillary

Aorta

Com. iliac

Radial

Ulnar

Greater saphenous

Femoral

Popliteal

Ant. tibial

Peroneal

Post. tibial

Dorsal venous arch of foot

Arteries

Veins

Tunica intima: endothelium

Tunica media Circular smooth muscle and elastic tissue

Tunica adventitia: White fibrous connective tissue

PLATE 4

RESPIRATION AND THE HEART

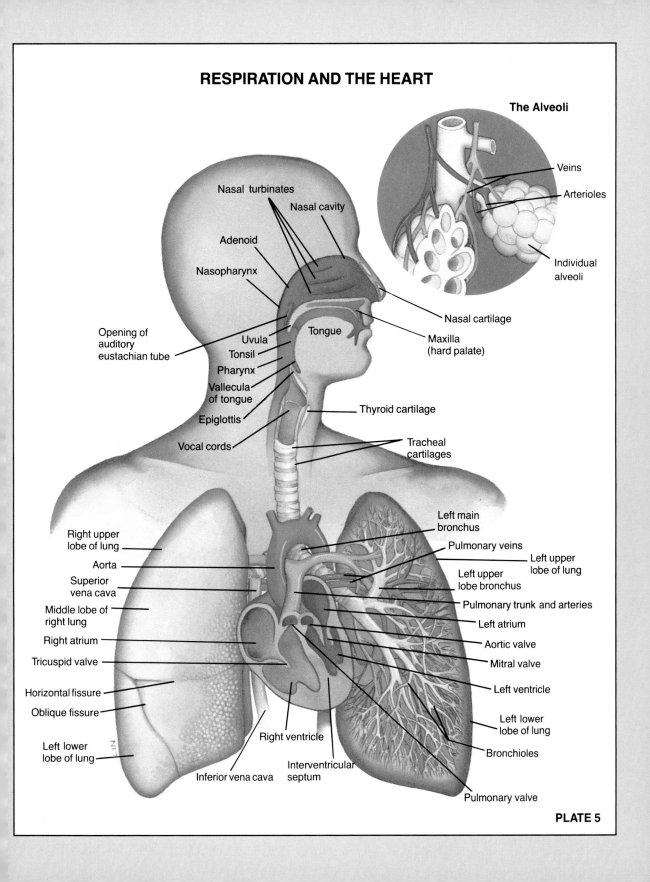

The Alveoli

Veins

Arterioles

Individual alveoli

Nasal turbinates

Nasal cavity

Adenoid

Nasopharynx

Opening of auditory eustachian tube

Uvula

Tongue

Nasal cartilage

Maxilla (hard palate)

Tonsil

Pharynx

Vallecula of tongue

Epiglottis

Thyroid cartilage

Vocal cords

Tracheal cartilages

Left main bronchus

Pulmonary veins

Right upper lobe of lung

Left upper lobe of lung

Aorta

Left upper lobe bronchus

Superior vena cava

Pulmonary trunk and arteries

Middle lobe of right lung

Left atrium

Right atrium

Aortic valve

Tricuspid valve

Mitral valve

Horizontal fissure

Left ventricle

Oblique fissure

Left lower lobe of lung

Left lower lobe of lung

Bronchioles

Right ventricle

Inferior vena cava

Interventricular septum

Pulmonary valve

PLATE 5

THE DIGESTIVE SYSTEM

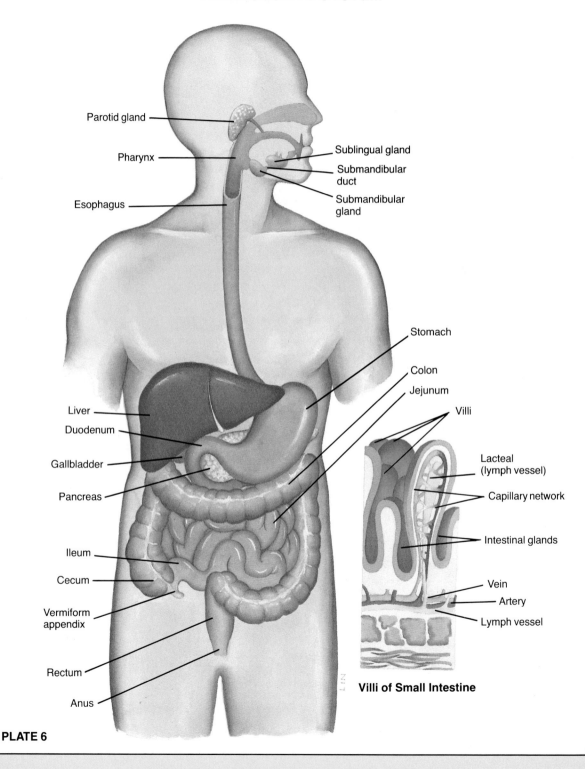

Parotid gland

Pharynx

Esophagus

Sublingual gland

Submandibular duct

Submandibular gland

Stomach

Colon

Jejunum

Villi

Lacteal (lymph vessel)

Capillary network

Intestinal glands

Vein

Artery

Lymph vessel

Liver

Duodenum

Gallbladder

Pancreas

Ileum

Cecum

Vermiform appendix

Rectum

Anus

Villi of Small Intestine

PLATE 6

THE EXCRETORY SYSTEM

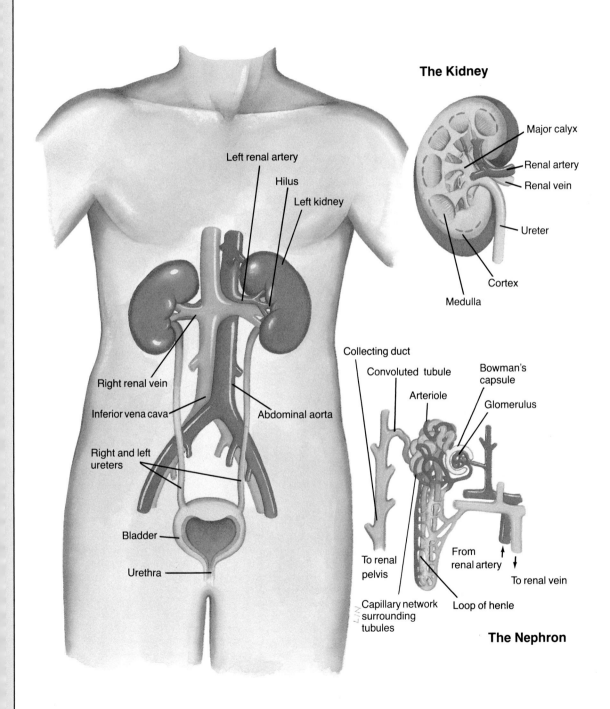

The Kidney

Major calyx

Renal artery

Renal vein

Ureter

Cortex

Medulla

Left renal artery

Hilus

Left kidney

Right renal vein

Inferior vena cava

Abdominal aorta

Right and left ureters

Bladder

Urethra

Collecting duct

Convoluted tubule

Arteriole

Bowman's capsule

Glomerulus

To renal pelvis

From renal artery

To renal vein

Capillary network surrounding tubules

Loop of henle

The Nephron

PLATE 7

THE ENDOCRINE SYSTEM

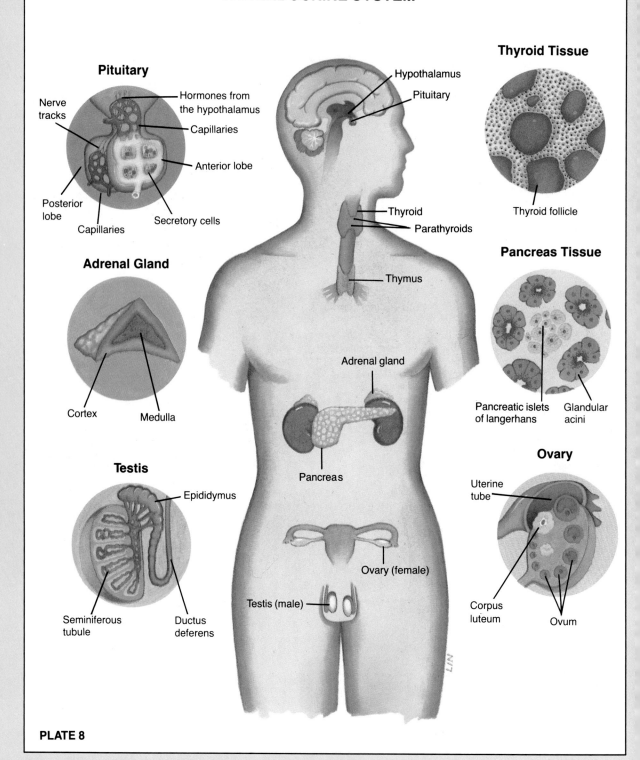

Pituitary

Nerve tracks

Hormones from the hypothalamus

Capillaries

Anterior lobe

Posterior lobe

Capillaries

Secretory cells

Hypothalamus

Pituitary

Thyroid Tissue

Thyroid follicle

Thyroid

Parathyroid

Thymus

Pancreas Tissue

Pancreatic islets of langerhans

Glandular acini

Adrenal Gland

Cortex

Medulla

Adrenal gland

Pancreas

Ovary

Uterine tube

Corpus luteum

Ovum

Testis

Epididymus

Seminiferous tubule

Ductus deferens

Ovary (female)

Testis (male)

PLATE 8

HEALTH
CAREERS

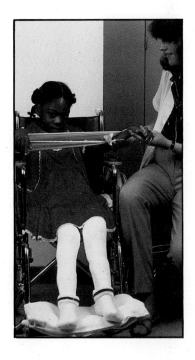

PHYSICAL THERAPIST

Wanted: people with special patience and compassion to work with the physically handicapped. Such people must have good manual coordination, average physical strength, good health, and an ability to communicate well with all age groups. Acting on a physician's prescription, therapists first evaluate the extent of a patient's disability. They then plan and direct a treatment program to restore as much body movement as possible. Assistant physical therapists work under the supervision of therapists and help with treatment. People who need physical therapy include young children with cerebral palsy learning how to walk with braces, stroke victims regaining the use of limbs, elderly persons stricken with arthritis, and many other people. Physical therapy treatment may include exercise, application of heat or cold, and use of water to change the patient's condition. To see if you like physical therapy, work as a hospital volunteer for the handicapped. To find out more about this field, write to the American Physical Therapy Association, 1156 Fifteenth Street, N.W., Suite 500, Washington, D.C. 20005.

OPTOMETRIST

Most of us take our eyesight for granted. One person who doesn't, however, is the optometrist. The eyes must be examined, not only for sight problems, but for other abnormalities and diseases. Since an optometrist may not use surgery or drugs, treatment may include the prescribing of corrective lenses or vision therapy, as well as exercise. An ophthalmologist is a physician specializing in the diseases and structure of the eyes. Since this person is a medical doctor, he or she may use surgery or drugs. How can you become an optometrist? You must have a four-year degree from a school of optometry and pass a state licensing exam. You need to learn about visual perception, optics, and eye diseases. Field work with patients would be another part of your training. After graduation, most optometrists work in a general private practice. Some of them specialize in contact lenses or vision therapy. Still others work as

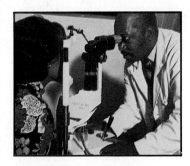

vision consultants for government and industry. For more information, write to the American Optometric Association, 243 North Lindbergh Boulevard, St. Louis, Missouri 63141.

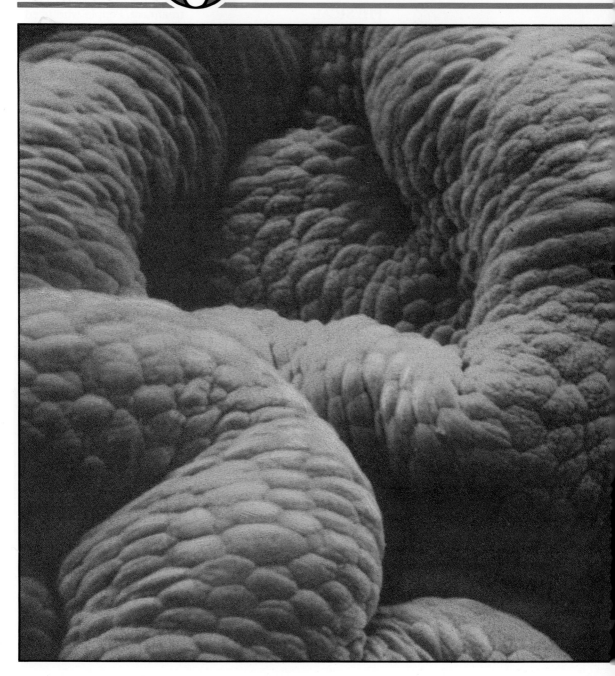

Your Supply Systems

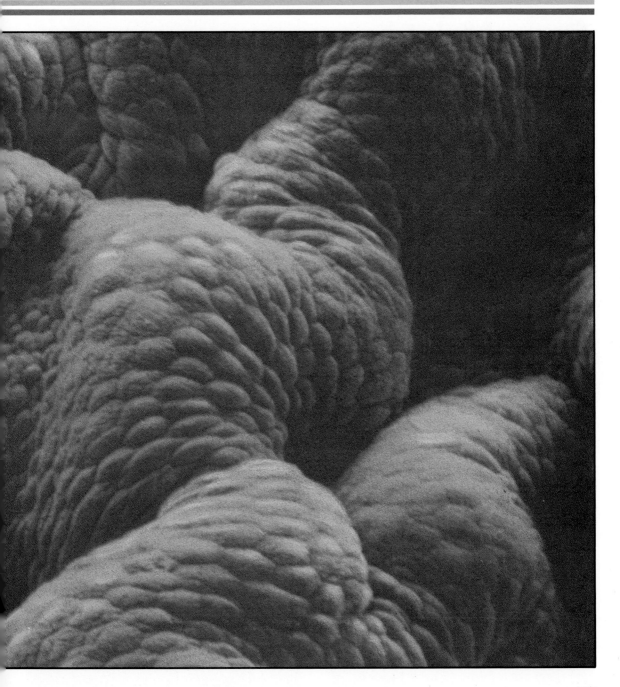

CHAPTER 18

Tissue Maintenance

OBJECTIVES

- DESCRIBE the chemical changes in food during digestion
- STATE the functions of the organs in the digestive system
- STATE the functions of the organs in the excretory system
- IDENTIFY the diseases of the digestive and excretory systems

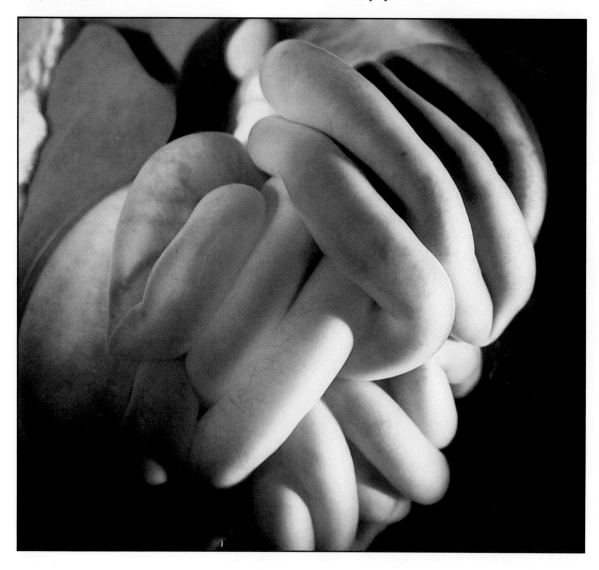

Think of all the time spent each day in purchasing, preparing, and eating food. But did you ever wonder what happens to food after you swallow it? After food is swallowed, digestion is no longer under your voluntary control. The food you eat begins a long journey through the digestive tract that takes at least two days. It is pushed by smooth muscles lining the digestive tract, which rhythmically relax and contract. As it passes through, it is digested along the way. In this chapter, you shall follow the journey that food takes through the digestive system, and find out where it goes from there.

STRUCTURE AND FUNCTION OF THE DIGESTIVE SYSTEM

Digestion is a step-by-step process in which many organs work together. We classify the organs of digestion into two groups: (1) those forming the **alimentary canal** and (2) those forming the accessory organs of digestion. The mouth, pharynx, esophagus, stomach, small intestine, and large intestine form the alimentary canal, which extends 9 meters (30 ft) through the body. As food is digested it moves through the alimentary canal. Indigestible and unabsorbed substances enter the colon, where they are disposed of as intestinal waste. The salivary glands, liver, gallbladder, and pancreas are classified as accessory organs of digestion. Food never enters these organs. However, these organs secrete **enzymes** that chemically break down and digest food. The photo on page 378 shows the small intestine, liver, and pancreas of a child.

OVERVIEW OF THE DIGESTIVE PROCESS

As food is digested, it is mechanically broken down and chemically split into small nutrient molecules. This is necessary since only small nutrient molecules enter the bloodstream. Food is mechanically broken down by being chewed in the mouth and by being churned in the stomach. Food is chemically broken down by being acted on by secretions of the digestive glands. These secretions contain enzymes and

THE DIGESTIVE SYSTEM

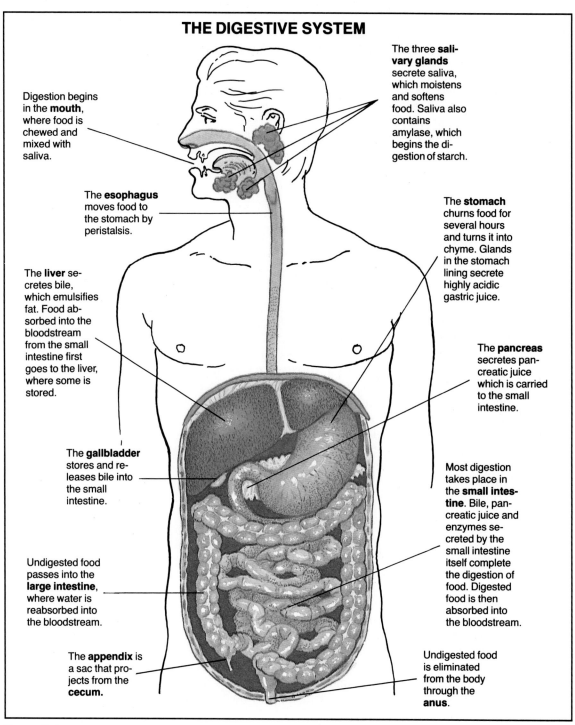

Digestion begins in the **mouth**, where food is chewed and mixed with saliva.

The three **salivary glands** secrete saliva, which moistens and softens food. Saliva also contains amylase, which begins the digestion of starch.

The **esophagus** moves food to the stomach by peristalsis.

The **stomach** churns food for several hours and turns it into chyme. Glands in the stomach lining secrete highly acidic gastric juice.

The **liver** secretes bile, which emulsifies fat. Food absorbed into the bloodstream from the small intestine first goes to the liver, where some is stored.

The **pancreas** secretes pancreatic juice which is carried to the small intestine.

The **gallbladder** stores and releases bile into the small intestine.

Most digestion takes place in the **small intestine**. Bile, pancreatic juice and enzymes secreted by the small intestine itself complete the digestion of food. Digested food is then absorbed into the bloodstream.

Undigested food passes into the **large intestine**, where water is reabsorbed into the bloodstream.

The **appendix** is a sac that projects from the **cecum**.

Undigested food is eliminated from the body through the **anus**.

Figure 18-1

other substances that cause specific chemical changes during digestion. Digestion of a meal requires the action of a series of enzymes.

There are six different kinds of nutrients: proteins, carbohydrates, fats, water, vitamins, and minerals. Water, vitamins, and minerals do not need to be digested, since they can enter the bloodstream as they are. *Proteins* must be chemically broken down into small molecules called *amino acids*. This is done by enzymes secreted by the glands in the walls of the small intestine and stomach. *Fats* are broken down into *glycerol* and *fatty acids*. Bile from the liver and enzymes secreted by the pancreas and small intestine accomplish this. *Starch* and *large molecules of sugar* are broken into *simple sugars* by enzymes secreted by the salivary glands, the pancreas, and the small intestine.

Once food is broken down into soluble form it is absorbed into the bloodstream and transported to the liver, where some of it is removed and stored. The rest is transported to the billions of cells that make up the human body.

DIGESTION IN THE MOUTH

Chewing is the first step in the process of digestion. Chewing breaks food into smaller particles. As food is chewed, it is thoroughly mixed with *saliva*, which moistens, softens, and lubricates it. Saliva also contains an enzyme, *amylase*, that changes starch into a form of sugar known as *maltose*.

THE ESOPHAGUS AND SWALLOWING

Swallowing is a complex, three-stage process. The tongue and cheeks push the food to the back of the throat and the person swallows. Contraction of the throat muscles forces the food into the opening of the esophagus. As this occurs the opening of the air passage to the lungs is closed by a small flap of tissue, the **epiglottis** (eh-pi-**glot**-is).

The esophagus is a tube about 30 centimeters (12 in.) long. Cells lining the esophagus secrete *mucus* that aids the movement of food. Two sets of muscles surround the walls of the esophagus. A wave of contractions of these muscles mechanically moves the food mass downward to the stomach. This mechanical movement is called **peristalsis** (pear-is-**stal**-sis). Gravity helps to move the food mass downward, but is not necessary. Even if you stand on your head, food would reach your stomach, however uncomfortably. If peristalsis reverses, vomiting occurs.

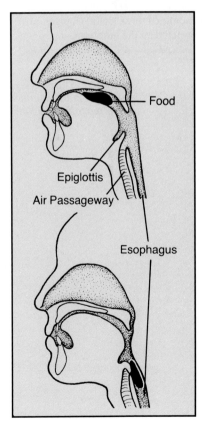

18–2. When you swallow, the epiglottis closes off the trachea, and a wave of muscular movements called peristalsis pushes the food to the stomach.

Food

Epiglottis

Air Passageway

Esophagus

18–3. Note the three layers of muscle in the stomach wall, magnified 29 times.

THE STOMACH

The stomach is in the left upper part of the abdominal cavity. The shape and size of the stomach vary with the amount of food and liquid it contains. Three layers of smooth muscle lie in the stomach wall. Each layer contracts in a different direction, causing the stomach to twist, squeeze, and churn its contents. These actions are important for the mechanical breakdown of food particles and for the thorough mixing of food with digestive secretions.

Solid food usually stays in the stomach for several hours. During this time the process of changing food into small molecules continues. Numerous glands within the walls of the stomach secrete the stomach juices, or *gastric juices*, necessary for digestion. Certain of these glands secrete highly acidic *hydrochloric acid.* Hydrochloric acid softens food and destroys some of the bacteria in it. Hydrochloric acid is also needed for the formation and chemical activity of the enzyme *pepsin.* Pepsin begins the digestion of proteins into simpler forms. Pepsin is secreted by other glands of the stomach wall.

A small muscle at the lower end of the stomach, the **pyloric sphincter** (pie-**lore**-ik **sfink**-ter), separates the stomach from the small intestine. The sphincter muscle is closed

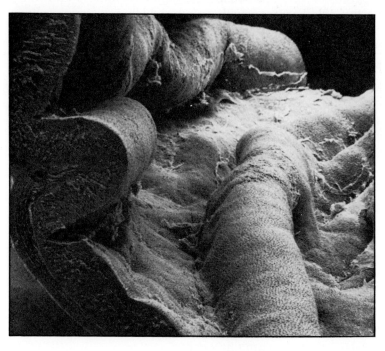

while food is undergoing digestion in the stomach. When the stomach completes its job, the pyloric sphincter opens and closes several times as the stomach gradually empties its contents into the small intestine.

DIGESTION IN THE SMALL INTESTINE

In the small intestine digestion of food is completed and the food is then absorbed into the bloodstream. The small intestine is a coiled tube about 3 centimeters (1.5 in.) in diameter and 7 meters (23 ft) long. The end of the small intestine joins the large intestine.

Secretions that act on foods in the small intestine come from the liver, the pancreas, and the intestinal glands. The intestinal glands also secrete four enzymes that act on protein and sugar (see Table 18-1).

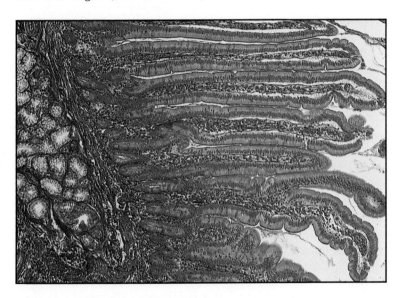

18–4. Villi of the small intestine, magnified 126 times. Note the brush borders around each villus.

THE LARGEST GLAND: THE LIVER. The liver, the largest gland in the body, has an average weight of 1.5 kilograms (3.4 lb). It lies just below the diaphragm in the upper right region of the abdominal cavity. This remarkable gland acts as:

1. a storehouse for digested food, especially carbohydrates, which are stored as glycogen
2. a regulator of the level of blood sugar
3. a chemical factory in which fats are changed and amino acids are split

4. a blood filter and regulator of blood volume
5. an organ of excretion, and
6. a digestive organ.

In its role as a digestive organ, the liver secretes up to 1 liter (1.06 qt) of *bile* each day. Bile is a brownish-green fluid that contains salt, blood pigment, and disintegrated red blood corpuscles. Bile flows from the liver to the gallbladder through a series of bile ducts. When food passes into the small intestine from the stomach, the gallbladder contracts, releasing bile into the intestine. Bile has no enzymes, but it is essential in the digestion of fats. Since fats do not mix with water, bile *emulsifies* them. This means that large globs of fat are broken into tiny globs. Detergent works in the same way to break up fats. This increases the surface area of the fats so that enzymes can work on them.

THE PANCREAS. The pancreas is an endocrine gland that secretes the hormone *insulin*. It is also a vital digestive gland. The pancreas is a whitish gland behind the stomach. It passes a digestive secretion called *pancreatic juice* into the small intestine. The pancreatic juice contains three vital enzymes, which act on proteins, fats, and carbohydrates (see Table 18-1).

ABSORPTION IN THE SMALL INTESTINE. The small intestine is ideally suited to the absorption of soluble, digested foods. Its walls are lined with millions of tiny, fingerlike **villi** (**vil**-lie) (see Figure 18-4) projecting from folds of the mucous membrane. These villi greatly increase the absorbing surface of the small intestine. Each villus has a *brush border*, which further increases the absorbing surface. Inside each villus there is also a small lymph vessel called a **lacteal** (**lak**-tee-al).

A single layer of cells separates the lacteals and capillaries from the contents of the small intestine. Amino acids and glucose enter directly into the capillaries. Digested fats first pass into the lacteals, and from there into the blood. By the time the food you have eaten reaches the lower end of the small intestine, only water and indigestible matter remain. The rest has been absorbed into the bloodstream.

THE LARGE INTESTINE

The small intestine ends in the lower right region of the abdomen, where it joins the **colon,** or large intestine. This junction that connects the small intestine to the colon is

384

called the **cecum** (**see**-kum). The appendix is a small, wormlike projection of the cecum.

The colon is about 1.5 to 1.8 meters (5 to 6 ft) long and 5 centimeters (2 in.) in diameter. Indigestible matter or wastes enter it from the small intestine. The colon ends in the muscular rectum. The feces in the rectum are held by a sphincter muscle until they are discharged through the anus.

Peristaltic movements in the colon are normally slower than those of the upper digestive organs. Bacteria have time to grow and reproduce there. Some are beneficial because they produce certain vitamins that are then absorbed into the blood. But the most important function of the large intestine is the absorption of water through its walls and into the blood. This is vital to the water balance in the body. Indigestible food enters the colon from the small intestine in a watery mixture. When the contents enter the rectum, they have become nearly solid because of water absorption.

Table 18-1

Place of Digestion	Organ or Gland	Secretions	Enzymes	Digestive Activity
mouth	salivary	saliva	salivary amylase	changes starch to maltose; lubricates
esophagus	mucous	mucus		lubricates
stomach	gastric	gastric juice	pepsin	changes proteins to polypeptides
		hydrochloric acid		activates pepsin; kills bacteria
	mucous	mucus		lubricates
small intestine	liver	bile		emulsifies fat; activates lipase
	pancreas	pancreatic fluid	trypsin chemotrypsin	changes polypeptides to tripeptides and dipeptides
			amylase	changes starch to maltose
			lipase	changes fats to fatty acids and glycerol
	intestinal	intestinal fluid	peptidases	changes tripeptides and dipeptides to amino acids
			maltase	changes maltose to glucose
			lactase	changes lactose to glucose and galactose
			sucrase	changes sucrose to glucose and fructose
large intestine (colon)	mucous	mucus		lubricates

SUMMARY OF DIGESTION

COMMON PROBLEMS
OF THE DIGESTIVE SYSTEM

INDIGESTION

The term "indigestion" can refer to a stomachache, heartburn, bloated feelings, nausea, vomiting, or pain in any part of the abdomen. Most people experience these symptoms at one time or another. Usually indigestion is a temporary condition. However, if it occurs frequently, it could be a symptom of a serious illness. Many times indigestion is due to poor eating habits. Eating too much, too little, too irregularly, or too quickly can cause stomach upsets. Emotional upset can also disturb the digestive process, resulting in gas, cramps, nausea, and vomiting. Food poisoning is another cause of digestive disturbances. *Heartburn* occurs when highly acidic gastric juices from the stomach spurt up through the esophagus. The esophagus becomes irritated, resulting in pain that seems to come from the heart.

EXCESS GAS

Gastrointestinal gas is a common ailment that is usually curable by a change in eating habits. A common cause of excessive belching is swallowing a lot of air. This may happen if you eat or drink too fast and don't chew thoroughly. Passing excessive amounts of gas can be caused by eating foods such as beans, bran, and broccoli. These foods contain carbohydrates and proteins that people cannot completely digest. The indigestible matter is passed on to the large intestine. Here bacteria feed on it, and produce excessive amounts of gas.

DIARRHEA

Diarrhea is the discharge of colon wastes in a watery condition. The colon becomes overactive, and produces extra mucus and contracts more frequently. The intestinal wastes are forced through so rapidly that water is not reabsorbed by the body in normal amounts. Laxatives produce the same effect.

Diarrhea can be caused by emotional stress and by various bacteria and viruses, which irritate the mucous lining. It is important to drink plenty of liquids during attacks of

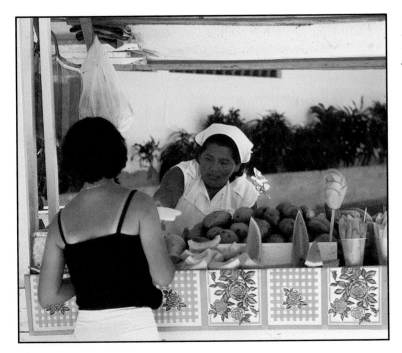

18–5. When visiting a foreign country, prevent traveler's diarrhea by peeling fresh fruit and vegetables before eating.

diarrhea. Otherwise, you may get dehydrated. Over-the-counter drugs that contain pectin or kaolin can also help. Seek medical advice if diarrhea is severe and prolonged, or if it alternates with constipation.

Traveler's diarrhea is a common ailment among visitors to other countries. This problem is most common in countries that have inadequate water treatment and unsanitary food preparation, but it can happen in other countries as well. It usually strikes travelers who are not accustomed to the particular strains of bacteria that are present in the country they are visiting. To prevent it, do not drink unchlorinated water. Also, peel raw fruits and vegetables before eating them.

CONSTIPATION PROBLEMS

Infrequent, hard, or difficult bowel movements are all termed *constipation*. The condition can be temporary or chronic. How many different advertisements do you know of that promise a quick remedy? Often the problem can be corrected without self-medication.

Constipation in young people is usually caused by a diet that is deficient in fiber. Foods that are rich in fiber include bran, whole wheat, leafy vegetables, and fruit. Without fiber to stimulate muscular activity in the colon, the contents move slowly, leading to dehydration of the colon contents. Eating too little fiber, not getting enough exercise, insufficient water intake, and postponing defecation can be other causes of dehydration.

Older people often develop constipation because of loss of tone in the muscles of the colon wall. This often results from frequent use of laxatives. If constipation persists or alternates with diarrhea, seek medical advice. The underlying cause may require medical treatment.

THE DANGER OF LAXATIVES. The laxative habit, acquired by millions, causes several health problems. Laxatives are classed as *purgatives*. They flush the intestine rapidly and act as irritants, leaving the lining of the colon inflamed. High fiber foods, such as bran, fruit, and vegetables, should be used instead. They stimulate peristaltic action without irritating the colon. Figure 18-6 shows some foods that are rich in fiber.

18–6. To help prevent constipation, eat foods rich in fiber, such as these.

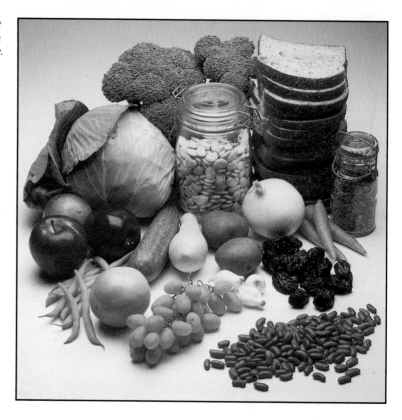

HEMORRHOIDS AND FISSURES

The rectum is richly supplied with veins. Straining during a bowel movement because of constipation may stretch them abnormally. We refer to these enlarged veins as **hemorrhoids**. Internal hemorrhoids are above the sphincter muscle of the rectum; external hemorrhoids are below it. Under strain, external hemorrhoids often bulge alongside the anal opening. Rectal bleeding may be due to a ruptured hemorrhoid, a condition that should be checked by a doctor.

A *fissure* is a crack in the membrane lining of the rectal opening, causing bleeding, smarting, and itching. Healing of a fissure can be difficult, because strain during a bowel movement tears it open again.

Various rectal suppositories (medicated lubricants that melt after insertion into the rectum) ease the stinging of hemorrhoids or fissures. Medications and foods containing fiber are valuable, because they soften the intestinal contents, preventing irritation and strain. Severe cases of hemorrhoids can be corrected surgically.

FOOD POISONING

Everyone brought a dish of food to the class picnic. That evening, several students became ill. The symptoms included severe stomach pains, nausea, vomiting, and diarrhea. What was the cause of their sickness? Upon questioning, it was discovered that those who had become ill had eaten potato salad. The salad had remained unrefrigerated for several hours before it was consumed. During this time, bacteria had grown and multiplied, contaminating the salad with toxins.

Bacteria that causes food poisoning can grow if food is improperly handled and cooked. Most of these bacteria are killed by normal cooking and do not grow if food is refrigerated. However, if food is left standing unrefrigerated, or if food is not cooked properly, the bacteria can grow and produce toxins. On picnics, be sure to keep cold foods cold and hot foods hot. Do not take foods containing eggs or milk on picnics unless they can be kept very cold until serving.

People recover from most cases of food poisoning within a few days. Eating a bland diet and drinking lots of fluids will help to speed recovery.

Botulism (**boch**-ah-liz-um) is a dangerous form of food poisoning. If these bacteria are not killed during canning, they start their deadly activity by releasing toxins into the canned food. If this food is eaten, the toxins begin acting on the nervous system, causing vision defects, headache, dizziness, and muscle weakness. Complete muscle paralysis and death can follow. Fortunately, botulism is rare today. Commercial canning companies process food sufficiently to kill bacteria and spores. However, botulism is still a danger in home-canned vegetables. If you do your own canning, be sure to follow safe canning techniques. Before you eat canned foods, look for signs of spoilage, such as bulging of the container, gas bubbles, or unnatural odor. To be safe, cook home-canned, low-acid foods for at least fifteen minutes in boiling liquids.

IRRITABLE BOWEL SYNDROME

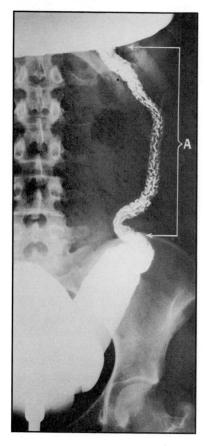

18–7. A spasm in the colon is shown in area A.

One of the most common gastrointestinal diseases among Americans is *irritable bowel syndrome*. It is caused by stress, and is more likely to attack tense, anxious people and those with irregular eating and sleeping habits. Attacks are usually triggered by emotional stress in combination with certain foods and drinks, such as coffee, alcohol, spicy food, and raw salads. The bowel contracts suddenly and violently, which causes a sharp or dull pain. This is called a *spasm*. The pain can be relieved by manual pressure or heat. Diarrhea and constipation may be other symptoms of this syndrome.

APPENDICITIS: A FREQUENT TROUBLEMAKER

Many intestinal infections are easily confused with appendicitis, since their symptoms (abdominal pain, nausea, vomiting, and fever) are similar.

Although the appendix is small, it can cause serious problems if infected. Swelling of the appendix indicates an infection. The swelling can cause the appendix to burst, spreading its infected contents onto the lining of the abdominal cavity, the *peritoneum*. This results in *peritonitis*, a dangerous infection. Fortunately, modern drugs have greatly reduced the mortality rate from this infection.

If you have any severe pain in the abdomen, combined with the symptoms just described, call the doctor at once. *Do not take a laxative.* This can cause an inflamed appendix to burst. A diseased appendix must be removed surgically as soon as possible.

CHRONIC DISEASES OF THE DIGESTIVE SYSTEM

GALLBLADDER DISEASE

Gallbladder disese is a common ailment among Americans. The gallbladder can get inflamed, stop working, and become filled with small particles called **gallstones.** If they get into the bile duct, they block it, and bile backs up in the blood. This produces a yellow color in the skin known as **jaundice**. Other symptoms include severe pain in the right lower ribs and in the right shoulder, with nausea, gas, and bloating, especially if fats are eaten.

More than 16 million Americans have gallstones. Gallstones are extremely common in our society, because our diets are high in Calories and cholesterol. X rays of the gallbladder will often show gallstones (see Figure 18-8). If gallstones cause problems, the gallbladder can be removed. Patients can live normal lives without a gallbladder. Bile is then delivered to the small intestine directly from the liver. Recently, drugs to dissolve stones have been developed. In the near future many gallbladder operations may be avoided by using these drugs.

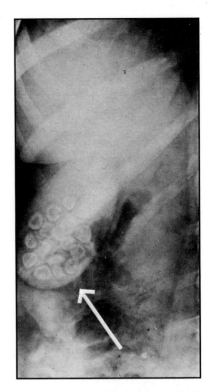

18–8. The arrow in this X ray points to gallstones.

LIVER DISEASE

Liver disease is the eighth leading cause of death. There are many causes of liver ailments, including viruses, drugs, toxins, and hereditary defects. Infectious hepatitis (type A) is caused by a virus that is transmitted through contaminated water and food. Serum hepatitis (type B) is spread by blood transfusions. Symptoms of both types of hepatitis include yellowing of the skin, loss of appetite, nausea, vomiting, and fever. Chapter 23 discusses hepatitis in more detail.

Cirrhosis is a chronic liver disease characterized by destruction of the liver cells and replacement with scar tissue. Liver circulation may also be obstructed. An individual with cirrhosis may feel weak, lack an appetite, and have an enlargement of the liver. Most cirrhosis in the United States is associated with excessive alcohol intake.

STOMACH AND DUODENAL ULCERS

About one in ten people gets an ulcer sometime during his or her life. What causes ulcers? How and why they occur is

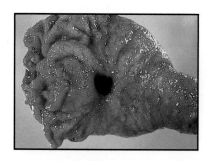

18–9. An open sore, or ulcer, in the stomach lining

not completely understood. It is known that emotional anxiety stimulates the flow of excess hydrochloric acid in the stomach. Alcohol, tobacco, and aspirin also cause an increased flow of stomach acids. The excess acid may actually begin to eat away at the stomach or duodenal lining; or, the stomach lining itself could be weak, in which case ulcers could develop even with normal amounts of hydrochloric acid. Ulcers in the stomach lining are called *peptic ulcers*. Ulcers in the *duodenum* (the first section of the small intestine) are called *duodenal ulcers*. They are much more common than stomach ulcers. Doctors recommend avoiding smoking, caffeinated drinks, alcohol, and aspirin for patients with ulcers. Eating small meals more frequently also helps the condition. Antacid preparations that contain gels absorb acid and carry it out of the stomach. A medication called *Cimetidine* blocks hydrochloric acid production. It has been shown to hasten the healing of duodenal ulcers.

DIVERTICULOSIS

The most common disease of the colon in older adults living in western countries is **diverticulosis** (die-ver-tik-you-**low**-sis). This disease causes the wall of the colon to pouch out and produce many small sacs, or *diverticuli*. These sacs may become inflamed or infected, causing diverticulosis. The sacs can occasionally burst and cause a problem as serious as that caused by a ruptured appendix. Diverticulosis is now thought to be the result of not eating enough fiber. A high-fiber diet is advised to prevent and treat diverticulosis.

ULCERATIVE COLITIS

Chronic bloody diarrhea from many ulcers in the colon is the primary symptom of **ulcerative colitis** (**ul**-sir-ra-tiv ko-**lie**-tis). The cause of this serious condition is unknown. Treatment consists of a bland diet, certain medications, a change in life-style, if possible, and in extreme cases, removal of part or all of the colon.

CANCER OF THE STOMACH

Stomach cancer begins as an open sore. As it spreads, it involves more and more of the stomach wall. The lining, muscle layers, and blood vessels are gradually invaded or destroyed. Persistent indigestion and changes in bowel habits can be symptoms of early stomach cancer. Unfortunately, people often waste valuable time trying various self-prescribed treatments. Cancer cells then spread through the circulatory system to other parts of the body. If the cancer is discovered before this happens, part or most of the stomach can be removed. It is amazing how well the small intestine can take over most of the stomach's functions when this operation is done.

CANCER OF THE COLON

Cancer of the colon is the second most common cancer. Rectal bleeding, changes in bowel habits that persist, and abdominal pain may be early warning signs. People with a history of ulcerative colitis or polyps (small growths in the large intestine) are at a higher risk for colon cancer. This cancer occurs most often after age 40. Therefore, those over this age should receive a yearly rectal examination. If detected early, it is easier to cure than any other internal cancer. Colon cancer has been related to diet. High-fiber, low-fat diets in some countries have been linked to low rates of colon cancer.

THE EXCRETORY SYSTEM

After nutrients leave the digestive system, they go first to the liver. Some of the nutrients are stored there. The rest are transported to all the cells in the body. Once the nutrients reach the cells, some are used as the raw materials for building and repairing cells and carrying on other cell functions. The rest are oxidized, or burned, to produce energy to carry on the cells' functions. Every cellular function requires energy. For example, each time a muscle cell contracts, energy is used. Each time an enzyme is made, energy is used. Oxygen from the lungs is needed for this process. When fats and sugars are oxidized, carbon dioxide and water are released as waste products. When proteins are oxidized, urea and uric acid are also released as waste products. These waste products pass through the cells' membranes into the bloodstream. Once in the bloodstream, the waste products are carried to the kidneys. The **kidneys** filter these waste products out of the blood, and produce urine. Urine excreted by the kidneys travels down two tubes called the **ureters** (**yur**-ee-terz), to the bladder. Here the urine is stored until it leaves the body through a tube called the **urethra** (**yur**-ee-thra).

STRUCTURE AND FUNCTION OF THE KIDNEYS

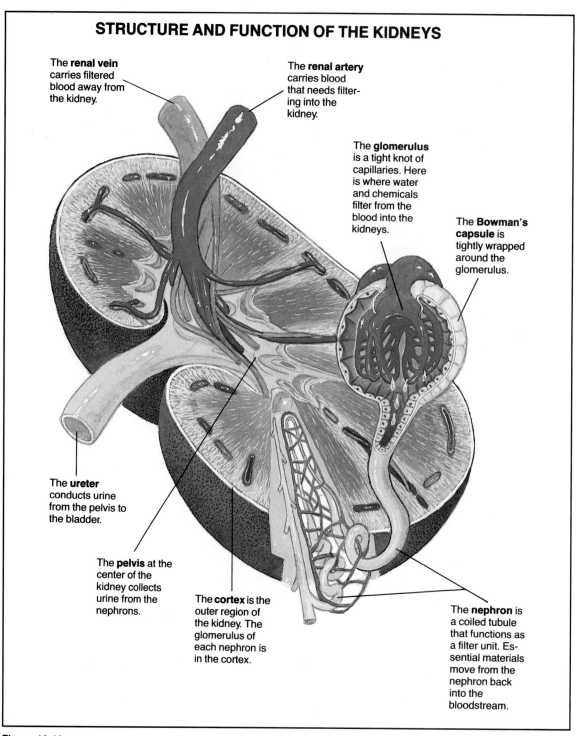

The **renal vein** carries filtered blood away from the kidney.

The **renal artery** carries blood that needs filtering into the kidney.

The **glomerulus** is a tight knot of capillaries. Here is where water and chemicals filter from the blood into the kidneys.

The **Bowman's capsule** is tightly wrapped around the glomerulus.

The **ureter** conducts urine from the pelvis to the bladder.

The **pelvis** at the center of the kidney collects urine from the nephrons.

The **cortex** is the outer region of the kidney. The glomerulus of each nephron is in the cortex.

The **nephron** is a coiled tubule that functions as a filter unit. Essential materials move from the nephron back into the bloodstream.

Figure 18-10

THE KIDNEYS

The kidneys are two bean-shaped organs located just above the small of the back. They serve to cleanse the blood and maintain the body's balance of salt and water. Blood enters the kidneys through the renal arteries and leaves through the renal veins. While circulating through the kidneys, blood passes through a remarkable filtering system. There the various substances transported in the blood are sorted. The blood retains the nutrients and some of the salts and water it is carrying. It is also cleansed of waste materials.

Look at the diagram of a kidney in Figure 18-10. The renal artery and vein pass into and out of the interior of each kidney on the concave side. Layers of fat protect each kidney. The kidney is composed of an outer layer, called the **cortex,** and an inner layer, the **medulla** (meh-**dull**-ah). The core of the kidney is called the **pelvis.**

The kidney contains about 1,250,000 tiny filters called **nephrons.** Nephrons remove wastes from the blood. Each nephron enlarges, twists, and ends up in a cup-shaped structure called a *Bowman's capsule*. Blood flows toward the capsule in a small arteriole, one of the millions of branches off the renal artery. Within the pocket formed by the capsule, the arteriole branches into a twisted network of tiny blood vessels, the **glomerulus** (glo-**mer**-you-lus).

In a day the blood pours large amounts of water, waste, and food materials into the kidney capsules. About 1.4 liters (3 pt) of urine per day pass from the body. The amount varies, however, depending on the amount of fluids a person drinks and the amount lost in the form of perspiration.

The kidneys have a large reserve capacity. During normal body activity only a portion of the glomeruli, capsules, and tubules function in the filtering of blood. If one kidney is badly damaged or removed, the other can take over its job.

NORMAL KIDNEY FUNCTION

A large amount of the water your body needs comes from the foods you eat and the liquids you drink. Water is lost through the skin as perspiration, from the lungs in exhaling, from the kidneys as urine, and from the large intestine in feces. Therefore, adequate fluid intake, at least five or six glasses a day, EVERY DAY, is necessary.

Did you ever notice that cold weather and nervous tension promote urine flow? The amount of urine flow also varies with how much fluid you drink. Some substances, called

RESULTS OF URINALYSIS

Finding	Possible Meaning
blood, pus, and bacteria in urine; urine alkaline	urinary tract infection
sugar (glucose)	diabetes mellitus
urine dilute	excessive fluid intake; use of diuretics; diabetes insipidus; kidney disease
casts (protein plugs formed in tubules)	always indicates kidney disease
crystals	amino acid crystals associated with liver disease; uric acid crystals associated with gout
protein	severe kidney disease; infection of urinary system

Table 18–2

diuretics, stimulate urine flow. Caffeine and alcohol are examples of diuretics. The color of the urine varies with the diet and with the amount of bile released from the liver.

The appearance of the urine is not usually an indication of the health of the body or of the kidneys. However, an analysis of the urine does reveal important facts about your general health, as well as the condition of your kidneys and bladder. *Urinalysis* should be a part of a routine medical examination. Table 18-2 summarizes some of the results of urinalysis and their possible meanings.

EXCRETORY SYSTEM DISORDERS

Interference with kidney function causes serious complications throughout the body. If the blood is not relieved of its waste products by the kidneys, the waste piles up, preventing removal of additional wastes from the cells. This condition is called uremic poisoning, or **uremia** (you-**ree**-me-ah).

The body's reaction to uremia is severe. There can be high fever and chills. Accumulation of wastes in the tissues causes extreme fatigue. Brain cells are slowed in their activity. Coma and death may follow unless the uremia is treated.

KIDNEY AND BLADDER INFECTIONS. Infection can reach the kidneys from the bloodstream, or bacteria can ascend the ureters from the urinary bladder. The usual site of infection, called *pyelitis*, is in the kidney pelvis. Symptoms are a sudden onset of chills and high fever, fatigue, and pain in the back above the kidneys. Sometimes the kidneys can be infected without producing any of these symptoms. Anyone who has a history of kidney infection should be checked periodically.

The urinary bladder can be infected by bacteria entering from the urethra. This condition is known as *cystitis*. It is usually accompanied by frequent and painful elimination of small amounts of urine containing pus, pain over the lower abdomen, fever, and chills. Bladder infections are more common among women than among men. This is due to a shorter urethra, which provides less protection for the bladder against bacteria.

Kidney and urinary bladder infections should be diagnosed and treated promptly by a physician. Neglect can cause permanent damage to one or both kidneys. Treatment, which includes antibiotics, is usually successful, especially if started early. Drinking lots of liquids each day, voiding frequently, and keeping the genitals clean can help to prevent both kidney and bladder infections.

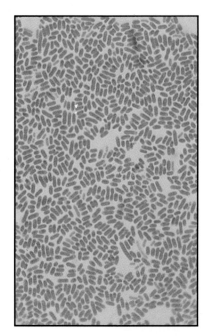

18–11. Cystitis, or bladder infection, is caused by these bacteria.

NEPHRITIS. **Acute nephritis** is an inflammation of the kidney cortex and medulla, usually caused by an infection elsewhere in the body. Glomeruli swell, and filtration of the blood is reduced. This in turn decreases the amount of urine produced. Fluid collects in the body tissues, causing swelling in the face, around the eyes, and in the ankles. Headaches, dizziness, and coma are other symptoms.

Blood and albumin in the urine are important signs in diagnosing the disease. However, since there is usually no permanent damage nor destruction in the glomeruli and tubules, the victims usually recover. Antibiotics are valuable in controlling bacterial infections.

Recovery from **chronic nephritis** is not as common. With this condition there is less inflammation than in acute nephritis, but much greater destruction of the glomeruli and tubules. Gradual accumulation of poisonous waste products causes poisoning and eventual death of the body tissues. Carefully regulated diet and adequate rest are essential in delaying kidney destruction from chronic nephritis.

KIDNEY STONES. For some unknown reason, various minerals, especially calcium compounds and nitrogen-containing waste products, sometimes form **kidney stones** in the kidney pelvis. The stones can be small and numerous, like gravel. In other cases, they can be large and branching.

Kidney stones are about three times as common in men as in women, and they most often develop in people between the ages of 30 and 50.

Small stones can pass through the ureter to the bladder. This usually causes extreme pain across the back, down the ureter, and into the thigh. Such pain is often severe enough to cause nausea, vomiting, sweating, faintness, and shock. Complete obstruction of the ureter by a large stone causes urine to back up into the kidney. Unless the stone is removed or dissolved, it can lead to complete destruction of the kidney.

PROBLEMS OF THE PROSTATE GLAND. The prostate gland, which adds fluid to semen, surrounds the urethra. **Prostatitis** is an inflammation of the prostate, which requires antibiotic treatment. In older males, enlargement or, less frequently, cancer of the prostate can cause obstruction to the flow of urine. If not treated, the urine backs up to the kidneys and can destroy their function. The prostate can be treated surgically to help restore urine flow.

KIDNEY FAILURE

Kidney failure due to infections, burns, injury or other factors requires prompt treatment. Once kidneys stop purifying blood, waste products will build up in the body. This can cause coma and death within a week unless treated. Kidney failure is treated by a process called *dialysis*. Blood from a patient's artery goes through a system of tubing that is made of a membrane similar to cellophane. The tubing is immersed in a bath of fluid, similar to blood but without blood proteins. Waste products in the patient's blood pass through the membrane of the tubing into the bath of fluid. The cleansed blood then flows back into the patient's body through a tube inserted into a vein. Dialysis can also be used to rid the bloodstream of certain drugs or poisons. Dialysis was formerly done only in hospitals three to four times per week, but now compact equipment makes home dialysis possible. A newer technique provides portable, continuous cleansing of the blood. A plastic bag worn around the abdomen delivers a filtering solution into the abdominal cavity. Wastes collect in this solution and four to six hours later, the fluid is drained back into the bag. Then a fresh solution is put in the bag. Should both kidneys fail completely through disease or injury, a person must continue on dialysis unless a kidney is transplanted from another person.

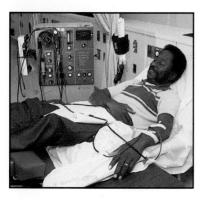

18–12. Dialysis acts as a normally functioning kidney by filtering wastes from the blood.

SUMMARY: The digestive system is divided into specialized organs. Each organ is adapted to perform a specific function in the digestive process. Food is broken down, mechanically and chemically, into a form that can be used by the body's cells. Cells need food to carry on their functions and to repair and reproduce themselves. Various waste products result from digestion and metabolism. These products are removed through the kidneys, lungs, skin, liver, and large intestine. A healthy diet and good eating habits will help maintain the normal functioning of the digestive and excretory systems.

CHAPTER REVIEW

words at work

Find the word in the left column that fits one of the definitions in the right column. DO NOT WRITE IN THIS BOOK.

a. alimentary canal
b. appendix
c. colon
d. cystitis
e. enzymes
f. hemorrhoid
g. jaundice
h. lacteals
i. peristalsis
j. villi

1. Lymph vessels that absorb food from the digestive organs
2. An enlarged vein in the rectum
3. Muscular action of the walls of digestive organs
4. A urinary bladder infection
5. A wormlike projection of the cecum
6. Food moves through it
7. Chemical secretions that act on food during digestion
8. Yellow coloration of the skin
9. Tiny projections from the inner wall of the small intestine
10. The large intestine

review questions

1. Why is digestion necessary?
2. Explain the function of enzymes in the process of digestion.
3. List the principal organs involved in the process of digestion.
4. Describe the stomach, and tell what it does to digest food.
5. Describe the small intestine. What part does it play in the process of digestion?
6. Outline the functions of the liver.
7. What happens if your pancreas fails to do its part in the digestive process?
8. What is the purpose of the absorption process?
9. Describe how the large intestine functions as an organ of elimination.
10. What causes indigestion?
11. Discuss the causes and symptoms of gallbladder disease.
12. List several causes of stomach ulcers.
13. Why is early detection of cancer of the stomach important?
14. Why should you never eat food from a can that is swollen or bulging?
15. Describe the usual symptoms of appendicitis.

16. Why are older people more likely to have chronic constipation than younger people?
17. Describe diverticulosis.
18. What are hemorrhoids?
19. Distinguish between ordinary diarrhea and ulcerative colitis.
20. Why is the so-called "laxative habit" dangerous to health?
21. List the parts of a kidney.
22. How does the kidney function as a filter?
23. Why is a urinalysis an important part of a good physical examination?
24. What are the causes and symptoms of uremia?
25. Describe the symptoms and discuss the treatment for cystitis.
26. Contrast acute and chronic nephritis.
27. Describe kidney stones. List some symptoms and possible treatment.
28. Discuss the treatment for kidney failure by the process called dialysis.

discussion questions

1. From what you have learned about digestion, discuss the organs or glands of the digestive system that could be removed, if necessary, and which are essential to life.
2. Discuss the effect of emotions and stress on the digestive system.
3. Outline a health program that would benefit the digestive system.
4. Discuss the effects of alcoholic beverages on the digestive system.

investigating

PURPOSE:
To demonstrate the digestion of starch by saliva.

MATERIALS NEEDED:
Soda crackers; 4 clean test tubes or other glass containers; Benedict's solution; a pan of water; a hot plate or Bunsen burner.

PROCEDURE:
A.   Label one test tube "chewed" and another tube "unchewed." Chew but do not swallow a piece of cracker. Place the chewed cracker in the correct test tube. Place a piece of cracker that has not been chewed into the other test tube. Add a few drops of Benedict's solution to each test tube.
B.   Place both test tubes in a pan of water and heat until there is a color change. A change in color to green, yellow, or red indicates the presence of sugar.
    1.   Did the solution with the unchewed cracker change color? Did the solution with the chewed cracker change color?
    2.   What did the saliva do to the cracker?

CHAPTER 19

The Respiratory System

OBJECTIVES

- **STATE** the structure and function of the organs of the respiratory system
- **DESCRIBE** the mechanics of breathing and conditions that affect breathing
- **IDENTIFY** some common respiratory ailments and their prevention and cure
- **DESCRIBE** some chronic respiratory diseases and their prevention and treatment

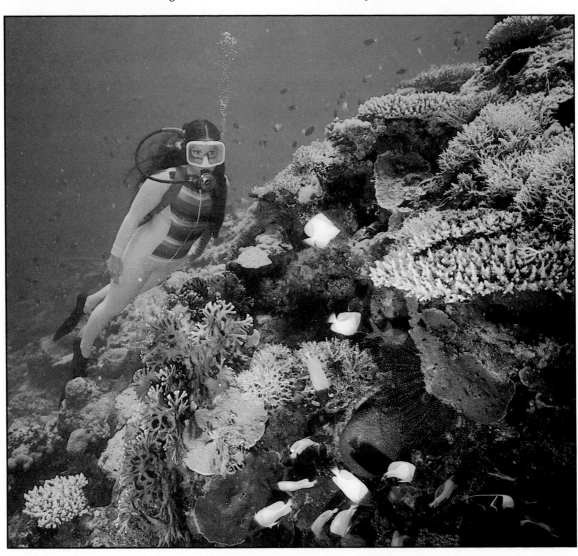

Your lungs weigh only a little over two pounds. Healthy lungs are bright pink and feel spongy to the touch. They contain thousands of tiny balloon-like structures, called alveoli, *that are filled with air. If you were to spread all of the alveoli in your lungs out flat, they would cover an entire tennis court! The membranes of these tiny structures are thinner than tissue paper. Can you guess the function of the alveoli? In the process of respiration, oxygen passes into them and carbon dioxide passes out of them as you breathe in and out.*

STRUCTURE AND FUNCTION

Each cell in your body requires energy to carry on its functions. Each time a muscle cell contracts or a cell divides, energy is used. The energy needed for these functions comes from the food you eat. But food must be burned in order to release the energy in it. This process, called **cellular respiration,** requires oxygen. Oxygen is used to burn food, and carbon dioxide is produced as a waste product.

How do your cells get a constant supply of oxygen and get rid of carbon dioxide? In your lungs, oxygen diffuses from the air into your blood, while carbon dioxide diffuses from your blood into the air. This process is called **external respiration.** Once oxygen is in your blood, it is carried to your cells. When oxygen diffuses from your blood into your cells and carbon dioxide diffuses from your cells into the blood, the process is called **internal respiration.**

THE INTAKE OF AIR

Without using conscious control, you normally inhale and exhale sixteen to twenty-four times per minute. During normal breathing, air enters the respiratory passages through the **nostrils.** The nostrils lead into the **nasal cavity.** A thin sheet of cartilage and soft bone, the *nasal septum*, divides the nasal cavity into a right and a left side. You can feel the cartilage portion of your septum between the nostrils. Nostril hairs and moist mucous membranes serve as an air filter to screen out dirt and foreign substances. Air is also warmed and moistened as it passes through the nostrils.

Air passes from the back of the nasal cavities to the throat. The throat cavity, or **pharynx (far**-inks), has an upper and

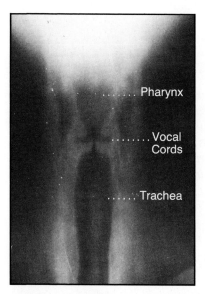

19–1. X ray of the pharynx, vocal cords, and trachea

lower portion. The upper cavity, the **nasopharynx,** lies in back of the nose and above the roof of the mouth. The lower cavity leads to the windpipe. Air reaches the pharynx either through the nasal passages or through the mouth. Notice how you open your mouth and pant when you are out of breath. When you do this, you are using both air intakes. Even though breathing through the mouth is more direct, breathing through the nose is more beneficial. When air passes through the nose, it is warmed, moistened, and filtered before it reaches the lungs.

The *sinuses* are air-filled cavities in certain facial and cranial bones. Short ducts connect the sinuses to the nasal cavity. The exact function of the sinuses is not known. They may aid in warming and moistening air during breathing. They may also add resonance to the voice by acting as sounding chambers. Another theory is that they lighten the weight of the skull. Unfortunately, they are often the cause of many complaints. The narrow passages that connect the sinuses to the nasal cavity often become obstructed. This leads to *sinusitis* (infection of the sinuses).

THE PHARYNX. You might compare the pharynx to a subway station where many tunnels converge. Seven tunnels enter the pharynx. The two nostrils open into the nasopharynx. Two **Eustachian tubes** connect the nasopharynx to the middle ears. The mouth cavity joins the pharynx farther down. The base of the pharynx opens into the esophagus and the windpipe. Food and water go down one opening into the esophagus, and air passes through another opening leading to the windpipe. Traffic becomes complicated during eating. Fortunately, traffic control is automatic. Try to swallow and breathe at the same time. It cannot be done.

TONSILS AND ADENOIDS. The back of the mouth cavity forms an arch leading into the pharynx. **Tonsils** are masses of soft lymph tissue, one mass on either side of the arch just behind the teeth. Healthy tonsils perform a valuable service by trapping and destroying bacteria. Under normal conditions tonsils rid themselves of bacteria they trap. In some cases, however, tonsils may become so infected that tonsillitis, sore throat, and other respiratory infections become frequent. Tonsillitis usually responds to antibiotics. In some cases doctors may recommend a *tonsillectomy* (removal of the tonsils), but this is not done often.

Adenoids are masses of lymph tissue that are on the back wall of the nasopharynx. Like tonsils, they serve to trap bacteria but can also become infected. Enlarged adenoids may block the openings of the Eustachian tube, preventing equalization of pressure in the middle ears. This can lead to deafness. When adenoids block the nasal passages, they force mouth breathing. This causes the mouth to be continually open. Adenoid removal is a simple operation. They are often removed with tonsils if they interfere with breathing or speech.

THE LARYNX: ORGAN OF SOUND. How is sound produced when you talk? The **larynx** contains the **vocal cords.** Air exhaled from the lungs is forced past the vocal cords, which causes them to vibrate. Muscles regulate the distance between the vocal cords and the amount of tension put on them. If you shout, the vocal cords are pulled apart. A lot of air is expelled from the lungs. This causes the cords to vibrate vigorously, which produces a loud sound. When you speak softly the vocal cords are closer together and only a small amount of air passes over them. Differences in pitch result from variations in the tension and length of the vocal cords. To produce a high note, the cords are tight and short. Relaxing the vocal cords produces lower sounds. The quality of the voice is modified by the cavities of the mouth, nose, sinuses, throat, and chest.

The larynx forms a triangular ridge, sometimes called "the Adam's apple," that bulges out at the front of the neck. This ridge is more prominent in males than in females. This is because the vocal cords that lie behind it are longer and thicker in men. The larger the larynx and the longer the vocal cords, the deeper the voice. Women have higher-pitched voices, since their vocal cords are shorter. During the teen years a boy's larynx grows rapidly and his voice deepens.

The larynx is made of nine separate pieces of cartilage. Muscles that attach to it can change its shape. A leaflike plate of flexible cartilage, the **epiglottis** (ep-eh-**glot**-tis), partially covers the opening of the larynx. When you swallow, the base of your tongue rolls back and your larynx comes up against the base. This action presses the epiglottis against the larynx and causes the opening of the larynx to close. As a result, food is prevented from entering the larynx.

THE TRACHEA. The trachea is a tube about 11.5 centimeters (4 1/2 in.) long and 2.5 centimeters (1 in.) in diameter. It extends from the bottom of the larynx through the neck and into the chest cavity. At its lower end it divides into two tubes, called the **bronchi,** which lead into the lungs.

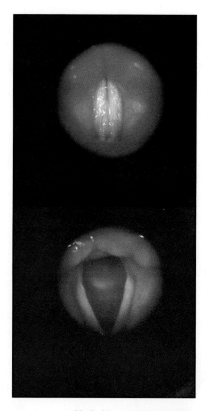

19–2. Vocal cords during respiration (bottom) and speaking (top). Notice how tightly they are held to produce a sound.

THE RESPIRATORY SYSTEM

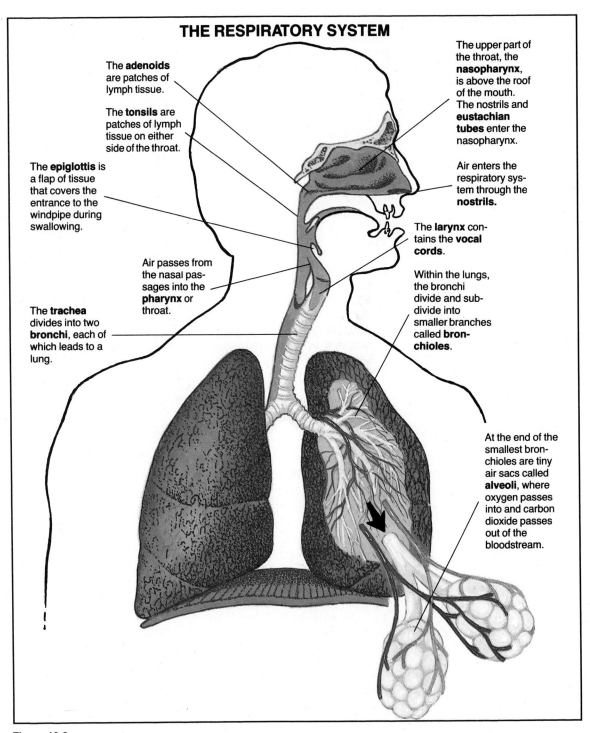

The **adenoids** are patches of lymph tissue.

The **tonsils** are patches of lymph tissue on either side of the throat.

The **epiglottis** is a flap of tissue that covers the entrance to the windpipe during swallowing.

Air passes from the nasal passages into the **pharynx** or throat.

The **trachea** divides into two **bronchi**, each of which leads to a lung.

The upper part of the throat, the **nasopharynx**, is above the roof of the mouth. The nostrils and **eustachian tubes** enter the nasopharynx.

Air enters the respiratory system through the **nostrils.**

The **larynx** contains the **vocal cords**.

Within the lungs, the bronchi divide and subdivide into smaller branches called **bronchioles**.

At the end of the smallest bronchioles are tiny air sacs called **alveoli**, where oxygen passes into and carbon dioxide passes out of the bloodstream.

Figure 19-3

DESIGN FOR GAS EXCHANGE

Each bronchus divides and then subdivides within a lung, forming a network of bronchial tubes resembling branches of a tree. The tiny divisions of the bronchial tubes are called **bronchioles** (**bron-**kee-ohls).

As the bronchioles branch and become smaller, their walls become thinner. Each bronchiole ends in a tiny chamber from which air sacs called **alveoli** (al-**vee-**oh-lie) extend in a cluster. A vast network of blood capillaries penetrates the lungs. Tiny capillaries surround each of the alveoli. Air in an alveolus is separated from the blood by two thin membranes: the wall of the alveolus and the wall of a capillary. These thin walls permit easy exchange of gases.

STRUCTURE OF THE LUNGS. The lungs are spongelike, cone-shaped organs. Deep fissures divide the right lung into three lobes. The left lung has two lobes. The heart lies in a deep cavity between the lungs.

The lungs are protected by two membranes, called **pleural membranes** (**plur-**al). One lies over the lungs; the other lines the chest cavity. The two membranes are separated only by a thin layer of pleural fluid. During breathing, the fluid prevents the two membranes from rubbing against each other. Inflammation of the pleura causes rubbing and pain. This condition is known as *pleurisy*.

THE MECHANICS OF BREATHING. The lungs themselves do not draw air in or push air out. This is the job of the **diaphragm** and the chest cavity. The diaphragm separates the chest and abdominal cavities. As you breathe in and out, the size of your chest cavity changes. This causes the air pressure inside your lungs to increase and decrease. In response to changing air pressure, air is drawn in and pushed out of your lungs. When you inhale, your rib muscles contract, pulling the ribs upward and outward. At the same time, the diaphragm contracts so that it is straightened and lowered. This enlarges the chest cavity, reducing air pressure in the lungs. Air rushes into the lungs to equalize the internal pressure with the outside atmosphere. When you exhale, the process is reversed. The ribs spring back by moving downward and inward, and the diaphragm rises. The chest cavity decreases in size, raising air pressure in the lungs. Thus, air is forced out of the lungs (see Figure 19-4).

Although you can regulate your breathing by conscious control, breathing is usually unconscious and automatic.

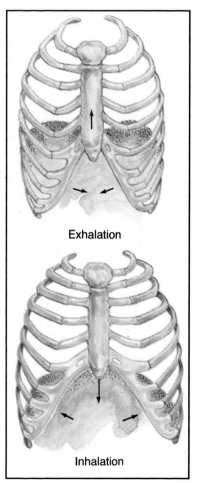

19–4. This is how the diaphragm and chest function during breathing.

Exhalation

Inhalation

The control center for respiration is in the medulla of the brain. This respiratory center is very sensitive to the concentration of carbon dioxide in the blood. When there is excess carbon dioxide in the blood, the respiratory muscles are stimulated to greater activity.

The amount of oxygen taken in and the amount of carbon dioxide released vary tremendously with the amount of energy the body requires. At rest, only about a half pint (250 cubic centimeters) of oxygen is absorbed per minute. A distance runner may use up more than a gallon (4,000 cubic centimeters) of oxygen each minute.

EXCHANGE OF GASES IN THE LUNGS. Oxygen composes nearly 21 percent of the air entering the lungs. The air you exhale is only about 16 percent oxygen. In other words, you utilize about one-fourth of the oxygen taken into the lungs. Air entering the lungs contains about .04 percent carbon dioxide. The air you exhale contains nearly 4.5 percent carbon dioxide. The increase represents carbon dioxide discharged from the blood into the lungs.

Regardless of how cold or how dry the atmosphere is, the air you exhale is saturated with moisture and is close to body temperature. The moisture exhaled in your breath totals about .47 liter (1 pt) of water daily.

CONDITIONS THAT AFFECT BREATHING

LOW PRESSURE. At 3,000 to 3,600 meters (10,000 to 12,000 ft) in altitude, the air is so thin that breathing becomes difficult. Lack of oxygen and low air pressure cause dizziness, light-headedness, increase in breathing rate, and fatigue. This is sometimes called *mountain sickness*. Above 6,000 meters (20,000 ft), air barely supports human life.

The low pressure of the atmosphere at high altitudes adds to the problem of low oxygen supply. When air pressure is low, it is more difficult for air to enter the lungs. Newcomers to a high-altitude region find breathing difficult. Yet those who live at such an altitude do not experience this difficulty. Their bodies have adjusted by producing extra red blood cells for delivering oxygen to the tissues. Athletes from an area near sea level are at a disadvantage at high altitudes. If athletic events are held at high altitudes, athletes sometimes move to these areas a week or more before competing. This gives their bodies a chance to produce extra red blood cells.

HIGH PRESSURE. The effect of high air pressure on breathing is the opposite of that of low pressure. Air rushes into the lungs with greater ease, and extra oxygen is forced into the bloodstream. In addition, nitrogen is absorbed by the blood. This does not cause a problem as long as a person stays in the high-pressure area. But if he or she returns to normal atmospheric pressure too rapidly, the blood releases its extra oxygen and nitrogen too quickly. Body cells can absorb the extra oxygen in the blood, but not the nitrogen. The nitrogen cannot pass from the blood to the lungs fast enough. As a result, nitrogen bubbles may form in the blood. The situation is much like what occurs when bubbles of carbon dioxide appear in soda pop when the bottle is opened and the pressure is released. Nitrogen bubbles block small blood vessels, especially in the joints, causing a condition referred to as "the bends." Symptoms include nausea, vomiting, abdominal pain, muscle spasms, dizziness, and nosebleed. In more severe cases, the person suffers from muscle paralysis and unconsciousness. The bends can be fatal in some instances. Deep-sea divers develop the bends if they are brought to the surface too quickly. It is also an occupational hazard among miners who work in tunnels deep in the earth. The bends can be avoided if miners come to the surface slowly or if they are put into special decompression chambers that gradually decrease pressure.

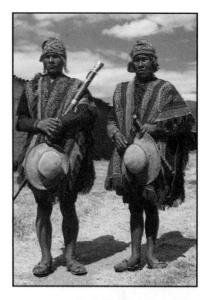

19–5. The Andes Indians have broad chests and large lungs that help them to breathe at high altitudes.

INDOOR POLLUTION. Is the air in your home and school safe to breathe? Many people may not realize that the air they breathe inside may be more polluted than the outside air in most polluted areas. Indoor pollution has been linked to a wide variety of illnesses, including headaches, respiratory problems, colds, sore throats, and chronic coughs.

How does the air get polluted inside? There are many commercial products that can be a source of indoor pollution. Formaldehyde is one of the worst of these. It is found in some types of foam insulation, in particle board, and in synthetic fabrics used for rugs, drapes, and clothing. Repeated exposure to formaldehyde can cause headaches, eye irritation, and respiratory problems.

Nitrogen dioxide and carbon monoxide are other indoor air pollutants that can be released into the air when substances burn. For example, coal- and wood-burning stoves and smoking cigarettes add these pollutants to the air.

Many household chemicals and cosmetics, especially sprays, may cause indoor pollution if used improperly. Always follow the directions when using these products.

Humidifiers can be helpful during the winter months. When indoor air is heated, it becomes very dry. However, it is very important to clean the inside of humidifiers with soap at least weekly. Otherwise, harmful bacteria can grow in them which can cause a wide variety of illnesses.

To minimize indoor air pollution, limit the use of formaldehyde products. Do not seal up a house tightly, and make sure there is good ventilation.

RESPIRATORY PROBLEMS
ASPHYXIATION

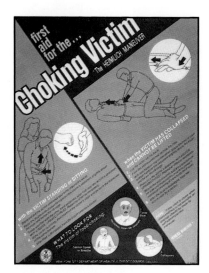

19–6. The international sign for choking

Obstruction of the air passages, interference with breathing movements, lack of sufficient oxygen in the air, or inability of the blood to deliver oxygen are all factors that can result in tissue suffocation, or **asphyxiation** (as-fik-see-**ay**-shun).

A chunk of food or a foreign object can block the passage of air if it wedges into the glottis or lodges in the trachea. This is especially hazardous among small children. This all-too-frequent emergency situation commonly occurs in restaurants. Drinking too much alcohol or swallowing food too quickly may result in food lodging in the trachea. Coughing may dislodge a foreign object and force it back up. When a choking spell fails to dislodge the food particle, death by suffocation occurs. Sometimes people think a victim is having a heart attack, when in fact the victim is suffocating due to a blocked air passageway. There is an international sign that must be posted in restaurants that describes the symptoms of food choking and emergency treatment for it (see Figure 19-6). Dr. Henry Heimlich discovered that sudden upward pressure on the diaphragm will force air out of the lungs, forcing out the obstructing particle. This technique, called the **Heimlich maneuver,** will be discussed fully in Chapter 27, "First Aid."

When asphyxiation occurs for any reason, artificial respiration should be started immediately after the airway is cleared of the obstruction. If the victim of asphyxiation has no pulse, cardiopulmonary resuscitation should be started. These techniques are also covered in Chapter 27.

Sometimes a small object can find its way into a bronchial tube of the lung. A doctor's attention is needed immediately. A doctor uses an instrument called a *bronchoscope* to view the lodged object so it can be removed.

HEALTH ACTION

Find out how to administer the Heimlich maneuver for choking victims. Practice the technique with a partner.

Drowning is the most frequent cause of asphyxiation. It is important to administer artificial respiration for drowning victims until medical help arrives. Abandoned wells and silos can also snuff out life because heavy gases, such as carbon dioxide, settle in them. As a safety measure, be especially careful when entering any closed, poorly ventilated place. Dizziness and light-headedness are the first warning signs of lack of oxygen.

COMMON RESPIRATORY AILMENTS

THE COMMON COLD. Colds are caused by several different viruses; thus, a cold is not any one specific disease. Organisms capable of causing a cold are present in your respiratory passages at all times. When your body's resistance is low or when a new strain of virus is introduced into your body, you may develop a cold. Colds usually last about a week. During the infection, viruses attack the mucous membranes, causing inflammation. The irritated membranes secrete an unusually large quantity of mucus, which is discharged through the nostrils. When the infection has run its course, the membranes shrink and heal. Although there are over 50,000 different products on the market for the common cold, the truth is that there is no cure for the common cold. Some products may relieve symptoms of running nose and sneezing. However, these products may do more harm than good, since they may also thicken mucus secretions in your lungs, leading to bronchitis. The best remedy for a cold is rest, warmth, and lots of fluids.

SINUSITIS. We refer to an infection of the sinuses as **sinusitis.** Since the membranes lining the nasal passages extend into the sinuses, a head cold infection can easily reach the sinuses. The mucous membrane of an infected sinus swells and may close off the drainage tube. This traps mucus, converting the sinus into an incubator for bacteria or viruses. Pressure from infection in the sinuses causes pain in the face and headache, usually on only one side of the head. Often the membrane shrinks, and the sinus drains without treatment. In severe cases a doctor may need to force water or a mild antiseptic solution through the clogged passage to clean out the sinus. A doctor may also prescribe antibiotics. To help prevent sinusitis, make sure you get adequate rest and exercise, and eat well-balanced meals. If you smoke, stop. When you blow your nose, do it gently so that you do not force mucus into the sinuses.

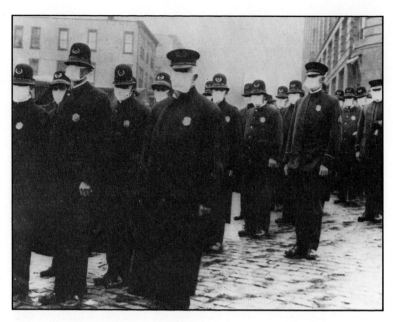

19–7. During an epidemic of influenza in New York City, police officers went to extremes to protect themselves.

INFLUENZA ("flu"). **Influenza** is a contagious viral disease, more commonly called the "flu." It usually begins in the respiratory tract, but also causes fever, headache, general aching, and sometimes nausea and vomiting. Like colds, the flu is much more common in winter. Do you know why? People spend more time indoors in winter. Since they are closer together they can more easily infect one another. Although the flu usually lasts only about a week, it can lower the body's resistance to viral and bacterial pneumonia, especially in older people. An annual vaccination is advised for people 65 years of age and older. The best remedy for flu is bed rest, warmth, and lots of liquids. If a secondary bacterial infection develops, antibiotics may be prescribed.

THROAT INFECTIONS. Among throat infections, strep throat is one of the most severe. Symptoms can include sore throat, swollen glands, fever, and headache. A doctor may take a throat culture to see if a sore throat is strep throat. Since strep throat is caused by a bacterium, it can be treated with antibiotics. Failure to do so could lead to rheumatic fever and damage to the heart and lungs.

Sore throats, often in conjunction with colds, can also be caused by viruses. There is no cure for these viral infections other than time. Antibiotics do no good against viruses. Gargling with half a teaspoon of salt in warm water or drinking warm liquids can help relieve the soreness.

LARYNGITIS. Colds and other kinds of upper respiratory infections may travel to the larynx, causing **laryngitis.** The mucous membrane of the larynx becomes inflamed. Often the swelling extends to the vocal cords and causes hoarseness, or complete loss of voice. Smoking or overuse of the vocal cords may also cause hoarseness.

If a person develops persistent hoarseness for more than two weeks, he or she should be examined by a doctor. Cancer sometimes develops on the vocal cords and other areas of the larynx. If found in time, cancer of this region can be successfully treated by radiation or surgery.

OTHER RESPIRATORY PROBLEMS

ACUTE AND CHRONIC BRONCHITIS. **Bronchitis** is an inflammation of the membrane lining the bronchial tubes. It may be acute or chronic. Acute bronchitis follows virus infections of the respiratory tract, like colds or influenza. The virus infection weakens the body and lowers its resistance to infection. This allows bacteria present in the nose and throat to invade the lower trachea and bronchi. Acute bronchitis usually causes a mild fever for one to three days, followed by a cough that may last several weeks.

Chronic bronchitis produces similar symptoms. However, the cough and spitting up of thick sputum from the lungs becomes chronic, meaning it persists for at least three months a year for two years in a row. The mucous membrane of the bronchi become thickened and produce excess mucus.

Several antibiotic drugs are effective in treating bronchitis in the early stages. However, chronic bronchitis is difficult to treat. Statistics show that most people suffering from chronic bronchitis are heavy smokers. The best preventive measure to take is to avoid smoking. People who suffer from chronic bronchitis should also avoid irritating fumes and dust as much as possible.

PNEUMONIA. We speak of several different lung infections as **pneumonia. Bacterial pneumonia** is caused by one of several types of bacteria within the respiratory passages. Most bacterial pneumonia is caused by *Pneumococcus* bacteria. It can occur as a secondary infection in people who have been weakened by the flu. Bacterial pneumonia centers in the bronchioles and alveoli, filling them with fluids and pus. An entire lobe of a lung or a whole lung may become almost solid. This disease strikes suddenly and can be fatal

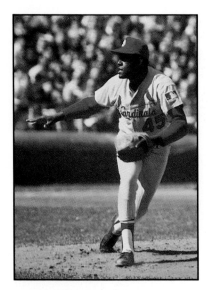

19–8. Many people who have asthma, including Bob Gibson, have become famous athletes.

HEALTH IN HISTORY

Since it was the leading cause of death in the nineteenth century, tuberculosis was known as the white plague. Many nineteenth-century writers used the symptoms of the disease as dramatic material in their novels. In this century, death from tuberculosis has steadily declined. The death rate per 100,000 population has fallen from about 400 in 1870 to 12.6 in 1953 and to 4.3 in 1964, and it has continued to fall, thanks to effective treatment and steadily improving sanitary conditions.

if not treated immediately. It usually starts with a chill, followed by high fever. The patient's breathing is rapid and shallow, and breathing movements are painful. Although bacterial pneumonia usually responds to antibiotics, it is still a leading cause of death in older people. A new vaccine has been developed that immunizes against several types of pneumococci for as long as five years.

Viral pneumonia often follows a severe, neglected cold. About three-quarters of pneumonia cases are caused by viruses. It is usually less serious and tends to involve only patches of the lungs rather than an entire lobe. Symptoms are not as serious as those of other pneumonias, and often go undetected. They include fever, headache, and weakness.

ASTHMA. As in other allergies, **bronchial asthma** may result from sensitivity to substances such as pollens, dusts, feather pillows, certain foods, and dog or cat hair. In some cases the allergic reaction is to products formed in the body during an infection, like a cold, sore throat, or bronchitis. Even emotional upset may bring on an attack of bronchial asthma.

The symptoms of bronchial asthma are difficult breathing and wheezing. Mucous membranes lining the bronchioles swell. The air passages are also obstructed with mucus. Muscle spasms constrict the walls of the bronchioles which further obstructs breathing. Although a person may think he or she is going to suffocate during an attack, bronchial asthma is rarely fatal, and damage to the lungs seldom occurs. Nevertheless, the condition is very distressing to the patient.

If possible, asthmatics should avoid exposure to substances that trigger an attack. A doctor can help to identify these triggering factors. Sometimes allergy desensitization over a period of several months can solve the problem. Lots of liquids, a healthful diet, and adequate rest and exercise can also help.

A doctor can relieve a patient suffering from a severe attack with injections of adrenaline or cortisone. However, this is usually not necessary. To prevent or treat milder attacks, certain medications can be taken by mouth or can be inhaled.

TUBERCULOSIS. Tuberculosis bacteria can attack the alveoli of the lungs, causing a lesion called a *tubercle* (see Figure 19-9). The lung walls off the lesion, cutting off circulation and causing death of the tissues within the wall. The

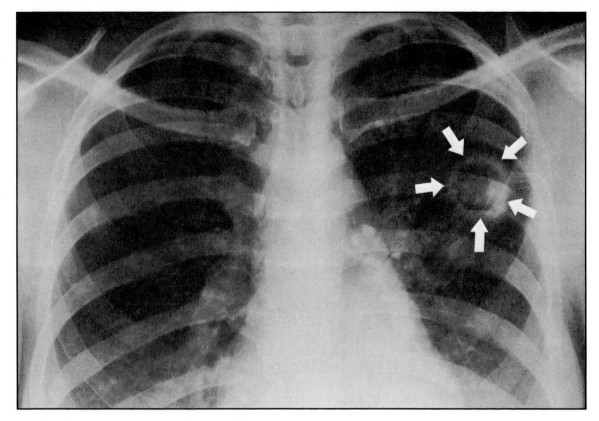

19–9. The arrows point to
a tubercle, caused by a
tuberculosis infection.

blood absorbs poisons and bacteria from the dead tissue, spreading them through the body. This results in fever, night sweats, general weakness, and loss of appetite and weight. Coughing may be severe, and sputum may contain blood. In some cases the walling-off of a lesion arrests the disease. In other cases, no wall forms and the disease is then usually fatal.

The lesions of early tuberculosis show up in X rays, and treatment at this stage is highly effective. Tuberculosis was formerly one of the greatest killers. Today it can easily be detected with a TB skin test or an X ray. Effective antibiotics, like streptomycin, in combination with other drugs can effectively arrest the disease.

EMPHYSEMA. **Chronic pulmonary emphysema** is a progressive disease of the lungs that usually develops over a period of several years. It occurs most frequently in middle-aged or older people. It may also appear in young people with chronic lung infections, asthma, or chest deformities.

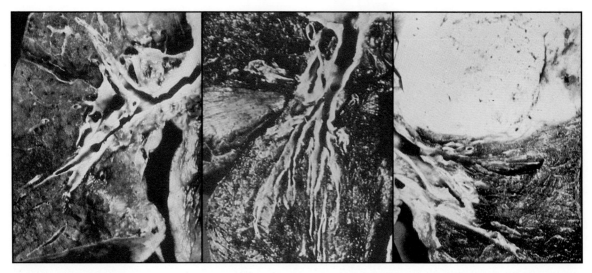

19–10. From left to right,
normal lung tissue,
emphysema (note
cavities), and lung cancer
(note abnormal cell
growth)

Emphysema is more common among heavy smokers than among nonsmokers. It is one of today's fastest growing causes of disability and death.

The characteristic symptom of pulmonary emphysema is shortness of breath. Alveoli become overinflated and are destroyed. This produces cavities that trap dead air. These cavities make *exhalation* difficult, accounting for the shortness of breath. *Elastin*, which normally makes the lung tissue elastic, is destroyed. As the lungs increase in size with the inflation of air cavities, the diaphragm becomes flattened and moves poorly, adding to the problem of exhalation. As the disease progresses, shortness of breath and difficulty in exhalation become more severe. Victims cannot get enough air into their lungs to sustain normal activities. Even eating and dressing are difficult.

Treatment of pulmonary emphysema is limited because the lung damage cannot be corrected. However, inhalation of oxygen several times a day brings a patient relief. The cough and congestion associated with the condition can be relieved with drugs. Anyone who has a chronic cough should stop smoking. The cough may be a warning of emphysema in its early stage.

LUNG CANCER. Lung cancer was considered a rare disease only 50 years ago. Today it is the most common cause of death from cancer in American men and is rapidly increasing among women. Smoking is responsible for three-fourths of all lung cancer cases.

One of the earliest symptoms of lung cancer is a chronic cough, producing mucus tinged with blood. There may also be chest pain, unusual fatigue, and loss of weight, although these symptoms usually appear later. Any of these symptoms should mean a visit to the doctor.

The doctor would begin with X-ray studies, followed by examination of the bronchi and microscopic examination of the sputum for cancer cells.

Depending on the type of cells found, a whole lung would need to be removed, or radiation and chemotherapy would be used. Only 9 percent of lung cancer patients live for five or more years after detection of the disease. If lung cancer is detected in its early stages, (20 percent of lung cancers are discovered that early), chances of recovery are better. The rate of recovery is then 39 percent. However, the best treatment is still prevention: avoid smoking!

WELLNESS WATCH

1. Do you exercise regularly to strengthen your diaphragm muscles and to improve the efficiency of your respiratory system?
2. Do you avoid the use of tobacco and minimize the amount of smoke you breathe in from other people smoking?
3. Do you try to minimize the use of products that cause indoor pollution, such as aerosol sprays and insulation and fabrics made from formaldehyde?
4. Does your home and school have proper ventilation so that indoor air is exchanged for outdoor air at least once per hour?
5. Do you get proper rest and eat a balanced diet to minimize your susceptibility to colds, flu, and other infections of the respiratory system?

SUMMARY: Respiration involves the intake of oxygen and the expulsion of carbon dioxide. As air is breathed in, it passes from the nasal passages through the pharynx, larynx, and bronchi into the lungs. Once the air reaches the alveoli, the oxygen in it passes into the bloodstream. Carbon dioxide passes from the bloodstream into the alveoli. Then it is breathed out of the lungs. Various respiratory diseases are caused by bacteria, viruses, and irritating particles such as tobacco smoke.

CHAPTER REVIEW

words at work

Find the word in the left column that fits one of the definitions in the right column. DO NOT WRITE IN THIS BOOK.

a. alveoli
b. bronchi
c. asphyxiation
d. adenoid
e. epiglottis
f. larynx
g. pharynx
h. pleurisy
i. sinus
j. tubercle

1. Soft tissue in the back arch of the nasopharynx
2. A small lesion in the lungs
3. Inflammation of the membranes covering the lungs and lining the chest
4. Tiny air sacs at the end of a bronchiole
5. The voice box
6. Lack of oxygen causing tissue suffocation
7. The leaflike plate of cartilage that covers the opening to the larynx during swallowing
8. An air-filled cavity in a facial bone
9. The throat cavity
10. Branches at the lower end of the trachea

review questions

1. What is the function of respiration?
2. Why does a distance runner require more oxygen?
3. Identify the seven openings that are connected to the throat or pharynx.
4. What is the function of healthy tonsils?
5. How can enlarged adenoids lead to deafness?
6. Explain how the vocal cords produce sounds of various frequencies and pitch.
7. Describe the trachea or windpipe.
8. Draw a diagram showing the organs of the respiratory system.
9. Explain the mechanics of the breathing process.
10. Compare the contents of the air you inhale with the air you exhale.
11. Why is breathing difficult at an altitude of more than 10,000 feet?
12. What causes "the bends"? How can "the bends" be avoided?
13. Why do you often feel drowsy in a poorly ventilated room?
14. Define asphyxiation. What are some common causes?
15. List and discuss three common respiratory problems.
16. Why are "strep throats" especially dangerous?
17. List some causes of laryngitis.

18. Distinguish between acute and chronic bronchitis.
19. What causes bronchial asthma?
20. Name and describe two types of pneumonia.
21. How has tuberculosis been brought under control?
22. What are the symptoms of pulmonary emphysema?
23. What can you do to reduce the possibility of acquiring lung cancer? Of acquiring emphysema?

investigating

1. Discuss some health habits that affect the respiratory system.
2. Discuss differences in air pressure inside and outside of the lungs when exhaling and inhaling.
3. Describe the path that air takes and how it changes as it is breathed in and out.
4. Discuss how the most common diseases of the lungs have changed over the last 100 years and why.

discussion questions

PURPOSE:
To measure your lung capacity.

MATERIALS NEEDED:
Gallon jar with top; dishpan; water; rubber tubing; liquid measurer.

PROCEDURE:
A.   Fill the dishpan so that the water reaches to a height of about 5 cm. Fill the gallon jar to overflowing with water. Cover the jar with the top, and invert into the dishpan without letting any water out.
B.   Insert one end of the rubber tubing through the mouth of the jar. Be careful not to admit any air into the jar while doing this.
C.   Take a deep breath and, through the tube, blow as much air as you can into the jar. Plug your nose when you do this.
D.   Pull the tube out, again being careful not to admit any more air into the jar. Carefully replace the top on the jar and invert, without letting any water out of the jar. Measure the amount of water it takes to refill the jar. This is your lung capacity.
   1.   What is your lung capacity?
   2.   How does your lung capacity compare to the lung capacities of other students in your class?
   3.   How do you think you could increase your lung capacity?
   4.   What would cause a decrease in lung capacity?

CHAPTER 20

The Cardiovascular System

OBJECTIVES

- DESCRIBE the structure and function of the cardiovascular system
- TRACE the path of blood through the heart
- DESCRIBE how blood pressure is measured

- IDENTIFY the components of blood and STATE the function of each component
- DESCRIBE some disorders of the cardiovascular system

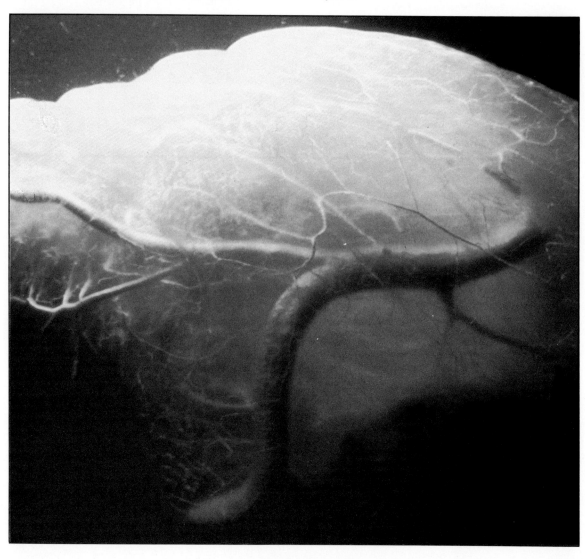

Your heart is a muscular pump about the size of your fist, which weighs well under a pound. No human-made machine has yet successfully duplicated the efficiency of this marvelous organ. Far from being delicate, it is the strongest muscle in your body. The average heart beats about 72 times per minute, 100,000 times each day, and 37 million times each year. In one day, it pumps about 18,175 liters (5,000 gal) of blood, enough to fill a railroad tank car.

Night and day, blood vessels carry nutrients and oxygen to trillions of cells in your body. If all of your vessels were placed end to end, they would reach 160,000 kilometers (96,000 mi).

STRUCTURE AND FUNCTION

Cardio means heart, and *vascular* means blood vessels. The cardiovascular system is made up of the heart and blood vessels. The heart receives oxygen-poor blood, and pumps it to the lungs. Here the blood gets rid of waste gas (carbon dioxide) and picks up oxygen. The bright red oxygenated blood returns to the heart, which pumps it back out to all parts of the body. The **arteries** are the vessels through which oxygen-rich blood is transported to all parts of the body. The **veins** are the vessels that carry blood from various parts of the body back to the heart. Arteries and veins are connected by tiny microscopic **capillaries.** Oxygen and nutrients diffuse from capillaries into body cells, and waste products diffuse from body cells into capillaries. The **lymphatic system** is also considered part of the cardiovascular system.

THE STRUCTURE OF THE HEART

The heart is a muscular organ lying under the breastbone and between the lungs. Most of the heart lies a little to the left of the midline of the chest cavity, with its point extending downward and to the left. Since the beat is strongest near the tip, many people have the mistaken idea that the entire heart is on the left side.

The heart is enclosed in a sac, or chamber, called the **pericardium** (pehr-ih-**kar**-dee-um). Fluid in the pericardium cushions the heart and prevents irritation of the heart wall. The muscle, or **myocardium** (my-oh-**kar**-dee-um), forming the heart wall is different from other muscles of the body. It contracts and relaxes rhythmically.

The four-chambered heart is composed of two sides, right and left. The two halves are entirely separated by an inner wall called the **septum.** Each half is composed of two chambers: a thin-walled upper chamber called the **atrium** (**ay**-tree-um) and a thick, muscular lower chamber called the **ventricle.** A tough membrane, the **endocardium** (en-doe-**kar**-dee-um), lines the four chambers.

The **atrioventricular valves** (ay-tree-oh-ven-**trik**-you-lahr) divide the atria and ventricles. These valves are like flaps. Blood passes freely from the atria to the ventricles through these valves. The valves cannot open from the lower side because of the tendons anchoring them. Therefore,

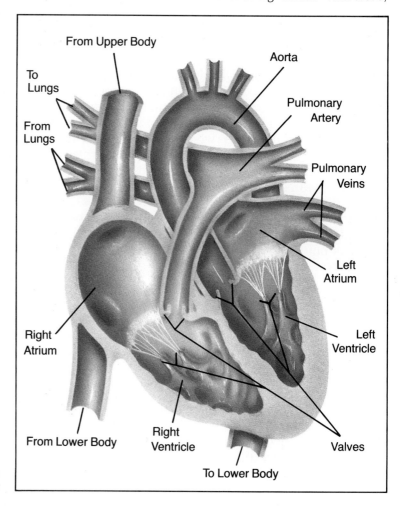

20–1. The structure of the heart

blood cannot flow backward into the atria during contraction of the ventricles. Other valves, called the **semilunar valves,** are located at the openings of the arteries. These cuplike valves open by the force of blood passing from the ventricles into the arteries. They prevent blood from returning to the ventricles.

THE PATH OF BLOOD THROUGH THE HEART

The heart is actually a double pump. The right side of the heart receives blood from the body and pumps it to the lungs. The left side of the heart receives blood from the lungs and pumps it to the body.

Blood from the body enters the right atrium of the heart by way of two large veins, the **superior vena cava (vee-nah kah-**vah) and the **inferior vena cava.** The superior vena cava returns blood from the head and upper parts of the body. The inferior vena cava returns blood from the lower body regions. From the right atrium, blood then passes through the right atrioventricular valve into the right ventricle. The circulation of blood through the lungs, **pulmonary circulation,** begins at the right ventricle. When the right ventricle contracts, blood is forced through a set of semilunar valves and into the **pulmonary artery.** This artery then carries the blood to the lungs. In the lungs oxygen enters the blood, and carbon dioxide and water are removed.

After the blood has passed through the lungs, it is returned to the heart through the right and left **pulmonary veins.** These blood vessels open into the left atrium. From here the blood passes through the left atrioventricular valve and into the left ventricle. Finally, blood passes out through the semilunar valves into the largest artery, called the **aorta,** and then to all parts of the body.

THE HEART IN ACTION

Since heart muscles are controlled by the autonomic nervous system, your heart beats without your conscious control. A series of nerve impulses stimulates the heart to contract rhythmically.

A nerve impulse from a small mass of nerve tissues in the right atrium, called the **sinoatrial node** (sy-no-**ay**-tree-al) starts a heartbeat. This node is the pacemaker of the heart.

The first major advance in our knowledge of the circulation of blood was made by an English physician, William Harvey. In 1628, he demonstrated that the blood is pumped by the heart through the arteries to all parts of the body and is returned by the veins.

20–2. Branches of the systemic circulation

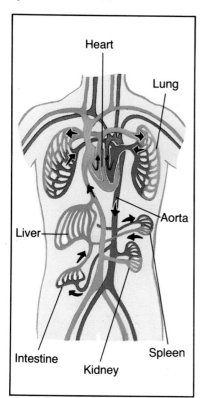

The contraction of the atria stimulates another node at the junction of the atria and the ventricles, the **atrioventricular node.** A branch from this node leads into each ventricle. Fine fibers from each of these branches form a network. A nervous impulse carried along the fibers causes contraction of the ventricles toward the tip of the heart.

The rate of a heartbeat varies. Age, body size, exercise, and surrounding temperature are some factors that affect the rate of a heartbeat. In an average healthy adult the heart beats about 72 times per minute. With strenuous exercise, it can increase to 180 times per minute.

If you listen to your heartbeat through a stethoscope, you would hear a sound often described as "lubb-dupp." The "lubb" is the sound caused by the closing of the atrioventricular valves between the atria and ventricles. The "dupp," which follows, is the sound of the closing of the semilunar valves at the base of the arteries. Some hearts have additional swishing or gurgling sounds, which are caused by blood flowing through the heart. These sounds are called *murmurs*. Usually a murmur is harmless, but it may indicate a serious heart condition. If you have a heart murmur, a heart specialist should examine you.

THE CIRCULATION OF BLOOD THROUGH THE BODY

The circulation of blood through the body tissues is called the **systemic circulation.** The aorta branches into the neck, the shoulders, and the arms. The aorta also forms an arch toward the left and runs downward along the spine. Then it forms a *Y* in the pelvic region, with a branch going into each leg. Veins of the systemic circulation system lead to the superior vena cava and inferior vena cava, which empty into the atrium.

There are several branches of the systemic circulation. The first branch is the **coronary circulation** (see photo on page 420 of coronary arteries). The blood passing through the chambers of the heart cannot nourish the heart itself. Just above the heart, the aorta sends a right and left branch down into the heart muscle. These branches encircle the heart and send smaller branches that lead to all parts of the heart muscle.

The **renal circulation** is the branch of the systemic circulation that carries blood from the aorta to each kidney. One artery goes to each kidney. Capillaries penetrate the kidney tissue. Blood nourishes the kidneys and removes water, salts, and nitrogenous cell wastes. In fact, blood in the renal veins is the purest blood in your body. Renal veins return blood from the kidneys to the inferior vena cava.

Portal circulation is the branch of the systemic circulation system that includes veins from the spleen, pancreas, stomach, small intestine, and colon. These *hepatic portal veins* transport digested food and water to the liver. The hepatic veins flow from the liver to the inferior vena cava. Blood in these veins is richly supplied with nutrients. This circulation supplies blood to all the body tissues.

THE STRUCTURE OF THE BLOOD VESSELS

Arteries have thick walls made of three layers. A membrane lines the inside of an artery. Its slick surface reduces friction as blood flows through an artery. A thick layer of muscle surrounds the membrane (see Figure 20-3). The walls of arteries are elastic so that each surge of blood from the heart causes their walls to bulge. Between beats the walls spring back. The third layer is connective tissue.

Large arteries branch throughout the body into smaller vessels. The finest branches of arteries, the **arterioles** (ar-**tee**-ree-ohls), are microscopic in size. They lead directly into the capillaries.

Capillaries have very thin walls. Nutrients and oxygen can diffuse from the capillaries into the cells. Also, waste products diffuse into the capillaries from the cells.

Capillaries lead into tiny branches of veins called **venules** (**ven**-yoolz). The venules empty into veins, which in turn empty into larger veins. Veins become larger in diameter as they approach the heart. The largest veins, the inferior vena cava and the superior vena cava, enter directly into the right atrium of the heart. Veins lack the thick, muscular walls of arteries. Although their walls are thinner, their cavities are much larger. Veins have valves that keep blood flowing in an upward direction. These valves open in one direction only. Blood flowing toward the heart can pass through these valves. But the valves close to keep blood from flowing backward.

LYMPH AND LYMPHATICS

As blood flows through the capillaries, some of its clear fluid oozes out through the capillary walls and enters the

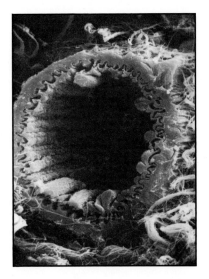

20–3. Cross-section of an artery. Note the thick layer of muscle and elastic fibers.

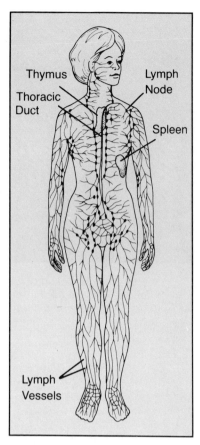

20–4. The lymphatic system

spaces between body cells. This fluid, which bathes all the cells in the body, is called **lymph.** The lymph is then absorbed by lymphatic capillaries. These are similar to regular capillaries, but are more permeable to allow the passage of larger particles. Lymphatic capillaries run together to form larger ducts that intertwine around arteries and veins. These larger lymph ducts are similar to veins. They have valves that prevent the backward flow of lymph. Along the lymphatic ducts are **lymph nodes** which filter out infections and toxic materials and destroy them. All lymph must pass through these ducts before it reenters the bloodstream. Thus, the lymphatic system is one way the body defends itself against disease. This function will be discussed further in Chapter 23. The lymphatics lead to the thoracic duct in the neck, the chief lymphatic vessel in the body. From here the lymph reenters the bloodstream through the **subclavian vein** (sub-**klay**-vee-an **vane**) and returns to the heart.

BLOOD PRESSURE

Blood leaves the heart's ventricles under a large amount of pressure. With each contraction of the ventricles, blood surges through the arteries with sufficient force to cause a bulging of their elastic walls. Arterial blood pressure is greatest at this point and is known as the **systolic pressure** (sis-**tol**-ik). The artery wall maintains part of this pressure while the heart is at rest. This is the time of lowest pressure in the arteries, or the **diastolic pressure** (die-a-**stahl**-lik). When you take a pulse, you are feeling the bulge in an artery wall caused by systolic pressure. The alternation of contraction and relaxation occurs at an average rate of about 70 times per minute.

MEASUREMENT OF BLOOD PRESSURE

An instrument called a *sphygmomanometer* is used for measuring blood pressure. This is a simple device consisting of an air bag, a small pump, and a pressure gauge attached to the bag. The bag is wrapped around your arm just above the elbow, and a stethoscope is placed against the bend of your elbow. The bag is inflated until blood flow through the artery is cut off. While releasing air from the bag, the return of a pulse in the artery can be heard through the stethoscope. At this point the gauge is read, and the *systolic blood pressure* is recorded. When the ventricles are contracted, the artery is exerting more pressure than the air bag, so blood can pass

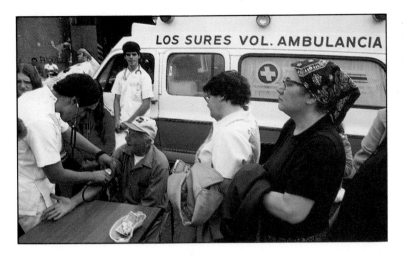

20–5. It is important to have your blood pressure checked at least once every year.

20–6. Capillaries seen through a microscope. Because they are so small, blood must pass through them in single file.

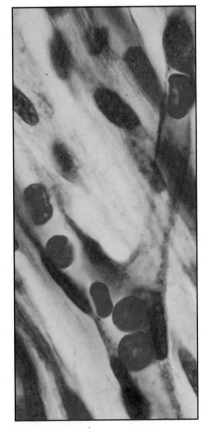

through. Air is released from the bag until there is a sudden change in tone or until the sound disappears completely. The reading of the gauge at this point is the *diastolic blood pressure*. At this point the artery is exerting more pressure, even when the heart is at rest, than the bag is exerting. The two blood pressures are recorded as a fraction, for example, 120 (systolic) over 80 (diastolic).

Blood pressure varies from one person to the next, and in the same person at different times. It is lowest during sleep, and is influenced by digestion, emotions, exercise, and drugs. Blood pressure is an important measure of the health of the cardiovascular system. Blood pressure may be too high or too low if the energy of the heart, the volume of blood, or the elasticity or muscle tone of the vessel walls is abnormal. Anything that has an effect on these factors also affects blood pressure. For example, the blocking of the arteries can cause high blood pressure. This is a dangerous and all too common disease in this country, called *atherosclerosis*, to be discussed further in Chapter 22.

HOW BLOOD MOVES IN THE CAPILLARIES AND VEINS. Arteries lead into millions of tiny capillaries. As blood moves into capillaries, blood pressure drops. If it were not for the sudden drop in pressure, blood would burst the thin walls of the capillaries and spill into the tissue spaces.

By the time blood reaches the veins from the capillary network, it has lost all but one-twentieth of its pressure. The pressure is reduced even more when veins increase in diameter. Therefore, blood pressure alone would not return blood to the heart. How can your blood flow from your fingers and toes upward to your heart, against the flow of gravity? One reason is the movement of muscles in your arms and legs, which squeeze the veins and push the blood toward your heart. The valves in veins also keep blood flowing in one direction only, as explained earlier.

BLOOD

The bloodstream functions as the lifeline of all body cells. Blood is the vital link between your body's cells and the outside world. Blood delivers nutrients, oxygen, hormones, and other substances to the living cells. Blood also receives carbon dioxide and other cellular wastes and transports them to the excretory system and lungs for disposal. Blood picks up heat in tissues and distributes it throughout the body. It also rids the body of excess heat in the body. When the body overheats, more blood goes to the surface of the skin, and heat radiates to the outside of the body. Blood also has special cells and chemicals that help to guard the body against infection.

THE COMPOSITION OF BLOOD

20–7. Red and white corpuscles seen through a microscope

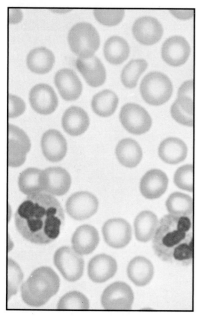

Blood is made up of **plasma** and blood cells. Plasma is the fluid part of the blood. Distributed throughout the plasma are red blood cells, white blood cells, and **platelets.** The average person has about 5.6 liters (6 qt) of blood. This supply is always maintained by the formation of new blood.

RED BLOOD CELLS.   The most numerous blood cells are **red corpuscles.** You have about 20 to 30 trillion red blood cells in your body. The main function of the red blood cells is to carry oxygen to the cells and carbon dioxide away from the cells. Red blood cells are shaped like tiny disks. Both sides of these disks are concave, or curved inward. This shape is ideal because the concave surfaces increase the red blood cells' oxygen-absorbing area.

The red pigment in blood cells is called *hemoglobin.* Hemoglobin is a protein substance combined with iron. When hemoglobin combines with oxygen in the lungs, it becomes bright scarlet. Thus, the blood flowing through arteries to the tissues is bright red. The red blood cells release oxygen to the cells and pick up carbon dioxide from the cells. The blood flowing through veins from the body cells is dark red,

428

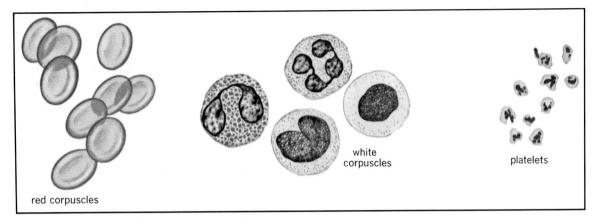

red corpuscles

white corpuscles

platelets

20–8. The solid components of blood

since it contains no oxygen. Carbon dioxide is carried to the lungs, where it is released, and the cycle is repeated.

The life span of a red cell is short. As it travels through the vessels at great speed, it bumps other blood cells and bounces off vessel walls. It is squeezed through tiny capillaries and subjected to great pressure changes in the arteries and the veins. The average red cell endures this hard life for about 30 to 120 days. Then it breaks up. The spleen, a small organ in the left upper abdomen, filters out much of the red-corpuscle remains. The bone marrow makes new red blood cells at a rate of 2 million or more per second. There is not enough iron from red blood cell remains to make new ones. This is why it is essential to include iron each day in your diet.

WHITE BLOOD CELLS. Whenever bacteria or other enemies invade your body, a microscopic army of white blood cells moves in to destroy them. There are several different kinds of white blood cells. Some white cells poison bacteria with chemicals. Others attack bacteria directly and ingest them. Certain kinds of white corpuscles are produced in the bone marrow. Others are formed in the lymph nodes. White blood cells are present in the blood in a ratio of about 1 to 600 red cells. Normally, there are between 5,000 to 10,000 white blood cells per cubic millimeter of blood.

Unlike red blood cells, white blood cells can move and change their shape. This ability enables them to move through tiny pores in the capillary walls and to travel through the tissue fluid. They can travel to the center of infection and surround it. During an infection, the bone marrow speeds up production, pouring an enormous number of white cells into the blood. This explains why the white-cell count rises rapidly during a serious infection.

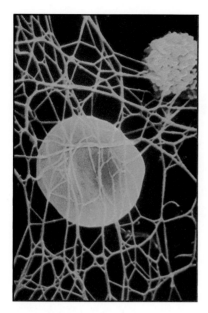

20–9. Fibrin catches red blood cells to form a clot.

HEALTH IN HISTORY

The first recorded blood transfusion was performed on dogs in 1665. At that time, there were many attempts to transfuse dogs' blood to humans, but these were almost always fatal, so, as a result, transfusions were outlawed for many years. In 1818, Dr. James Blundell performed several successful human blood transfusions for hemorrhage in children.

THE PLATELETS.   Blood platelets are smaller and less numerous than red cells. They total about 1 1/2 trillion. Platelets are essential in the clotting of blood. When a blood vessel is cut and bleeding occurs, platelets break up and give off a substance needed for the blood to clot.

PLASMA.   A pale yellow fluid called plasma makes up about 55 percent of whole blood. About 92 percent of plasma is water with dissolved nutrients, mineral salts, and waste products. The remaining 7 or 8 percent is composed of proteins. The proteins are of three types. **Albumin** (al-**bew-**min) helps to keep blood pressure normal by regulating the amount of water in the plasma. **Globulin** (**glob-**you-lin) contains antibodies, which are chemical substances that are effective against specific diseases. **Fibrinogen** (fi-**brin-**oh-jin) works with platelets in the clotting process. Plasma from which fibrinogen has been removed is called **serum.** Plasma carries nutrients to the tissues and transports cell wastes and heat. It is also vital in giving blood sufficient volume to maintain blood pressure.

THE CLOTTING OF BLOOD.   When blood flows out of a cut or ruptured vessel, a chemical process takes place. A clot forms, and blood flow is blocked. Clotting is a complicated process involving platelets and fibrinogen. Platelets and injured body cells give off chemicals that start a series of changes. Fibrinogen changes to solid threads called **fi-brin.** Fibrin catches red blood cells to form a clot.

BLOOD TYPES

Many people died from blood transfusions until it was learned that not all blood was alike. One type of blood may cause the cells of another type to clump, a reaction called *agglutination*. There are four blood types in the world's population: types A, B, AB, and O. Although blood types vary from one region to another, tests indicate that about 45 percent of the world's population has type O, 41 percent type A, 10 percent type B, and 4 percent type AB. Before a patient is given a whole-blood transfusion, the blood must be typed. When the type is determined, a donor's blood of the same type is used in the transfusion, provided that certain other blood factors described below are compatible. When the wrong bloods are mixed, clumping of blood cells results. For example, type A blood mixed with type B blood would cause clumping. If the clumps passed through the heart to the lungs or brain, they could cause death.

THE Rh FACTOR IN BLOOD. One other important factor must be considered in matching blood. The blood of about 85 percent of the human population contains one of several proteins termed **Rh factors,** the most important of which is the Rh(D) factor. We refer to these people as **Rh positive.** The 15 percent who lack the Rh(D) factor are called **Rh negative.** If an Rh-negative person receives Rh-positive blood, the person's own blood will make a substance called *antibodies*. These antibodies will act against the Rh-positive blood.

Suppose a patient with Rh-negative blood mistakenly receives a transfusion of Rh-positive blood. The transfusion causes production of Rh antibodies in the bloodstream. Later the patient receives another transfusion of Rh-positive blood. The blood, which already contains the antibodies, attacks the added red blood corpuscles immediately. Clumping of the added corpuscles may cause serious complications and even death.

Rh disease of babies develops in a baby who has inherited Rh-positive blood from the father and whose mother has Rh-negative blood. If the mother has become sensitized to the Rh factor by a previous pregnancy or by a blood transfusion, her blood develops antibodies that destroy the Rh-positive cells that the child inherited from the father.

20–10. When an Rh negative mother has a child who is Rh positive, she develops antibodies against the Rh factor. If she becomes pregnant with a second Rh positive baby, the baby could develop Rh disease.

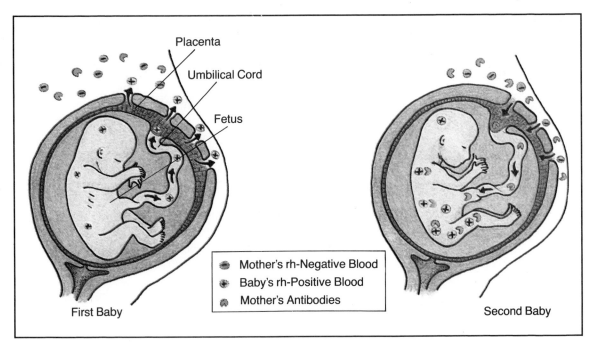

Placenta

Umbilical Cord

Fetus

⊛ Mother's rh-Negative Blood
⊛ Baby's rh-Positive Blood
⊛ Mother's Antibodies

First Baby

Second Baby

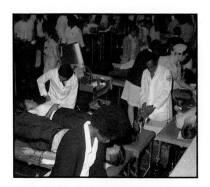

20–11. The Red Cross and other organizations sponsor blood drives when there is an acute shortage of blood.

All women of childbearing age should be tested for Rh factor. If a mother is Rh negative and the father is Rh positive, Rh disease can be prevented by giving her a vaccine called *Rh-immune globulin.* When this is injected into an Rh-negative woman immediately after a pregnancy, she does not produce antibodies if a next child is Rh-positive.

BLOOD BANKS AND BLOOD TRANSFUSIONS

There is a constant need for blood, which often outstrips its supply. To meet this need, blood banks have been established all over the United States, many by the American Red Cross. They depend on donors to replace the blood used in hospitals. Donors must be carefully screened to be sure that they have a normal pulse; adequate hemoglobin, blood pressure, and temperature; and, insofar as possible, that they have no disease that could be passed on to a receiving patient. Hospitals and blood banks are required to test all blood to rule out hepatitis. Donors may give a pint of blood as often as every two months.

The whole blood is drawn into a sterile container. The blood is typed, a preservative is added, and the blood is then stored in a refrigerator at about 10 degrees above freezing. It may be kept for up to 21 days. It is also possible to separate the red cells, white cells, platelets, and plasma from the whole blood, so that each may be given separately, according to need.

TRANSFUSIONS. Whole blood transfusions are used in cases of severe hemorrhage. Plasma transfusions are given when the need is for blood volume rather than for blood cells. This is the case with many burn and accident victims. Plasma can be frozen or dried and kept for up to two years. Red-cell transfusions are used in over 80 percent of patients needing transfusions. Such patients do not need extra plasma but do need the extra oxygen-carrying capacity of the red cells. Red cells may be frozen and stored for at least two years. Platelet transfusions are used to treat bleeding in patients who lack platelets due to bone-marrow damage from chemotherapy or radiation treatment of leukemia or other types of cancer or due to other diseases. White blood cell transfusions may be used for patients who lack them due to bone-marrow damage or disease.

Plasma can be divided into many useful products including albumin (to increase resistance to infection) and fibrinogen (to aid in diseases in which clotting is deficient).

ROUTINE BLOOD TESTS		Table 20-1
Test	Description	
Hemoglobin	Test for anemia; concentration of hemoglobin is measured	
Hematocrit	Test for anemia; percentage of red blood cells per unit of blood is determined	
White blood cell count	Test for bacterial infection and certain diseases such as leukemia	
Red blood cell count	Test for anemia and other blood disorders; number of red blood cells per unit of blood is counted	
Platelet count	Used in diagnosis of bleeding disorders	
Clot formation time	Used when a clotting disorder is suspected	

BLOOD TESTS. Blood tests are physical or chemical examinations of the blood to detect disease. Formerly, the counting of red cells, white cells, and platelets was a time-consuming task. Now, with the aid of computers, more than 30 tests on one sample can be run in a matter of minutes with a much greater degree of accuracy. Table 20-1 describes some of the tests that are performed on blood. Tests for white blood cell count and anemia are usually done as part of a routine physical exam.

DISORDERS OF THE CARDIOVASCULAR SYSTEM

VARICOSE VEINS.   When valves in the veins weaken, they leak and no longer aid in moving blood toward the heart. Blood forms pools in these veins, stretching their walls. **Varicose veins** almost always occur in the legs, where they appear as bulging, bluish cords standing out under the skin. The circulation of the skin about the ankles may become so poor that ulcers form and fail to heal. If discovered early, cases may be treated by raising the legs or by applying elastic bandages or stockings. These collapse the varicose veins, sending blood into deeper veins.

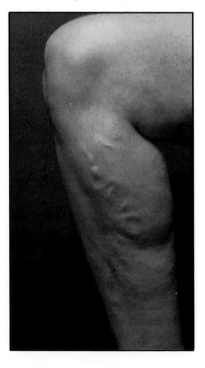

20–12. How can you help prevent varicose veins?

Varicose veins often result from an occupation that requires standing for many hours at a time. They can also be caused by excessive overweight or even by the use of constraining clothes, such as tight socks.

ANEMIA. Diseases of the blood may involve any of its cells. The most common ailment is **anemia.** This condition results either from lack of sufficient red blood cells or from lack of sufficient hemoglobin in the cells. In all kinds of anemias, the body tissues suffer from lack of oxygen.

Naturally, sudden loss of blood through a hemorrhage or an injury brings on an anemic condition. Certain infections result in the invasion of the bloodstream and the destruction of red corpuscles. Whole blood transfusions are important in correcting both of these conditions.

In pernicious anemia the red cell forming centers of the bone marrow fail to function properly. The greatest advance

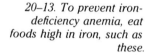

20–13. To prevent iron-deficiency anemia, eat foods high in iron, such as these.

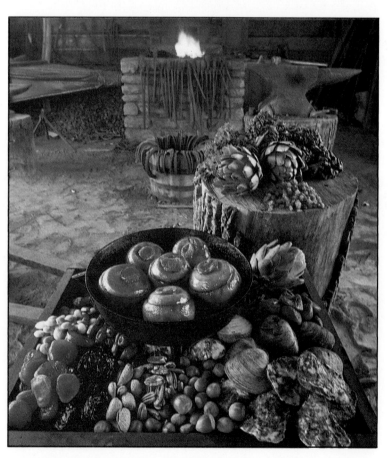

in the treatment of this disease was the discovery of vitamin B-12. This vitamin is normally stored in the liver and acts as a stimulant of the red cell forming elements in marrow. People with pernicious anemia can maintain a normal red blood cell count with only one injection of B-12 monthly.

In iron-deficiency anemia, red cells are present in sufficient quantity, but they are small and lack normal hemoglobin content. Symptoms include pale color and easy fatigue. This kind of anemia is more common in children than in adults. Iron-deficiency anemia is also common during the teenage years, especially among girls. Since women need more iron during pregnancy, it is especially important to include enough iron in the diet during this time. Iron-containing foods, such as liver, lean meat, and leafy green vegetables, and iron supplements help correct this kind of anemia.

SICKLE CELL ANEMIA.   Sickle cell anemia is an inherited blood disease that can cause pain and damage to vital organs. Its effects vary greatly. Many people with sickle cell anemia can enjoy reasonably good health most of the time. However, under certain conditions, the red blood cells of these people change from being disk shaped into being a sickle shape (see Figure 20–14). These sickled cells can become trapped in the spleen where they are destroyed. This leads to a shortage of red blood cells (anemia). Sometimes sickled cells become stuck in tiny blood vessels causing these vessels to become totally blocked. This can be very painful and can destroy areas of tissue.

How is sickle cell anemia acquired? Since it is an hereditary disease, a person must inherit the genes for this trait from his or her parents. If a person inherits only one gene for sickle cell trait from either parent, he or she is called a *carrier*. Carriers do not develop the disease. If a person inherits two genes for sickle cell trait (one from each parent), this person will have the disease. This is explained in more detail in Chapter 21.

Do we all have the same chance of inheriting sickle cell anemia? No. In the United States, most cases of sickle cell anemia occur among blacks and Hispanics of Caribbean origin. About one in every 400 to 600 blacks inherits sickle cell disease. The disease also affects some people of Mediterranean ancestry. There is no cure for sickle cell disease, but it can be treated with blood transfusions.

LEUKEMIA.   **Leukemia,** a cancer of the blood-forming tissues, strikes both sexes and all ages. There are two major

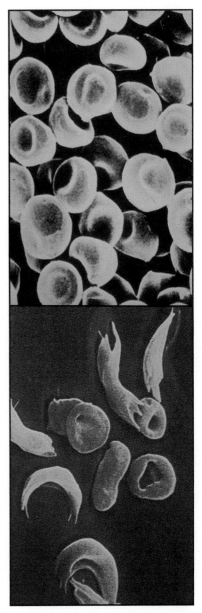

20–14. Top: normal red blood cells Bottom: sickled red blood cells

types of leukemia, acute and chronic. Acute leukemia appears suddenly. Symptoms may include fatigue, paleness, weight loss, and bleeding. Chronic leukemia progresses slowly and without warning signs. Symptoms may not appear for years.

When leukemia strikes, millions of abnormal, immature white blood cells are produced. Because they are immature, they cannot carry on their basic function of fighting infection. The uncontrolled production of abnormal cells crowds out the production of red blood cells and platelets. As a result, anemia and hemorrhaging occur.

The causes of most cases of leukemia are unknown. It has been linked to excessive exposure to radiation. Studies indicate that viruses may also be involved.

Chemotherapy is by far the most effective treatment. Continuing research is yielding new and better drugs for treating leukemia. There has been a dramatic improvement in the survival of patients with acute leukemia in the last ten years.

HEMOPHILIA. **Hemophilia** is an inherited disease in which blood fails to clot or clots very slowly. Minor injuries may result in dangerous bleeding. In cases of severe bleeding, a substance called Factor VIII can be given. Fortunately, this condition is uncommon. Hemophilia rarely appears in females but, since females are carriers, it is usually transmitted from mother to son (see Chapter 21).

RHEUMATIC FEVER AND HEART DISEASE. If untreated, a strep throat can develop into **rheumatic fever.** This serious fever may affect the heart, joints, brain, or skin. Rheumatic fever may permanently damage the heart valves, a condition called **rheumatic heart disease.** With this disease, the damaged valves fail to fully close or open. This places an extra load on the heart. The heart labors to keep sufficient blood flowing. As the damaged heart labors over a period of years serious effects are seen. A person can experience severe shortness of breath, quick fatigue, swelling of body tissues, and chest pain. Eventually the heart may fail. It is estimated that almost two million people of all ages in the United States have had rheumatic fever. Some are now affected with rheumatic heart disease.

One bright side to rheumatic heart disease is that it can be prevented. If you have a sudden sore throat, particularly if it is accompanied by fever, swollen neck glands, nausea, and vomiting, promptly seek medical attention. Laboratory tests can confirm whether or not you have a strep throat.

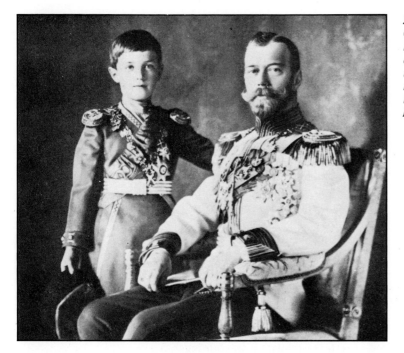

20–15. The son of Russian Czar Nicolas had hemophilia. Hemophilia is a hereditary disease, which was inherited by many princes due to many intermarriages among European royalty.

Penicillin or other antibodies can control the infection, thereby preventing rheumatic fever. Most people can recover from an initial bout of rheumatic fever without permanent heart damage if they receive proper medical care. People who have had rheumatic fever are at greater risk of developing the fever again and then suffering heart damage. A more continuous treatment program may be prescribed to prevent repeated infections.

CHRONIC DISEASES OF THE HEART AND BLOOD VESSELS

Diseases of the heart and blood vessels account for 53 percent of all deaths in the United States each year. Cardiovascular disease strikes 28 million Americans, one out of every seven people. The number of fatalities from cardiovascular disease is over 1 million per year, more than the deaths from all other diseases combined, including cancer.

The major underlying cause of cardiovascular disease has been associated with atherosclerosis. This is the buildup of fatty deposits within the walls of arteries that restricts the flow of blood. These diseases will be discussed in full in Chapter 22, Major Health Problems Today.

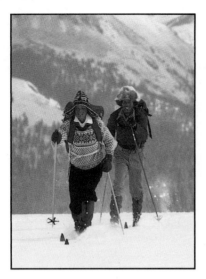

20–16. Positive health habits, such as doing aerobic exercises regularly, is the best way to keep the cardiovascular system healthy.

KEEPING YOUR CARDIOVASCULAR SYSTEM HEALTHY

If you follow positive health habits, you can keep your cardiovascular system healthy. You can greatly reduce your risk of acquiring heart or blood vessel disease by making the effort to eat wisely, get regular exercise and rest, and avoid smoking.

A physically fit person has more hemoglobin and blood plasma than someone who is not physically fit. A physically fit person also has a stronger heart that can pump more blood with each beat. The blood vessels in a physically fit person are more efficient at transporting blood to body cells.

WELLNESS WATCH

1. Do you eat wisely, and include low-fat, iron-rich foods in your diet each day?
2. Do you get regular exercise to keep your cardiovascular system in good shape?
3. Do you avoid wearing tight socks and other clothing that restrict circulation in your legs?
4. Do you avoid standing or sitting for long periods without walking or otherwise moving around?
5. Do you have your blood pressure checked at least once a year?
6. Do you avoid all forms of tobacco?
7. Do you maintain your ideal body weight?
8. Do you seek medical attention promptly when you have symptoms that are related to strep throat?

SUMMARY: The heart is a pump that delivers blood to all parts of the body. It has two atria and two ventricles. The atria receive blood from the veins. The contractions of the ventricles force blood through the arteries. Arteries carry blood from the heart to the body tissues. Veins return blood to the heart. Blood is a fluid made up of liquid plasma, red blood cells, white blood cells, and platelets. Red blood cells transport oxygen to all cells. White blood cells help fight disease. Platelets are needed for the blood to clot. It is important to know your blood type, which can be A, B, AB, or O, and either Rh positive or RH negative. Disorders of the blood and blood vessels include varicose veins, anemia, leukemia, hemophilia, and rheumatic heart disease.

CHAPTER REVIEW

words at work

Find the word in the left column that fits one of the definitions in the right column. DO NOT WRITE IN THIS BOOK.

a. atrium
b. diastolic
c. hemoglobin
d. systemic
e. leukemia
f. myocardium
g. plasma
h. pulmonary
i. sinoatrial node

1. Lowest blood pressure in an artery
2. Upper chamber of the heart
3. Circulation to and from the lungs
4. A mass of tissue in which the impulse for a heartbeat originates
5. The liquid portion of the blood
6. Muscular heart wall
7. A disease in which a great excess of white corpuscles is formed
8. The blood substance that carries oxygen
9. The principal circulation of blood in the body

review questions

1. Describe the heart.
2. Trace a drop of blood through the heart and lungs.
3. Identify the largest artery in the body.
4. Name and describe three different types of blood vessels.
5. Describe the lymphatic system.
6. How is the rate of the heartbeat controlled?
7. Explain how blood pressure is measured.
8. What are systolic pressure and diastolic pressure.
9. What does the blood system deliver to the cells?
10. Describe the structure and function of red corpuscles.
11. What is the main function of white corpuscles?
12. Why are platelets necessary?
13. Describe plasma. What percentage of blood is made up of plasma?
14. Name the four types of blood.
15. What happens when a person with Rh-negative blood receives a transfusion of Rh-positive blood?
16. Distinguish between pernicious anemia and iron-deficiency anemia.
17. Describe the nature of the sickle cell trait.

discussion questions

1. Blood pressure is much greater in the arteries than in the veins. Where is the pressure lost, and why? Explain how blood gets back to the heart even though there is low blood pressure in the veins.
2. Describe the various routes that blood takes through the body.
3. Discuss the importance of the work of blood banks in providing blood for transfusions. How can people be motivated to donate blood? Do you think they should be paid?

investigating

PURPOSE:
To compare the heart rates of different people.

MATERIALS NEEDED:
Watch or clock with second hand; paper; and a pencil.

PROCEDURE:
A.   Sit quietly for 15 minutes. Then count your pulse rate for 15 seconds. Take three different counts and find the average of the three counts. Multiply your average by 4 to get your heart rate per minute.
    1.   What is your resting heart rate?
B.   On the chalkboard, write your resting heart rate under one of these categories: Male, exercises vigorously for 20 minutes at least 3 times per week; Male, does not exercise; Female, exercises vigorously for 20 minutes at least 3 times per week; Female, does not exercise. Find the average resting heart rate for each group.
    2.   Which group had the slowest heart rate? Which group had the fastest?
    3.   The heart works harder, faster, and less effectively in the nonexerciser. The average resting heart rate of a physically fit person is between 50 and 60 beats per minute. The average for a typical inactive person is between 70 and 80 beats per minute. Do your class results agree with these findings?
C.   Hop up and down on one foot 50 times. Then sit down and immediately take a pulse count. Take a pulse count after 2, 3, and 4 minutes of sitting quietly. If you are physically fit, your pulse count should not increase more than 20 to 30 beats, and it should return to normal in 2 to 3 minutes.
D.   At home measure the resting rate of at least three different people of different ages. Ask each person if they exercise regularly or not. On the blackboard, record your results by age, sex, and whether or not the person exercises. Age categories should be 0 to 12, 13 to 29, 30 to 50, and over 50. Find the average resting heart rate for each group.
    4.   Does average heart rate change with age?
    5.   Is the average heart rate of females different from that of males?
    6.   Do your findings indicate that exercise slows down the resting heart rate?

HEALTH
CAREERS

MEDICAL LABORATORY SPECIALIST

Medical laboratory specialists conduct tests on body tissues and fluids. These tests help determine the presence, absence, or extent of disease. Every part of the human body, its secretions and excretions, can now be analyzed. The presence and percentage of proteins, trace metals, hormones, drugs, and other substances can be detected. To become a medical technologist, you must complete a four-year college program. To work as a laboratory technician, you must have a two-year college degree. If you want to be a laboratory assistant, you'll need one year of special training. As a technician you would perform simpler tests than the technologist. As an assistant you would carry out routine lab work. Although a specialist may perform the same test several times in one day, each time it must be done with care and accuracy. For more information, contact either the American Society of Clinical Pathologists, 2100 W. Harrison Street, Chicago, Illinois 60612, or American Medical Technologists, 710 Higgins Road, Park Ridge, Illinois 60068.

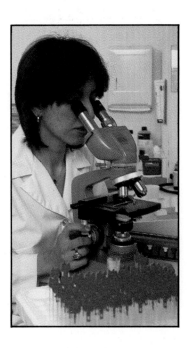

PHYSICIAN ASSISTANT

Meet the physician assistant, PA for short: one of the newest members of the

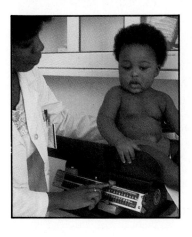

health care team. The PA is trained to perform many tasks that traditionally were done by doctors alone. They perform tasks like giving complete physical examinations, carrying out simple patient treatments, prescribing certain drugs, and suturing (stitching) wounds. What prepares the PA for these medical responsibilities? Generally two years of college and another two years of intensive special training are needed. The program is much like an abbreviated version of medical school.

Students briefly study all basic areas of medicine from anatomy and physiology to surgery and emergency care. Classroom knowledge is also combined with practical work experience with patients in hospitals. After graduation PAs can work in hospitals, clinics, and physicians' offices: wherever people seek health care. Find out more about PAs from PAs themselves. You can do this by writing to the American Academy of Physician Assistants, 2341 Jefferson Davis Highway, Suite 700, Arlington, Virginia 22202.

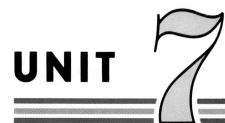

UNIT 7

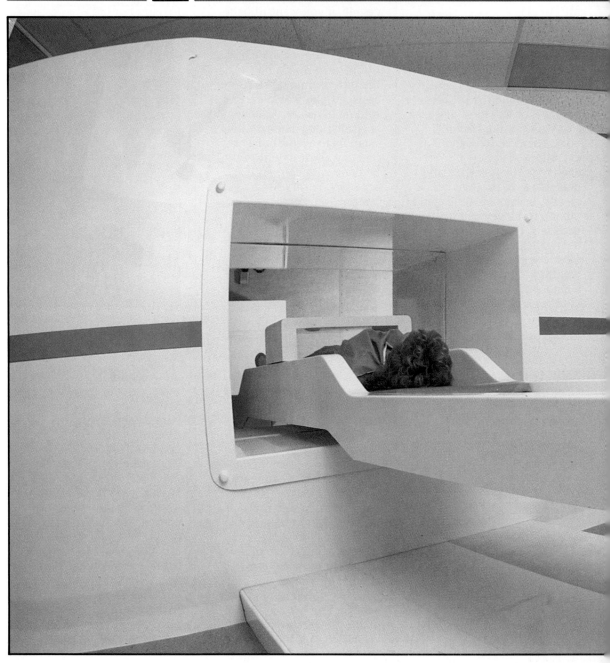

Health Promotion and Protection

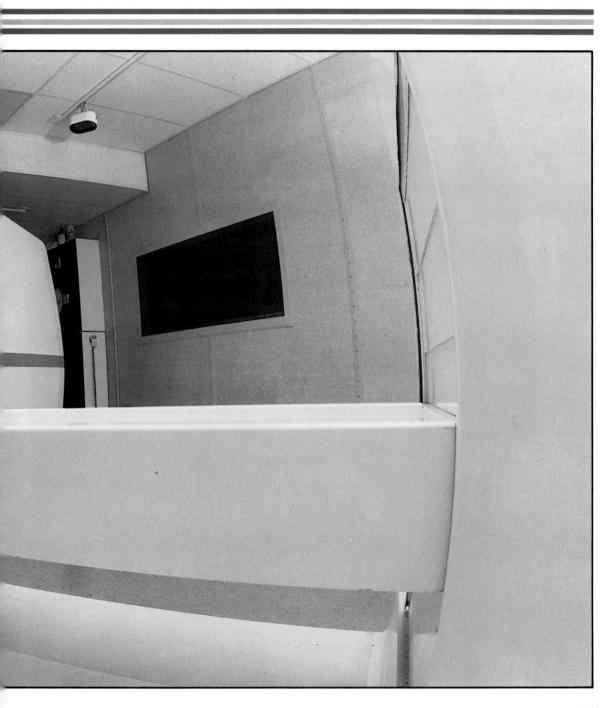

CHAPTER 21

Heredity and Health

OBJECTIVES

- STATE how genetic traits are passed from one generation to the next
- DESCRIBE recessive and dominant inheritance
- EXPLAIN some of the causes of birth defects

- DESCRIBE the importance of prenatal care for the health of the baby
- RELATE the techniques used in genetic counseling and prenatal diagnosis

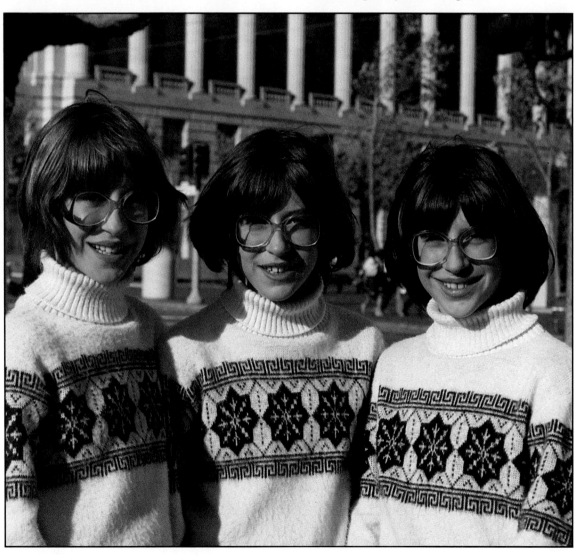

Gary and Bertha Wilkins wished to have a child, but were afraid that the child might inherit sickle cell disease. Neither of them had the disease, but Gary's brother Mike did. Mike was seriously ill with the disease. He had severe anemia and his internal organs were damaged.

Did Gary and Bertha carry the disease? If so, what were the chances that their child would inherit the disease? Should they risk having a baby at all? Years ago, they would have had to make this decision without the benefit of genetic counseling. Today screening tests are available to identify carriers of sickle cell and other genetic diseases. Luckily, Gary and Bertha had heard about these tests. They decided to see a genetic counselor to find out more about the tests. Later in this chapter you will learn what the Wilkinses found out.

HOW ARE TRAITS INHERITED?
GENES AND CHROMOSOMES

How are traits passed from one generation to another? The answer begins with heredity factors called **genes,** which are the blueprints for all new life.

Genes are chemical units found in the cells of all living things. Genes perform two functions: (1) They carry heredity traits; and (2) they give cells the day-to-day instructions for reproduction, growth, and development.

Each gene is a small section of a larger structure known as a chromosome. The word **chromosome** means "colored body." Chromosomes are dark, rodlike bodies found in the nucleus, or center of a cell. Each chromosome is composed of a long complex molecule known as DNA (deoxyribonucleic acid). Figure 21-1 shows the structure of DNA. As you can see, DNA looks like a twisted ladder with interlocking chemicals called bases forming each rung. DNA has only four different chemical bases. Yet these bases can be arranged in countless combinations along DNA's winding ladder. Each combination of three bases forms a chemical code that acts like a word in a sentence. You can think of a gene as a chemical "sentence" that conveys information to the cell. A chromosome can contain hundreds of genes, or "sentences." Therefore, each chromosome contains much information that controls cell structure and function.

Have you noticed differences among members of the same species of plant or animal? Though each species has

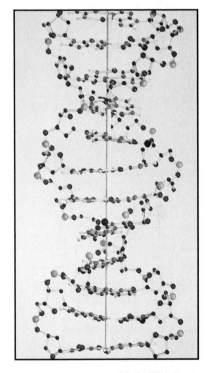

21–1. DNA is an interlocking, twisting ladder that is composed of four different chemical bases.

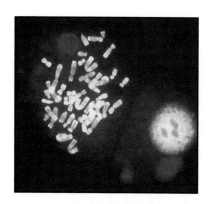

21–2. The 46 chromosomes of a human cell

its own specific genetic code, there are individual genetic variations that make a particular member of that species unique. Not all members of one species carry exactly the same information in their genes.

Though every cell of your body carries your own unique genetic code, particular cells respond only to the genetic code words that have meaning for them. For example, the genes that produce your eye color are not "active" or "switched on" in your skin cells. This is why as cells reproduce each day they maintain their particular structure and function. Skin cells remain skin cells; they do not change into eye cells or muscle cells. Likewise, you maintain the genetic traits that make you a unique individual. If you have brown eyes today, you will always have brown eyes.

The cells of the normal human body each contain 46 chromosomes arranged in 23 pairs (see Figure 21-2). The reproductive cells, the female egg cell and male sperm cell, are an important exception. The egg and sperm cells contain only half the usual number of chromosomes, or 23 chromosomes. These cells are formed when cells with 46 chromosomes divide into two cells with 23 chromosomes each. When these two reproductive cells are united they form a new cell. This new cell, called a **zygote** (meaning "joined together"), then contains the complete set of 46 chromosomes. Thus, new life begins.

Whether the zygote has the genetic potential to develop into a male or female depends on a pair of chromosomes called the sex chromosomes. One type of sex chromosome is called an X chromosome; the other is called a Y chromosome. Females have an XX chromosome pair. Males have an XY chromosome pair. Have you ever heard that the father determines the sex of the child? In a sense this is true. The female egg cell always contains an X chromosome. This is because females do not possess any Y chromosomes. The male sperm cell may contain either an X or a Y chromosome. When the egg is united with an X-bearing sperm, the XX pair results. This will produce a female offspring. If the egg is joined with a Y-bearing sperm, the XY male combination occurs.

GENES IN ACTION. Can two parents with brown eyes produce a child with blue eyes? It is possible because of the way genes act in nature. When new life is conceived, half the chromosomes, and, therefore, half the genes, are passed on from the mother and the other half from the father. The genes of the resulting cell work in pairs, one gene from each

HEALTH IN HISTORY

An Austrian monk, Gregor Mendel, first studied how unknown "factors" control inheritance in garden peas. In 1866, he worked out the laws of inheritance for garden peas. These same laws apply to all sexually reproducing organisms, including humans. Mendel's "factors" are what we now call genes.

parent, to produce specific inherited traits such as eye color.

When the genes from both parents contain the same information, there is little doubt about the trait that will result. What happens when the genes do not contain the same information? The outcome then depends on which parent's gene has a "stronger" effect over the other. The gene that "shows up" is called the **dominant** gene. It masks or "hides" the information carried by the other gene of the pair. This gene that is "hidden" is called the **recessive** gene.

In the case of eye color, the gene for brown eyes (represented as B) is dominant over the gene for blue eyes (represented as b). Therefore, the gene for blue eyes is recessive. If a person has two genes for brown eyes (represented as BB), then he or she will have brown eyes. If a person has one gene for blue eyes and one gene for brown eyes (represented as Bb), then he or she will also have brown eyes.

Now let's consider a father who has two genes for brown eyes (BB) and a mother who has blue eyes (bb). What color eyes would the children have? Look at Figure 21-3. The sperm cells have genes only for brown eyes (B). The eggs have genes only for blue eyes (b). The children would all have brown eyes, since the only possible gene combination they could have is Bb.

Let's now consider two parents, each of whom has one gene for blue eyes and one gene for brown eyes. Therefore, half of the egg cells and half of the sperm cells will carry the gene for blue eyes. The other half will carry the gene for brown eyes. Each offspring has a 50-50 chance of receiving either gene (B or b) from either parent. What possible combinations of genes for eye color could the children of these two parents have? As you can see in Figure 21-4, the possible combinations are Bb, BB, and bb. There is a 75 percent (three out of four) chance that these parents will have a brown-eyed child (Bb or BB), and a 25 percent (one out of four) chance that they will have a blue-eyed child (bb). Each is as likely to happen as any other. What are the chances that their child will have two B genes?

OUR HEALTH HERITAGE

Following conception, the zygote divides and redivides thousands of times. As it does so, the cells become more highly organized. They develop into an **embryo** surrounded by a sac called the **placenta.** The placenta carries nutrients to and removes wastes from the developing embryo. After eight

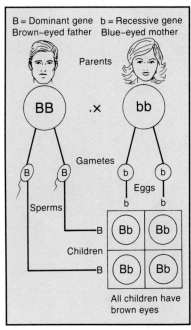

Figure 21–3

Figure 21–4

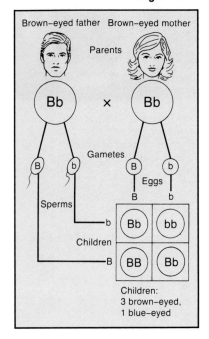

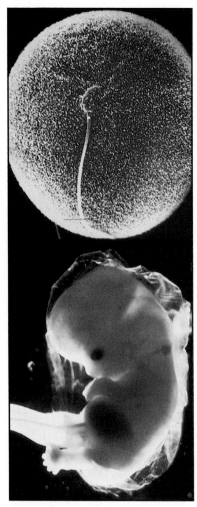

weeks of growth, the developing baby is referred to as a **fetus.** After nine months of pregnancy, a healthy baby is usually born.

However, 1 in 14 newborns (7 percent) has a birth defect. What causes birth defects? Sometimes they are due to defective genes or chromosomes. For example, a mistake may occur during cell division. The resulting egg, sperm, or zygote may have too much or too little chromosome material, which may cause abnormal development. Sometimes the egg and sperm cells contain defective genes. It is estimated that everyone carries eight to ten defective genes. Usually they do not produce any harmful effects and the fetus develops normally. However, in some cases they do cause birth defects and health problems. When very serious genetic errors occur, the body often aborts the embryo spontaneously. This often occurs before the woman even knows she is pregnant. However, many genetic errors are not fatal, but do cause birth defects and health problems.

Not all birth defects are due to genetic factors. The majority are caused by environmental factors or a combination of genetic and environmental factors. During pregnancy, oxygen and nutrients are transferred from mother to fetus. Thus, a healthy mother and a healthy prenatal environment are essential for the development of the normal baby. The early months of pregnancy are especially crucial because this is when the brain and major body structures are developing.

First you will learn about some disorders caused by heredity. Later you will learn how a healthy prenatal environment can help to ensure the health of newborns.

21–5. Top: A sperm fertilizing an egg Bottom: The embryo at 6 weeks, hardly bigger than a pea

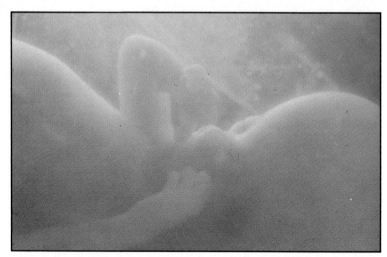

21–6. The fetus at 20 weeks

HEREDITY AND HEALTH PROBLEMS

CHROMOSOME ABNORMALITIES. Down's syndrome is the most well-known example of a defect caused by a chromosome abnormality. People with Down's syndrome have an extra chromosome. The risk of Down's syndrome increases with the age of the mother, and possibly, the age of the father as well. The risk is 1 in 3,000 if the mother is under 29 years of age. The risk increases to 1 in 40 after age 44. Down's syndrome is characterized by mental retardation, increased susceptibility to infection, heart defects, and folding eyelids that give the eyes a slanting look (see Figure 21-7).

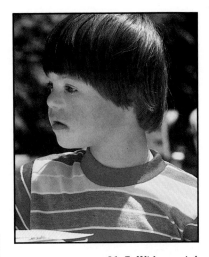

21-7. With special education, Down's syndrome children can lead much more productive lives.

GENETIC DISORDERS

Dominant Inheritance

Achondroplasia – A form of dwarfism
Chronic simple glaucoma – Blindness if untreated
Huntington's disease – Progressive degeneration of nervous system, fatal
Hypercholesterolemia – High blood cholesterol, propensity to heart disease
Polydactyly – Extra fingers or toes

Recessive Inheritance

Cystic fibrosis – Abnormal function of mucous and sweat glands; the most common genetic disease among white Americans
Galactosemia – Inability to metabolize milk
Phenylketonuria (PKU) – Essential liver enzyme deficiency
Sickle cell disease – Blood disorder (sickling of red blood cells); primarily affects blacks, Mediterraneans, and Caribbeans
Thalassemia – Blood disorder; primarily affects persons of Mediterranean ancestry
Tay-Sachs disease – Fatal brain damage; primarily affects persons of Eastern European, Jewish ancestry

Chromosome Abnormality

Down's syndrome – Extra chromosome, mental retardation, increased susceptibility to infection, heart defects, folding eyelids

Sex-linked Inheritance

Agammaglobulinemia – Lack of immunity to infections
Color blindness – Inability to distinguish certain colors
Hemophilia – Defect in blood-clotting mechanism
Muscular dystrophy – Progressive wasting of muscles

Table 21–1

DOMINANT INHERITANCE. Sometimes a defective gene may be dominant. In this case, only one defective gene causes a disorder. The other normal gene cannot compensate for the defective gene. If a parent has a dominant defective gene, then there is a 50 percent chance that each child will also have the defective gene (see Figure 21-8). Huntington's disease, a fatal disease of the nervous system, is inherited in this way.

RECESSIVE INHERITANCE. Sometimes a defective gene is recessive. If someone carries a defective recessive gene, the normal gene of the pair can compensate for the defective gene. Therefore, the defective gene does not cause any harmful effects. People who possess a recessive gene for a genetic disease but do not have the disorder are called **carriers.** However, if a carrier marries someone who has the same defective gene, there is a 25 percent (one out of four) chance that their children will inherit the defective gene from both parents and have the disease (see Figure 21-8). Fortunately, the chances of this happening are slight. *Cystic fibrosis, sickle cell anemia, Tay-Sachs disease,* and *PKU (phenylketonuria)* are examples of diseases caused by recessive defective genes (see Table 21-1).

Cystic fibrosis is the most common genetic disease among the American population of European descent. This condition causes a thick, sticky mucus to collect in the lungs and intestinal tract, resulting in difficulty in breathing and digestion, and often a shortened lifespan. At present there is no cure for the disease.

Sickle cell disease is the most common genetic disease among black Americans. See pages 435 and 452 for more information.

Figure 21–8

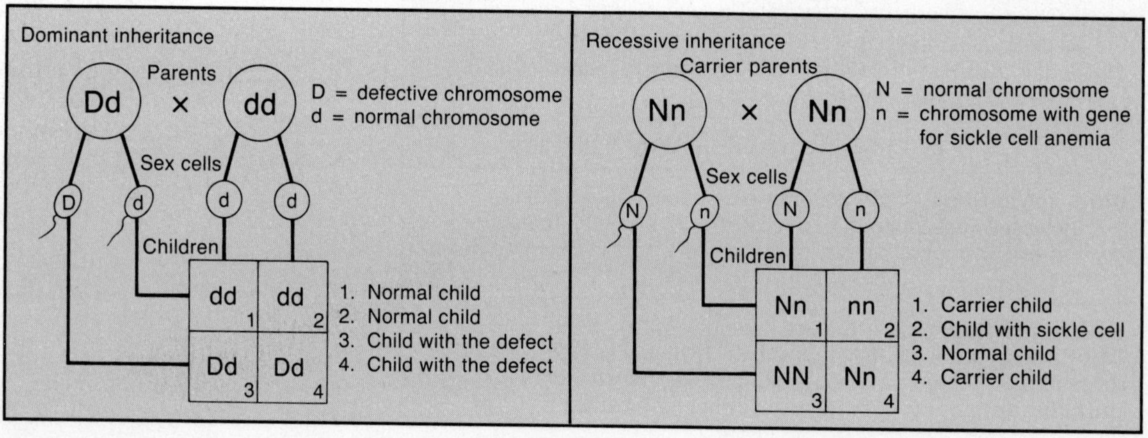

Dominant inheritance

Parents

Dd × dd

D = defective chromosome
d = normal chromosome

Sex cells

D d d d

Children

dd	dd
1	2
Dd	Dd
3	4

1. Normal child
2. Normal child
3. Child with the defect
4. Child with the defect

Recessive inheritance

Carrier parents

Nn × Nn

N = normal chromosome
n = chromosome with gene for sickle cell anemia

Sex cells

N n N n

Children

Nn	nn
1	2
NN	Nn
3	4

1. Carrier child
2. Child with sickle cell
3. Normal child
4. Carrier child

SEX-LINKED INHERITANCE. As you learned, women have two X chromosomes, and men have one X chromosome and one Y chromosome. What if there were a gene disorder carried on an X chromosome? Would men or women be more likely to be affected by it? Women are seldom affected because they have another X chromosome that is likely to have a normal gene that will compensate for the defective gene. Since men have only one X chromosome, they will be affected if they inherit a defective gene on that X chromosome. If a woman carries a defective gene on one X chromosome, there is a 50 percent chance that each son will inherit the disorder. There is also a 50 percent chance that each daughter will be a carrier. Can you explain why? Hemophilia and color blindness are two disorders that are inherited in this way. Figure 21–9 shows how a mother, who is a carrier for hemophilia, can pass her defective gene on to her children.

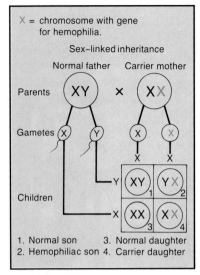

Figure 21–9

PREGNANCY AND PARENTHOOD

Do you think that you will have children some day? If so, some planning and extra care on your part can help ensure the health of your children. You do not have much control over the genes you inherit or the genes you pass on to your offspring. However, you can control environmental factors that affect your health and the health of your future children.

The health and life-style of both parents play a role in the development of a healthy infant. For example, sexually transmitted diseases can be passed on to the baby during the birth process. The use of certain drugs can cause sperm abnormalities. Ideally, a woman should have a complete medical exam before conceiving. This will ensure that she has no infections, nutritional deficiencies, or other conditions that could impair the baby's development. Being either overweight or underweight places the mother and infant under higher risks of many problems during pregnancy. Hypertension and diabetes are also high risk factors. They should be under control before pregnancy.

Both parents should be tested for blood type before pregnancy. If a mother is Rh negative, and a father is Rh positive, then there is a possibility that the baby could develop Rh disease. A serum has been developed that can be given to women immediately after pregnancy to prevent this condition in future births. This is described in greater detail in Chapter 20.

21–10. The health of both parents affects the health of the infant.

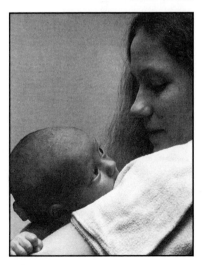

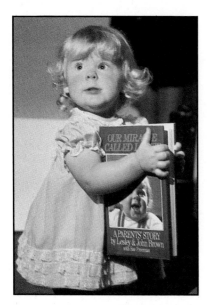

21–11. Louise Brown is the first baby conceived by in vitro fertilization.

Some viruses contracted by the mother may cause the baby to be born with certain defects. For example, if the mother contracts German measles (rubella) during the early stages of pregnancy, physical defects and/or mental retardation may result. Other viruses may cause similar defects. Prior to pregnancy, a woman should be sure she is immune to rubella. This can be determined with a simple blood test. If she is not immune, a vaccine should be given at least three months prior to conception.

Your age is a factor you may wish to consider when planning a family. Mothers under 20 are at higher risk of anemia and low-weight babies. Mothers over 40 have a high risk of Down's syndrome babies and of pregnancy complications.

GENETIC COUNSELING. The Wilkenses had an interview with Mr. Scott, a genetic counselor. "There is a possibility that you are both carriers for sickle cell," Mr. Scott told them. "But there is also a good chance that at least one of you is not. One in ten black Americans are carriers of sickle cell. If both of you are carriers of sickle cell, then you have a 25 percent chance of having a child with sickle cell disease. Another way of looking at this situation is that you could have a three in four chance of having a healthy child. If neither or only one of you is a carrier, then none of your children could inherit the disease."

Gary and Bertha both had the screening test. The tests showed that Gary did have the sickle cell trait, but Bertha did not. They could be assured that none of their children would inherit sickle cell disease.

If there is a possibility that either parent is a carrier of a genetic disease, then it is wise to seek genetic counseling. Accurate carrier detection tests have been developed for a number of potentially damaging genetic traits, such as sickle cell and Tay-Sachs disease. *Tay-Sachs disease* is a fatal, brain-damaging disorder found primarily in infants of Eastern European, Jewish ancestry. A person with Tay-Sachs disease lacks a gene and thus cannot produce a necessary protein. Children with this condition die early in childhood.

Genetic tests are recommended for those who are at high risk of carrying serious genetic disorders. Persons at high risk include those who belong to ethnic groups that have a high rate of a particular genetic disorder, or those who have a family history of a certain genetic disorder. The information that these tests provide can help people to make their own decisions about having children.

452

INFERTILITY. Two methods can help infertile women have children. **In vitro** fertilization is fertilization outside the uterus. This procedure is used when a woman's fallopian tubes, through which the egg travels to the uterus, are blocked. An egg is withdrawn from the mother's ovary and sperm from the father is used to fertilize the egg in a small dish. The zygote is then implanted into the uterus. In **embryo transfer,** a woman donor is needed. Her egg is fertilized artificially with sperm from the infertile woman's husband. After conception, the embryo is removed and reimplanted into the infertile woman. With either method, there is a good chance that normal pregnancy and delivery will occur.

PRENATAL CARE. As soon as a woman suspects she is pregnant, she should see a doctor. Regular medical visits during pregnancy are necessary to ensure the health of the mother and help prevent the birth of low weight infants. Low weight babies are at higher risk of premature death, birth defects, and other health problems.

Nutrition during pregnancy is one of the most important factors affecting the baby's health and weight. Diet fads and unbalanced diets should be avoided. Weight reduction should not be attempted during pregnancy.

Drugs of any kind, including aspirin and vitamins, should never be taken by the mother during pregnancy unless advised by a doctor. Some drugs, such as Accutane, are known to cause birth defects. Excessive use of alcohol and tobacco by the mother is known to cause low-birth-weight babies. An expectant mother who drinks an excessive amount of alcohol also has a very high risk of having a baby with "fetal alcohol syndrome." This syndrome causes mental retardation and other problems.

Expectant women who smoke one pack of cigarettes per day cut the oxygen supply to the fetus by about 10 percent. Two packs decrease the supply by more than 20 percent. Women who smoke have more miscarriages, stillborns, and premature babies.

X rays may be very harmful to a developing fetus, especially during the early stages of pregnancy. A woman who suspects she is pregnant should try to avoid X rays.

Pregnant women should guard against exposure to infectious diseases. Avoid eating improperly cooked meat or handling cat litter. Both can be a source of a *toxoplasmosis* infection that seriously affects the normal development of the fetus. If the couple has a cat, it is wise to bring it to a veterinarian, who can test the cat to see if it is infected.

HEALTH TIP

Many young couples are attending natural childbirth programs. These programs combine classes on the birth process, deep breathing exercises, and relaxation exercises to make the birth process more comfortable. During childbirth, the father or other interested family member serves as a coach to help guide the mother through the techniques learned.

21–12. Special exercises can help make pregnancy and delivery less physically stressful.

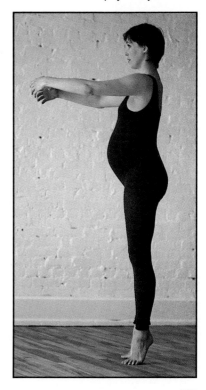

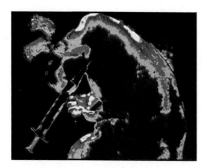

21–13. This ultrasound image of a fetus is used to help guide a syringe in a prenatal surgery technique.

PRENATAL DIAGNOSIS. Prenatal diagnosis is a way of detecting certain problems before birth. These procedures often help doctors better plan for labor and delivery and give parents added information about their child.

Ultrasound and *amniocentesis* are two of the most useful prenatal diagnostic techniques (see Figures 21-14 and 21-15). In ultrasound, high frequency sound waves produce an image of the developing fetus that is projected onto a small television screen, which provides valuable information on fetal development but does not carry the risk of X rays. It involves the insertion of a hollow needle through the mother's abdominal wall, and into the placenta. The ultrasound image helps guide the needle insertion, so the procedure is generally safe. The risk of miscarriage due to this procedure is less than one-half of one percent. A small amount of fluid surrounding the fetus is withdrawn for analysis. The fluid contains cells (therefore chromosomes) from the growth of the fetus. Over 100 genetic disorders and some structural birth defects may be detected through this procedure. This procedure is usually performed during the fourteenth to sixteenth week of pregnancy.

Amniocentesis is usually recommended in the following situations:

1. Parents age 35 or over, who are at higher risk for having a child with Down's syndrome.
2. History of a previous child with Down's syndrome.
3. Either parent having an unusual chromosome arrangement.

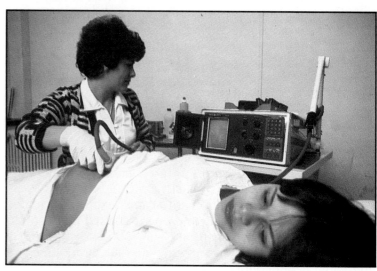

21–14. Ultrasound is used to produce an image of the fetus that is projected on a screen.

454

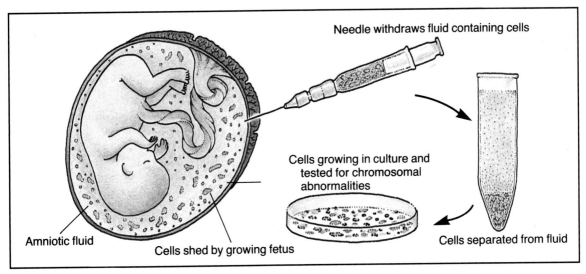

4. Both parents being known carriers for a disease.
5. Mother being a known carrier of a sex-linked defect, such as hemophilia.

NEWBORN SCREENING. Testing babies at birth for genetic disorders is called **newborn screening.** All states have testing programs for newborn infants but the number of conditions included in the test varies. One common genetic disorder included in newborn screening is PKU (phenylketonuria). People with PKU cannot metabolize certain chemicals in a normal diet. This condition can result in mental retardation if it goes undetected. Newborn screening can detect this problem and a modified diet can prevent mental retardation.

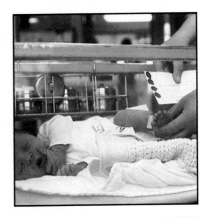

21–16. Infants with PKU can be identified shortly after birth by a PKU screening test.

<u>SUMMARY:</u> Human cells contain 46 chromosomes. Each chromosome contains many genes. Genes, composed of DNA, are the blueprints for all life. When new life is conceived, half the chromosomes, and, therefore, half the genes, are passed on from the mother and the other half from the father. The genes of the resulting cell work in pairs, one from each parent, to produce specific inherited traits. Genes that are dominant have a stronger effect, and therefore mask genes that are recessive. Birth defects are due to genetic errors and/or environmental factors. Those who are at high risk of carrying defective genes should seek genetic counseling. Prenatal care and new techniques such as ultrasound and amniocentesis can help assure the health of the baby.

CHAPTER REVIEW

words at work

Find the word in the left column that fits one of the definitions in the right column. DO NOT WRITE IN THIS BOOK.

a. recessive
b. chromosomes
c. Down's syndrome
d. ultrasound
e. amniocentesis
f. fetal alcohol syndrome
g. dominant
h. genes
i. sex-linked
j. carrier

1. A technique for diagnosing genetic defects before birth
2. Caused by excessive alcohol intake by the mother
3. Composed of DNA chains
4. Genes that are not expressed if their pair is stronger
5. Caused by an abnormal chromosome number
6. Masks the effects of its gene pair
7. A technique for viewing the fetus
8. There are two of them for each genetic trait
9. A gene on the X chromosome
10. Has a recessive gene for a genetic disorder

review questions

1. List two functions of genes.
2. What is a chromosome?
3. What is the importance of the molecule known as DNA?
4. How is genetic information stored, used, and passed on?
5. How many chromosomes are normally present in human cells?
6. Distinguish between X and Y sex chromosomes.
7. How is the sex of the fetus determined at conception?
8. What is the difference between a dominant and a recessive gene?
9. Explain sex-linked inheritance traits.
10. Explain why a father cannot transmit a sex-linked disorder to a son.
11. List some factors in the prenatal environment that may be harmful to the health of the baby.
12. Identify three diseases that result from recessive genes.
13. What groups of people are at a higher risk of having a child with a recessive genetic disorder?
14. List some disorders that result from the inheritance of dominant genes.
15. What increases the risk of Down's syndrome?
16. Why is prenatal diagnosis important?

17. Explain how ultrasound and amniocentesis are used in prenatal diagnosis.
18. Why is newborn screening required in every state?
19. Outline some precautions that should be taken by prospective mothers before pregnancy.
20. How does cigarette smoking affect a developing fetus?
21. What is meant by fetal alcohol syndrome?

discussion questions

1. Discuss the environmental hazards to which many expectant mothers expose their babies.
2. Should a couple at risk consider genetic counseling before considering having a baby? Why or why not?
3. Discuss questions that you as a prospective parent might want to ask during a genetic counseling session.

investigating

PURPOSE:
To demonstrate the effects of dominant and recessive genes in families and populations.

MATERIALS NEEDED:
Paper and pencil.

PROCEDURE:
A.   The ability to curl the tongue into a U-shape is governed by the dominant gene code C. Persons able to curl the tongue carry genes CC or Cc; those who cannot carry genes cc. Ask a family of at least four members to participate in your experiment. Instruct family members to try to curl their tongues into a U-shape.
B.   Observe and record your results on a chart with these headings: subject, family relationship (mother, etc.), tongue curl (yes or no), genes.
C.   As a class, compute class percentages of trait-carriers and nontrait-carriers. Compare your class average with national averages estimated at 65 percent carriers, 35 percent noncarriers for both traits.

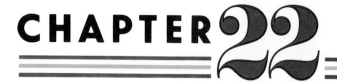

CHAPTER 22

Major Health Problems Today

OBJECTIVES

- DESCRIBE some of the causes of the major chronic diseases
- IDENTIFY the symptoms and treatment for cardiovascular diseases
- IDENTIFY cancer symptoms and treatment
- STATE the risk factors for chronic diseases
- DESCRIBE positive ways that aging and death can be viewed

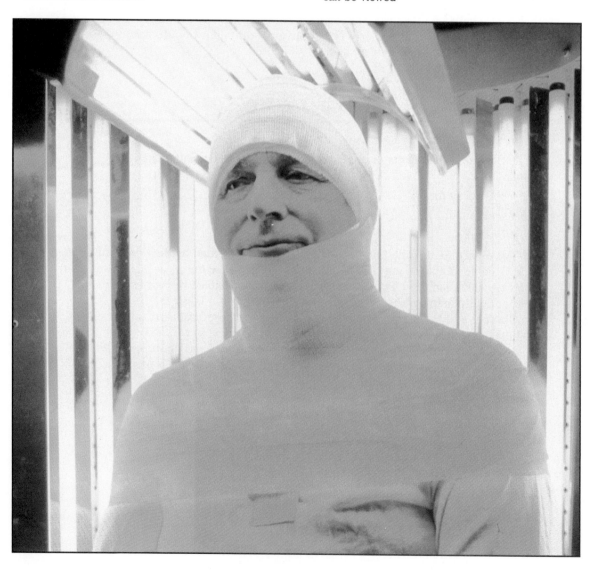

Jonathan's father, at age 50, was a hard-working, hard-driving salesman of a large insurance company. He smoked two packs of cigarettes daily, was about 20 pounds overweight, and got almost no exercise because "he didn't have time for it." He collapsed one day in his office and was rushed to the hospital. His doctor, who had previously warned him to "slow down," stop smoking, exercise, and lose weight, *found that he had suffered a heart attack. After several weeks of treatment in a coronary care unit, he recovered. As he left the hospital, his doctor recommended a complete change of lifestyle with a reduction in stress, a reducing diet, a fitness program, a low-salt diet, and no smoking. This time he heeded his doctor's advice. Now at age 55, he told Jonathan: "At last, I have learned how to live."*

THE MAJOR CAUSES OF DEATH TODAY

Most of us have known someone who has been stricken with cardiovascular disease or cancer. Cardiovascular disease, the leading cause of death, accounts for 51 percent of total deaths each year. Cancer, the second leading cause of death, accounts for another 20 percent of all deaths each year. In 1900, infectious diseases, such as tuberculosis, were the leading causes of death. Today there are effective treatment and prevention measures for infectious diseases and people are living longer. Cardiovascular diseases and cancer are usually chronic, that is they develop over long periods of time. Therefore they are more commonly seen in middle and old age. Partly because Americans are living longer than before, chronic diseases have become the leading causes of death. However, the incidence of chronic disease has also increased due to changes in life-styles.

Is there anything that can be done to combat the major killers of today? This is one of our national health goals, as stated in the Surgeon General's 1979 report on health promotion: "Goal: To improve the health of adults and, by 1990, to reduce deaths among people ages 25 to 64 by at least 25 percent...." How can this goal be reached? Deaths from cardiovascular disease have continually declined since the 1960s. One reason for the decline is the advances taking place in medical care. Another reason is that there has been

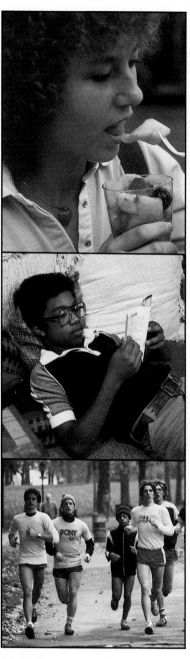

a change in life-styles. People are more interested in assuming responsibility for their health. As the Surgeon General's report states, "There is every reason to believe that the downward trend not only can be maintained but accelerated with increased efforts on behalf of such preventive measures as high blood pressure detection and control, reduction of smoking, prudent diet, increased exercise and fitness and better stress management."

In this chapter you will learn about the causes of today's major killers. You will also learn what measures you can take, starting today, to decrease your risks of developing these diseases.

CARDIOVASCULAR DISEASES

It has been estimated that more than 42 million people in the United States suffer from cardiovascular diseases. Every day 4,000 people have heart attacks and 1,000 have strokes. These diseases cause more than 700,000 deaths each year.

Cardiovascular disease develops when the normal flow of blood through the heart and through the body is stopped in some way. Something may go wrong with the heart or the blood vessels may become blocked. As a result, the heart, brain, kidneys, and other vital body organs may be damaged. Some common forms of cardiovascular disease include heart attack, stroke, congestive heart failure, and high blood pressure.

HYPERTENSION: HIGH BLOOD PRESSURE

Blood pressure is the force of blood against the vessel walls as the heart pumps blood (see Chapter 20). **Hypertension** may be defined as blood-pressure levels consistently above 140/90. If high blood pressure continues for a very long time without treatment, the heart has to work harder than it should to pump blood. This can result in heart disease, strokes, and/or kidney failure. It is estimated that 37 million people in the United States have high blood pressure. Another 25 million have borderline hypertension. Most people think that high blood pressure is a disease of old age, but doctors now realize that the problem often starts during childhood.

What causes hypertension? One type of hypertension is due to an excess of thyroid or adrenal hormones, which can

22–1. Good health habits, such as eating properly, relaxing, and exercising can help prevent chronic diseases.

be corrected by surgery or medication. Another rare type of hypertension, due to an abnormal circulation in the kidneys, can be corrected surgically. However, in most cases the causes of hypertension are unknown.

Since there are no real warning symptoms of hypertension, it is often referred to as the silent disease. Everyone should have their blood pressure taken periodically as a preventive measure.

Doctors today have a growing list of drugs that are effective in controlling high blood pressure. Proper diet including cutting down on the amount of salt used, is also an important measure to take to control blood pressure.

ATHEROSCLEROSIS

Atherosclerosis (ath-err-row-skleh-**row**-sis) is a disease that, in time, can narrow or block arteries to the heart, brain, and other parts of the body. This disease can begin in childhood. The linings of arteries become thickened by fatty deposits called **plaque.** The artery walls become hard and thick as these deposits build up. Then arteries lose their ability to expand and contract. Blood cannot move through them as easily. If a clot of blood or plaque becomes lodged in one of these arteries, then the artery may become completely blocked. Then the body tissues that the artery supplies are deprived of needed oxygen and nutrients. When this happens, the tissue begins to die. If a blocked artery is to the heart, a heart attack may occur. If a blocked artery is to the brain, a stroke may occur.

ANGINA

Arteries that supply the heart with blood may become narrowed due to artherosclerosis. This condition is called **coronary artery disease.** People with this condition may not have any symptoms. In more severe cases, chest pain called **angina pectoris** (an-**ji**-na pec-**tor**-is) can be caused by narrowed arteries. Narrowed arteries can deliver enough blood to meet the normal heart needs. However, during excitement, physical exertion, exposure to cold, or digestion of a heavy meal, the heart requires additional blood. Then the blood supply to the heart muscle is insufficient to meet these demands. Angina pectoris may occur suddenly. The pain is under the breastbone but may also be present in the neck or arms. It is usually relieved by rest and medication.

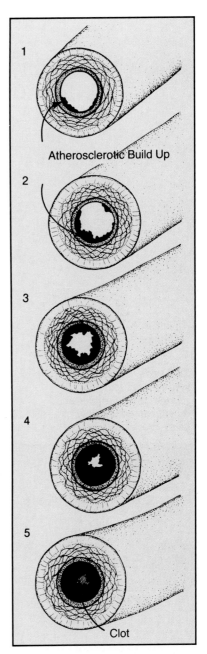

Atherosclerotic Build Up

Clot

22–2. The progression of atherosclerosis on artery walls

HEART ATTACK

The heart muscle, like other body tissues, needs an adequate supply of blood to stay alive. If a blood clot in a narrowed artery blocks the flow of blood to part of the heart muscle, a heart attack occurs. The section of heart muscle that does not receive blood begins to die. Doctors refer to this as **myocardial infarction** (mi-o-**car**-de-al in-**fark**-shun), or M.I. As a result of M.I., heart action can be seriously impaired. A heart attack may be a sudden episode. However, the condition that leads to an attack, coronary artery disease, develops over a long period of time.

Often the symptoms of heart attack are confused with those of indigestion. Signs of a heart attack include uncomfortable pressure, fullness, squeezing or pain in the center of the chest, and sometimes in the arms and shoulders, lasting for two minutes or more. Sweating, dizziness, nausea, fainting, or shortness of breath may also occur. The dying area may upset normal electrical activity. The heart starts a wild, twitching movement called **ventricular fibrillation** (ven-**trik**-u-lar fi-bri-**lay**-shun). Then the heart is no longer pumping blood effectively. If this happens, CPR, as described in Chapter 27, should be administered immediately.

Many people deny that they are having a heart attack and think, "This can't be happening to me." Without proper treatment, most people who die of heart attacks die within 2 hours of the first signals. Last year, 350,000 died before reaching the hospital. Many could have been saved if they had reached the hospital in time. Know the warning signs of a heart attack. If someone is having a heart attack, get him or her to a hospital at once.

Treatment for heart attacks may include drugs, surgery, and physical therapy. If a person survives a heart attack, the healing process begins almost immediately. Scar tissue begins to form and gradually replaces the destroyed heart muscle. Small arteries bordering on the damaged area enlarge to provide a sufficient supply of blood to the heart.

The time necessary for recovery from a heart attack depends on the extent of the damage. Victims of heart attacks have a good chance of returning to normal life. Overwork, tension, worrying, emotional episodes, lack of rest, excess weight, and smoking must be avoided. Many who have heart attacks never have second ones because they learn to live a healthy lifestyle. As soon as the critical period is over, most doctors recommend a supervised gradual return to moderate physical activities, such as walking, jogging, or swimming.

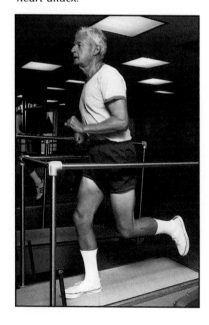

22–3. Many victims of heart attacks learn to change their life-styles in order to avoid another heart attack.

STROKE

If brain tissue does not receive adequate oxygen and nutrients, it begins to die. As a result, a **stroke** occurs. Once this happens, there may be severe losses in mental and bodily functions. A blood clot lodging in one of the arteries to the brain is the major cause of strokes. However, strokes can also be caused when a diseased artery in the brain bursts. This is called a **cerebral hemorrhage.** Cells nourished by the artery are deprived of blood and cannot function. The blood from the burst artery soon forms a clot that can also destroy brain tissue.

Sometimes several small strokes occur before a major stroke. Signs of a small stroke include sudden, temporary weakness or numbness of the face, arm, and leg on one side of the body, temporary loss of speech, temporary dimness or loss of vision, and unexplained dizziness. Prompt medical attention to these symptoms may prevent a fatal stroke from occurring.

Treatment for stroke may include surgery, drugs, and physical therapy. With proper therapy, victims of strokes can often fully recover.

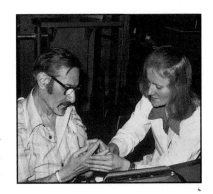

22–4. Physical therapy helps this stroke victim recover the use of his hands.

CONGESTIVE HEART FAILURE

Prolonged high blood pressure, heart attack, and other cardiovascular diseases can cause **congestive heart failure.** The heart muscle may then lack the strength to keep blood circulating normally through the body. Blood flow slows and is inadequate to supply all the body's needs. Blood returning to the heart is backed up, causing swelling, mostly in the ankles and legs. Kidneys may not be able to work properly and fluid may collect in the lungs.

Congestive heart failure requires rest, a low salt-diet, and drug therapy. Sometimes the underlying cause of heart failure can be corrected. For example, if defective heart valves can be replaced, then symptoms of congestive heart failure will disappear.

CONGENITAL HEART DEFECTS

According to statistics of the American Medical Association, between 30,000 and 40,000 children are born in the United States each year with **congenital** (existing at birth) heart defects. These physical defects usually involve the structure of the heart chambers and the heart valves.

Congenital heart defects may show up at birth or become noticeable as the child matures. Deficient blood circulation resulting from a congenital heart defect causes easy fatigue and retarded growth. Until recent years many people with congenital heart defects were forced to live as semi-invalids. Because of the advances in medical care, most people with congenital heart defects can now be restored to normal or near-normal health.

IS THERE ANY WAY TO PREVENT CARDIOVASCULAR DISEASE?

Extensive studies have identified several risk factors that contribute to cardiovascular disease. The more risk factors a person has, the greater the chance of cardiovascular disease. Some risk factors can be changed, others cannot.

Major risk factors that cannot be changed include heredity, sex, race, and age. The tendency for cardiovascular disease seems to run in families. If your parents or grandparents have these diseases, then you are more likely to develop them also. Men have a greater risk of heart attack than women. But, after the child bearing years the rate for women sharply increases. Black Americans have almost a 45 percent greater chance of developing cardiovascular disease than whites. Age is another risk factor. Three out of 4 heart attacks and strokes occur after age 65.

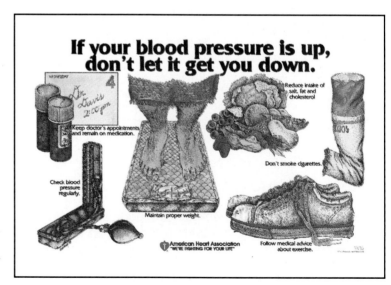

22–5. Tips for controlling high blood pressure from the American Heart Association

A healthful life-style is the foundation for preventing heart attacks and strokes. The three major risk factors that can be changed are cigarette smoking, high blood pressure, and high blood cholesterol levels. Other contributing factors include diabetes, obesity, lack of exercise, and uncontrolled stress. Cigarette smokers have a 70 percent greater chance of developing heart disease than people who do not smoke.

Blood pressure should be monitored and kept under control. High blood pressure is the single most common risk factor associated with stroke, and it is also an important risk factor for heart diseases. Weight loss and reduction of salt in the diet also can help prevent high blood pressure. Americans, especially teenagers, commonly consume too much salt (see Chapter 2 for more tips about salt). Aerobic exercise can help to keep blood pressure low (see Chapter 4 to learn more about aerobic exercise). For many people with moderate hypertension, following this advice can reduce their blood pressure to normal levels. However, drugs are sometimes necessary for those with severe hypertension.

Too much cholesterol can cause buildups on the walls of arteries. There are simple tests that can measure cholesterol levels in the blood. A diet low in animal fat can help lower blood cholesterol levels.

Diabetes, which usually appears during middle age, can sharply increase a person's risk of heart attack. A change in eating habits, weight control, exercise, and in some cases drug therapy can keep it in check. Obesity places a heavy burden on the heart, and also contributes to high blood pressure and blood cholesterol levels.

In your study of stress, you learned that anxiety and tension can cause narrowing of the arteries. The narrowing causes an increase in blood pressure. This is not damaging if it occurs occasionally and for a short time. However, many people may be under stress for long periods of time. This can contribute to hypertension. For this reason, it is important to learn how to cope with stress effectively (see Chapter 8).

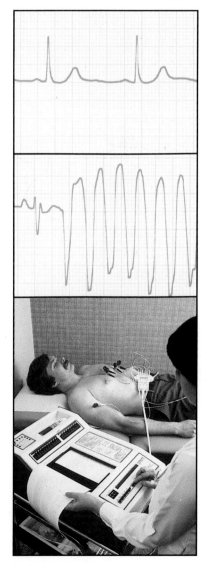

22–6. EKG of a normal heartbeat (top) and abnormal heartbeat (bottom). An EKG can detect heart attack and pre-heart attack conditions.

BASIC TESTS AND TREATMENT FOR CARDIOVASCULAR DISEASE

EKG. An **electrocardiograph** (ee-lek-tro-**kard**-ee-oh-graph) is a delicate instrument used to analyze heart action. Electrical waves, impulses formed in the heart, travel to the instrument through wires attached to the patient. The instrument magnifies the impulses, making a record of them in a line picture, called an **electrocardiogram** (EKG). Damage to a portion of the heart muscle following a heart attack causes an abnormal line tracing.

DRUG THERAPY. Heart disease can be treated with drugs that affect the supply and demand of the heart for oxygen. *Vasodilators* improve blood flow, thus supplying more oxygen to the heart. Other drugs reduce blood pressure, or slow heart rate, to reduce the heart's demand for oxygen. *Digitalis* increases the force of heart contractions. *Aspirin* has been found to reduce blood-clot formation.

Nitroglycerine is the principal medicine used to relieve attacks of angina pain. A small tablet placed under the tongue soon dissolves and reaches the coronary arteries. The coronary arteries dilate, increasing the blood supply to the heart muscle. If the tablet does not quickly relieve the pain, seek medical help. The pain may be due to a heart attack rather than angina.

HEART SURGERY. Before the modern heart-lung machine was available, a surgeon's time was limited in a heart operation. Extensive repair of a damaged heart was impossible. Today a surgeon can perform open-heart surgery that lasts for hours. The heart-lung machine bypasses both the heart and lungs and assumes their functions. This remarkable machine allows a surgeon to correct congenital heart defects, repair structural heart damage, replace damaged valves with plastic valves, and repair defects in the coronary arteries, aorta, and other major blood vessels.

Coronary bypass surgery is a common operation for improving blood supply to the heart. When coronary vessels are found to be blocked, a vein is removed from the patient's leg, and the two ends of the vein are inserted above and below the blocked area. This procedure restores the flow of blood. It also reduces and in some cases eliminates anginal pain.

Several methods have recently been devised to clear the blockage in coronary arteries without surgery. A clot-dissolving drug can be delivered by means of a tube into a recently clogged vessel of a heart-attack victim. In another technique, a tube carrying a tiny balloon is pushed through an arm or leg artery into a blocked coronary vessel. The balloon is inflated, which pushes the blocking material against the arterial wall, thus opening it, at least temporarily.

Many **heart transplants** have been performed in various parts of the world. The success of the transplants has greatly

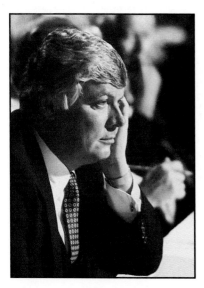

22–7. Governor Brown of Kentucky is one of millions who has returned to normal activity after coronary bypass surgery.

HEALTH IN HISTORY

A new and dramatic chapter in medical history was written in Cape Town, South Africa, in December 1967. The first human heart transplant was performed. This historic heart transplant operation was accomplished by Dr. Barnard and a team of doctors. Surgeons had removed the heart from a young woman's body immediately after her death. The heart was kept alive with a mechanical pump. After transplantation, electric shocks from electrodes started the heart beating. This was a historic milestone in heart surgery.

improved due to the development of drugs that suppress the body's natural rejection of foreign tissue.

Rheumatic fever or a blood clot in a coronary artery sometimes damages areas of the heart regulating the heartbeat. As a result, the heartbeat rate can drop, reducing blood supply to the brain, and causing unconsciousness or death.

Today an implanted electronic device, called an artificial **pacemaker,** can supply the electrical stimulus needed to keep the heart beating at the proper rate. A small pacemaker is inserted under the skin of the abdomen. The wires are inserted into or near the heart. The pacemaker stimulates the heart to beat when the pulse drops below normal. Otherwise it does not interfere with normal beating of the heart.

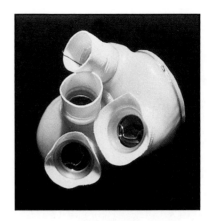

22–8. The artificial heart

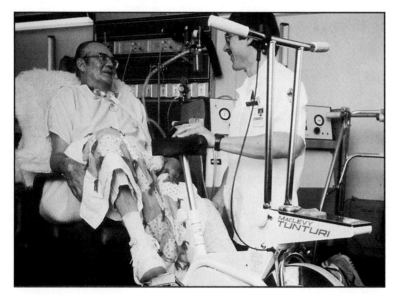

22–9. Barney Clark was the first person to have an artificial heart.

CANCER

The word **cancer** produces more fear in people than any other disease. It is estimated that it kills 440,000 people in the United States annually. Cancer can attack people of any age. Although people over 40 are most susceptible, cancer causes more deaths in young adults between the ages of 15 to 34 than any other disease. However, more than a third of all cancer victims are cured today. It is estimated that there are more than a million cured cancer patients in the United States. Many more cancer patients could have been cured if their cancer had been detected and treated earlier.

WHAT IS CANCER?

Cancer is a group of diseases that cause rapid uncontrolled growth of cells in body tissue. Normal cells usually divide and grow in a very orderly manner. The rate at which this happens is usually carefully controlled by each cell's genes. In this way, worn-out tissues are replaced, injuries are repaired, and body growth proceeds normally. When something goes wrong with the controlling mechanism, cell division and growth become more rapid. Then a growing mass of cancerous cells, referred to as a **malignant tumor,** crowds out normal tissue and absorbs vital nutrients.

Cells of a cancerous growth often break off from a mass and travel through the blood and lymph to other body regions. This spread to new areas is referred to as **metastasis** (meh-**tas**-tah-sis).

Some cancers are very slow-growing. Others may double in size within a month. Regardless of the rate of growth, many cancers can be cured if they are found before vital tissues are destroyed or metastasis has occurred. Thus, early detection and treatment are extremely important.

WHAT CAUSES CANCER?

The basic causes of cancer are unknown. However, scientists have discovered several factors that are often connected with cancer. For years evidence has accumulated to indicate that many agents in our environment seem to cause cancer. Any agents that cause cancer in animals and/or humans have been called **carcinogens.** They include prolonged overexposure to tobacco tar, ultraviolet radiation, X rays, certain food additives, and viruses. Their effects are long term and vary from one individual to another.

There is no proof that cancer can be inherited. However, because higher cancer rates are found among some families, the tendency to develop cancer may be inherited.

How do carcinogens cause cancer? Research now shows that most carcinogens seem to work in pairs. Each partner is needed in order to cause cancer, at least in animals. In a two-stage process, one partner acts as an **initiator;** the other acts as a **promoter.** Cancer develops in animals only when they are first exposed to an initiator, and then to a promoter. This same mechanism may induce cancer in humans. Research is underway to identify initiators and promoters. Researchers are also trying to find ways to interfere with the two-stage process.

22–10. Abnormal cancer cells (top) compared to normal cells (bottom), both from a Pap smear

Recent evidence indicates that cells contain **oncogenes,** or tumor-producing genes, that are usually inactive. Oncogenes may be activated by carcinogens such as radiation, chemicals, or even viruses. The oncogenes direct the cells to become cancerous. Researchers are trying to learn how to suppress these oncogenes.

It is believed that normally we all have cells in our body that become cancerous. When a cell becomes cancerous, the body's immune system usually goes into action. Antibodies attach to the cell, and special killer cells and chemicals dispose of it. However, if the immune system is deficient, cancer cells continue to multiply out of control. Scientists are trying to find ways to bolster the immune system in order to fight cancer.

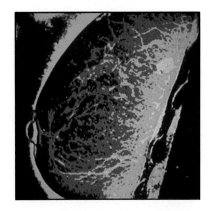

22–11. Thermography is used to detect breast cancer.

SITES OF CANCER

Although cancer may develop in nearly any body tissue, certain organs are attacked more than others (see Figure 22-11).

SKIN CANCER.   Skin cancer ranks first in the number of new cases reported each year. Skin cancers are easily detected and are usually easily cured. In fact, most skin cancer is nearly 100 percent curable if treatment is started in time. Fair-skinned people, especially those who overexpose themselves to the sun, are more likely to develop skin cancer than darker-complexioned people.

COLON AND RECTUM CANCER.   This cancer ranks second only to lung cancer in number of cases reported (excluding common skin cancers). The death rate could be cut in half if the cancer were detected early by colon and rectal examinations.

BREAST CANCER.   Breast cancer is the most common form of cancer in women. Over 100,000 new cases are reported annually. Yet most deaths can be prevented if discovered in time. Every woman should learn how to examine her breasts monthly to detect any unusual lumps or other abnormalities (see Appendix for examination techniques). These should be reported to a doctor at once. In most cases such lumps are noncancerous. Other methods of finding breast cancer early include X ray (mammography), thermography, and ultrasound. Should there be any doubt as to whether or not a lump is cancerous, a **biopsy** is performed. In a biopsy, some of the tumor cells are surgically removed for closer examination.

LUNG CANCER. This is the most common cancer in men, and it has increased steadily in recent years in both men and women. Lung cancer is frequently fatal. The lung cancer risk among heavy cigarette smokers is much higher than in non-smokers. Because more women are smoking, experts predict it will soon be the leading cancer among women.

CANCER OF THE UTERUS. This was once the most frequent cause of death in women. However, the death rate has been reduced to one in four because more women are getting pelvic exams on a regular basis. Part of this examination is a **Pap smear,** in which the doctor painlessly removes some tissue from the cervix. Microscopic examination of this tissue can reveal cancer in an early, curable stage.

PROSTATE CANCER. This disease appears most frequently in older men and causes difficulty in urinating. There are several methods of treating the condition if it is detected in its early stages. Prostate cancer can almost always be detected by a rectal exam, which should be a part of the regular physical exam after age 40.

TESTICULAR CANCER. Cancer of the testes is one of the most common cancers in men 15 to 34 years of age, accounting for 12 percent of all cancer deaths in this age group. If discovered early, testicular cancer can be treated effectively. All men should learn how to do the simple monthly self-exam, as described in the Appendix.

CANCERS OF THE KIDNEY AND BLADDER. These cancers are more common in men than in women and result in difficulty in urinating and blood in the urine. Blood can be detected by a urinalysis. This form of cancer can be treated effectively if discovered in time.

CANCER OF THE STOMACH. Stomach cancer has decreased steadily, but it is still a major medical problem. More than half the deaths could have been prevented if the person had gone to the doctor in time. Often the victim is convinced that the indigestion, nausea and vomiting will respond to home remedies, and does not see a doctor until it is too late for medical help. An X ray may reveal a tumor in the stomach wall in time for surgical removal.

CANCERS OF THE MOUTH, THROAT, AND LARYNX. These cancers are usually curable if detected in the early stages. Warnings include persistent hoarseness, continuing sore throat, difficulty in swallowing, or a sore in the mouth.

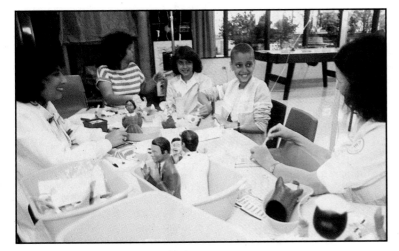

22–12. Today, chemotherapy is very effective in treating leukemia. Play therapy helps these leukemia patients keep their spirits up while undergoing treatment.

LEUKEMIA AND HODGKIN'S. Leukemia is the most common cancer in children. It affects the bone marrow which produces blood cells (see Chapter 20). Victims become pale, tired, anemic, and easily prone to infection. Hodgkin's disease is a cancer of the lymph nodes. Symptoms may include weight loss, fever, night sweats, and anemia. Today, most cases of leukemia and Hodgkin's disease can be effectively treated.

Figure 22–13

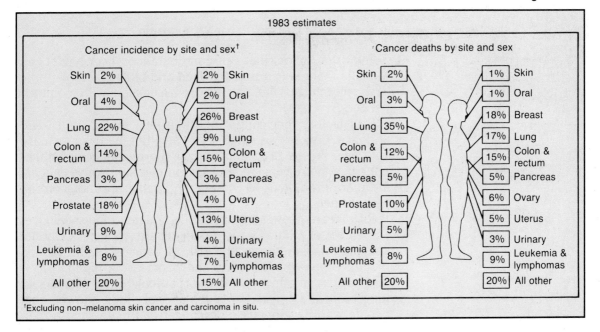

1983 estimates

Cancer incidence by site and sex[†]

	Male		Female	
Skin	2%		2%	Skin
Oral	4%		2%	Oral
			26%	Breast
Lung	22%		9%	Lung
Colon & rectum	14%		15%	Colon & rectum
Pancreas	3%		3%	Pancreas
Prostate	18%		4%	Ovary
			13%	Uterus
Urinary	9%		4%	Urinary
Leukemia & lymphomas	8%		7%	Leukemia & lymphomas
All other	20%		15%	All other

Cancer deaths by site and sex

	Male		Female	
Skin	2%		1%	Skin
Oral	3%		1%	Oral
			18%	Breast
Lung	35%		17%	Lung
Colon & rectum	12%		15%	Colon & rectum
Pancreas	5%		5%	Pancreas
Prostate	10%		6%	Ovary
			5%	Uterus
Urinary	5%		3%	Urinary
Leukemia & lymphomas	8%		9%	Leukemia & lymphomas
All other	20%		20%	All other

[†]Excluding non–melanoma skin cancer and carcinoma in situ.

RISK FACTORS FOR COMMON CANCERS

Type of Cancer	Risk Factors
Lung cancer	Heavy cigarette smoking, history of smoking for 20 or more years, exposure to certain industrial substances, such as asbestos, particularly for those who smoke
Breast cancer	Over age 50, personal or family history of breast cancer, never had children, first child after age 30
Uterine cancer	For cervical cancer, early age at first intercourse, multiple sex partners; for endometrial cancer, history of infertility, failure of ovulation, prolonged estrogen therapy, late menopause, and the combination of diabetes, high blood pressure, and obesity
Colon and rectal cancer	Personal or family history of colon and rectal cancer, personal or family history of polyps in the colon or rectum, ulcerative colitis, low fiber diet
Skin cancer	Excessive exposure to the sun, fair complexion, occupational exposure to coal tar, pitch, creosote, arsenic compounds, and radium
Oral cancer	Heavy smoking and drinking, use of chewing tobacco

Table 22–1

CAN CANCER BE PREVENTED?

Several risk factors that can contribute to cancer have been identified. Some can be controlled and others cannot. Table 22-1 summarizes the risk-factors associated with common cancers.

Risk factors that cannot be controlled include age, sex, and race. Cancer can strike at any age, but the risks increase with age. Figure 22-13 summarizes the incidences of different types of cancers by sex. As you can see, some cancers are more prominent in women, and some are more prominent in men.

Risk factors that can be controlled relate to life-style. Over 75 percent of all lung cancer patients are smokers. Cigarette smoking also increases the risk of cancers of the larynx, mouth, esophagus, bladder, and pancreas. A high-fat, low-fiber diet is another risk factor, particularly for cancers of the colon and breast. An international study showed that people who developed colon cancer had many fats in their diets. Consider eating more fish, chicken, grains, beans, fruits, vegetables, and low-fat dairy products and fewer meats, eggs, and high-fat dairy products. Foods rich in vitamins C and A also seem to reduce the risks of cancer. It would also help to avoid drinking an excessive amount of alcohol. Heavy drinkers have a higher risk of developing cancers of the esophagus, mouth, throat, larynx, and liver.

A number of carcinogens are found in our environment. Asbestos, an insulation material, is a known cause of a cancer of the lining surrounding the lung. Sometimes carcinogens are found in the workplace. Overexposure to X rays increases risk of cancer. Experts suggest that you should try to minimize the number of X rays you receive. Overexposure to the sun has been linked to skin cancer. Shield yourself from the sun to avoid overexposure. You can read more about carcinogens in the environment in Chapter 24.

EARLY DETECTION

Early detection and treatment of cancer will greatly increase your chances of survival. It is estimated that cancer cures could be increased by 50 percent, saving an additional 128,000 lives a year, if everyone diagnosed as having cancer were treated early enough. For every six people who get cancer, two will be saved. One will die needlessly of a cancer that might have been cured if treated in time.

What are some warning signs of cancer? Table 22-2 lists the American Cancer Society's seven warning signs of cancer. *Caution* means be careful. These signals do not mean that you have cancer. In fact, 9 times out of 10, these signals are caused by a very minor illness. However, if you have a warning signal, see a doctor.

HOW IS CANCER TREATED?

Treatment of cancer is steadily improving. Some cancers can be treated more successfully than others, depending on the site. For example, cervical cancer can be detected in the early stages and cured. Lung cancer, on the other hand, is hard to detect early. Most often it is discovered after it has spread. Therefore cure rates for treatment are very low.

Surgery is often used to treat cancer. It is used for cancers of the breast, lung, digestive system, ovary, prostate, urinary system, and skin.

Table 22–2

CANCER'S SEVEN WARNING SIGNALS

Change in bowel or bladder habits
A sore that does not heal
Unusual bleeding or discharge
Thickening or lump in breast or elsewhere
Indigestion or difficulty in swallowing
Obvious change in wart or mole
Nagging cough or hoarseness

Radiation kills cells that are dividing rapidly. Therefore, it kills cancer cells. Radiation therapists give patients the exact dosages they need to kill cancer cells but not cause extensive damage to normal tissues.

Chemotherapy is becoming increasingly effective in stopping the progression of cancer. Some drugs block certain chemical changes in cancer cells. Others prevent cell division. Drugs often increase the effectiveness of radiation therapy and surgery.

A diagnosis of cancer often fills victims with fear and a sense of desperation. Because of these feelings, many are lured by promises of quick and easy cures. Do not let yourself or anyone you know fall into the hands of a cancer quack. They only sell false hopes and, tragically, many people who have cancer lose precious time when they turn to quacks for miracle cures.

OTHER MODERN HEALTH HAZARDS

DIABETES

Melanie has diabetes. Because her body cannot oxidize glucose normally, she must take daily injections of insulin. But Melanie is an honor student, class president, and a cheerleader. No one would suspect that she, along with an estimated 10 million other Americans, has **diabetes.**

TYPES OF DIABETES.   There are several types of diabetes. The most severe type is called **juvenile** or **insulin-dependent diabetes.** This type of diabetes can appear at any age, but usually first appears in childhood. It is due to a deficiency or failure of the pancreas to secrete insulin. Insulin is needed to burn glucose, which is needed by the body cells for energy. In some cases there can be an immune reaction, which blocks the action of insulin.

Most cases of diabetes are called **adult-onset** or **insulin-independent diabetes.** As the name implies, this type of diabetes usually appears between the ages of 40 and 60. It can usually be controlled by diet and exercise, and does not require insulin injections.

DETECTING DIABETES.   The symptoms of severe diabetes are loss of weight, excessive hunger and thirst, weakness, and frequent urination. All of these symptoms result from excess sugar in the blood. Water moves out of the body cells to dilute the levels of sugar in the blood. Kidneys work hard to remove this excess sugar and water. This leads to extreme thirst and frequent urination. In cases of severe diabetes, atherosclerosis and circulation problems in the feet and legs may occur. Mild diabetes is the most difficult to detect, because there are no obvious symptoms. Moderate and severe diabetes may be detected by the presence of glucose in the urine. In the case of milder diabetes, glucose often does not show in the urine. A blood glucose test, two hours after a meal, is valuable in detecting mild diabetes. Diabetes is a hereditary disease. If there are diabetics in your family, they should have periodic blood tests.

CONTROLLING DIABETES. With proper care, people with diabetes can live normal lives. Most young diabetics require insulin injections. Scientists have now produced a synthetic human insulin, a significant breakthrough that could benefit millions of diabetics. This insulin is superior to present animal insulin. It does not contain the impurities that cause allergic reactions in some diabetics.

For those who do not need insulin, diet, exercise, and weight loss alone will control diabetes. In fact, all cases of diabetes can be improved by following these suggestions. Exercise stimulates the production of insulin by the pancreas. In all cases, diet is important in controlling diabetes. Diets high in fats should be avoided. Diabetics are at higher risk of developing atherosclerosis, which is aggravated by a diet high in fats. In moderate or severe diabetes, a dietician or doctor can plan properly balanced meals that are low in sugar content. Recent studies have shown that a diet very high in fiber and complex carbohydrates (such as dried peas and beans and whole grains) is ideal for helping to control diabetes.

ARTHRITIS

Arthritis is not a major killer, but it is the nation's leading chronic disease that causes loss of normal function. Almost all of us will develop arthritis in at least one joint, if we live long enough.

Various arthritic conditions result in inflammation, swelling, aching, pain, and stiffness, most often in the joints. The many kinds of arthritis are difficult to diagnose and usually require extensive laboratory tests for proper identification.

Correct diagnosis is very important, since treatments vary with the cause and nature of the disorder.

RHEUMATOID ARTHRITIS.   We usually associate arthritis with older people, but **rheumatoid arthritis,** the most serious of the arthritic diseases, frequently appears in young people. This condition can become steadily worse, resulting in joint deformity and loss of function. Various drugs, such as aspirin, drugs related to cortisone, and gold injections, are prescribed to relieve symptoms. In addition to medication, there should be a period of rest each day, alternating with exercise of the joints involved. Rest is important in reducing inflammation, while exercise prevents deformity of the joints. Surgery on affected joints has been successful in restoring useful motion. Evidence is mounting that rheumatoid arthritis is an autoimmune disease. In other words, the body produces an antibody that acts against joints. Measures to counteract this antibody may lead to a cure.

OSTEOARTHRITIS. **Osteoarthritis** most often occurs beyond middle age. It often causes knobby enlargements of the end and middle joints of the fingers, and can also involve the hips, knees, and spine, resulting in pain, stiffness, and crippling in severe cases. The cause of osteoarthritis is not known. It seems to be an inherited condition in which cartilage is gradually destroyed and replaced with thickened bone deposits. The latest findings suggest that arthritis can be prevented by exercise. This builds strong bones, ligaments, and cartilage. Early medical treatment is necessary to prevent permanent damage to the joints. Treatment consists of aspirin and other drugs, and special exercises. Weight control is important to reduce strain on the hips, knees, and spine. In severe cases, joints may be replaced surgically.

GOUT.   **Gout** is a disease in which uric acid, an end product of amino-acid metabolism, accumulates in the blood. The uric-acid deposits settle in the kidney and form stones. Crystals of uric acid also deposit in and around joints, causing acute attacks of painful arthritis. Drug therapy is very effective for treating gout.

AGING

What does the term "old person" mean to you? "Young" and "old" are relative. You are old to a young child. A 60-year-old man may seem young to a person who is 85. Aging is a normal process that begins the moment we are born. After about age 27, the human body becomes less efficient and needs more care to keep it healthy. The heart, lungs, eyes, and ears become less efficient and the muscles, bones, and skin tissue begin to break down. But the way a person ages depends, in part, on their life-style and attitude toward living. There is growing evidence that people who remain physically and mentally active age much slower. Regular exercise is as important for the elderly as it is for other people. Arthritis, brittle bones, cardiovascular disease and other problems associated with old age can be improved through exercise, as well as other positive health habits.

Some people have the mistaken belief that senility, or loss of mental function with age, is unavoidable. Yet only 10 percent of people over 65 are afflicted. What causes senility? About 50 to 60 percent of people who are senile suffer from a disease known as **Alzheimer's disease.** It is an irreversible condition that is characterized by tangled nerve fibers and deposits in the brain, and a lack of a certain enzyme. It can strike both middle-aged and elderly people, usually causing death within 10 years. At present there is no cure for Alzheimer's disease, but research is underway to find effective treatments.

Small strokes, usually associated with high blood pressure, account for another 20 to 25 percent of all senility cases. Senility caused by small strokes can be prevented by detecting and treating high blood pressure. The remaining 10 to 20 percent of people who are senile have conditions that can be corrected. Their senility may be due to depression, reactions to drugs, nutritional deficiencies, and disease. People who are senile should be thoroughly examined by a doctor who specializes in aging. Relatives can benefit from counseling to help them care for a senile family member.

Loneliness and depression are feelings that many old people have to contend with. Physical ailments prevent many old people from leaving their houses. After retirement older people may feel useless, even though they still have a lot to contribute. These problems are made worse by the fact that we live in a youth-oriented society. Many people prefer to avoid older persons, and often they are kept hidden away. Activist groups of older citizens are calling attention to this situation. Since people are living longer today, there is a growing number of older citizens in this country. It is important that these growing numbers of elderly people continue to be valued and valuable members of society.

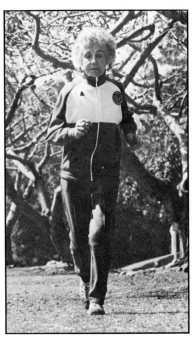

22–14. Eula Weaver, age 87, jogs a mile each day. Seven years ago she could only walk 100 feet.

FOCUS ON HEALTH

ORGAN TRANSPLANTS

About 25 human organs and tissues can now be transplanted. Transplants have saved the lives of thousands of people. Kidney transplantation is the most frequently performed organ transplant. Each year over 5,000 kidneys are transplanted. Corneal, heart valve, bone marrow, and cartilage transplants also have been performed successfully for the last 20 years. Corneal transplants have restored the sight of many whom have undergone cataract surgery. Bone marrow transplants have cured those with blood and immune deficiency diseases.

Survival rates of transplant patients have been steadily improving. This is due partly to advances in surgical techniques as well as the development of new antirejection drugs. Tissue rejection is one of the main problems in transplanting organs. Sometimes the tissues of the organ donor are not compatible with the tissues of the organ recipient. The recipient's immune system reacts to the donated organ as if it were an invader by producing antibodies against it. Antirejection drugs suppress the immune system to prevent rejection of the new organ.

There is a continuing shortage of donated organs that prevents many transplants from taking place. Tens of thousands of more lives could be saved if there were more donors. Every state has an Anatomical-Gift Act that allows people 18 and older to make provisions to donate their organs. This can be done in many states by filling out the donor card that is on the back of a driver's license.

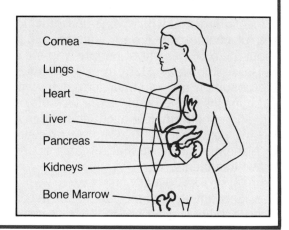

Cornea
Lungs
Heart
Liver
Pancreas
Kidneys
Bone Marrow

DEATH AND DYING

Part of living involves the experience of death: of losing our friends and relatives. This separation is a very difficult one and brings with it the feeling of grief, and sometimes anger because the person has left us. Though extremely painful, these feelings are very normal. Sometimes people try to avoid this pain by refusing to accept the separation. When not expressed, grief can then become a physical ailment, literally making the person sick. When grieving, it's hard to believe that the feeling will ever go away. It does leave with time.

People who are terminally ill have to learn how to face their own deaths, their own separations from those they love. A pioneer in the psychology of dying, Dr. Elizabeth Kubler-Ross, learned that there are 5 emotional stages that

478

UNIT 7   HEALTH PROMOTION AND PROTECTION

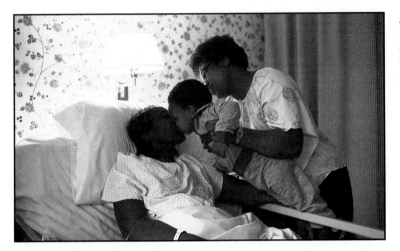

22–15. This woman, who has a terminal illness, is staying in a hospice where she can receive medical care while living in a more homelike setting.

dying people typically pass through. When survivors pass through the same stages, death is much more peaceful for all concerned. The stages she identified are: (1) denial: the person feels, "This can't be happening to me"; (2) anger: the person feels, "Why me?" and may feel angry and resentful and express this anger and frustration by lashing out at others; (3) bargaining: just as a child hopes to gain a special favor by being good, the dying patient bargains for a bit more time in return for the promise to change or alter one's life; (4) depression: the patient experiences grief and sorrow over the inevitable separation from life and loved ones that death brings; (5) acceptance: if death does not come suddenly and unexpectedly, the patient finally comes to grips with death and achieves a quiet acceptance and peace.

SUMMARY: Many major modern health hazards may begin in young people. Later in life, especially among people who engage in an unhealthy life-style, these hazards often result in cardiovascular diseases, including atherosclerosis, high blood pressure, heart attacks, and strokes. Although there have been major medical breakthroughs in curing these diseases, a wellness life-style is a better safeguard for your health. Cancer is the uncontrolled growth of cells which eventually crowd out normal cells. Treatments for cancer, including drugs, radiation, and surgery, are becoming more effective all the time. Diabetes and rheumatic diseases are other health hazards that affect a growing number of people. Understanding the natural processes of aging and death can make these experiences easier to handle.

CHAPTER REVIEW

words at work

Find the word in the left column that fits one of the definitions in the right column. DO NOT WRITE IN THIS BOOK.

a. angina pectoris
b. atherosclerosis
c. cancer
d. carcinogen
e. plaque
f. electrocardiogram
g. diabetes
h. hypertension
i. metastasis
j. osteoarthritis

1. Spread of cancer fragments from a large mass
2. Knobby enlargement of fingers, hips, and knees
3. Cancer-causing substance
4. High blood pressure
5. A severe pain around the heart
6. Caused by a buildup of plaque in vessel walls
7. An instrument that records heart impulses
8. A chronic disease resulting from insulin deficiency
9. A disorderly growth of body cells
10. A fatty, waxy substance

review questions

1. Cite statistics to illustrate the extent of cardiovascular disease.
2. Give some reasons why heart and blood-vessel diseases are the leading cause of death.
3. List five possible causes of high blood pressure.
4. What can you do to prevent high blood pressure?
5. Describe the causes and symptoms of atherosclerosis.
6. How does nitroglycerine relieve attacks of angina pectoris?
7. Explain what happens when a heart attack occurs.
8. What is an electrocardiogram?
9. How can you help to avoid a heart attack?
10. Describe stroke, give possible causes, and list measures for preventing strokes.
11. Outline possible treatments for heart failure.
12. Explain the meaning of congenital heart defects.
13. What is the principal significance of the use of the heart-lung machine?
14. Describe the function of the pacemaker.
15. To what do you attribute the remarkable reduction in the rate of death from cardiovascular disease?
16. How are cancer cells different from other body cells?

17. List several frequent sites of cancer.
18. Describe cancer's seven warning signals.
19. Review the possible causes of cancer.
20. How is cancer treated?
21. Explain how diabetes is detected.
22. Describe how diabetes can best be controlled.
23. Explain, in general, the term, "rheumatic disease."
24. Define *osteoarthritis* and list possible treatments.
25. Describe the process of aging and some of the changes that take place.

discussion questions

1. Discuss the importance of health education and individual responsibility in dealing with modern major health hazards.
2. Discuss the importance of early detection of these major health hazards.
3. Give several possible reasons for the advance of heart and blood-vessel diseases to first place among causes of death.

investigating

PURPOSE:
To play a game that explores risk-reduction measures for chronic diseases.

MATERIALS NEEDED:
Textbooks.

PROCEDURE:
A.   Review the risk factors associated with chronic diseases.
B.   Write the following categories on the chalkboard: nutrition, exercise, early detection, environment, and drug habits (smoking and drinking).
C.   As a class, divide into two teams, A and B. First team A should name a chronic disease, such as lung cancer. Then team B should choose one of the categories on the chalkboard, for example, drug habits. Then team B should state a drug habit that is a risk for lung cancer, and a measure that can be taken to reduce the risk. For example, "Smoking increases your risk of lung cancer. Quitting smoking can reduce this risk."
D.   If team B cannot answer correctly, team A has a chance to do so. Whichever team answers correctly first gets one point. Your textbook or other resource information can be used to document the correct answers.
E.   The team that loses chooses the next category.

CHAPTER 23

Infectious Diseases and the Immune System

OBJECTIVES

- STATE organisms that cause disease
- COMPARE methods of disease transmission
- DESCRIBE some common infectious diseases
- EXPLAIN body defenses against disease

- DESCRIBE the use of immunization and chemotherapy against disease
- LIST some autoimmune and immune-deficiency diseases

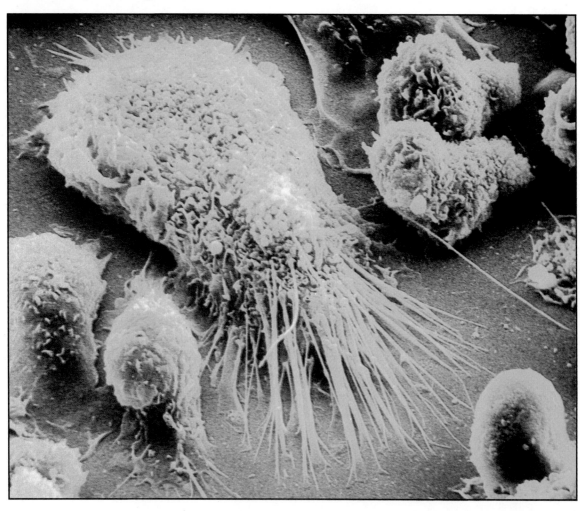

In the fourteenth century, an epidemic of the bubonic plague or "Black Death" caused 25 million deaths, about one-third of the world's population at that time. In 1665, another plague epidemic struck London causing more than 30,000 deaths. It is now known that the fleas from infected black rats carried the plague bacteria to humans.

Plague is rare today, as are cholera and yellow fever. Better sanitation, vaccination, and medication have helped to nearly eradicate these diseases.

Have we won the battle against infectious diseases? Not yet. Pneumonia is still one of the ten leading causes of death. The number of cases of sexually transmitted diseases has been rising throughout the world. Recently a new mysterious disease called AIDS has been in the headlines. These facts demonstrate the impact that infectious diseases still have in today's world.

INFECTIOUS AGENTS

The body is engaged in a constant battle against trillions of tiny invaders. Most of them are so small that they cannot be seen without the aid of a microscope. Thus, they are called *microorganisms*, or "microbes." These invaders that cause disease are also known as **pathogens.** They are always ready to attack by way of the air we breathe, the water we drink, the food we eat, and through the slightest break in our skin.

BACTERIA

Bacteria outnumber all other forms of life combined. They can live anywhere that life can exist. They can even live in some places where other organisms cannot exist. Bacteria float in the upper atmosphere and are found in the ocean depths. They are abundant in the soil, water, air, food, and in the bodies of other organisms. Fortunately, MOST bacteria are harmless, and many are even beneficial to humans. For example, they are used to make cheese, yogurt, wine, and vinegar. Only a few bacteria invade our bodies and cause disease. Typhoid fever, pneumonia, and botulism are some examples of diseases caused by bacteria.

A single bacterial cell consists of a small mass of living substance enclosed in a thin protective cell wall. They do not have a definite nucleus. Their genetic material is distributed throughout the cell.

23–1. Bacteria are used to make a wide variety of cheeses.

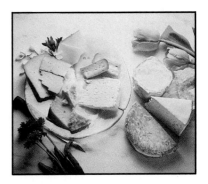

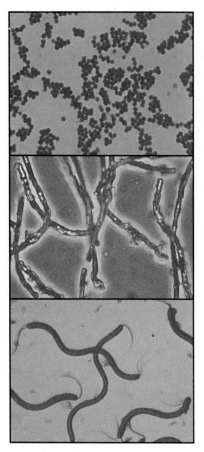

23–2. From top to bottom, coccus, bacillus, and spirillum bacteria, magnified about 600 times.

There are three basic shapes among bacteria: (1) **Coccus** bacteria are spherical. These may be grouped in long chains like beads, joined in pairs, or clustered like grapes. (2) **Bacillus** bacteria are rod-shaped and may form chains of rods, resembling strings of sausages. (3) **Spirillum** bacteria cells are in the form of twisted rods, like corkscrews (see Figure 23-2).

One of the most amazing facts about bacteria is the rate at which they multiply. A cell, after reaching full size, divides and forms two new cells. Under ideal conditions, divisions may occur every 30 minutes. Consider what this rate of multiplication actually means. If we start with a single bacterial cell, in 30 minutes this cell divides and becomes two. A half hour later, this number becomes four. At this rate there would be 16,777,216 bacteria at the end of 12 hours! Fortunately, this rate of multiplication continues for only a short time. Bacteria in a growing mass compete with each other for food and other requirements for life. Many bacteria are eliminated in the competition. If bacteria did not compete, they would soon cover the earth.

When temperature, moisture, and other environmental conditions are not suitable for growth, some species of bacteria can survive by becoming inactive or dormant. Some bacteria become *spores* by surrounding themselves with a tough, resistant wall. Spores can endure such extreme conditions as dryness, low temperature, and even boiling water. When conditions are again favorable for growth, they begin growing and multiplying.

Have you ever gone to the doctor for a puncture wound? The doctor probably gave you a tetanus shot. Tetanus bacteria can form spores. These spores are common on many objects, such as rusty nails. If an object contaminated with these spores punctures your skin, the spores will quickly begin to grow and release poisons into your body. A tetanus shot contains an *antitoxin* that neutralizes these poisons.

VIRUSES

The common cold is an example of a disease caused by a virus. Viruses are the smallest of the disease-producing organisms. They must be magnified 100,000 times in order to be seen.

Are viruses living organisms or nonliving particles? Like nonliving particles, a virus has no nucleus, cytoplasm, nor cell membrane. But, like living organisms, virus particles do

484

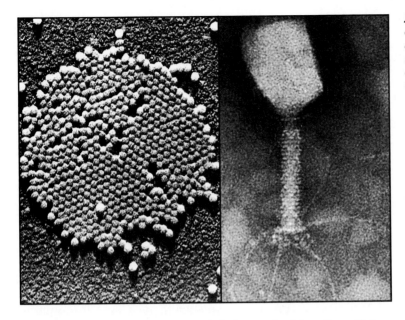

23–3. *Two different types of viruses as seen through an electron microscope: left) a type of polio virus, and right) a bacterial virus, or phage*

have a core of genetic material. Once inside other living cells, they can grow and reproduce. Therefore, they are usually classified as living.

All viruses are parasites since they can only survive inside living cells for their growth and reproduction. When a virus invades a living cell, it takes control of the cell. For example, if a virus cell gains entry into a bacterial cell, the bacteria will stop producing its own substances. Amazingly, the bacteria will become a virus factory and produce new virus particles (see Figure 23-3).

Each type of virus is highly specific in the kind of cell it attacks. Certain kinds of viruses invade only bacteria, while others require the cells of plants as their hosts. Still others invade animal and human cells.

Most types of viruses only invade a specific kind of tissue in their hosts. Altogether more than 50 viruses are known to cause infections in the human body. Many types of virus particles appear to be harmless, even though they are present in bacteria, plants, animals, and humans.

PROTOZOA AND FUNGI

Protozoans are one-celled animals. They are much larger than bacteria and more complex in their cellular structure. Many protozoans are harmless. Those that cause disease thrive in tropical areas that have poor sanitation.

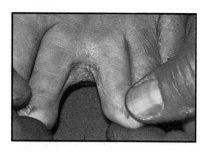

23–4. Athelete's foot is a common fungus disease.

23–5. The tapeworm head (top). What is the purpose of the hooks? One kind of tapeworm can reach a length of 3 meters (10 ft).

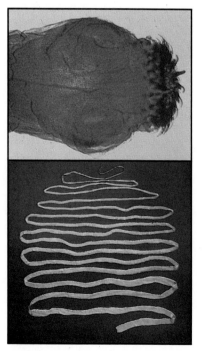

A severe disease of the intestinal tract, **amoebic dysentery,** is an example of a disease caused by a protozoan. Another protozoan causes malaria. This organism, carried by the female *Anopheles* mosquito, lives in the blood of humans, destroying red blood corpuscles.

Fungi are primitive plants that include yeast and molds. Pathogenic fungi affect nails, skin, hair, and lungs. **Ringworm** is one of the most common infectious fungal diseases. Ringworm gets its name from its ringlike growth when it infects the scalp. Another common fungus causes **athlete's foot.**

PARASITIC WORMS

The agents of disease mentioned so far are all microscopic. A discussion of causative agents of disease would not be complete, however, without reference to a group of larger, many-celled animals: the parasitic worms.

Parasitic worms are severe health problems in countries and areas with poor sanitation and contaminated food and water. Even in some areas of the United States, these organisms are a serious health problem.

The **hookworm,** a round worm of the southern states and all semitropical and tropical regions, is a serious health menace. Young worms develop in the soil from eggs, which are in the feces of infected animals. The worms enter the human body by boring through the skin of bare feet. They find their way to the intestine, where they fasten themselves to the wall and grow to adult worms. The worms suck blood from the intestine and inflict wounds in the intestinal wall. Loss of blood lowers the victim's strength, producing a characteristic fatigue. Rectal itching is caused by female hookworms that lay their eggs at night in the rectal area. It is reported that more than 1 million persons in the United States, mostly children, are infested with hookworm.

The **tapeworm** is the best known of the parasitic flatworms. An adult tapeworm has a flat, ribbonlike body, grayish white in color. The small knob-shaped head is equipped with suckers and hooks. Tapeworms enter the human body when a person eats insufficiently cooked pork or beef. In the human intestine, digested food is absorbed directly into the tapeworm, robbing the person of nourishment. If human wastes containing tapeworm eggs are eaten by hogs or cattle, the eggs become worms, which burrow into the muscles of these animals.

The **trichina worm** is one of the most dangerous of the parasitic roundworms. It passes its first stage in the muscles of the pig, dog, rat, or cat. Pork is infested when pigs are fed uncooked garbage, or if pigs eat rats that are also infested. The worms reproduce in the intestine, producing as many as 10,000 from a single worm. The young bore through the intestine and enter the bloodstream. Later they leave the blood vessels and enter the muscles, producing the painful and often fatal disease *trichinosis*. The best way to prevent this disease and other parasitic worm infestations found in meat is to cook all meat thoroughly, especially pork.

SPREADING DISEASES

Do you know what an **epidemic** is? Whenever the number of new cases of disease incidence exceeds the normal average, an epidemic exists. Most outbreaks of infectious diseases do not become epidemics. Today, doctors have highly effective weapons for fighting infectious diseases once they have struck. However, it is far better to prevent infections. Many infectious diseases can be avoided by understanding how microbes are spread and how they enter the body. Precautions can then be taken.

AIRBORNE INFECTIONS

Microbes that infect the nasal passages, sinuses, throat, trachea, and lungs are present in saliva and mucus. A sneeze or a cough can spray a mist of germ-laden droplets into the air. **Droplet infection** is a serious health problem. In nearly every public place, people cough and sneeze. A situation like this is difficult to control.

The number of respiratory infections could be reduced greatly if everyone realized the danger of droplet infection. When you have an infection, you should try to protect others from it. During a sneeze or a cough, the nose and mouth should be covered with disposable tissue. It has been found that when droplets get on the hands, they can infect others through hand-to-hand contact. Washing hands frequently during a cold may prevent infecting others with the virus. Neglecting a severe cold or sore throat is hazardous to you as well as to those around you. A neglected cold can progress to pneumonia. A sore throat may become tonsillitis. Strep throat can be followed by rheumatic fever, acute nephritis, or other serious complications.

23–6. To prevent droplet infection, always cover your mouth when you sneeze.

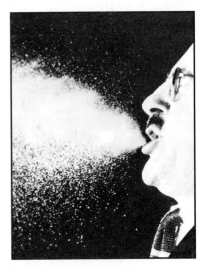

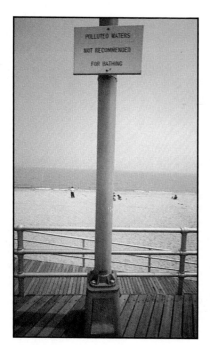

23–7. Swimming in polluted water can lead to typhoid fever, dysentery, and other intestinal infections.

WATERBORNE INFECTIONS

Typhoid fever, dysentery, and other intestinal infections are spread through water polluted with sewage. Fortunately, most cities and towns in our country supply drinking water safe from microbes. Chemical treatment and improved community sanitation have made this possible. However, large numbers of people in suburban and rural areas depend on wells for their water supply. If contamination is suspected in wells, water should be tested by the Public Health Department to be sure that it is safe to drink.

Many cities prohibit swimming in nearby streams and rivers because of water pollution. Some inland lakes are posted as unfit for swimming. The water in public swimming pools is regularly filtered and chlorinated. Even then, summer crowds may raise the bacterial content of the water to a dangerous level. Infections of the ear, nasal passages, sinuses, and throat are commonly spread in swimming pools. For this reason, public health officials frequently check chlorine levels in municipal swimming pools to help prevent the spread of disease.

FOOD-BORNE INFECTIONS

Diseases such as typhoid, dysentery, and other intestinal infections can be caused by eating contaminated foods. Many advances in the food industry have greatly reduced the danger of food-borne infections. Sanitary packaging, freezing, drying, canning, and other methods of preservation have reduced the danger of contamination and spoilage during transportation and storage. Even cooking destroys many infectious microbes. Fresh foods eaten raw should always be washed thoroughly.

Milk, in addition to being an ideal food for humans, is also an ideal food for many pathogens. Disease-causing organisms can get into milk in various ways. They may be present in milk taken from infected cows. Others are introduced by flies, contaminated milking equipment, or infected handlers. Mastitis and a form of tuberculosis can infect cattle and can be spread to humans through milk.

Pasteurization, a heating process, destroys most of the bacteria present in milk. Immediately after pasteurization, the milk is cooled and placed in bottles or cartons. Pasteurized milk is not entirely free of bacteria. However, the few organisms surviving the process do not cause human infections. Pasteurized milk is healthful, easy to digest, and far safer than raw milk. Since many milk-souring bacteria are destroyed by heat, pasteurized milk also sours more slowly than raw milk.

DISEASES BORNE BY INSECTS, TICKS, AND MITES

Insects, ticks, and mites carry diseases in many different ways. In one method, the pathogenic organism undergoes a complicated life cycle involving an insect in certain stages and a human in others. The insect involved is referred to as an *intermediate host*. Malaria is an example. The malaria organism, a protozoan, is transmitted to humans by the bite of an infected female *Anopheles* mosquito. As the mosquito pierces the skin, malaria organisms are injected into the blood of the victim. Certain stages of the life cycle of the malaria organisms then occur in the blood of the human victim. Red blood cells are destroyed, causing the characteristic chills and fever. To complete the life cycle, a mosquito must draw blood from an infected person. Then the malaria organisms spend the other stages of their life cycle in the mosquito.

The African sleeping sickness organism undergoes a similar life cycle, involving an intermediate stage in the tsetse fly. This is also the manner in which the *Aëdes* mosquito transmits yellow fever, the rat flea carries bubonic plague and typhus, the body louse carries epidemic typhus and trench fever, and the tick transmits Rocky Mountain spotted fever.

The housefly and the cockroach are examples of mechanical carriers of various infectious organisms. In this method, the insect travels from a source of infection, like sewage and garbage, to a person or to foods and articles that the person handles. Microbes are carried on the sticky feet or on the bodies of mechanical carriers.

Control of insect-borne infections depends on getting rid of the insects that carry them.

HUMAN CARRIERS

Many infections are transmitted from one person to another by direct contact through an infection on the body surface or a body opening. Among diseases spread in this way are boils and abscesses, impetigo, pinkeye, and sexually transmitted diseases.

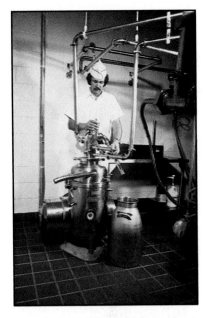

23–8. Milk processing is necessary to destroy disease-causing organisms.

Certain other infectious diseases may be transmitted by human carriers who do not have symptoms of the disease. Typhoid is a well-known example. Asymptomatic carriers of typhoid are immune to the disease, but they harbor typhoid organisms in their gallbladders. Without knowing it, they may spread the disease to others who are not immune. In the mid-1800s one such carrier, known as "Typhoid Mary," was responsible for at least 10 outbreaks of typhoid fever that involved 100,000 people. She worked in restaurants and spread the disease through the food that she handled. Dysentery, another intestinal infection, may be spread by human carriers. Other infectious diseases associated with immune carriers include polio, diphtheria, and scarlet fever. Sometimes it is difficult for the public health department to locate immune carriers of these diseases.

SOME INFECTIOUS DISEASE PROBLEMS

In Table 23-1, you will find some important information about the most common infectious diseases today. Some of those that are especially important to know about are reviewed below.

INFLUENZA AND PNEUMONIA

As the sixth leading cause of death, **influenza** and **pneumonia** are the most serious infectious diseases today. They take their highest toll among the very old, the very young, and those suffering from chronic diseases such as heart, lung, and liver diseases. Among these high-risk populations, an attack of the flu is likely to lead to pneumonia. This is because the flu can weaken their bodies, opening the way for infections such as pneumonia. Those in the high-risk groups are advised to receive influenza vaccinations at least once each year.

HEPATITIS

Hepatitis is a serious viral infection of the liver. The virus destroys liver cells, causing bile to enter the bloodstream. This produces a jaundice, or yellowing of the skin. Other symptoms include fever, general weakness, headache, nausea, vomiting, and tenderness in the liver area.

UNIT 7   HEALTH PROMOTION AND PROTECTION

One form, caused by virus A, is known as *infectious hepatitis*, or hepatitis A. Symptoms, such as jaundice and severe fatigue, appear in 18 to 40 days after infection. The infection is transmitted through direct human contact or by food (such as shellfish) or water that has been contaminated with the intestinal wastes of a person harboring the virus. During the infection, the virus is in the bloodstream and intestines of the patient. Active virus can remain in the body for an indefinite period after recovery, thus producing a dangerous carrier situation.

Treatment for infectious hepatitis consists of bed rest, often for several weeks, and a diet high in carbohydrates and proteins but low in fats. Although the mortality rate is less than .5 percent, recovery is very slow. The liver often remains enlarged and tender for many weeks. Adequate sewage disposal and protection of the food and water supply are important in preventing this infection. Personal cleanliness is another important preventive measure.

Another form of the infection, caused by virus B and classified as *serum hepatitis*, or hepatitis B, results from a transfusion of contaminated human blood. The infection usually appears within 60 to 120 days. This problem has been partially controlled today by rejecting any blood donor who has ever been jaundiced. However, serum hepatitis is prevalent among drug addicts who use needles passed from one person to another.

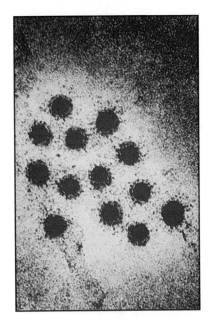

23–9. The hepatitis A virus, magnified 166,600 times

MONONUCLEOSIS

Mononucleosis, or mono, is a common viral disease among teenagers and young adults. It is sometimes called the "kissing disease" since kissing is one way it is transmitted. But it can also be transmitted through the communal use of cooking and eating utensils and by blood transfusions. Symptoms may include aching joints, fever, swollen glands, weakness, fatigue, and general discomfort. Mono does not usually cause permanent damage. Contrary to what many people think, recuperation usually requires only a few weeks. The only way to be sure that you have the disease is by getting a diagnostic laboratory test.

SEXUALLY TRANSMITTED DISEASES (STD)

The incidence of STDs has been rising throughout the world, especially in this country. People at high risk for STDs are those who are sexually active with multiple partners. There

INFECTIOUS DISEASES

Disease	Cause	How Spread	Usual Infection Site
Athlete's foot	Various fungi	Contact with contaminated floors	Feet, especially between toes
Chicken pox	Virus (Varicella Zoster)	Direct contact droplets or airborne	General and skin
Diphtheria	Toxigenic strain of C. Diphtheria	Droplets infected articles	Throat, upper trachea
Dysentery bacillary	Bacillus	Infected food and water	Intestinal tract
Gonorrhea	Bacterium Neisseria gonorrhea	Direct sexual contact with infected person	Mucous membranes, genital organs
Hepatitis	Viruses of hepatitis A and B	Contaminated food, water, syringes, or blood	Liver and bloodstream
Herpes simplex	Herpes simplex viruses I and II	Contact	Lips (HSV-I) Genitals (HSV-II)
Impetigo	Streptococcus or staphylococcus	Contact with lesions or infected articles	Face, less often hands
Influenza	Virus, usually A or B	Droplet infection	Respiratory organs
Malaria	Protozoan (four distinct species of Plasmodia)	Bite of infected female Anopheles mosquito	Bloodstream, especially red blood corpuscles
Measles, red (rubeola)	Virus	Droplets and nasal discharge, contact	Upper respiratory tract
Measles, German (rubella)	Virus	Droplet infection, contact	Respiratory organs
Meningitis	Variety of organisms	Droplet and contact with discharges	Brain; meninges or lining
Mononucleosis infections (glandular fever)	Virus, probably	Droplets from nose and throat and direct contact	Lymph glands
Mumps (epidemic parotitis)	Virus	Droplet infection and direct contact	Parotid salivary glands
Pneumonia(s)	Bacteria, several viruses	Droplets; may follow other virus infections	Lungs
Poliomyelitis	Virus types 1, 2, 3	Contact with discharges from nose and throat	Spinal cord and motor nerve roots
Rabies (hydrophobia)	Virus	Saliva of infected animals	Central nervous system and brain substances
Scarlet fever and other streptococcal diseases	Beta Hemolytic streptoccoli Group A	Direct and indirect contact with discharge	Throat (portals of entry)
Syphilis	Spirochete (Treporema pallidum)	Sexual contact	Genitals, then blood, then any organ in body
Tetanus (lockjaw)	Bacterium (Ci tetani)	Puncture wound	Wound
Tuberculosis	Bacterium (mycobacterium tuberculosis)	Droplet infection, sputum	Lungs
Typhoid fever	Bacterium (Salmonella typhi)	Contaminated water, food, carriers	Large intestine, bloodstream
Whooping cough (pertussis)	Bacterium (Bordetella pertussis)	Droplet infection, contact	Lower respiratory organs

Table 23–1

UNIT 7 HEALTH PROMOTION AND PROTECTION

Symptoms and Signs	Treatment	Immunity
Cracks and itching, sores	Fungicides, change socks frequently	None
Mild fever, skin eruptions in different stages	Relief of itching and prevention of infection	Permanent after recovery; no immunization
Sore throat, pain, fever	Antitoxin and antibiotics	Permanent after recovery; toxoid
Abdominal pain, severe diarrhea	Antibiotics and fluid replacement	Immunity after recovery
Burning on urination, pus discharge from genitalia	Antibiotics	None
Jaundice, fever, nausea, pain over liver	Rest, fat-free diet, high in carbohydrates and proteins	Gamma globulin (passive)
Painful blisters	Acyclovir ointment	None
Circular, raised, crusted lesions, usually on face	Antibiotic creams	None
Fever, sore throat, aching	Bed rest, force fluids, aspirin	Vaccine effective few months only
Attacks of chills, high fever and sweats	Quinine Chloroquine	Possible temporary to one type after recovery
Fever, cough, red swollen eyes, rash	Bed rest, eye care, antibiotics for complications	Permanent after recovery; vaccine could eliminate
Slight fever, swollen glands, rash	Bed rest until rash has faded	Permanent after recovery; vaccine
Headaches, fever, nausea	Depends on organism; antibiotics when indicated	Strain specific; vaccine for some forms
Enlargement of lymph glands, spleen, fever	Bed rest, antibiotics	None
Swelling of parotid glands and complications	Local applications; gamma globulin	Permanent after recovery; vaccine
Fatigue, muscle pain, cough, chills, fever	Antiobiotics if bacterial; none if viral	Vaccine for pneumonia
Headache, stiff neck, fever, paralysis of limbs	Therapy to regain use of limbs	Permanent after recovery; Sabin (oral) vaccine
Convulsions, spasms, general paralysis	Series of injections	Vaccine
Sore throat, fever, chills, bright scarlet rash second day	Antibiotics effective	Usually permanent after recovery
Primary lesion in form of sore	Antibiotics	None
Muscle spasms	Antitoxin	Toxoid gives protection 10 years
Cough, weight loss, fever, chest pain	Antibiotics, especially streptomycin; chemotherapy	BCG vaccine in special cases
Fever, abdominal pain, bloody diarrhea	Antibiotics	Permanent following recovery; vaccine
Cough followed by a "whoop"	Antibiotics, bed rest	Permanent after recovery; vaccine

are at least 20 infectious diseases that are sexually transmitted. Those of major importance in the U.S. are syphilis, gonorrhea, chlamydia, and herpes simplex type II. Until now there has been little understanding of the significance of STDs. All are preventable and most are curable. One of the big dangers of STDs is that people do not report it. Therefore, they have become more widespread. Only 10 to 20 percent of all venereal diseases are reported. The initial symptoms of syphilis, chlamydia, and gonorrhea disappear in the normal course of the disease. People then mistakenly believe that they are cured. The diseases themselves do not disappear. They can cause severe damage unless treated.

Untreated gonorrhea and chlamydia can cause sterility, arthritis, heart disease, and blindness. Untreated syphilis can cause sterility, crippling, paralysis, heart disease, blindness, severe brain damage, and death. Genital herpes may be the cause of cervical cancer in women. Sexually transmitted diseases have devastating effects on unborn children. A mother's untreated gonorrhea can infect a baby's eyes during birth, and cause blindness. Chlamydia is the most common cause of infant eye infection and infant pneumonia. An unborn child can be infected with syphilis. The baby may appear healthy at first, but heart defects and deformity may appear in childhood. A baby can be infected with herpes simplex during birth. A baby who survives a severe infection suffers physical and mental damage.

GONORRHEA. Gonorrhea is a very common bacterial infection in adults. Since 1957 there has been a rapidly increasing incidence of the disease. It is estimated that it strikes some 3 million Americans each year.

Gonococcus, the bacteria that causes gonorrhea, cannot live outside of the human body. Therefore, intimate sexual contact is the only way in which it is transmitted. Initial signs usually develop within 3 or 4 days following contact. Men usually experience a burning sensation when urinating. A pus-like discharge from the penis may also be observed. The burning when urinating is also a symptom of a urinary infection. A lab test is the only way to determine whether or not the infection is gonorrhea. Eighty percent of women who are infected do not experience any early symptoms. They usually do not experience any discomfort until several months after contact, when pelvic organs become inflamed. This serious condition is called *pelvic inflammatory disease* (PID). If untreated, PID can lead to scarring of the female reproductive organs and sterility.

The treatment for gonorrhea requires penicillin injections. Other antibiotics are used for those who have developed an allergy to penicillin.

CHLAMYDIA.   Until recently, the incidence of chlamydia was unknown because there was no simple, inexpensive test to detect the infection. Now that a simple diagnostic test is available, it has been found that chlamydia is even more common than gonorrhea. Symptoms resemble mild gonorrhea and appear from one to five weeks after contact. If untreated, it can also cause pelvic inflammatory disease in women, and sterility in both men and women.

SYPHILIS.   Syphilis is not as common as gonorrhea, but it is a much more severe disease. The spirochete bacterium that causes syphilis dies in about 30 seconds outside the human body. Direct sexual contact is almost always the method by which it is transmitted.

There are several different stages of the infection. The symptoms of *primary syphilis* are usually evident about 3 weeks after contact. A *chancre*, or open sore, appears on the skin or mucous membrane, where the spirochete first entered the body. Many infected people pass through this stage of the infection without being aware of it. The chancre disappears by itself, but the disease is still present in the body. The symptoms of *secondary syphilis* appear as early as three weeks or as late as six months after the primary symptoms. Symptoms vary from one person to the next, but the most common are a non-itchy rash, headache, mild fever, sore throat, and loss of hair. Also, infectious lesions may appear on the mucous membranes of the body. These symptoms eventually disappear, but the infection continues its course of destruction. In *latent syphilis*, the spirochete settles down into clusters in various parts of the body. No symptoms are evident and the person infected may feel normal for years. However, during this stage syphilis does the most damage to the internal organs, nervous system, and bones.

If syphilis is untreated, chronic disabling conditions develop during the stage called *late syphilis*. Paralysis, blindness, mental disturbances, and cardiac disorders may result. Whenever an infection is suspected, seek medical treatment at once. The earlier stages are much easier to treat than the late stages. Penicillin is the preferred medication for all stages of syphilis.

HERPES SIMPLEX, TYPES I AND II.   Herpes simplex type I is a very common virus. In fact, a large percentage of the

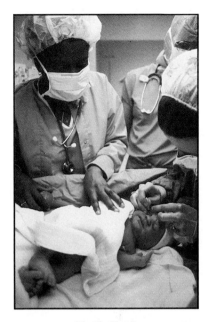

23–10. Newborns receive silver nitrate eye drops to prevent blindness caused by possible gonorrhea infection.

23–11. The respiratory tract has cells with hair-like structures called cilia that move mucus up toward the throat.

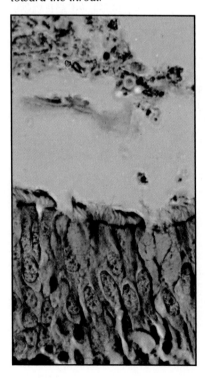

population harbors this virus in their bodies. It is usually in a dormant state until the body becomes rundown, due to a cold or other infection. Then the virus becomes active, and cold sores appear.

Symptoms of herpes simplex type II appear about 1 week after sexual contact with an infected person. There is usually minor itching or rash in the genital area. Later, blisterlike lesions may form, causing intense itching and pain. Other symptoms may include painful urination, swollen lymph nodes, and general fatigue. The symptoms last 2 to 3 weeks and then disappear. The virus then becomes dormant. Periodically the disease becomes active again, causing lesions to reappear. The virus can easily be transmitted from open blisters. If you have open blisters, be very careful not to infect others or to infect other sites of your own body. Do not touch the blisters, unless applying medicine. Then immediately wash your hands. A new medicine called *Acyclovir* does not cure herpes, but can shorten the duration of the blisters.

BODY DEFENSES

As you have learned, your body constantly battles with pathogens that seek to invade it, thereby causing disease. However, if you come in contact with pathogens, you do not necessarily become ill. You have three lines of defense against pathogens that keep you from becoming their victim.

STRUCTURAL DEFENSES: THE FIRST LINE

Before pathogens cause disease, they must gain entry into your body. You have several built-in structural defenses to prevent this. Your skin provides a protective shield over most of your body. Unless it is broken by a wound, insect or animal bite, or burns, it is practically germ-proof.

Body openings, especially the mouth and nose, are strategic points of entry for invading pathogens. They are protected by mucous membranes, which prevent pathogens from entering the body. Mucus secreted by the lining of the respiratory passages forms a sticky coating. When pathogens are breathed in, they are trapped in this sticky mucus. The invading pathogens can then be forced out by coughing or sneezing, before they reach the lungs.

The lining of the windpipe is also equipped with tiny hairs called *cilia*. Cilia beat together and carry mucus from the lungs up the windpipe. Pathogens stuck in the mucus are also carried up to the throat, and then are swallowed along with the mucus.

If pathogens reach the stomach, most are destroyed by stomach acid. However, some pathogens may survive and enter the intestines. Digestive enzymes and mucus in the intestines usually prevent the pathogens from growing. The presence of many non-pathogenic bacteria also prevents the growth of pathogens. When an infection does develop in the digestive tract, it is often accompanied by vomiting, diarrhea, or both. These reactions are the body's effort to rid itself of the invading pathogens.

Tears also play an important defensive role. They contain antibacterial substances that destroy many bacteria and wash them from the eyes.

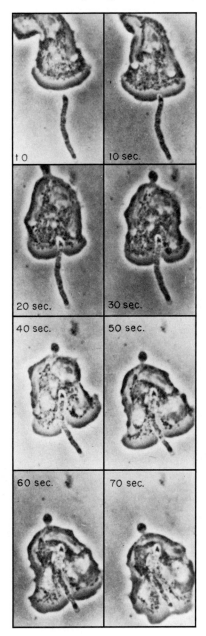

23–12. A phagocyte injesting a bacterial cell

CELLULAR DEFENSES: THE SECOND LINE

When pathogens penetrate the first line of defense, they invade body tissues, and the body responds by calling forth its second line of defense. Blood vessels dilate, causing an increased blood flow to the infected area. This causes the reddening you see around the infection. The increased flow of blood brings white blood cells to the area. The first white blood cells to arrive at the scene are *phagocytes*, which devour the bacteria (see photo on page 482). The area becomes filled with pus, a mass of living and dead pathogens and white blood cells. The lymph system, made up of lymphatic vessels and lymph nodes, also plays a part in destroying invading pathogens. Tissue fluid around an infection is picked up by lymph vessels. Then the lymph vessels transport this fluid, containing pathogens, to the lymph nodes. Here phagocytes capture and destroy the pathogens, thus preventing them from entering the bloodstream.

When a doctor checks your lymph glands for swelling, he or she is looking for infection somewhere in your body. Healthy tonsils, which are actually lymph glands, are valuable filters for clearing infected materials from nose and throat infections.

You can see why second-line defenses are so important. If an infection can be conquered in the tissues, your body is spared a more serious struggle. On the other hand, if these defenses are overpowered, the third line of defenses enters the battle.

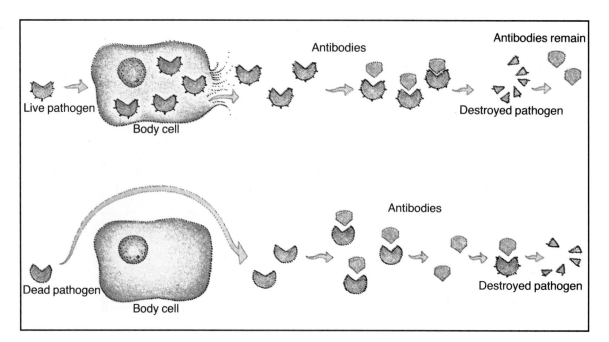

23–13. *Natural immunization occurs when an infectious pathogen enters the body cells. The pathogen multiplies and attacks other cells. The body responds by producing antibodies to destroy the invader. Artificial immunization occurs when a dead or weakened pathogen is introduced into the body by vaccination. The body responds by producing antibodies to destroy the invader. These antibodies remain to destroy live pathogens of the same type that might later enter the body.*

In the diagram: Live pathogen, Body cell, Antibodies, Antibodies remain, Destroyed pathogen; Dead pathogen, Body cell, Antibodies, Destroyed pathogen.

CHEMICAL IMMUNITY: THE THIRD LINE

Your body's third line of defense involves the production of **antibodies.** Antibodies are chemicals that the body produces in the presence of foreign substances, called **antigens.** Antigens can be toxins released by pathogens, or parts of the outside surfaces of the pathogens. Antibodies attach themselves to these antigens, which inactivates or destroys the pathogen. Each antibody will only react to its specific antigen (see Figure 23-13).

After the invading pathogen is destroyed, some antibodies remain in the body. If the pathogen ever gains entry into the body again, the antibodies for it are already present in the body. They immediately attach to their antigens, which prevents the disease from developing. Thus, your body has developed an **immunity** to this specific pathogen.

LYMPHOCYTES.   The chemical immune system is one of the most complex organizations within the human body. In recent years, scientists have been trying to unravel how this defense system works, in order to better understand the causes and cures of several diseases.

It is known that chemical immunity to specific pathogens is made possible by the **lymphocytes,** another kind of white

498

blood cell. They are the principal warriors of the immune system. There are about 15 billion lymphocytes in your body. They are made in the bone marrow and the thymus, but most of them then migrate to the lymph nodes. Besides the staggering number of lymphocytes present in your body, there are also several different types. Most are in an inactive state. When a specific antigen enters the body, some are activated. They begin multiplying and then they change into several different types of lymphocytes. Many scientists are studying the complex interactions of the immune system. Many are convinced that the key to using the immune system to fight cancer and other diseases lies in understanding how the whole system works.

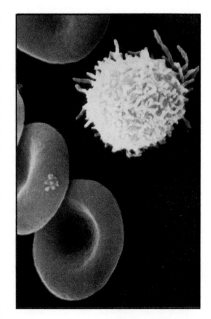

23–14. A human lymphocyte and red blood cells

IMMUNITY

If you are immune to a disease, your body has the power to resist the disease. Fortunately, we do not have to worry about being infected by diseases that affect other plants and animals. For example, the virus for canine distemper kills half the dogs it infects, but does not infect humans. Our bodies do not support the growth of these organisms. We have what is known as an **inborn immunity** to this disease.

Passive immunity is acquired when antibodies are introduced into your body. In other words, your own body does not produce the antibodies. A baby receives antibodies from its mother's blood before birth. These antibodies protect the baby from infection while in the womb and for a few months after birth. Breast-fed babies are also protected by *colostrum*, a fluid produced by the mammary glands of the mother immediately after childbirth. Colostrum contains antibodies that protect the newborn's digestive tract from infection and disease.

Passive immunity can also be induced medically. If a person's own immune system cannot fight an infection, the person can sometimes be protected temporarily by injections of antibodies produced by other animals. Usually horses are injected with small amounts of the disease organism, such as the bacterium that causes tetanus. Then the horse's blood, which contains antibodies to the tetanus bacteria, is collected. These antibodies can then be injected into the patient's body. However, these antibodies eventually disappear and passive immunity is lost.

Artificial *clones* of cells that produce antibodies have now been produced, which may someday make it possible to manufacture antibodies commercially. These clones are produced by combining a lymphocyte from a mouse spleen that makes a specific antibody with a cancer cell. A cancer cell is used because of its unique trait of growing much more rapidly than a normal cell. The resulting new cell has the traits of the two parent cells. It produces huge amounts of the desired antibody and multiples readily. As this cell multiplies, it produces a *clone*, a colony of cells all of the same kind. The clone produces **monoclonal antibodies.** Scientists hope that some day monoclonal antibodies will be a safe and an inexpensive substitute for horse serum. They may also be used in the future for destroying cancer cells.

People contract diphtheria, scarlet fever, mumps, chicken pox, and certain other infectious diseases only once. Recovery from the infection establishes **acquired active immunity.** During the infection, the body produces antibodies against the specific organisms or toxins. If the pathogen should enter your body again, antibodies are already present to destroy them. However, having a disease is a dangerous way to establish immunity. Active immunity can also be acquired artificially. Vaccines contain weakened or dead pathogens. When they are injected into your body, antibodies are formed but the pathogen does not cause sickness.

VACCINATION. In 1796, Edward Jenner discovered the first vaccine. He noticed that dairy workers who had a mild disease known as cowpox seemed to be immune to the deadly disease called smallpox. Jenner found that rubbing the pus from cowpox sores into scratches in the skin prevented people from coming down with smallpox. Although he did not know why it worked, he had introduced cowpox antigens, which are very similar to smallpox antigens, into these people's bloodstreams. Thus the bodies of those who had been infected with cowpox developed antibodies that were also effective against smallpox.

Since Jenner's time, scientists have developed vaccines for a number of diseases, including polio, influenza, and measles. "Booster shots" serve to jog the immune system's memory into producing more antibodies, so that enough are present should these pathogens invade.

You have probably received a **patch test** for tuberculosis at one time or another. **Tuberculin,** prepared from dead

HEALTH IN HISTORY

It is interesting to note that smallpox was the first disease to be prevented by vaccination, and also the first to be eradicated. The last known cases occurred in India and Africa in the 1970's. International vaccination programs succeeded in wiping out the last pockets of infections.

tuberculosis organisms, is used in this test. A small amount of tuberculin is placed in contact with the skin. A red, raised spot develops within a few days if the patient is sensitive. A positive reaction to tuberculin does not indicate that a person has active tuberculosis. It means that at one time the person had the infection, in most cases very mild. However, a positive patch test should always be followed by further testing.

AN IMMUNIZATION PROGRAM. Children should have the benefit of an immunization program started early in life. Control and prevention of infectious diseases have greatly reduced infant and childhood mortality. In addition, it has improved the general health of young people by sparing them the weakening effects and possible permanent damage of childhood diseases. Figure 23-15 illustrates how the incidence of several diseases has decreased after the introduction of vaccinations against these diseases.

Nevertheless, recent nationwide surveys show that, although almost 98 percent of children entering school have had at least one dose of vaccine, fewer than 40 percent of

HEALTH ACTION

Prepare an immunization schedule for yourself. See if you can trace the date and type of vaccine you received during childhood and if you need to be revaccinated. You may have to consult your parents or family doctors for these dates. Keep this information as a part of your permanent health record.

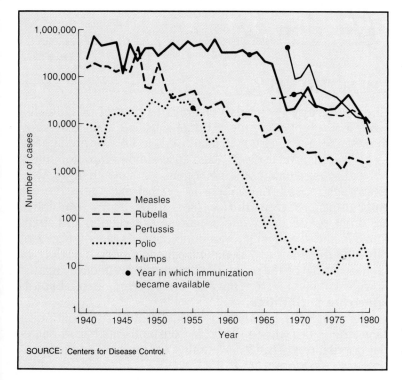

SOURCE: Centers for disease control.

Figure 23–15

these children have completed the recommended series of immunizations. This has caused concern regarding the possibility of nationwide epidemics of vaccine-preventable diseases. If all children were vaccinated, many more diseases would be eliminated, just as smallpox has been. Yearly vaccinations for influenza are recommended for those in high-risk groups. This includes the very old, the very young, and those suffering from chronic disease.

RECOMMENDED SCHEDULE FOR ACTIVE IMMUNIZATIONS	
Age	Type of Immunization
2 months	Diphtheria-tetanus-pertussis whooping cough vaccine (DTP) Trivalent oral polio virus vaccine (polio)
4 months	Same as above
6 months	Same as above
15 months	Measles, rubella, mumps
18 months	DTP, polio
4 to 6 years	DTP, polio
14 to 16 years after	Combined tetanus-diphtheria toxoids, adult type (TD)
Every 10 years	TD

Table 23–2

CHEMOTHERAPY

Chemotherapy is the use of drugs to control or cure disease. To be effective, these drugs must be able to destroy disease-causing agents, yet ideally cause little or no damage to body cells. Most drugs used in chemotherapy for infectious diseases either kill pathogens or slow their growth. The drugs most commonly used against pathogens are the sulfa drugs and **antibiotics** (see Table 23-3). Antibiotics are drugs produced by microorganisms. Penicillin and streptomycin are the best-known antibiotics. Large numbers of other antibiotics have been introduced under a variety of names. Some of these new antibiotics are effective against a wide variety of bacteria and are referred to as **broad-spectrum antibiotics.**

The search for new and better antibiotics still continues. New strains or forms of bacteria constantly appear in bacterial populations. These new strains are resistant to many antibiotics in current use.

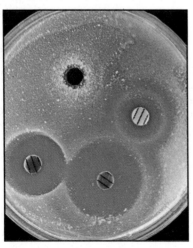

23–16. In screening for antibiotics and to determine antibiotic resistance in pathogens, scientists use small discs of blotting paper saturated with an antibiotic solution. The discs are placed on the surface of Petri dishes "seeded" with germs. The clear area around the disc indicates that the antibiotic prevented the growth of pathogens.

CHEMOTHERAPY COMMONLY USED TODAY				
Drug	How Produced	Used for	First Discovered	Possible Side Effects
Sulfa drugs	Produced chemically	Urinary infections	1935	Can damage blood cells, kidneys, or other organs if used improperly
Penicillin	Produced by green molds	Many coccus type bacteria such as pneumococcus, gonococcus, staphylococcus, streptococcus, and the spirochete causing syphilis	1929	Many people are allergic to it, suffering severe and even fatal reactions, penicillin-resistant bacteria can develop
Streptomycin	Produced by soil fungus	Tuberculosis, plague, cholera, dysentery	1944	Streptomycin-resistant bacteria can develop

Table 23-3

Eileen had a mild urinary infection. Her doctor prescribed a sulfa drug for her to take for 12 days. Since her symptoms had disappeared after 6 days, she quit taking her pills. A week later her infection returned, only it was even worse than before. What had happened? Although her symptoms had disappeared after 6 days, there were still bacteria present in her urinary tract. Those that had survived were those that were more resistant to the sulfa drug she had taken. They continued to grow and multiply until her symptoms reappeared. Her doctor had to prescribe an even stronger dose of the sulfa drug in order to kill these bacteria.

One of the main causes of bacterial resistance to antibiotics is inadequate treatment. Like Eileen, many people stop their antibiotics as soon as the symptoms of their infection subside, instead of heeding their doctor's advice to take the full prescription.

INTERFERONS. Drugs used in chemotherapy have brought many bacterial diseases under control. Unfortunately, there are no drugs other than vaccines that are effective against viruses. However, a discovery in recent years may prove to be a breakthrough in the control of viral diseases. When infected by a virus, certain cells secrete chemicals called **interferons.** Interferons are carried to other cells by the blood stream and act as messengers to warn them of danger. These messengers may trigger the production of antiviral chemicals by other cells. Interferons can now be produced artificially in labs. In experimental trials, it has successfully boosted people's immunity to some viral

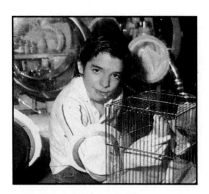

23–17. David, who died at age 12, survived longer than anyone else with severe immune deficiency disease. For most of his life he lived in a germ-free bubble. He died after undergoing an unsuccessful bone marrow transplant.

diseases. Some scientists are optimistic that interferons combined with other therapy may also prove to be more effective in treating certain kinds of cancers.

PROBLEMS WITH THE IMMUNE SYSTEM

Two things can go wrong with the immune system. It may fail to function, resulting in *immune-deficiency diseases*, in which the body cannot react to the invasion of pathogens. Or, it can turn against the body and attack various organs, causing a number of serious conditions known as *autoimmune diseases*.

IMMUNE-DEFICIENCY DISEASE. Some infants are born without a normal immune system. They may lack a thymus and certain kinds of lymphocytes. Therefore, their immune systems can neither produce antibodies nor combat pathogens directly. Frequent and severe infections of all kinds are common. This condition is known as immune-deficiency disease, and it is sometimes inherited. In the past, these infants usually died within the first year of life. Now, the transplantation of the thymus gland or bone marrow, where needed in the infants, can restore normal immunity in many cases.

ACQUIRED IMMUNE-DEFICIENCY SYNDROME (AIDS). In June 1981, a rare type of pneumonia was reported in five young men. Next, clusters of a rare cancer also were reported. The victims of these rare diseases also had fallen prey to a host of other infections. This suggested to doctors that these victims had somehow acquired a problem with their immune systems. Doctors named this condition *acquired immune-deficiency syndrome*, or *AIDS*. Within the two years following the first reported cases, the Center for Disease Control received reports of 1,641 more cases. These included 644 deaths, an usually high mortality rate for an infectious disease. An analysis of these cases found 71 percent to be homosexual males, 17 percent to be intravenous-drug abusers, 5 percent to be Haitian immigrants, 1 percent to be hemophilia patients receiving blood products, and 6 percent not to fit into any of these groups.

AIDS patients have been found to have too few lymphocytes. Thus, they are at high risk for any number of infectious diseases. A virus that is transmitted by blood or sexual contact is the suspected cause of AIDS. The disease does not seem to be contagious in any other way. It is hoped that

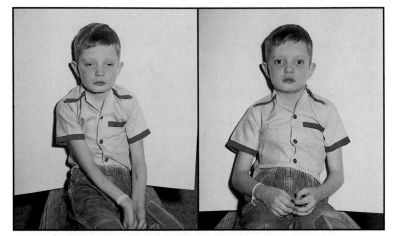

23–18. *Left: A 5-year-old boy whose eyelids, face, and shoulders droop because of severe myasthenia gravis. Right: The same boy immediately after a vein injection of Tensilon. His muscle power was brought close to normal.*

research will find a way to restore cellular immunity and cure the victim. Discovery of an AIDS virus could lead to the development of a specific AIDS vaccine.

AUTOIMMUNE DISEASES.   At times, the immune system turns against certain specific body cells, causing severe damage. The resulting diseases are called **autoimmune,** which means "immunity against one's self." Normally, the body learns to recognize its own proteins and cannot produce antibodies against them. Occasionally this self-recognition system breaks down. In most cases, it is not known why this happens. Scientists believe that people with autoimmune diseases have defective genes, which produce antibodies against their own body tissues. Among the first autoimmune diseases discovered were rheumatoid arthritis, thyroid diseases, and *myasthenia gravis.*

Myasthenia gravis is a disease of neuromuscular transmission, producing fluctuating weakness and rapid tiring of voluntary muscles. It may cause drooping eyelids, double vision, and difficulty in smiling, swallowing, speaking, and even breathing in severe cases. Victims with milder cases are often accused of laziness. It may affect anyone from birth to advanced old age, but the largest number of cases occur in young women.

The cause of myasthenia gravis is an antibody that damages receptors on the muscle for *acetylcholine*, the chemical that initiates muscle contraction. Acetylocholine levels can be raised by certain drugs. Figure 23-18 shows the remarkably rapid effect on a person with this disease after receiving a drug called *Tensilon*. This improvement can usually be

HEALTH IN HISTORY

Myasthenia gravis was first described in 1675. Since there was no effective treatment, 90 percent of its victims died. However, 10 percent did mysteriously recover.

In 1934, Dr. Mary B. Walker, an English doctor, noted the similarity between the effects of **curare,** a South American arrow poison, and the symptoms of her myasthenic patient. She knew that there was an antidote for curare called **neostigmin.** She injected her patient with this drug and observed improvement within minutes. Thus, a treatment for myasthenia gravis was found.

maintained by longer lasting drugs, taken by mouth. In more severe cases, a cortisone-like drug suppresses the antibody, giving even more effective treatment. In some cases, removal of an overactive thymus gland results in improvement.

Other diseases that have now been found to be autoimmune include insulin-dependent diabetes and multiple sclerosis. Experiments aimed at turning off the defective genes that produce the harmful antibodies give hope that a cure may someday be found for all autoimmune diseases.

WELLNESS WATCH

1. Do you keep up your resistance against infectious diseases by following positive health habits, such as eating well, getting proper rest, and handling stress effectively?
2. When antibiotics are prescribed, do you carefully follow the directions for use?
3. Do you have good hygiene habits, such as washing your hands often and covering your mouth when you sneeze?
4. Do you help prevent the spread of an infection by not exposing others to your own illness?
5. Do you avoid eating raw or improperly cooked meats? Also, when advised by local public health authorities, do you avoid eating shellfish from contaminated water?
6. Have you received all of your necessary immunization shots?
7. Do you seek medical help at the first sign of a serious infectious disease?

SUMMARY: Bacteria and viruses are the most common types of invaders of the human body. Diseases can be transmitted in various ways: by air, by water, by food, or by indirect or direct contact. Many communicable diseases can be controlled by individual concern and responsibility in seeking preventive measures or treatment.

The body has three lines of defense against infectious diseases: structural, cellular, and immune. Immunity may be inborn or acquired. Thanks to vaccines and chemotherapy, infections that once would have been fatal are now curable. The immune system may turn against the body and cause autoimmune diseases. Or, it may fail completely, resulting in immune-deficiency diseases.

CHAPTER REVIEW

words at work

Find the word in the left column that fits one of the definitions in the right column. DO NOT WRITE IN THIS BOOK.

a. droplet infection
b. antibody
c. chemotherapy
d. immunity
e. virus
f. lymphocyte
g. pathogenic
h. structural
i. protozoa
j. STDs

1. A protein substance that attacks antigens
2. A type of white blood cell that fights infection
3. Capable of causing disease
4. The ability of the body to resist certain diseases
5. A method of treating diseases by certain drugs
6. The smallest agent of infection
7. Transmittal of bacteria through discharges from the nose and throat
8. One-celled animals
9. Diseases transmitted through sexual contact
10. The body's first line of defense against infection

review questions

1. Identify three basic types of bacteria by their shape.
2. Describe the method and rate of growth of bacteria.
3. Describe a virus particle.
4. Name several well-known infections caused by viruses.
5. Name two skin diseases caused by fungi.
6. List several methods of controlling airborne infections.
7. What precautions should be taken to prevent waterborne infections?
8. Identify four sexually transmitted diseases.
9. Why is it important to cook pork well?
10. Describe the body's first, second, and third lines of defense against infection.
11. Explain the difference between active and passive immunity.
12. List several diseases for which vaccination has been effective in producing active immunity.
13. Define chemotherapy.
14. List several diseases for which penicillin has been used effectively.
15. Identify two things that may go wrong with the immune system.
16. Explain immune-deficiency diseases.
17. Name some autoimmune diseases.
18. List some of the symptoms of myasthenia gravis.

discussion questions

1. Viruses may or may not be living organisms. What characteristics of a virus raise this question?
2. Discuss water pollution as a major health hazard.
3. Discuss the possible cause of the spread of STDs in the United States.
4. Will we ever be able to eliminate infectious diseases?
5. Discuss possible measures that could be taken to control or eliminate infectious diseases.
6. If you have ever had the mumps or chicken pox, it is unlikely that you will ever get it again. Explain why.
7. Discuss new breakthroughs in the study of the immune system, such as the function of different types of lymphocytes, monoclonal antibodies, and interferon. What could these discoveries lead to in the future?

investigating

PURPOSE:
To find out if the incidence of measles and mumps has decreased since the introduction of vaccinations.

MATERIALS:
Graph paper.

PROCEDURE:
A.   Conduct a survey of at least five people of different ages. Ask: (a) Did you ever get vaccinated for the measles? the mumps? (b) Did you ever get the measles? the mumps? (c) What is your age?

B.   As a class, compile your results by age group as follows: 0-10 years; 11-20; 21-30; 31-40; 41-50; 51-60; over 60. Count the number of people who were vaccinated for measles and the number of people who were vaccinated for mumps in each age group. Next, count the number of people who had the measles and the number of people who had the mumps in each age group.

C.   Draw two bar graphs, one for measles and one for mumps, of your results. Record the number of cases in one color and the number vaccinated in another color along the vertical axis. Record age group along the horizontal axis.

D.   Look at the graph of reported cases of diseases before and after availability of immunization on page 501 (Figure 23-15).

    1.   How many years ago were vaccines against measles and mumps first available?

    2.   Did the incidence of these diseases decrease after the vaccines became available?

E.   Compare the results of your survey with those in Figure 23-15.

    3.   Are your results similar to the results recorded on this graph?

    4.   If your results are not similar to this graph, can you suggest why?

HEALTH
CAREERS

REGISTERED NURSE

If Florence Nightingale, the founder of nursing, could see this profession today, she would be astounded. White caps are disappearing, and men have joined the nursing profession. After high school you can choose to follow one of three routes to become a nurse. The choices include a two- or three-year hospital diploma program, a two-year college program, or a four-year college program. Graduation from any of these programs allows you to take the state licensing exam to become a registered nurse (RN). Hospital and two-year college programs emphasize technical nursing skills such as administering drugs. Four-year college programs enable graduates to work in expanded roles, performing such duties as screening and counseling patients. Some specialized nursing careers require advanced training after a basic nursing degree. If nursing interests you, begin now by taking science and math courses. Hospital volunteering will also help you decide whether this career is for you. For more information, write to the National League for Nursing, 10 Columbus Circle, New York, New York 10019.

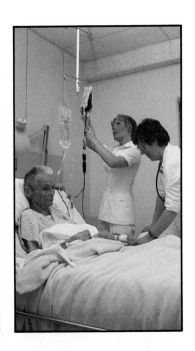

MEDICAL RESEARCH SCIENTIST

Contrary to popular belief, disease is not just fought in hospitals or physicians'

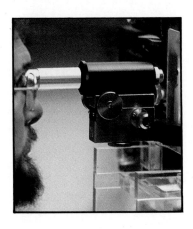

offices; it is also fought behind the scenes in medical research laboratories. Scientists are searching for new vaccines to prevent disease; they are developing new drugs to combat illness; they are studying basic cell processes which will unlock the mysteries that heredity, growth, or other factors may play in sickness. The world of medical research is vast. It covers many different sciences: biology, chemistry, physics, engineering, and math are just a few. To become a part of this special world, you'll need special preparation. First, four years of college in your chosen science and then additional study, usually four to five years, to earn a Ph.D., a doctoral degree. So, a strong math and science program in high school is a must. Good communications skills and a foreign language, particularly French, German or Russian, are also important. Medical researchers must be able to write reports and share their research with other scientists worldwide. Interested? Then write to the American Institute of Biological Sciences, 1401 Wilson Boulevard, Arlington, Virginia 22209.

UNIT 8

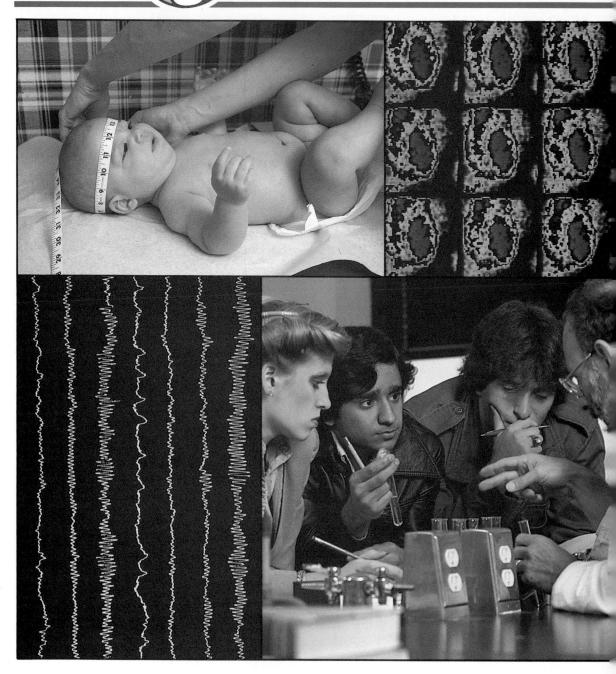

Safeguarding Your Health

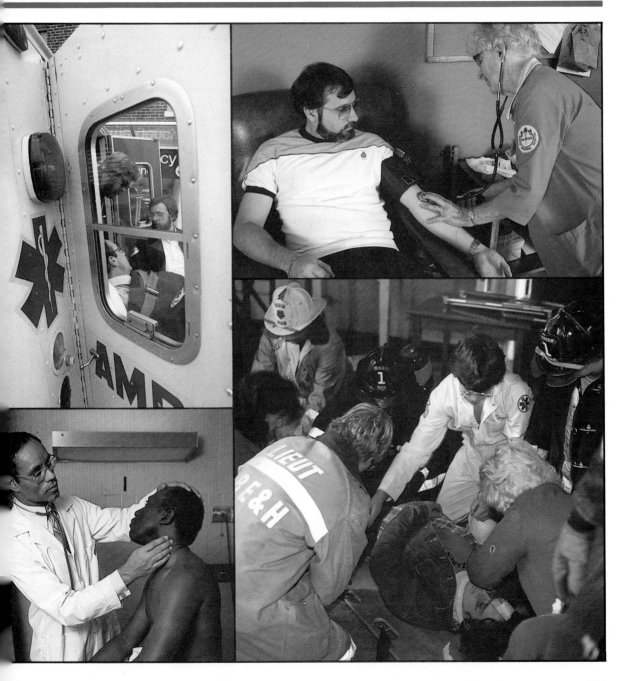

CHAPTER 24

Public Health and the Environment

OBJECTIVES

- DISCUSS the role of public health at local, state, national, and international levels
- EXPLAIN health risks related to the environment

- IDENTIFY major sources of environmental health hazards
- OUTLINE societal and individual action to safeguard health

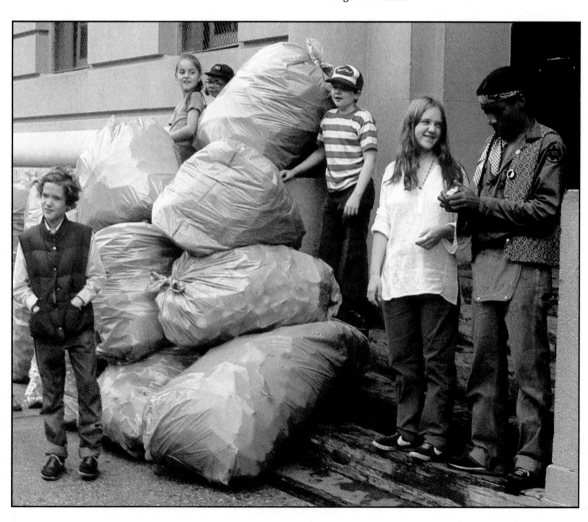

Do you know the story of the "Love Canal?" Love Canal is a small community near Niagara Falls, New York. It is not a honeymooning resort. In 1976, heavy rains soaked the earth and flooded basements in the area. Soon afterward, gardens began to die. Pets became sick, then people. Over the next two years the residents suffered high rates of miscarriages, birth defects, cancer, and other ailments. Why did this happen? The Love Canal community had been built on a forgotten toxic dumpsite. During the flooding, the water mixed with chemicals seeping from toxic wastes buried there over twenty years earlier. In the end, state health officials evacuated the area. The President declared Love Canal a disaster area.

Love Canal is but one example of how the environment can affect public health. Tragedies such as this can be prevented if the environment and public health become everybody's business.

WHAT IS PUBLIC HEALTH?

Public health involves efforts to prevent disease and to promote total well-being on an individual, local, state, national, or international level. Organized teams of doctors and other health professionals, scientists, public officials, and consumers are working together to achieve better health for every person.

STATE AND LOCAL HEALTH DEPARTMENTS

Boards of health are found at the city, county, and state levels. It is their responsibility to plan, provide, and evaluate community health services. The state health department handles health problems that are more widespread. The activities of all health departments fall into five main categories: medical care, disease detection, environmental health programs, facilities and services for patients, and support services (see Figure 24-1).

NATIONAL HEALTH DEPARTMENTS

In 1798 Congress authorized a federally operated marine hospital for the care of American merchant seamen. This marked the beginning of our national government's involvement in public health. Today the federal government is involved in every phase of public health through the Department of Health and Human Services and other agencies.

PUBLIC HEALTH DEPARTMENT FUNCTIONS

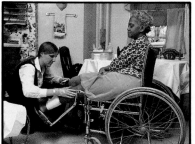

Medical Care Programs
Immunization: control of infectious disease; *screening:* testing for chronic disease, sexually transmitted disease, tuberculosis; *nursing:* in-home care for new mothers, ill or elderly; *dental:* prevention and treatment; *occupational health and safety:* on-the-job inspections for worker protection.

Disease Detection
Investigation of any unusual outbreaks of illness whether common diseases like food poisoning or measles or mysterious problems like Acquired Immune Deficiency (AIDS). Victims and their personal contacts may be questioned to track down causes and find prevention measures.

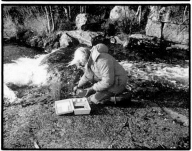

Environmental Health Programs
Sanitation: protection of drinking and recreational waters from disease-causing microbes and toxic chemicals; *food and drug control:* safety of food, drugs, cosmetics; *vector control:* prevention of disease carried by insects and rodents; *radiologic health:* protection against excess radiation; *air pollution control:* safeguards air quality; *housing and urban planning:* elimination of slums or housing conditions that contribute to ill health.

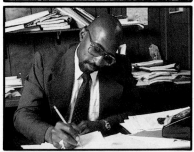

Patient facilities and Services
Inspection, licensing, and monitoring of facilities such as hospitals, nursing homes, and laboratories; licensing of health professionals; administration of government health insurance programs for elderly (Medicare) and low-income persons (Medicaid) to prevent fraud and abuse.

Support Services
Social work: identifies and coordinates health and social programs; *nutrition:* food assistance and education for low-income mothers, children, and elderly; *health statistics:* accurate recording of birth, death, and disease to study health trends from one generation to the next and compare trends among geographical areas; *laboratory services:* testing of water, food, and human specimens to detect disease-causing agents; *health education:* providing knowledge and teaching practical skills.

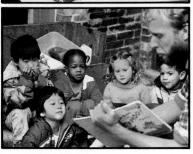

PUBLIC HEALTH SERVICE. In April 1953 the Department of Health (now Health and Human Services) was created. The Public Health Service is the division within this department that is concerned with every phase of the health of Americans. There are five branches within the Public Health Service: the Centers for Disease Control; the Health Resources and Services Administration; the National Institutes for Health; the Alcohol, Drug Abuse, and Mental Health Administration; and the Food and Drug Administration.

OTHER FEDERAL AGENCIES. Because so many factors affect health, several other Federal agencies have a public health role, too.

- The United States Department of Agriculture (U.S.D.A.) inspects and approves meat found free from disease or parasites. It supervises meat packing and processing.
- The Department of Labor has a branch called the Occupational Safety and Health Administration (OSHA). OSHA develops, promotes, evaluates, and enforces standards to protect workers from all job-related health hazards.
- The Environmental Protection Agency (E.P.A.) protects our environment from pollution.
- The Department of Transportation is concerned with safety on our nation's highways.

NONGOVERNMENT HEALTH AGENCIES. Voluntary health agencies like the American National Red Cross, American Heart Association, National Foundation-March of Dimes, and the American Cancer Society are concerned with specific health problems or health services. They raise funds for medical research, alert the public to specific health problems, and provide health education programs. Through their state and local chapters, health services are made available to the communities they serve.

Professional health associations represent health professionals or types of health facilities, such as hospitals and nursing homes. Well-known examples of these organizations are the American Medical Association (AMA), the association for physicians, and the American Hospital Association.

PUBLIC HEALTH AT THE INTERNATIONAL LEVEL

WORLD HEALTH ORGANIZATION (WHO). In 1948 the United Nations formed the World Health Organization

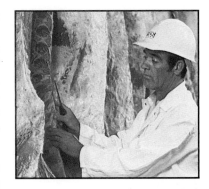

24–2. The United States Department of Agriculture inspects meat to make sure it is free from disease and parasites.

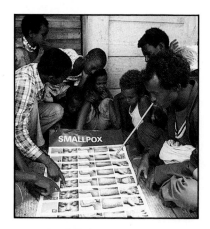

24–3. The WHO worldwide campaign against smallpox helped to eliminate this disease.

(WHO) to "raise the physical and mental health of all people." WHO sponsors projects for infectious disease control and immunization in developing countries. It is also concerned with improving nutrition and sanitation, as well as training public-health personnel.

ENVIRONMENT AND HEALTH

Think about what life would be like without cars and planes, electricity, and running tap water. These are only some of the conveniences of twentieth-century American life. However, technology has brought many problems as well as benefits. Once our air was pure, but now it contains many pollutants. Our water and food may contain hazards such as toxic chemicals from industrial wastes. Nuclear power has brought the promise of cheap energy but the risk of radiation danger too.

Just 100 years ago, microbes were the major cause of sickness. Today most causes of disease are related to modern living. But these causes are much harder to prove for two reasons. A great deal of time, 20 years or more, may elapse between exposure to **environmental hazards** and the onset of illness. Also, since we are exposed to many substances each day, it is much harder to pinpoint the exact causes of illness. Therefore, we have been slow to realize the full impact of our environment on health.

Yet scientists now estimate that 20 percent of all premature deaths, plus countless cases of disease and disability, could be prevented if stronger action were taken to safeguard health against environmental hazards. This is the major challenge of public health now and in the years ahead.

ECOLOGY AND HUMAN HEALTH

What does **ecology** have to do with human health? Ecology is the science that studies the relationship of all living things to one another and their environment. A living community and its environment are interdependent. They form what is called an **ecosystem.** When one link in the ecosystem is disrupted, a chain reaction can occur, affecting other links.

Humans are interdependent with other living things and their environment. The natural process of **biomagnification** demonstrates this point. Biomagnification is the increasing concentration of some toxic chemicals in the food chain.

For example, before the chemical DDT was banned in the United States, it was sprayed on crops to control insects. This pesticide then entered the food chain through the water or soil. Here it was absorbed by microscopic plant and animal life. Tiny fish and insects that feed on these organisms then became contaminated. These small animals in turn were preyed upon by larger fish and birds. Eventually these larger animals became food for humans. At each step in the food chain, the DDT concentration increased. This magnification problem is compounded by another fact. DDT, like many other toxic chemicals, also **bioaccumulates.** This means that once these chemicals enter living cells they are not broken down. Instead they accumulate in cells, particularly fat cells, so their concentration grows with each exposure. What effects does DDT have on humans? No effects have been seen yet, but there is a possibility of long-term consequences.

THE HEALTH EFFECTS OF ENVIRONMENTAL HAZARDS

Since World War II an astounding number of new chemicals have been created. Today more than four million chemical compounds exist. Just these numbers alone make it hard to investigate their effects. Also, many chemicals interact, so you can see why there is much that is not yet known.

We do know how hazards enter the body. They may be ingested, inhaled, or absorbed through the skin. Once inside, they can cause problems ranging from simple skin rashes to sudden death. When the brain is affected, mental and emotional problems may result. The harmful effects depend on such factors as the dose received, the frequency and length of exposure, and the properties of the hazard.

Some hazards, like chemicals, may cause toxic reactions right away, even in very small doses. Other hazards, like radiation in small amounts, may have less severe or no immediate effects. But with repeated exposure over a long period of time, they may cause slow, subtle damage to body tissues. Symptoms may develop gradually until disease or disability occurs. Cancer, birth defects, and hereditary changes are some of the worst effects of these hazards.

CANCER. Over the last decade scientists have observed a rise in cancer rates. Most cancer cases are now believed to be related to our life-style and/or hazards in our environment. For instance, poor health habits, such as smoking, and certain hazards in the environment, such as radiation, are known to increase the risk of cancer. Anything that causes cancer is called a **carcinogen** (kar-**sin**-o-jen). Some environmental hazards cause cancer directly. Others are not carcinogens themselves, but they promote the development of cancer when a person has been exposed to a carcinogen.

BIRTH DEFECTS. At one time people thought the fetus was protected from environmental hazards while in the womb. We now know that many toxic substances reach the fetus when the mother is exposed to them. These agents, known as **teratogens** (**ter**-ah-to-jen), may cause damage any time during pregnancy. However, exposure during the first three months of pregnancy, when the limbs and major organs are forming, often causes the most serious effects. One big problem with teratogens is that their potential for damage is rarely known in advance.

HEREDITARY CHANGES. Hazards called **mutagens** (**mu**-tah-jen) change the genetic structure of cells. When the egg or sperm cells are affected, these changes can be passed from one generation to another. Sometimes these changes do not appear for two generations, which makes them difficult to trace. Some chemicals found in our environment are known to be mutagens for some species. It is not known if low doses of these chemicals over long periods of time also cause mutations in humans.

HIGH-RISK GROUPS

What are the odds that a person will become ill or disabled from environmental hazards? Each person's odds vary. Much depends on a person's inherited sensitivity. Other factors play a part, too. The young and old are at greater risk as well as those who are already weakened by illness.

Risks also vary by occupation. For instance, people who work with asbestos have eight times the risk of getting *mesothelioma* than the general working population. This is a deadly form of cancer of the lining surrounding the lung. Where and how you live also affect your risks. As shown in Figure 24-4, cancer rates vary across the country. Higher rates are often found around heavier industrial areas. But when you add a poor life-style habit such as smoking to already existing risks your odds multiply. The chances of getting mesothelioma increases by 92 times for smokers who work with asbestos.

518

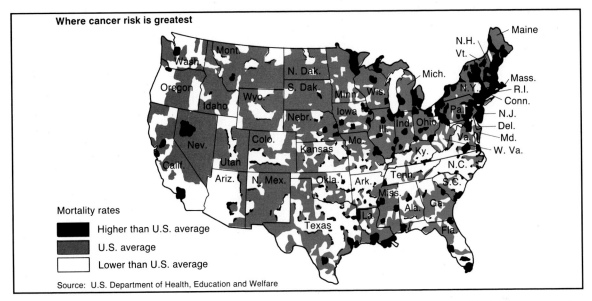

Where cancer risk is greatest

Mortality rates
- Higher than U.S. average
- U.S. average
- Lower than U.S. average

Source: U.S. Department of Health, Education and Welfare

24–4. Incidence of cancer nationwide

SOURCES OF ENVIRONMENTAL HAZARDS

HAZARDOUS WASTES

How would you handle a container labeled "Discarded Product: flammable, corrosive, and explosive in reaction and toxic to human and animal life"? According to the E.P.A. such products are seldom disposed of carefully. The label states the E.P.A. definition of **hazardous wastes.** These wastes come from industrial processes that produce goods like plastics and paints. Where do these wastes go?

In some cases they are deliberately dumped into waterways. Some are carelessly burned, sending chemical fumes into the air. Later these chemicals return to earth in rain or snow. Some are poorly recycled. Often they are packed in drums and discarded in dumpsites. Eventually many dumpsites are covered with earth and are forgotten. These landfills may then become the sites for homes. In time, these wastes can seep through rusted drums and foul the air, water, and soil. Their potential for environmental disaster is great. Few are **biodegradable.** If they were, they would decompose in the environment. Once they enter the environment they persist for years and can cause problems as in the case of the Love Canal.

24–5. Public health officials ask that everyone watch for signs of toxic wastes: leaking drums, dead or dying plant or animal life, stained soil or water, and irritating fumes. Do not explore these areas but report them to your local health department.

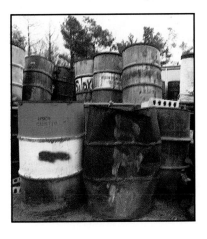

The most deadly episode of air pollution occurred in London in December 1952. For 5 days the city was enveloped in stagnant air, intense fog, and smoke from coal-burning homes and factories. Four thousand more people died than was normally expected for that time of year. The majority were those already suffering from heart or lung disease.

Since the Love Canal incident, other toxic dumpsites have been located. But, without a doubt, there are many more as yet undiscovered. Drums of toxic wastes have also been found in empty warehouses, in fields, and in vacant lots.

WHAT IS AIR POLLUTION?

Air pollution can result from natural forces or from modern living. Air normally contains four main gases: *nitrogen, oxygen, argon,* and *carbon dioxide.* Typical urban air has an excess of carbon dioxide plus *sulfur dioxide, nitrogen oxide, ozone,* and a group of compounds called *hydrocarbons.* Also present are *lead, mercury,* and **particulates.** Particulates are small particles or liquid droplets that are suspended in air, including fumes, smoke, and mist. Air pollution is mostly due to the burning of fossil fuels by cars and factories.

Certain weather conditions can make air pollution worse. Are you familiar with the term **smog?** Sometimes air pollutants form a thick, visible haze called smog. It often blankets large cities where there are more cars and industry. Under normal weather conditions, this haze rises toward the cooler air in the upper atmosphere where it diffuses. Sometimes, however, an unusual condition called a **temperature inversion** occurs. A layer of cold air becomes trapped under warmer air. It seals the smog over the city and prevents it from rising (see Figure 24-6).

Polluted air makes the eyes burn and tear, irritates the throat, and can cause coughing or breathing difficulties. It also promotes the development of a wide range of respiratory and other health problems. Asthma, emphysema, and bronchitis are just a few examples. For people with existing heart and lung ailments, pollution can be life-threatening.

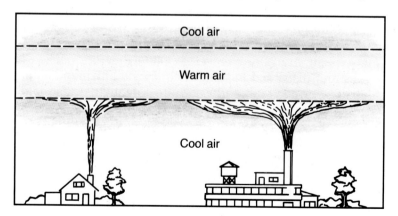

24-6. A temperature inversion

Cool air

Warm air

Cool air

OTHER AIR ATTACKS. Health effects aside, air pollution attacks our environment in other ways. When sulfur-rich fuels like coal are burned, the toxic gas sulfur dioxide fills the air. It then combines with water to form an acid strong enough to erode building surfaces and statues (see Figure 24-7). When it rains, this acid falls to the earth. This **acid rain** upsets the normal acid balance of the water and soil and kills water plants and animals. As fish and birds lose their food supply, they too die. Acid rain also damages crops and kills trees.

Air pollution also raises the temperature of the air. Normally carbon dioxide in the air absorbs some of the heat radiated from the earth. But pollution increases carbon dioxide levels in the air. Scientists worry that in time these high levels may hold too much heat in the atmosphere, and thus raise the earth's temperature. On a global scale a rise of just a few degrees could melt the polar ice caps. This would raise sea level by as much as 120 meters (400 feet). Coastal states would be flooded and cropland destroyed.

WATER POLLUTION

Modern sewage treatment has brought water-borne diseases under control. But most modern plants are not equipped to deal with chemical contaminants. Where do we get our drinking water? Rivers, lakes, and reservoirs supply water or wells are dug to tap groundwater for drinking. Over 300 chemicals, some suspected carcinogens, have been found in local water supplies. Where do these chemicals come from? The chemical **chlorine** is added to water to kill disease-causing organisms. At high levels, it can combine with other chemicals in water to produce toxic chemicals. Some chemicals are pesticides that have washed into the water supply. Others are toxic industrial wastes that have been improperly dumped into waterways.

Improperly dumping human wastes and phosphate detergents has created pollution problems too. Phosphates and sewage provide extra nutrients for rapid growth of bacteria and algae, which deplete the normal oxygen level in the water. Once-blue waters turn green with algae growth. If nothing reverses this process, rapid **eutrophication** (you-tro-fi-**kay**-shun), or aging, of the waterway occurs. Normally this process occurs over thousands of years. But with pollution it can happen within a person's lifetime. As a lake ages, it becomes choked with weeds and a marsh forms.

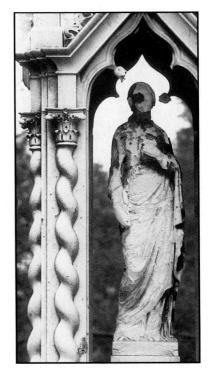

24–7. This statue has been damaged by acid rain.

HEALTH TIP

In soft water areas, let the tap water run a few minutes when the faucet has been unused for several hours. This helps flush out toxic metals that may have leaked from pipes.

OUR FOOD SUPPLY

Water pollution often leads to pollution of our food supply. For instance, the industrial chemicals known as PCBs have polluted the Great Lakes and Hudson River. A 1968 disaster in Yusho, Japan, underscored the dangers of PCBs. Villagers who ate rice accidentally contaminated with PCBs quickly came down with severe nervous system disorders. PCBs are now banned.

Pesticides are chemicals that are used to control unwanted plant and animal life, such as insects, rodents, fungi, and weeds. The use of pesticides has made it possible to greatly increase food supply. But pesticides need to be used properly in order that we may reap their benefits yet avoid needless harmful effects. There has been an expanded use of pesticides in the last 20 years. Today about 90,000 different pesticides exist. As of 1972, all pesticides sold in this country must be registered by the E.P.A. Some highly toxic pesticides are restricted to commercial use. Yet even with these controls many concerned scientists believe that some of the pesticides in use today may have as yet unknown harmful effects on our health. *Dioxin* is a case in point. It is one of the most poisonous substances ever developed by man. It was discovered that dioxin was a contaminant in some pesticides. A defoliant called *Agent Orange* was used extensively during the Vietnam War. Agent Orange contains dioxin. What was the effect on the American soldiers and Vietnamese civilians in Vietnam at that time? No one knows the answer yet.

RADIATION

Have you observed a microwave oven in action? Microwaves are one example of *nonionizing radiation*. This form of radiation has a low energy level, and only produces heat. *Ionizing radiation* has high energy, and can injure cells and cause genetic damage. You cannot escape from some exposure to this radiation. Ionizing radiation from outer space constantly strikes the earth. Also, certain radioactive substances in the earth, like uranium and radium, constantly give off this radiation. Other sources include X-ray devices used in medicine, luminous watches and clocks, nuclear power plants, and fallout from aboveground nuclear tests.

X rays penetrate all body tissues. Some tissues, such as breast tissue and the reproductive organs, are more sensitive than others. The cells of the young, particularly the unborn,

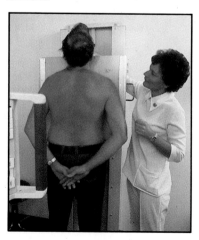

24–8. Radiation can be useful. It can also be harmful.

can easily be damaged by radiation. The amount of damage depends on the radiation dose, the size of the area exposed, and the length of exposure. For instance, 500 **roentgens** (**rent**-genz) of radiation can be fatal when applied to the whole body at once. Yet ten times this amount can be given to small areas of the body over a period of time to kill cancer cells.

The effects of radiation are cumulative over a lifetime. The population's overall exposure to radiation has been quite low. But very little is known about the long-term effects of exposure to low-level radiation. Most scientists believe that there is no absolutely safe level of radiation.

Many people are very worried about radiation from nuclear power plants. Yet, short of an accident, the risks from this source of radiation are quite low. The greatest radiation risks by far come from medical and dental X rays. Many of these X rays are needed and can benefit health. For instance, an annual X ray of the breast is advised for women over age 50. This can detect breast cancer very early, when it is most curable, long before a tumor could ever be felt. But few X rays are advised routinely. As a general rule, X rays should be used only when symptoms are present and no other tests can provide the doctor with the needed information. Studies show that many X rays given each year are not necessary. When X rays are ordered, patients in doubt about their value should ask why they are needed.

SOLID WASTES

When you finish drinking a canned beverage, do you merely toss out the can? If so, your container becomes part of the 4.7 billion metric tons (4.3 billion tons) of solid waste that must be disposed of each year. This amounts to 2.7 kilograms (6 pounds) of refuse per person daily. Figure 24-8 shows the typical composition of household refuse. Notice that paper is the largest single item. Disposable packaging is the source of much of this paper.

What happens to these solid wastes? They can only end up in one of three places: our earth, our water, or our air. The cost of solid waste disposal is the third largest item in local municipal budgets. But solid wastes cost us more than money. They destroy the beauty of our land. Open dumps can also become the breeding grounds for rats, flies, and other disease carriers. Improper burning of solid waste increases air pollution.

24–9. Typical composition of household refuse

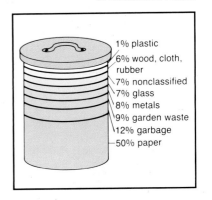

1% plastic
6% wood, cloth, rubber
7% nonclassified
7% glass
8% metals
9% garden waste
12% garbage
50% paper

TESTING FOR CARCINOGENS

Have you seen the warning label on saccharin-sweetened diet drinks? It cautions that the product has caused cancer in lab animals. Therefore, it may be hazardous to your health. The mice and rats used in these scientific studies had consumed the human equivalent of 250 cans of soda a day. When this fact was made public, many people dismissed the warning as ridiculous. After all, they reasoned, "No one drinks so much soda. Besides, rats and mice are very different from human beings." Other people thought, "What's the use of avoiding saccharin? It seems that everything causes cancer if the doses are high enough." Are these consumers right? Let's look at the facts.

Though rats and mice are very different from people, they also share similiarities. Both are made of cells, the basic units of life. These cells undergo the same biologic processes and are affected by factors in the environment. In fact, almost all the substances known to cause cancer in humans also cause cancer in animals.

Why give animals such large doses? Higher doses help to compensate for the differences in animal versus human life span, (2 to 3 years versus 70 years or more). We are exposed to potential carcinogens in low doses over a lifetime. If an agent causes cancer eventually in only one out of every 10,000 people, this may not seem very worrisome. But in our population of over 220 million, this would mean 22,000 extra cases: a public health epidemic! We cannot run an experiment with 220 million mice. Even an experiment with 10,000 mice could fail to detect the problem. So, to compensate for this research problem the doses are increased.

As for the claim that "everything causes cancer in high doses," this is simply not true. Of all the thousands of chemicals tested, only about 5 percent are proven carcinogenic. Given these scientific facts, would you consume foods and beverages that have warning labels?

LOW-CALORIE
GRANULATED SUGAR SUBSTITUTE
A BLEND OF NUTRITIVE AND NON-NUTRITIVE SWEETENERS

USE OF THIS PRODUCT MAY BE HAZARDOUS TO YOUR HEALTH. THIS PRODUCT CONTAINS SACCHARIN WHICH HAS BEEN DETERMINED TO CAUSE CANCER IN LABORATORY ANIMALS.

CONSUMER PRODUCTS

Our constant quest for better living brings new consumer products to our homes. They too carry potential health risks that must be weighed against their benefits.

Cosmetics are a mix of chemicals, some of which can be toxic. Red Dye No. 2, for example, was once used to color food and lipsticks. It has now been banned as a carcinogen. Some commercial hair dyes have been proved to be mutagenic in laboratory tests. Tests also show that these dyes do not remain in the hair, but circulate through the body.

THE WORKPLACE

Have you heard the expression "mad as a hatter"? At one time hatmakers breathed in toxic mercury while making felt hats. As a result they often became irrational. Many workers come into contact with unknown hazards such as toxic chemicals, noise, or radiation.

ENVIRONMENTAL ACTION

The problems of pollution may seem overwhelming. Yet some progress has been made. For example, between 1960 and 1979, particulate levels in the air decreased by 32 percent. This change in air quality shows that, if we take action as a society, the environment can improve.

LEGISLATIVE ACTION

Why haven't some industries taken stronger action to safeguard the environment and health? High profits have often outweighed environmental concerns. Therefore, federal, state, and local laws have been enacted for protection. These laws have helped set basic standards for environmental safety and penalties for pollution. But to be effective, laws must be strictly enforced. Often they are not. Environmentalists argue that penalties must be stiff enough to deter the crime. Many industrial offenders view pollution fines as part of the cost of doing business.

OTHER SOLUTIONS

Is pollution an inevitable part of modern living? It need not be. Science and creative minds can help solve the pollution problems of our planet. But we must be committed to this task. Some basic methods and technology already exist to fight pollution problems. They only need to be used.

AIR IMPROVEMENT.   Can you think of any ways to improve air quality? Control devices are available that can curb industrial and car pollution. Simple energy conservation measures could produce impressive results. If Americans who drive alone to work would carry just one other passenger, 400,000 barrels of oil could be saved each day!

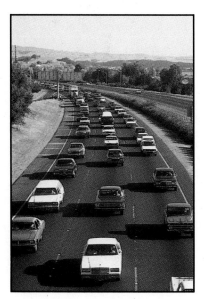

24–10. How can car pollution be reduced?

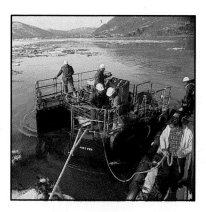

24–11. Cleaning up the effects of an oil spill

The long-term answer to pollution is the development of new technology and new ways of living. More and better public transportation and more energy-efficient buildings, homes, cars, and appliances are needed. Alternative, non-polluting energy sources such as solar energy are also needed.

FOOD AND WATER QUALITY. Two simple steps could improve our food and water quality today: reduction of pesticide use and proper toxic waste disposal.

Research is currently underway to find pesticides that are effective and not poisonous. Biological control methods are also being developed. For example, plant breeders are developing new varieties of crops that are resistant to pests.

Basic solutions also exist for toxic waste disposal. Wastes can be stored in concrete block containers that will not erode. Or they can be destroyed in unclosed, high-heat processes. Some can be chemically changed to make them harmless. Municipal water plants can install charcoal filtering systems to screen out most toxic wastes.

SOLID WASTE CONTROL. Do you discard refuse properly or are you a litterbug? When you compact your empty packages or flatten them before discarding, you can reduce solid waste volume. Do you buy products that have been or can be recycled? Do you practice recycling yourself? Think twice about an item before tossing it out. Many communities have started active recycling programs. Support them!

SAFER WORKPLACES AND CONSUMER GOODS. Researchers, employees, and unions must work together to achieve safer workplaces and consumer goods. At present protective standards for many workplace hazards have not yet been set. More research must be done. To safeguard health, better ventilation systems may be installed or protective clothing issued. Also, employees may be screened regularly to detect health problems early.

The products of the workplace end up in consumers' hands. The Consumer Product Safety Commission (CPSC) helps monitor and control product hazards. The federal Food and Drug Administration is also involved in consumer safety. One way consumers can help ensure greater safety is to use consumer action. Learn all you can about the products you use. There are excellent guides that evaluate products. When in doubt about safety, don't buy, and let companies know why.

YOUR PERSONAL PROGRAM

When you read about environmental hazards, how do you feel? Often people feel that there is nothing they can do. But there is much you *can* do personally to reduce your risk of environmental hazards.

YOUR LIFE-STYLE. First, think about your general health habits. When you follow a wellness life-style, you are likely to be healthier and more able to resist health hazards. When you avoid alcohol, nicotine, and other drugs, it is less likely that these chemicals will interact harmfully with pollutants in the environment.

Do you remember the guidelines for good nutrition discussed in Chapter 2? They also make good sense from an environmental viewpoint. As you have seen, toxic substances often bioaccumulate in fat cells. For this reason, a low-fat diet naturally contains fewer toxic substances.

PROTECTIVE PRACTICES. Do you always wash your fruits and vegetables carefully before eating? Just a quick rinse is not enough to remove pesticide residue. Thoroughly scrub or peel them. A charcoal filter on a water faucet can screen toxic chemicals. However, it must be changed often enough to prevent bacterial growth inside it. Unless the medical reasons are clear, avoid needless exposure to X rays. Finally, when you use household pesticides, use extreme care. Read and follow all instructions carefully. Spray pesticides only in well-ventilated areas. Wear protective clothing. Afterward, always wash your hands and face. Keep children and pets out of the way when you use these products. Store these products safely.

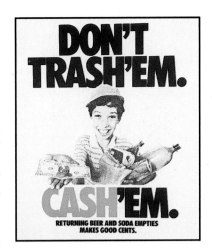

24–12. *Can you think of a reason why deposit cans and bottles can help keep parks and roadsides clean?*

SUMMARY: Public health includes all efforts, from the individual to the international level, to prevent disease and promote well-being. Environmental health hazards have replaced infectious disease as a major public health problem. These hazards may cause cancer, birth defects, or hereditary changes among other health problems. Sources of environmental hazards include hazardous wastes; polluted air, water or food supplies; radiation; solid wastes; consumer products; and the workplace. To safeguard health and protect the environment, legislative action has been and is, needed. The use of existing technology and conservation measures can help solve this problem, too. Individuals can reduce their risks through a healthful life-style.

CHAPTER REVIEW

words at work

Find the word in the left column that fits one of the definitions in the right column. DO NOT WRITE IN THIS BOOK.

a. biodegradable
b. carcinogen
c. bioaccumulation
d. mutagen
e. particulates
f. ecosystem
g. entrophication
h. teratogen
i. dioxins
j. roentgen

1. Causes birth defects
2. Substances suspended in the air
3. Aging of a waterway
4. A measure of radiation
5. Group of pesticides
6. Causes genetic cell changes
7. A living community and its environment
8. Causes cancer
9. Increasing concentration in body cells
10. Capable of decomposing in the environment

review questions

1. What is meant by the term "public health"?
2. Cite the five major categories in which all activities of health departments may be categorized.
3. Give three examples of the federal government's involvement in public health.
4. Describe professional and voluntary health agencies. Give examples of each.
5. Name three missions of the World Health Organization.
6. Cite two reasons why it is harder to trace illness to environmental hazards than to infectious microbes.
7. Define *ecology* and *ecosystem*.
8. Compare biomagnification and bioaccumulation.
9. How can environmental hazards enter the body?
10. Define the terms *carcinogen, teratogen,* and *mutagen.*
11. What factors affect the risk of environmentally related health problems?
12. What are hazardous wastes?
13. Explain the effects of smog and temperature inversion on air quality.
14. Cite the effects of acid rain on an ecosystem.
15. Why are some pesticides environmental health hazards? Give an example.
16. Compare ionizing and nonionizing radiation and contrast their effects.
17. Cite two reasons why solid wastes are considered health hazards.

18. Why is legislative action necessary to safeguard the environment and health?
19. Name two actions that would improve the quality of our food and water.
20. Why is a low-fat diet advised to reduce environmental health risk?
21. Outline protective practices for home pesticide use.

discussion questions

1. Justify the statement "Public health is everybody's business." Give examples of public health action on every level.
2. Is modern living hazardous to health? Discuss its benefits and risks and cite examples to support your position.
3. Discuss the problem of solid waste disposal. Identify changes that people could make in their life-styles to help overcome this growing problem.
4. How can a person's occupation affect his or her health? Would health concerns be a factor in your choice of occupation?
5. Outline personal action that individuals can take to safeguard their health from environmental risks.
6. Discuss actions that citizens might use to safeguard or improve the environment.

investigating

PURPOSE:
To observe the presence of pollution in the environment.

MATERIALS NEEDED:
Three petri dishes or plastic coffee can covers; petroleum jelly; tape; graph paper; paper; pencil; magnifying glass.

PROCEDURE:
A.   Tape graph paper to the inside of the petri dishes or plastic coffee can covers. Then grease the paper with petroleum jelly, making a thin film over the entire surface.
B.   Place the dishes or covers in various locations such as window sills or outdoor locations.
C.   Check your dishes each day for a week. Record the first day you observe particulates collecting. Then collect each dish (be sure you have marked its location). Use a magnifying glass to examine the dishes.
    1.   How many different types of particulates do you observe in each dish? Where do you think they came from?
    2.   Count and average the number of particles per square centimeter on each dish. Are some more heavily soiled than others? Which ones? Why?

CHAPTER 25

Using Health Services

OBJECTIVES

- IDENTIFY the warning symptoms of disease
- DETERMINE how to select good medical care
- EXPRESS your needs as a patient
- EXPLAIN the difference between types of medical specialists
- DESCRIBE some of the functions performed in hospitals and other health-related fields
- RECOGNIZE "quacks" and false advertising claims for health-care products

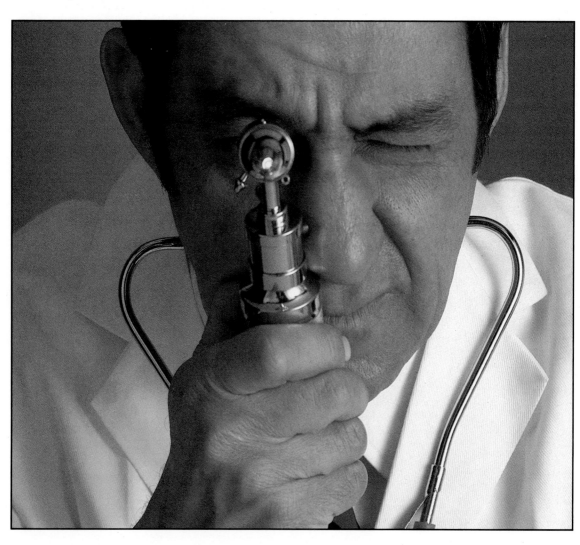

"You've had that stomachache for a week, Anna, and now you're nauseous. Don't you think you should go to a doctor?"

"No, I don't want to go."

"Why not? You can't go on taking aspirins and hoping it'll go away."

"The last time I went there I just ended up feeling silly. I guess I didn't have a good reason to go to a doctor."

"Well, this time I think the situation is different. I'll go with you if it'll make you feel better."

Do you know the difference between symptoms that need professional treatment and those that don't? If you need medical help, do you know how to find it and how to choose among available alternatives? This chapter will help guide these decisions.

WELLNESS: YOUR RESPONSIBILITY

A healthy and balanced life-style is the first step toward feeling well and being well. It is your responsibility to prevent sickness and accidents through positive action. In that way, you are less likely to become ill. Illness can strike even a normally healthy person, however. When that happens, knowing how to get appropriate medical care is essential.

BASIC SELF-CARE

Do you listen to your body? Do you know what is normal for you and what is abnormal? It is important to become aware of your body's signals. Each person has a different energy level. Sometimes you may feel more tired than usual. Then you should be able to ask yourself, "Have I been eating regularly and getting proper rest? Could my fatigue be due to emotional stress?" If none of these factors seems to be the cause, then you should listen to your body more carefully. Notice if your fatigue persists without explanation for more than a few days. If so, your body is telling you that something is wrong. Then you should see a health professional so that together you can find out if there should be cause for concern.

HOME TREATMENT. It has been estimated that, out of every ten patients in a doctor's waiting room, six don't need

Table 25–1

COMMON AILMENTS AND THEIR HOME-TREATMENT MEDICATIONS

Ailment	Medication
Allergy	Antihistamines; nose drops and sprays
Colds and coughs	Cold tablets/cough syrups
Constipation	Milk of magnesia; bulk laxatives
Dental problems (preventive)	Sodium fluoride
Diarrhea	Preparations that contain pectin
Eye irritations	Eye drops and artificial tears
Hemorrhoids	Hemorrhoid preparations
Pain and fever in adults	Aspirin; acetaminophen
Pain and fever in children	Liquid acetaminophen; aspirin
Poisoning for which vomiting should be induced (when in doubt, call Poison Control)	Syrup of ipecac
Fungus	Antifungal preparations
Sunburn (preventive)	Sunscreen agents
Sprains	Elastic bandages
Stomach, upset	Antacid; nonabsorbable
Wounds	
Minor	Adhesive tape; bandages
Antiseptic	Hydrogen peroxide; iodine
Soaking agent	Sodium bicarbonate (baking soda)

to be there. Those six have minor illnesses, such as colds, backaches, headaches, occasional insomnia, itching, minor cuts, constipation, or diarrhea. Most of these conditions could be treated effectively at home with rest, simple over-the-counter medications, and a minor change in life-style. Table 25-1 gives a list of OTC preparations useful in common home-treatment situations. They should be on hand, but well out of reach of children. Every home should also have a clinical (oral) thermometer, which can be purchased from any pharmacy.

SEEKING MEDICAL CARE
WHEN MEDICAL CARE IS NEEDED

Chapter 27 outlines first aid for emergency situations. These obviously require medical assistance urgently. Symptoms of serious illness, such as a fever over 38.9 degrees centigrade (102°F), sudden shortness of breath, sudden headaches, coughing that cannot be controlled or coughing up blood, diarrhea or vomiting that cannot be controlled, mental disorientation, and blood in the stool require prompt medical attention.

Other symptoms should not be overlooked, but do not call for a trip to the hospital emergency room. An *appointment* for medical care should be sought for:

1. Fever over 37.8 degrees centigrade (100°F) for several days.
2. Chronic shortness of breath.
3. Episodes of rapid or irregular heart action.
4. Night sweats not associated with the weather or known illness.
5. Fatigue without apparent cause.
6. Loss or gain in weight without change in diet or activity.
7. Pain that does not go away under any circumstance.
8. Marked change in bowel habits without change in diet or exercise.
9. Any lesion of the skin or mucous membranes that is slow to heal.
10. A swelling that does not go down or increases in size.
11. Unexplained bleeding from any body opening.
12. Unexplained depression or insomnia.

FINDING MEDICAL CARE

Most people want a **primary-care physician,** that is, a medical doctor who can give a thorough overall examination, make a diagnosis, and prescribe care and treatment for most illnesses. Your needs should determine which of the following you choose.

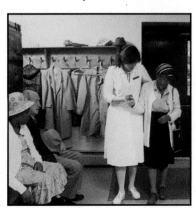

25–1. Today, people can choose from a wide variety of medical services.

1. **Private practice:** a physician alone with a nurse or receptionist. If you choose a physician in private practice, find out who "covers" for the doctor (that is, who takes his or her place) in times of vacation, illness, or business trip.
2. **Group practice:** several doctors who join together in one location. When you visit a group practice you may have to see whichever doctor is available. The advantage is that there is always someone "on call."
3. **Health Maintenance Organization** (HMO): has a full medical staff (doctors, nurses, and technicians). It provides most medical care, including minor surgical

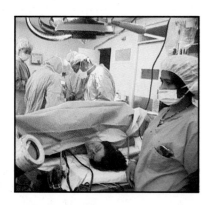

25–2. Obstetricians take care of expectant mothers and deliver babies.

procedures, on the premises. A family or individual pays a monthly fee to belong. This covers all services the HMO can offer. (Find out exactly what services they provide.)

4. **Hospital clinics:** clinics that provide a wide variety of services. Cost generally depends on the type of hospital it is. In a public hospital the fee may be based on income. The lower your income, the lower the fees charged.

To make your choice, consider the kinds of services provided and the kind of situation in which you'd feel most comfortable. Ask a medical person you trust who or what facility they would recommend. Ask someone who has used that same service what kind of care they received. You should do your research while you are well. It will also help to go to a medical facility that has your health records.

MEDICAL SPECIALISTS

If your primary-care physician thinks you need more specific or advanced care than he or she can provide, you may be referred to a specialist. Medicine has become specialized because the field of medicine has greatly expanded. Without specialization it would be difficult to keep up with all the latest developments, research, and treatment. Within the AMA (American Medical Association) there are currently about 25 medical specialties, with subspecialties under them (see Table 25-2).

Find out whether the specialist you choose has extra education and training in his or her specialty. Any licensed physician can legally practice any surgical or medical specialty. These physicians do not have to have extra training in a specialty to call themselves specialists. You should ask: Is the doctor *board-certified*? (*Yes* means he or she has passed an exam in the specialty.) Is the doctor *board-eligible*? (*Yes* means that he or she has the training and has not taken the specialty exam.) Is the doctor on staff at a hospital? (*Yes* means that he or she has the opportunity to be familiar with a wider variety of patients and treatments and is usually available in private practice.)

THE DOCTOR-PATIENT RELATIONSHIP

Finding medical care is the first step, but when you get there you must know how to communicate with the medical personnel.

534

MEDICAL AND SURGICAL SPECIALISTS

Name of Specialist	Areas in Which They Specialize
Medical Specialists	
Allergist	Allergic conditions, such as asthma, hay fever, hives, etc.
Cardiologist	Heart disease
Dermatologist	Skin disorders (which may include skin cancer)
Endocrinologist	Disorders of endocrine glands
Gastroenterologist	Gastrointestinal disorders
General internist (primary care)	Diagnoses by thorough history of the illness, complete physical examination, and often laboratory and X-ray studies
Gerontologist	Ailments and disorders of the aged
Gynecologist	Pelvic organs
Hematologist	Blood diseases
Nephrologist	Kidney disorders and diseases
Neurologist	Structural diseases of brain, spinal cord, and nerves
Obstetrician	Expectant mothers and delivery of babies
Oncologist	Cancer
Opthalmologist	Eyes, including eye surgery
Otolaryngologist	Ear, nose, and throat problems
Pediatrician	Children
Proctologist	Rectum, anus, and sigmoid colon
Psychiatrist	Emotional and mental disorders
Radiologist	Examination and treatment by means of X ray and radiation
Rheumatologist	Rheumatic diseases of joints and muscles
Urologist	Ureters, bladder, urethra, and prostate gland
Surgical Specialists	
Anesthesiologist	Anesthetic drugs for painless surgery; checks patient before and after surgery (does not do surgery)
Cardiovascular surgeon	Heart and blood vessels
General surgeon	Most kinds of surgery, especially abdominal
Neurosurgeon	Brain, spinal cord, and nerves
Ophthalmologist	Eye surgery
Orthopedic surgeon	Bones and joints
Plastic surgeon	Skin and soft tissue deformities
Thoracic surgeon	Chest and lungs

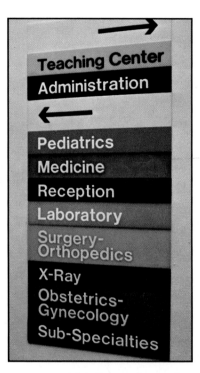

25-3. Do you know what the words on this sign mean?

Table 25-2

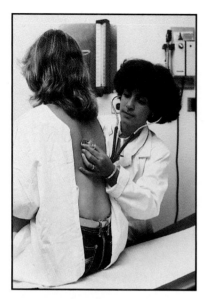

25–4. *Do you know how to communicate with medical personnel?*

COMMUNICATION. Sometimes doctors use a medical term to describe a disease without realizing that the patient isn't familiar with it. They may say *hypertension* instead of high blood pressure, or *myocardial infarction* instead of heart attack. If you do not understand what is being said, do not hesitate to say so. If you do not understand the nature of your illness, speak up. Ask for clarification.

You must learn to use appropriate words and labels as well. "It sort of hurts" doesn't tell a doctor very much. Be prepared to describe any pain in a variety of ways:

1. Where is it?
2. Is it dull, sharp, pressing?
3. When do you feel it and how long does it last?
4. Does it stay in one place, or is it spreading?
5. Does anything make it better?
6. What makes it worse?

Before calling or visiting a doctor, make a few notes describing your symptoms as clearly and precisely as possible and also jot down questions you want to ask. If you have medical records or a list of medicines you are taking, bring them along.

A doctor may need to know about personal habits that have contributed to your illness. Do not be embarrassed about telling a doctor something personal. The more open you can be, the more exact your doctor can be about his or her diagnosis.

If it is your first visit to a particular doctor, you will be asked a variety of questions about your health history, including questions about chronic diseases that other members of your family may have. When the diagnosis is made, that is, when you are told what is wrong, you should receive a full explanation of your symptoms and what the treatment will be.

SECOND AND THIRD OPINIONS. If a doctor prescribes surgery for your condition, you should ask about alternative possibilities and what risks are involved with each. Some surgery is necessary because of life-threatening emergencies; most surgery is elective. **Elective surgery** is non-emergency surgery performed to relieve pain, to prevent a more serious problem from developing, or to otherwise improve a patient's condition. The risks involved in the surgery have to be weighed against those involved in not having the surgery. If you have doubts about the necessity of the operation, you have a right to go to another specialist for a second opinion.

HEALTH ACTION

Briefly describe your medical history. Include family history of chronic diseases (heart disease, cancer, diabetes, etc.), infectious diseases you have had, dates and kinds of vaccinations, hospitalizations, operations, allergies, and present physical disorders. Keep this information so that it will be available at any time you need medical care.

Medical insurance usually covers the cost of getting a second opinion and sometimes a third if the first two doctors disagree. You may also wish to obtain a second opinion if your doctor says that you have a serious disease or if your doctor has not made a diagnosis after two or three visits.

MEDICATION.   Medication may not always be prescribed for you. Do not necessarily expect it. If the doctor does feel that medication is the best remedy, TAKE IT EXACTLY AS PRESCRIBED: NO MORE, NO LESS, AND AT THE TIMES INDICATED. If you don't understand the directions, ask your pharmacist or doctor to explain them. Sometimes you'll feel better after taking only part of the prescription. If the directions say to stop taking the medication when the symptoms disappear, stop taking it. However, if the directions say to continue until all the medication is gone, then continue.

OTC drugs can be dangerous to your health, especially if not used properly. Therefore, when using OTC medications in self-care, follow the directions on the label. For example, "cold remedies" contain antihistamines and cause sleepiness. If you drive while taking them, you may have an automobile accident. Be sure to read the label *completely* on every OTC drug that you take and do not mix OTC medications with prescribed drugs or alcohol.

DENTISTS

It is just as essential to choose a good dentist as a good physician. Besides helping to save your teeth, your dentist should be able to diagnose other problems. A good dentist can recognize oral cancer and other serious illnesses.

Follow the same procedure for finding a dentist as a doctor. (Remember: dentists have different kinds of practices, too.) If you find that you have special problems, your dentist may refer you to a dental specialist.

BEING A HOSPITAL PATIENT

If you need surgery, extensive medical testing, or special treatments, you may have to enter a hospital. You are most likely to be in the hospital with which your doctor is affiliated. Or you may have a choice or be sent to one that specializes in the treatment of your particular condition. There are children's hospitals; ear, nose, and throat hospitals; hospitals for cancer patients; and orthopedic hospitals.

HEALTH TIP

When your doctor prescribes a medication, ask if it is available in **generic** form, rather than a brand name. The generic name comes from the chemical name of the drug. If your doctor feels that the generic drug is equal in effectiveness to the brand-name drug, he or she may prescribe it instead. Generic drugs are usually much cheaper, because they are not advertised and the packaging is usually simpler.

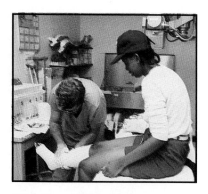

25–5. You should go to an emergency room only if you have a sudden illness or injury.

HEALTH IN HISTORY

Since the dawn of history, people have provided shelter and care for the sick and injured. Gradually these shelters evolved from simple lodging houses for the terminally ill to true hospitals with medical staffs and nursing care. However, for many years hygienic conditions in these hospitals were deplorable, and nursing care was poor, so that many were called "pesthouses."

In response to rapid advances in medical knowledge and improving social and economic conditions, the modern hospital came into being within the past hundred years. Before this century, millions of people died because they could not obtain the kind of care that is now available in the modern hospital.

In order to make a judgment about the quality of care and services you might receive in a hospital, you should ask a few questions. Is the hospital accredited? This means it has received approval through examination by the Joint Commission on Accreditation of Hospitals, or JCAH. About two-thirds of the general hospitals in the U.S. are accredited. Is it a teaching hospital? This usually, though not necessarily, means that it is affiliated with a medical school. It may also be a medical training center for nurses. Is it a voluntary, nonprofit hospital or is it a privately owned, profit-oriented hospital? Neither choice guarantees quality treatment, but knowing the difference tells you what to look for. If it is a nonprofit hospital, who operates it? If it is a private hospital, how much profit is made and on what is the profit made? Answers to these questions will help you choose a hospital in a non-emergency situation.

Should you have an emergency condition, you may be transported to the hospital by ambulance. The **emergency room** (ER) of a hospital receives victims of accidents and sudden illnesses. Many private-practice physicians may advise their patients to go to an emergency room in the event of sudden illness or injury. Even though you are brought to an emergency room you should not necessarily expect to receive immediate attention. The procedure followed in an ER is called **triage.** This means that injuries or illnesses are judged to be one of three kinds: (1) an emergency; (2) serious but stable; or (3) not serious. Life-threatening emergencies are treated first. If you are not treated at once that doesn't mean your injury is not considered serious. It means that someone else's injury or illness is even more serious.

Many hospitals have **outpatient clinics** that treat people who do not require admission to a hospital. This extends hospital services and all their modern equipment to more people in the community and saves the expense of in-hospital care. This also cuts the cost of some surgery. Surgery that formerly required a hospital admission is now performed in many of these outpatient clinics. Hernia repair and even cataract surgery are now done in hosptial outpatient clinics.

OTHER HEALTH CARE FACILITIES

FREE CLINICS.   In some cities *free walk-in clinics* exist for anyone with a specific medical problem, no matter what their income. Sometimes these are especially geared toward young adults who have a question or potential problem with drugs or sex-related diseases. These clinics are usually run by private, nonprofit organizations and are staffed by qualified medical personnel who volunteer their time.

There are also many types of free clinics provided by local health departments for low-income people. These include mental health, dental, and maternal health care clinics, as well as venereal disease clinics, cancer clinics, and clinics for general checkups and health care.

NURSING HOMES. Over 1 million Americans live in 25,000 nursing homes in the United States. Ninety percent of these people are over 65. Most are unable to care for themselves without help. Many are too ill to be cared for at home and need constant medical supervision.

A good nursing home provides recreational activities, medical care, physical therapy, and skilled nursing care. It is estimated that only one-half of the currently available homes provide adequate nursing care. The rest merely provide custodial care.

Home care provides an alternative to the hospital and nursing home. The American Public Health Association has estimated that up to 25 percent of institutionalized people could live at home if adequate care could be furnished. "Meals on Wheels," visiting nurses, homemakers, and all sorts of physical and emotional therapies are available in many communities. The cost is generally less than the same service in a nursing home, especially if medical insurance furnishes coverage. The most important advantages of home care are the psychological benefits. Many people, such as accident vicitms, often recover faster when they receive treatment in their own homes.

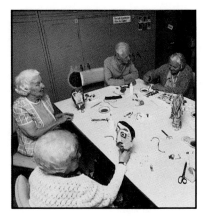

25–6. Good nursing homes provide recreational activities.

CHOOSING ADEQUATE HEALTH INSURANCE

For most people a serious illness, without the protection of health insurance, would mean financial disaster. The cost of hospital stays, treatments, medication, and nursing and doctors' fees are staggering. To prepare for possible medical expenses, about 85 percent of the U.S. population have some form of medical insurance.

Two types of health insurance are provided by the government. **Medicare,** which is for people over 65 years of age, covers part of the expense of hospital care and some outpatient expenses. **Medicaid** is insurance provided by the government for low-income individuals or families.

The HMO (health maintenance organization) is an alternative to traditional insurance. The monthly fee acts as prepayment for medical services you might need.

Private health insurance may be purchased by the consumer individually or as group policies through an employer, union, or other organization. Some insurance policies provide only minimum coverage. Others cover a wide range of expenses, such as dental fees and prescribed medications. The important thing to consider in choosing health insurance is type and amount of coverage. When choosing insurance, make sure you have all the information you need to make your choice. *Read the policy carefully,* and find out the following:

1. Does the insurance pay for these services: hospital stay; outpatient follow-up; in-hospital doctor's/medical staff fees; doctors' care outside hospital; medications; X rays; special treatments (for example, occupational therapy, dialysis)?
2. If insurance covers hospital stay, is there a limit to how many days it pays for?
3. What is the deductible, that is, how much of the bill do you pay before the insurance starts to pay?
4. What percentage of the bill does the insurance pay after the deductible? 100 percent? 80 percent? Less?
5. Under what conditions can the insurance company cancel the policy or refuse to pay for treatment?
6. Does the insurance pay for services such as mental health care or dental care?

BEWARE OF "QUACKS"

During the eighteenth and nineteenth centuries, there were very few doctors on our frontiers. This was a golden opportunity for traveling medicine shows, which claimed cures for all illnesses, real or imagined. They sold sugar pills and "elixirs," usually consisting of colored water or alcohol. The medicine show is still with us, although in a different form. With advertising in newspapers, direct mail, radio, and television, the medicine show reaches millions of people.

There are still **quacks** for every illness that exists. There are even some who claim to cure even incurable diseases

Table 25–3

INDICATORS FOR SPOTTING FRAUD
1. Does the sale of the pills, device, or equipment make a great deal of money for someone?
2. Does it offer a "quick" and "simple" or "painless" cure?
3. Do they use testimonials rather than research reports as evidence of the effectiveness of the cure?
4. Do they claim that all of the medical profession is out to get them?

or diagnose and treat a disease where none is present. These people may have little or no medical knowledge or training. They use worthless and sometimes harmful medicines. Odd-looking machines, equally ineffective, may be used to impress the patient.

It has been estimated that Americans spend $1 billion each year on useless gadgets, medicines, and food preparations. Arthritis victims alone pay more than $250 million every year on worthless or harmful treatments. They buy seawater concentrates and so-called electronic devices at very high prices. Meanwhile, their joints become more damaged, and their pain increases.

Cancer patients are also targets for fraudulent and "get better fast" schemes. Grapes and apricot pits have been recommended as cancer cures and preventive medicines. A victim of cancer may delay proper medical treatment until it's too late by relying on one or more "quick cures." Early diagnosis and proper treatment of cancer can be effective. Delaying treatment can be fatal.

Should you find evidence of quackery or fraudulent claims, report it to one of the federal agencies created to protect consumers. The federal Food and Drug Administration (FDA) monitors the testing of new drugs before they can be marketed. The FDA requires that all drugs be of standard strength, and that labeling be truthful and informative. The FDA prosecutes manufacturers of drugs and appliances found to be harmful or worthless. The Federal Trade Commission (FTC) monitors deceptive or false advertising of all health products. The United States Postal Service is constantly on watch for mail-order claims of fraudulent products. Fraud and quackery can be decreased through the watchful eye of the consumer.

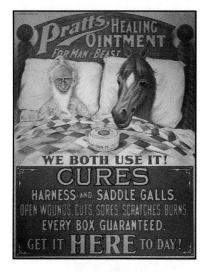

25–7. Advertisement from the late nineteenth century for healing ointment. In your opinion, would this ointment work?

SUMMARY: You are solely responsible for following a life-style aimed at good health. However, in spite of your best efforts, illness may strike. In this chapter, you have learned how to recognize signs of illness and how to choose the medical care you need. You have also learned how to get the best out of medical care by being aware of your symptoms and by being able to communicate with your doctor. You should now know how to detect worthless medical care, quackery, and drugs that do not work or are harmful. Above all, you know the importance of treating your body in a way that will ensure that you continue to have the best possible health.

CHAPTER REVIEW

words at work

Find the word in the left column that fits one of the definitions in the right column. DO NOT WRITE IN THIS BOOK.

a. generic
b. Medicare
c. Medicaid
d. quackery
e. HMO
f. triage
g. elective surgery
h. primary care physician

1. Unscrupulous medical practice
2. Government medical insurance for most people over 65 years of age
3. Government medical insurance for some low-income patients
4. The chemical name of a drug
5. Non-emergency surgery
6. System by which the seriousness of an emergency is judged
7. Diagnoses and treats most illnesses
8. Organization to which you pay a monthly fee to belong and get most medical services

review questions

1. What symptoms should mean an immediate call for medical help?
2. What conditions indicate a need to make an appointment with your doctor?
3. List the minimum contents of a home medicine cabinet.
4. How would you choose a doctor?
5. What communication problems arise between a doctor and a patient?
6. Identify six medical specialists whose services you might need in the future.
7. What is the purpose of the emergency room of a modern hospital?
8. Why do hospitals have outpatient clinics?
9. Identify the two types of medical insurance provided by the federal government today.
10. How does going to an HMO differ from going to a physician who is in private practice?
11. What is meant by a "generic" drug? How do generic drugs save the patient money?
12. Why is it important to use caution when taking over-the-counter drugs?
13. Why do people fall for "quackery" and fraud?
14. What are some of the ways in which you can spot quacks and fraudulent schemes?
15. What protection against quackery is provided by the federal government?

542

discussion questions

1. Discuss the role of the modern hospital.
2. Discuss the problems of medical costs and insurance needs.
3. Investigate quackery and fraud in advertising. Report your findings.
4. Find out if your community has a freestanding outpatient surgery clinic. Discuss the advantages and disadvantages of such clinics.
5. Discuss the opportunities and advantages of health services as a career.

investigating

PURPOSE:

To compare different methods of taking the body temperature.

MATERIALS NEEDED:

Different types of thermometers, including oral, mercury and strips for measuring skin temperature; sterile cotton; alcohol; cool water; and soap.

PROCEDURE:

A.   Examine an oral mercury thermometer. Look at the column of mercury and the temperature scale.
    1.   What are the lowest and highest degree markings on the thermometer?
    2.   How many degrees does each line on the scale represent?
B.   With the bulb end down, shake the thermometer to at least 96°F (35.5°C).
C.   Clean the thermometer. Dip the cotton in alcohol, and thoroughly wipe the thermometer. Then, wash it with cool water and soap. (Hot water may ruin the thermometer.)
D.   Place the thermometer under your tongue for at least three minutes. To read the thermometer, hold the glass end, and slowly twirl until you can see the column of mercury.
    3.   What is your body temperature under your tongue?
    4.   How does your body temperature compare to those of your classmates?
    5.   What were the highest and lowest temperatures recorded?
E.   Now, take your body temperature by holding the thermometer under your armpit. (This method works well for a baby or a very young child.)
    5.   What is your body temperature under your armpit?
F.   Examine a skin temperature strip. Get instructions for its use. Hold the strip against your forehead until the color stops changing.
    6.   What is the skin temperature on your forehead as measured by the skin strip?
G.   Measure the skin temperature of your hands, arms, and legs.
    7.   Does the skin temperature differ from one part of your body to the next?
    8.   Compare the two methods of obtaining body temperature. What are the advantages and disadvantages of each?

CHAPTER 26

Safety and Accident Prevention

OBJECTIVES

- EXPLAIN the National Safety Council's classification of accidents
- IDENTIFY major causes of automobile accidents
- IDENTIFY hazardous areas in the home
- SUGGEST what to do in case of a fire
- DESCRIBE the hazards of swimming, firearms, and certain occupations
- STATE how to protect yourself when a tornado, an earthquake, or lightning strikes

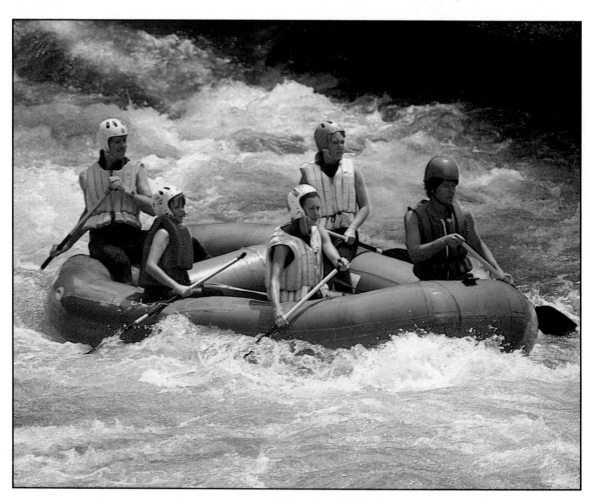

Two of Jan's friends piled into the car to go swimming.

"Seat belts everyone!" she said.

"Come on," answered Sean. "I'm not going to fall out the door. What do you think I am, a baby?"

"Hey, are we picking up Maria and Tyrell?"

"Definitely. That's our next stop."

"Where will they sit?" asked Barbara.

"Who knows? We'll stuff them in somewhere. Maria will probably have to bring her little sister, too."

Everyone groaned.

"I thought Tyrell couldn't swim."

"He can't, but a few dunkings will solve that problem," Andrew laughed.

"Say, it looks like rain. Maybe we shouldn't go."

"What's a little rain? It's only water. Swimming in a summer rain can be exciting."

This group is about to take a number of unreasonable risks, endangering their lives in the process. Can you point them out? How might they organize things differently?

THE CAUSES OF ACCIDENTS

Accidents are the leading cause of death among people under 44 years of age. In fact, accidents rank fourth among all causes of death, following heart disease, cancer, and stroke. In addition, millions suffer disabling accidents each day. The **National Safety Council** estimates that the total cost of accidents each year exceeds $87 billion. But most accidents can be prevented and you can learn how. The National Safety Council divides all accidents into four general classifications:

1. MOTOR VEHICLES. Motor vehicle accidents account for 50 percent of all fatal accidents and 20 percent of all disabling injuries. When you are involved in a motor vehicle accident, the chances of your being killed rather than seriously injured are far greater than in any other type of accident.

2. HOME. The home is a high-risk area accounting for over 20 percent of the fatalities and about 36 percent of the disabling injuries.

3. PUBLIC. Public places include public transportation, recreational swimming areas, hunting grounds, and athletic fields. About 18 percent of all fatal accidents and 27 percent of all disabling injuries occur in public places such as these.

The **National Safety Council,** a nonprofit organization founded in 1913, has spearheaded the safety movement in the United States. Headquarters are located at 444 North Michigan Avenue, Chicago, Illinois 60611. Each year they publish a book entitled *Accident Facts,* as well as a number of other publications. Their membership includes industrial organizations and institutions of all types, including high schools and colleges.

Thanks to their efforts, our country has developed safety consciousness. It is now a safer place to live and to work than any other place in the world. Much still remains to be done.

26–1. Is having a few drinks more important than someone's life?

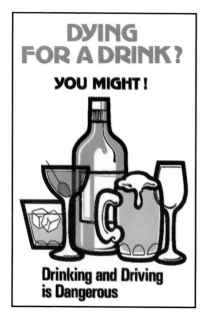

4. WORK. Accidents at work account for less than 12 percent of all fatal accidents and about 20 percent of all disabling injuries.

Pinpointing safety hazards in the home, at school, at work, and during recreation is the first step toward decreasing accidents. Accidents are not inevitable. They may involve an element of surprise, but there is always a reason why an accident occurs. Many can be prevented through individual and group awareness. The objectives of safety education include (1) promoting **safety awareness,** which is consciousness of safety problems (2) preventing accidents, and (3) preparing for emergencies.

Are some people accident-prone? A small percentage of people are involved in a large number of accidents. This group is referred to as **accident-prone,** and their accidents occur in the home, on the job, at school, and at play. Under physical, mental, or emotional stress, people are liable to be involved in an accident. Some have personality disorders or other traits that keep them in a state of turmoil. Recently, programs have been developed to help accident-prone individuals. The programs help people to improve self-concept, change attitudes, recognize and reduce stress, and experience success in daily activities.

AUTOMOBILE SAFETY

Each day about 130 people die as a result of automobile accidents. What causes automobile accidents? A look at all the factors suggests an answer. Weather and road conditions are responsible for some accidents. Poorly functioning cars and the design of the cars are occasionally at fault. However, careless, inefficient, reckless, and drunk drivers cause most accidents. Car manufacturers have been under pressure to produce safer cars. But the fact remains that preventing accidents is largely up to the driver.

THE CAUSES OF CAR ACCIDENTS

THE DRIVER.   Nearly half of all fatal automobile accidents involve a driver or a pedestrian who has been drinking. More than 8,000 young people are killed annually due to drinking and driving. Barbiturates also distort vision and slow down reaction time. Marijuana distorts perception of time and space and impairs judgment. Pep pills, used to reduce fa-

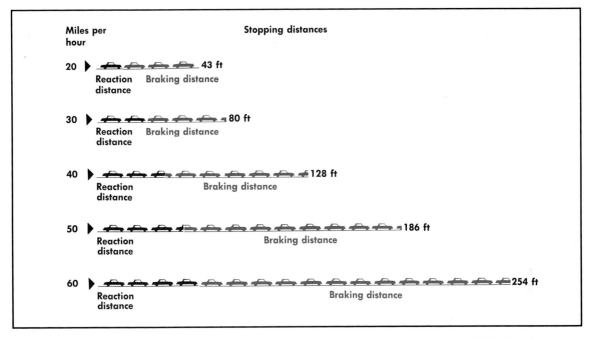

Stopping distances

20 ▶	Reaction distance	Braking distance	43 ft
30 ▶	Reaction distance	Braking distance	80 ft
40 ▶	Reaction distance	Braking distance	128 ft
50 ▶	Reaction distance	Braking distance	186 ft
60 ▶	Reaction distance	Braking distance	254 ft

tigue and keep drivers awake, are dangerous as well. All drugs that alter the mind are hazardous when taken by a driver.

In about one-half of all fatal automobile accidents, a driver was exceeding the speed limit. The national speed limit of 55 miles per hour, imposed as an energy-saving measure, has reduced the number of accidents on our nation's highways. Other speed regulations are set for safety reasons and should also be observed.

Too many people drive as if their car had an automatic pilot. They do not think. For example, over 1,000 people are killed each year at railroad crossings. Because they seldom see a train on the track, they disregard the warning signal. Most of these drivers are killed fewer than 25 miles from home.

Driving on long stretches of highway with little traffic can become boring and a person may start to daydream without realizing it. On long trips, it's best to travel with someone who can share the driving. Stopping frequently for ten-minute breaks will also help relieve boredom and maintain mental alertness.

One out of fifteen accident reports shows that a driver's physical condition was a contributing cause. General illness, going to sleep at the wheel, poor eyesight, and defective

26–2. The faster a car travels, the greater the distance needed to stop. Excessive speed, bad judgment, and defective brakes considerably increase the chance of an accident.

HEALTH TIP

Driving experts suggest that every 5 to 7 seconds drivers should glance into the inside and outside rear-view mirrors to see what is going on around them.

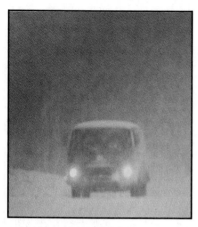

26–3. If possible, avoid driving in hazardous weather conditions. If you must drive in bad weather, drive very slowly and carefully.

hearing can all cause accidents. All states require a license to drive. Most states check for impaired eyesight and hearing, and for physical handicaps. Depending on the extent of impairment, the driver may be required to wear glasses, wear a hearing aid, use a knob on the steering wheel, or have other special devices.

No one should drive when under severe stress. It impairs judgment, self-control, and physical reactions. Accidents may be caused by the driver who, suffering from stress, just doesn't care what happens or is concentrating on something else. Don't be afraid to say you won't drive.

ROAD CONDITIONS. Ice, snow, rain, and fog create hazardous driving conditions. All drivers must make allowances for changes in weather conditions by driving slowly and watching the road more carefully, and, if necessary, using headlights. Slippery surfaces require greater stopping distances. Start with an easy foot on the gas so the wheels won't spin.

Another cause of car accidents is **traffic congestion.** Whenever traffic increases, the accident record climbs. Holidays always present special driving problems, and the accident rate soars. To help prevent accidents, plan to drive when the highways are less congested if at all possible.

PREVENTING AUTOMOBILE ACCIDENTS: THE EXPERT DRIVER

Expert drivers recognize their responsibilities to themselves and to others. They accept the car as a powerful machine that is fun to drive as long as it is under control. The expert drivers realize that regulations are designed for the protection of all. The expert drivers think ahead to avoid accidents. They follow these rules:

1. Obey all speed limits all the time.
2. Signal when changing directions.
3. Come to a full stop whenever a sign indicates that you should do so.
4. Think ahead and get in the proper lane.
5. Don't drink or take drugs when driving.
6. Stay in line with other cars; don't weave in and out.
7. Watch for pedestrians; children are especially liable to dart from between parked cars.
8. Don't compete with the other traffic; the street isn't a race track. Automobile races have special locations and rules of their own.

26–4. Anyone who wants to drive should learn how to drive safely.

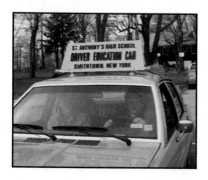

548

9. Reduce speed at night.
10. Keep your car in top condition. Don't just polish the outside. Make sure the inside is in safe working order.
11. Keep your distance and don't tailgate. A short stop can mean a dead stop.
12. Watch for all traffic signs.
13. Drive defensively.
14. Do not drive to "think things out" or to work out your anger.

PROTECTIVE DEVICES

SEAT BELTS. Safety belts are now available on all automobiles, but still many people do not use them. It is estimated that if everyone "buckled up," 16,000 lives would be saved annually. Safety belts help prevent passengers from being thrown through the windshield or against the dashboard. The use of safety belts reduces the chances of being killed in a car accident by as much as 60 percent.

CAR RESTRAINTS FOR CHILDREN. Children should be "buckled up." Many people think it is safe to hold a child on their laps. But a crash or sudden stop makes it impossible to hold on to a child. Children can be thrown about like flying objects. When a car moving 30 miles per hour crashes, unrestrained children hit the dashboard with a force equal to that of falling from a three-story building. Having car restraints for children is now a law in many states.

Small children, under 20 pounds, should be transported in a carrier, held in place by an adult's seat belt. The child should be secured in the carrier by means of a harness. The child should ride in a semi-upright position, usually in the back seat where it is safer. Toddler seats should be used for children too large for infant seats, but still too small for regular seat belts.

MOTORCYCLE SAFETY. We are witnessing a tremendous increase in the number of motorcycles on the road. In 1982 there were about 5,000 deaths and 480,000 injuries caused by motorcycle accidents. Riding a motorcycle requires more skill than driving a car. It is more hazardous because the rider is more exposed. Good protection usually includes an approved safety helmet, eye protectors, gloves, and boots or heavy footwear. The most important piece of protective equipment is the helmet.

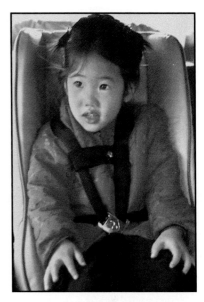

26–5. When traveling with children always buckle them up in car restraints.

SAFETY CHECKLIST FOR THE HOME

Stairs and Steps
- Stairs should be well-lighted, equipped with hand rails, free of all objects (toys, books, clothing).
- Bar steps with a gate on top if small children are in the house.
- Small rugs should be kept away from the foot and head of stairs.
- Treads and carpeting should be kept in good repair.

The Kitchen
- All electrical appliances should be in good working order and in good repair.
- The kitchen should be well-lighted.
- All household cleaners and insecticides should be kept separately from the food and out of reach of small children.
- Store matches in a closed metal container and away from heat.
- Make sure that handles of pots and pans are turned away from the edge of the stove.
- Cooking should not be done in flammable clothing or clothing with billowy sleeves or dangly ties.
- Have handy and visible the instructions for putting out grease and electrical fires.
- Take special care when frying or cooking with oil or grease.

The Bathroom
- There should be a handrail above the tub that you can reach to prevent falling.
- There should be a nonslip mat or a nonslip surface in the bathtub or shower stall.
- All medicines should be kept in the medicine cabinet properly labeled and out of reach of children.
- The area should be well-lighted.
- Keep electrical fixtures away from the bathtub so that they cannot be touched.

The Basement and Attic
- Keep close track of what is being stored there.
- All flammable items (paint rags, paint thinners, gasoline) should be stored safely in closed containers and preferably away from the living

area. Keep them tightly closed and away from any source of fire or heat.
- Do not use electrical power tools while standing on a wet surface.
- Dangerous mementos are often stored away and forgotten. Guns, rifles, and swords are brought back by soldiers returning home and simply put away and forgotten until a curious child rediscovers them.

Garden and Lawn Safety
- Before mowing, clear the lawn of rocks, nails, sticks, and other objects that the blade might pick up. These objects can strike the operator or a nearby person.
- When starting the mower, be sure to keep your feet away from the blade.
- Wear your sturdiest footwear.
- Keep gasoline in a tightly sealed container painted red. If possible, fill the gasoline tank when the engine is cold.
- Never attempt to remove any object from the mower until the motor and the blade have stopped running and the spark plug has been disconnected.
- When using an electric motor, be sure the grass is dry. Be extremely careful not to damage or cut the cord.

Safety Hazards in the Living and Sleeping Quarters
- A fireplace should have a screen to prevent sparks from popping out on the floor or rug.
- Highly polished floors may look attractive and be easy to clean, but they are slippery, too.
- Small rugs placed on slick floors are also dangerous. It makes good sense to use nonslippery wax.
- The backs of throw rugs can be treated with a nonslippery substance to prevent falls.
- Furniture should be kept away from walking spaces in rooms.
- There should be a light switch near the bed.
- Radio and television receivers should be disconnected during storms or when you are away for a long time.

Table 26-1

SAFETY AROUND THE HOME

Approximately 20 percent of all fatal accidents occur in and around the home. About 21,000 people annually lose their lives at home, and 13 million others are injured. The causes of home accidents that result in death, listed in the order of their frequency, are falls, fires and burns, poisoning, suffocation, firearms, drowning, **electrocution** (death by a charge of electricity), and explosion. Use the checklist in Table 26-1 to make your home safer.

FIRE PREVENTION

Fires account for more than 20 percent of the deaths in home accidents. About 1 million fires strike in this country every year, resulting in enormous financial loss estimated in the billions of dollars.

To help prevent fires in the home, keep electrical wiring inspected and repaired. Use flammable liquids with care, and use good judgment. Every smoker should make sure that a cigarette, cigar, or pipe is completely extinguished before retiring. No one should ever toss a burning match, cigarette, or cigar from the window of a moving vehicle.

Fires occur spontaneously where there are oil mops, dust rags, and other oil materials. These substances absorb

---

BASIC RULES FOR REDUCING RISKS IN CASE OF FIRE

- A fire extinguisher in good working order should be available.
- If in a burning building, never open the door until you feel the doorknob to make sure it is not hot.
- If it is hot, leave it closed. Find another way to escape, if possible. If you must stay in the room, plug the open airway under the door to prevent smoke from entering.
- Even though the door is not warm, use extreme care in opening it.
- If you do leave a room, close the door behind you. This helps stop the fire from spreading. Use stair exits, never elevators.
- If you must exit through a smoke-filled hallway, remember that the freshest air is close to the floor. Hold a blanket or something else over your mouth to decrease smoke inhalation.
- If clothing ignites, roll over on the floor.
- Never sleep in a hotel or motel until you have checked the location of the fire escape and know how to get out should a fire occur.
- Avoid panic and keep calm. Don't waste time trying to save personal belongings.
- Never take chances unless a life is involved. Do not jump from an upper-story window except as a last resort.

Table 26–2

26–6. Do you have escape routes planned from every area of your home in case of a fire?

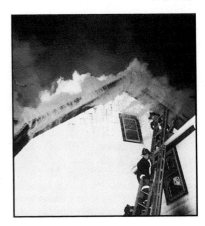

oxygen from the air so rapidly that they generate enough heat to ignite. This kind of fire is called **spontaneous combustion.** Store such materials in airtight containers. This guards against spontaneous combustion because the oxygen supply is decreased.

One or more properly installed **smoke detectors** should be in place in every home. The detectors should be installed near the ceiling on each level of the home where smoke is likely to rise. Near the top of a stairway is usually an excellent place. Most detectors are battery-powered and are equipped with a warning device that activates when the battery becomes weak. However, batteries should be replaced each year. If a fire should occur, learn the basic rules listed in Table 26-2 to minimize your risks.

WATER SAFETY

About 6,200 persons drown each year in this country in swimming and boating accidents. To decrease the risk of drowning:

- Learn how to swim.
- Learn the technique of keeping afloat called "drown proofing." This is a very simple technique that can be learned by anyone, even those who cannot swim. Since

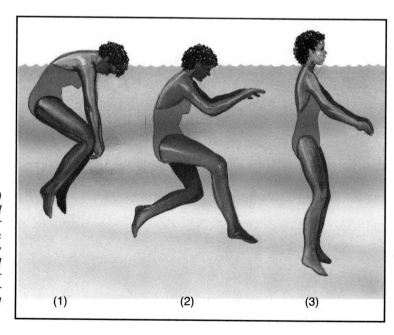

26–7. (1) Take a deep breath and hold it. Place face in water with arms and legs dangling. (2) When ready to breathe, raise arms and spread legs. (3) Lower arms, bring legs together quickly, exhale, raise head to clear water, and inhale.

(1) (2) (3)

it is less tiring than swimming, you can stay afloat longer until help arrives (see Figure 26-7).

- Always swim with a companion.
- If you get a cramp while swimming, don't panic. Flex the leg through the heel and kick to work it out.
- When boating, always heed weather conditions. Know the waterways where you are boating so that you do not get caught in currents. Always wear life jackets.
- If your boat overturns, you are safer to stay with it. An overturned boat seldom sinks, and you will have something to cling to until help arrives.

REDUCING FIREARM RISK

Approximately 1,900 people lose their lives in the U.S. every year in firearms accidents. Some of these are hunting accidents, but more than half of these happen in and around the house, and one-third cause the death of a child under 15.

Many people in the U.S. have legal firearms in their households. If there is a firearm in your house, make sure it is being stored properly. No one, except the person with the license to use it, should be able to get to it. It should be unloaded when stored. When practicing, do so at an official target range. Backyard target practice is always dangerous. Shooting at hard surfaces is hazardous because bullets can bounce back. Be sure the ammunition is suitable for your gun. The wrong ammunition can cause a serious accident. Never lean loaded guns against walls, fences, or stumps.

Always treat guns as though they were loaded. When handling one, keep the muzzle pointed down. Before loading a gun, inspect the barrel for any obstructions. You should never carry a loaded gun in a car. When hunting with a loaded gun, keep the safety lock on until you are ready to fire. If you fall, the gun could discharge, or a twig or branch might hit the trigger. When climbing over a fence, play safe by opening the breech, or "breaking" the gun.

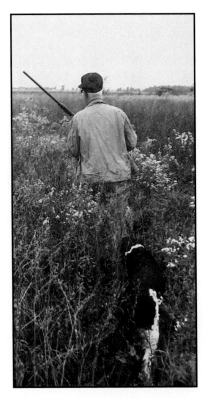

26–8. Hunting accidents can be avoided by following proper safety measures.

PREVENTING CRIME

PREVENTING HOMICIDE

Most, though not all, homicides are committed with guns. The handgun, or "Saturday Night Special," is the most common weapon used. There are approximately 52 million

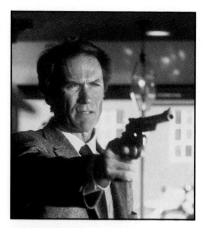

26–9. Do not try to imitate TV and movie heroes if faced with an assailant. Never argue with a gun.

handguns in the U.S., and about 22,500 Americans die from these handguns each year. Among young black men between the ages of 15 and 24, homicide is, in fact, the leading cause of death.

What if you found yourself in a situation where a firearm was being used in a threatening or irresponsible manner? If your presence is voluntary, you should leave immediately. If your presence is not voluntary, that is, if the person with the firearm is forcing you to stay or is asking for your possessions, do not argue with the gun. In spite of all the movies and TV shows you may have seen, bullets move faster than people can run. If you are faced by an assailant, your first impulse may be to fight back. Try to remain calm, and do not try to provoke a person with a gun.

RAPE PREVENTION

Rape is defined as sexual intercourse without consent. The assailant may threaten or inflict physical harm on the victim, or use emotional coercion to commit the crime. A person can also coerce others by threatening to ruin their reputations or harm their friends. In other words, psychological threats may be used. Rape is considered a crime of violence because it is an act of aggression by one person against another. It is not motivated by affection for or physical attraction to the victim.

It is estimated that 1 out of every 2,000 women is the victim of a reported rape. The very old as well as the very young are among the victims. Men are also raped, particularly young men and male children.

If you travel alone at night in unpopulated areas, if you hitchhike, or if you walk alone in secluded areas after dark, you are taking an unreasonable risk. Decrease the risk and avoid these situations.

If you find yourself being followed on a street, go up to a nearby house. Ring the doorbell, bang on the door. Do not be afraid to make noise and arouse attention. If attacked, scream loudly. Some self-help groups suggest screaming "fire" instead of "help." If your attacker has a weapon the situation poses greater danger. Try not to panic. Being calm will help you to judge the situation clearly and think of possible means of escape.

Police advise that if your attacker does not have a weapon, it is safer to fight back. Women sometimes need to practice fighting back. Sometimes they even hesitate to hurt people who are hurting them. Many community centers and

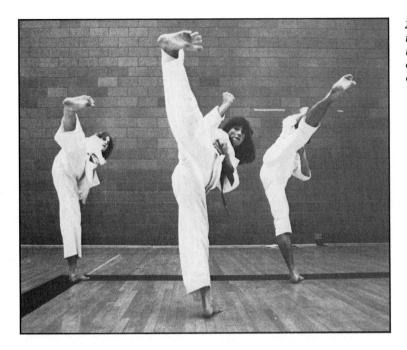

26–10. Many women are taking self-defense classes in order to feel more confident and more in control.

groups offer self-defense classes. You may never need to use what you learn, but you may feel more confident and in control if you have learned some skills for self-defense.

OCCUPATIONAL SAFETY

Workers spend about one-third of their time at work. Most accidents on the job are caused by unsafe conditions, unsafe acts, or a combination of both. The major causes of injuries are the mishandling of materials, falls, failure to wear protective equipment, and machinery mishaps. The need for **occupational safety** (safety on the job) cannot be overemphasized.

The Occupational Safety and Health Administration of the Department of Labor makes and enforces regulations to protect workers in factories, plants, and other work facilities. It helps insure that there are no health or safety hazards. There are stiff penalties if rules are broken. Occupational safety is a constant concern of both labor and industry.

26–11. Since working people spend one-third of their time on the job, occupational safety is essential.

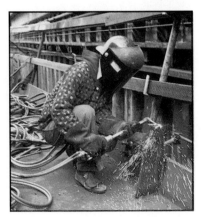

SAFETY ON THE FARM

In a recent year there were 1,800 farm-related fatalities and 180,000 farm-related injuries. Many farmers have accidents while working with farm machinery. Some of the most dangerous machines on the farm are tractors, power saws, corn-pickers, fertilizer spreaders, threshing machines, and mowers. Most of the accidents involve carelessness or misuse of the machinery. Farm workers should always use electrical power equipment safely and drive safely.

DANGEROUS WEATHER

LIGHTNING

The risk of injury or death from lightning varies from one area to another. Lightning usually strikes the tallest object in the area, if it is a conductor of electricity. If you live in an urban area, you are hardly ever likely to be the tallest or only object standing in an open area. If you live in the country, you are more likely to be near the tallest or only object in the area. To reduce the risk of being struck by lightning:

- Go indoors if possible. Stay away from windows and metal fixtures. Unplug the televisions and do not speak on the phone.
- If you must stay outdoors seek shelter in thick woods, *not* under an isolated tree.
- Stay away from fences and metal objects, such as golf clubs. Since they conduct electricity, they are frequently struck by lightning.
- If caught in an open area, drop to your knees, and bend forward. Place your hands on your knees.
- If in a boat, get to shore as soon as possible.

TORNADOES

A tornado is a funnel-shaped, rotating cloud, extending toward the ground from the base of the cloud. It varies in color from gray to black, spins like a top, and may sound like the roaring of an airplane. These storms are of short duration but are violent and destructive over a small area.

A *tornado watch* means that tornadoes are expected to develop. A *tornado warning* means that a tornado has actually been sighted or has been indicated on a radar weather screen. Once a tornado watch is announced, keep informed through the TV or radio. Watch the sky. If you sight such a cloud, report it to the police or the weather service.

The safest place to be is in an underground shelter or a steel and concrete reinforced building. If these are not available, take shelter in the basement if available. If none of these options is possible, take cover under heavy furniture

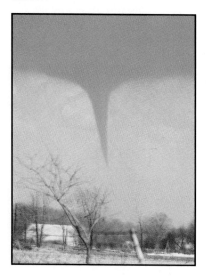

26–12. If you sight a tornado, report it to the police, and then take shelter.

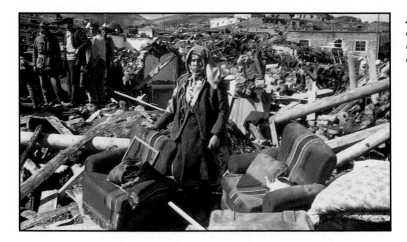

26–13. Strong earthquakes can be extremely destructive to buildings and human life.

on the ground floor, away from outside walls and windows. Stay away from all windows and doors. Do not remain in a trailer or mobile home when a tornado is approaching, since they do not provide enough protection. If you are in open country in a car, try to drive away from the tornado by driving at a right angle to the approaching storm. If there isn't time or you are walking, take cover and lie flat in the nearest ditch or depression.

EARTHQUAKES

Those who live in earthquake zones should follow these safety measures:
- Bolt down and provide support for water heaters and gas appliances.
- Stay away from windows, mirrors, and chimneys.
- Stay under a table, desk, or bed, or in a strong doorway.
- If in a vehicle, park and stay in it.
- If outside, move to an open area if possible.

SUMMARY: Accidents cause a terrible death toll, particularly among young people. Safety education aims to stimulate safety awareness, prevent accidents, and provide emergency plans. The automobile accounts for the largest number of accidental deaths and injuries. Seat belts can help prevent serious injury. The home is a high-risk area, accounting for about 20 percent of all fatal accidents. The number of accidents can be reduced. It is important to plan for emergencies. By following safety rules and using caution, risks can be reduced. Safety is everybody's business.

CHAPTER REVIEW

words at work

Find the word in the left column that fits one of the definitions in the right column. DO NOT WRITE IN THIS BOOK.

a. accident-prone
b. congestion
c. electrocution
d. smoke detector
e. National Safety Council
f. occupational safety
g. safety awareness
h. spontaneous combustion

1. A fire-safety measure
2. Consciousness of a safety problem
3. Fire caused by heat generated by rapid absorption of oxygen
4. Susceptible to accidents
5. Death from a charge of electricity
6. Wearing protective equipment at work
7. A concentration of vehicles, especially during holidays
8. An organization whose mission is accident prevention

review questions

1. Why should safety be a concern of everyone?
2. Into what four classes does the National Safety Council divide all accidents?
3. What is the approximate percentage of fatal accidents attributable to each class of accidents?
4. In most car accidents, who is to blame: the driver or the car?
5. What is meant by an accident-prone driver?
6. List several rules that expert drivers follow.
7. Make a list of the usual causes of automobile accidents.
8. How can the number of accidents caused by alcohol abuse be reduced?
9. Explain how weather conditions affect safety on the highways.
10. Why is it more dangerous to drive on weekends and holidays?
11. Give some examples of improper driving.
12. How can stress affect driving?
13. What are the advantages of wearing seat belts?
14. Explain how small children should be restrained in car seats.
15. Make a list of possible safety hazards in your home.
16. What can be done to decrease fire hazards in your home?
17. What articles in the home might cause spontaneous combustion?
18. What precautions should be taken when using a power mower?

19. List some safety precautions that should be followed when swimming.
20. Outline a safe procedure for handling firearms.
21. What are the most common hazards on the farm?
22. List the principal causes of on-the-job accidents.
23. Outline a safety procedure that should be followed during tornado threats.
24. What can you do to improve your personal safety?

discussion questions

1. Discuss the drunken driver as a public menace. How can the public be protected from drunken drivers?
2. Are young people safe drivers? If so, why are their insurance rates higher?
3. Why do some people refuse to wear seat belts? Since it is estimated that a fatal accident can cost others approximately $90,000, is it other people's business if some fail to "buckle up"?
4. Discuss escape plans to cover the possibility of a fire in your home. Do you have fire drills at home? Why or why not?
5. Discuss the safety features of today's automobile and suggest additional safety features.
6. Discuss how emotions and stress can affect a person's susceptibility to accidents.

investigating

PURPOSE:
To reduce the safety hazards in your home.

MATERIALS NEEDED:
Textbook; paper; pencil.

PROCEDURE:
A.   Make a list of the safety checkpoints listed in Table 26-1 for each area of your apartment or house.
B.   With the help of an adult, check each area of your home and note any hazards you find. Correct as many hazards as you can. As you correct each hazard, cross it off your list.

CHAPTER 27

First Aid

OBJECTIVES

- OUTLINE first-aid priorities
- IDENTIFY respiratory emergencies
- CITE the symptoms of heart attack

- DEMONSTRATE first-aid skills for control of bleeding, poisoning, shock, CPR, mouth-to-mouth breathing, and other emergencies

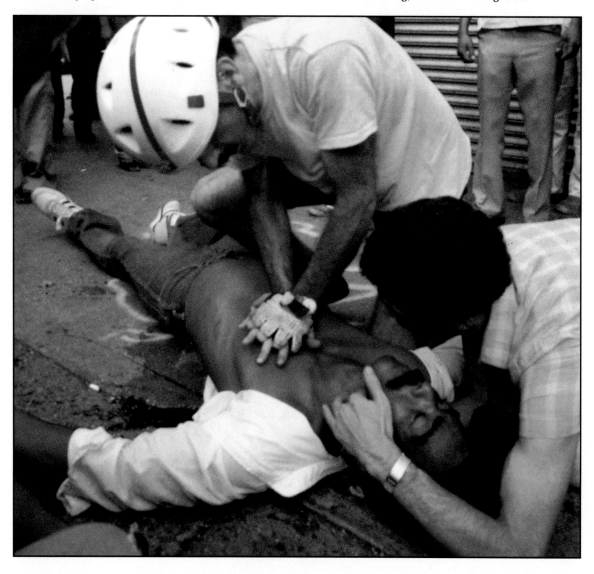

Several friends got together for a picnic. Everyone was having a great time, especially watching Joe who, as usual, was showing off, this time by hanging upside down on a branch. He was laughing so hard he lost his balance, and fell headfirst to the ground. He lay there moaning. He couldn't move his right arm, and his left leg was bent in a strange position.

"Quick. Help him!" shouted Renee.

Nick went over to pick him up.

"No, wait!" yelled Pam. "Go get help and we'll stay with Joe and watch him."

What would your reaction be to this situation? Would you know what to do?

FIRST AID PRIORITIES

First aid is the immediate, temporary care given to a person in case of an accident or sudden illness. When such emergencies arise, fast action may prevent serious injuries and even death. For example, if a major artery is cut, blood loss can cause death within a minute if first aid is not administered. If breathing stops for four to six minutes, the oxygen loss can cause permanent brain damage. First-aid givers should have a calming influence in an emergency. Fear and panic can increase injuries.

First aid is as much a matter of knowing what *not* to do as knowing *what* to do (see Table 27-1 for a list of first-aid priorities). The first-aid giver must be prepared to take charge if no other help is available. Certain skills are necessary for appropriate first-aid treatment. This chapter will give you some basic information about first aid. However, first-aid skills cannot be learned without supervised practice. The American Red Cross and many other organizations offer training in emergency first aid. Be prepared. Be trained.

WOUNDS

A wound is any break in the skin or mucous lining of the body. The most serious problems resulting from wounds are severe bleeding and infection. There is always danger of infection. The deeper the wound, the greater the chance of infection. Types of open wounds are classified as follows:

1. *Abrasions* are scrape-type wounds.
2. *Incisions* are cuts made by any sharp object.

HEALTH TIP

Emergency numbers should be kept by the phone. Your doctor, the emergency section of a hospital, the Poison Control Center, and the Suicide Hotline should all be listed for quick reference.

When reporting an emergency be prepared to tell the operator (1) the nature of the emergency; (2) your location and the location of the injured person; and (3) your name. It is essential that you speak clearly and stay calm.

A LIST OF FIRST-AID PRIORITIES

1. Check the scene of the accident for signs of immediate danger both to yourself and to the victim.
   - Check for escaping gas, live wires, fire, rising water, possible explosion, falling structures (walls, ceilings), and thin ice. All present the possibility of further injury to the victim and possible injury to yourself.
   - Be careful. Move the victim from danger without risking injury to yourself.

2. **Assess the condition of the victim.**
   - Check the ABCs: airway, breathing, and circulation.
     Is the airway obstructed?
     Is the person breathing?
     Is there a pulse?
   - Check for bleeding.
     Keep in mind the possibility of internal injury even if there is no sign of external bleeding.
   - Check for shock.
     Can the person speak?
     Is the skin warm or cool, dry or moist?
     Are the eyes focused?
     Are the pupils the same size?
   - Check for poisoning.
     Are there burns around the mouth?
     Are there empty bottles or containers lying around?
   - Check for broken bones.

3. Start first-aid procedures that are needed immediately, such as:
   - Artificial respiration.
   - Cardiopulmonary resuscitation.
   - Control of bleeding.

4. Contact help, for example:
   - Call 911 or the Operator.
   - Ambulance and medical assistance.
   - Fire department.
   - Police.
   - Poison Control Center.
   - Suicide Prevention Hotline.

5. Resume first-aid procedures.
   - If the injured person is conscious, talk to him or her as calmly as possible. Your own confidence and calm will help to keep the victim calm. A frightened person can be extremely difficult to care for.
   - If you need the victim's cooperation for a first-aid procedure (such as to induce vomiting, to keep him or her awake, moving, or still) direct him or her with your voice.
   - Try to keep the victim as comfortable as possible.
   - If you must move the victim, immobilize the areas of the body that appear to be broken.

Table 27–1

3. *Lacerations* are tears in tissue usually made by blunt instruments.
4. *Punctures* are deep-piercing wounds, such as those made by a pointed object.
5. *Avulsions* are wounds that result from a forceful tearing of tissues from the body.

CONTROL OF BLEEDING

The first priority is to stop great blood loss. A person can bleed to death in a few minutes. If an artery has been cut, it spurts great amounts of blood rhythmically. Blood loss is very rapid when an artery has been cut. Blood loss from a large vein can also be rapid.

Three methods may be used to control severe bleeding: (1) direct pressure and elevation; (2) pressure on pressure points; and, *only* as a last resort, (3) use of a tourniquet.

Direct pressure and elevation of an injured arm or leg will usually stop serious bleeding. When applying direct pressure, use a clean pad or cloth if available as a dressing and apply pressure directly on the wound. Don't worry if blood soaks through the pad. Do *not* remove it, since the blood may have started to clot. Just add additional layers of padding. If nothing is available to act as a dressing, place your hand or fingers directly on the wound. Apply a dressing as soon as possible. Apply a pressure bandage to hold pads over the bleeding wound.

If direct pressure on the wound does not control the bleeding, apply pressure against the nearest pressure point. These points are located next to main arteries. Pressure applied here greatly decreases blood flow and usually stops severe bleeding. Pressure points can be difficult to find unless you've had practice in first-aid skills. Figure 27-1 shows the pressure points that should be used to control severe bleeding.

USE OF A TOURNIQUET.   A **tourniquet** is a constricting band that is tight enough to cut off blood circulation. It should **never** be used unless severe bleeding **cannot** be controlled by any other means. Use a tourniquet only as a last resort if life is endangered. A tourniquet is dangerous because it cuts off the blood supply to the injured area of the body. This causes tissue death and often results in loss of a limb.

Place the tourniquet just *above* the wound, but always between the shoulder and elbow or the hip and the knee. Tourniquets are ineffective on the forearm or foreleg and *never* necessary on fingers, thumbs, or toes. It should not touch the edges of the wound. Once the tourniquet is applied, try to get the victim to a doctor as soon as possible. *Do not* loosen the tourniquet. Note the time the tourniquet was applied to the leg or arm.

TREATING WOUNDS.   Once severe bleeding has been controlled, first aid may be applied to the wound to prevent infection. Wounds that bleed freely, such as incisions, are less likely to become infected because the blood washes bacteria and dirt out. Wounds that bleed only a little, such as abrasions (scrapes) and punctures, can easily become infected if not cleaned well. If the area around the wound is dirty, wash it with soap and water. Then cover it with a sterile cloth or dressing and secure this in place. A dressing, sometimes called a compress, is applied over a wound to

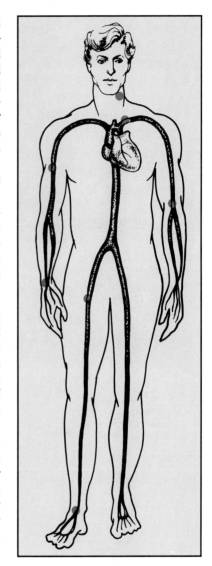

27-1. Pressure points for control of arterial bleeding

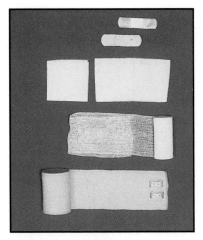

27–2. Small bandages for minor wounds, gauze dressing, gauze bandage, and elastic bandage

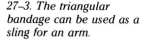

27–3. The triangular bandage can be used as a sling for an arm.

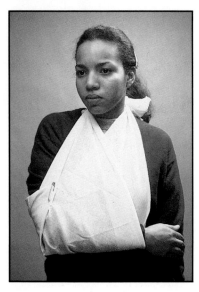

control bleeding, absorb blood and secretions, ease pain, and prevent added contamination. Bandages are never placed directly over wounds but are used to hold a dressing in place, to apply pressure, or to give support. Figures 27–2 and 27–3 show some common bandages.

Puncture wounds often require special care. They close quickly, sealing off the oxygen present in air. These conditions are favorable to the growth of tetanus and other bacteria. A physician should *always* be consulted if someone receives a puncture wound. The doctor will know whether or not the patient should have a tetanus antitoxin or a booster injection. If the object that made the puncture is still in the wound and you are expecting medical assistance, *do not remove* the object. This may cause severe internal bleeding.

BONE, JOINT, AND MUSCLE INJURIES

Bone, muscle, and joint injuries are common in all types of accidents. **Fractures** are breaks in the bones (see Chapter 3). It is important to immobilize fractures, since moving broken bones could cause further injury. This is especially important in the case of spinal fractures. Wrong handling can injure the spinal cord and cause death and paralysis. A fracture may be hard to detect. It is difficult to tell the difference between a sprain, a dislocation, and a possible fracture. For this reason, a doctor should always check all sprains and dislocations, as well as fractures. Table 27-2 summarizes first aid procedures for bone, muscle, and joint injuries.

HEAD INJURIES

The seriousness of head injuries is not always easy to detect. Seek help immediately. In the meantime, keep watch over the victim and take note of his or her general condition.

The most common serious head injuries are skull fractures and **concussions.** A concussion means that the blow causes loss of consciousness. A concussion must always be suspected if the head receives a hard blow. Signs of a concussion include unusual drowsiness, forceful or repeated vomiting, a convulsion, clumsy walking, a bad headache, or one pupil larger than the other. Clear fluid or blood running from the ear, nose, or throat indicates a possibly more serious head injury, such as a skull fracture. Do not move injured victims. Keep them warm and quiet. Stay with them until help arrives.

FIRST AID FOR BONE, JOINT, AND MUSCLE INJURIES

Injury	Treatment
Simple and Compound Fractures (symptoms include intense pain, swelling, evidence of a bruise, deformity, loss of movement)	1. If there is bleeding, try to control it. 2. Treat for shock. 3. If needed, splint to keep injured part from moving. A padded thin board or several thicknesses of newspaper can be used. Splint in position limb is found. Do not tie so tight that circulation is cut off. *Do not try to reset.*
Spinal Fractures (common in car or motorcycle accidents. Victims may have no feeling in fingers or may not be able to move toes.)	1. *Do not move* victim unless victim's life is endangered. 2. Immobilize entire body. Do not let head turn. 3. Get medical help at once.
Dislocation (bones out of joint, cause of swelling, pain)	1. Do not try to put bone back in place. 2. Support joint with bandage and apply cold cloth to prevent swelling. 3. Seek medical help.
Sprains (swelling, pain)	1. Apply ice to keep swelling from increasing. 2. Get to a doctor. Elevate sprained joint while waiting for doctor.
Strains (overstretched or torn muscles cause soreness)	1. Rest, gentle massage, and heat are usually sufficient treatment. 2. See a doctor if pain persists for several days.
Bruises (small blood vessels ooze blood that turns dark)	1. Apply cold cloth or ice bag at once to reduce swelling.

Table 27–2

UNCONSCIOUSNESS

A person may become unconscious for any number of reasons. Do not assume the worst. Quickly assess the condition of the victim and the situation for the probable cause in order to apply the appropriate treatment. Sometimes the color of the face can give a clue as to the cause of unconsciousness (see Figure 27–4). Check the condition of the victim: airway, breathing, and circulation. Stay calm.

27–4. Face color can indicate the type of problem as well as the kind of first aid needed.

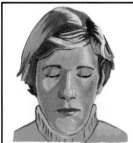 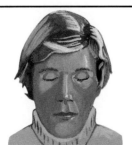 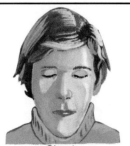 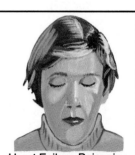

Heat Stroke   Carbon Monoxide Poisoning   Shock Heart Attack   Heart Failure, Poisoning Asphyxiation

RESPIRATORY EMERGENCIES

Drowning, choking, heart failure, suffocation, electric shock, collapsed lung, depressant drugs, and carbon monoxide poisoning are the leading causes of stoppage of breathing. Deprived of oxygen, cells suffocate. The process is referred to as **asphyxiation.**

To check for breathing, look, listen, and feel. With the victim on his or her back, place one hand under the neck, gently apply pressure on the forehead, and tip the head back, so that the chin points skyward. This action is often enough to clear the air passage and start the victim breathing again. Listen for breathing, your ear close to the mouth. Look and feel to see if the chest is moving. If there is no breathing, give artificial respiration.

ARTIFICIAL RESPIRATION

In respiratory emergencies, the most effective method for **resuscitation,** that is, restoring breathing, is the mouth-to-mouth or mouth-to-nose technique. It is direct and easy to administer. Mouth-to-mouth breathing provides air pressure to inflate the victim's lungs immediately. Time is vital. Without oxygen the person will die. The object is to keep the airway open. The steps shown in Figure 27–5 outline the correct procedure for mouth-to-mouth breathing for an injured person *without* neck or spinal injuries.

27–5. For mouth-to mouth breathing
A. *Clear the mouth of foreign material with a sweep of your finger. Be sure the tongue is not blocking the airway. Tilt the head back.*
B. *Pinch the victim's nose between fingers and thumb.*
C. *Take a deep breath and, making a tight seal around victim's mouth, blow air into victim's lungs.*
D. *While taking another breath, allow victim to exhale. Give one breath every 5 seconds (one every 3 seconds for an infant and one every 4 seconds for a child). Continue until medical help arrives.*

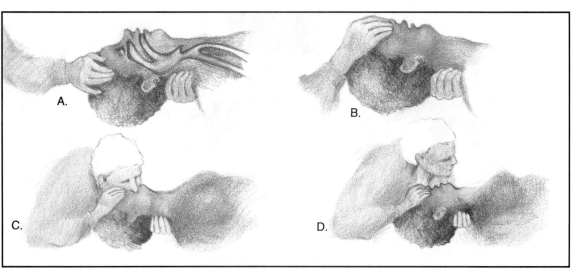

CHOKING

For adults, choking is the sixth leading cause of accidental death; for children, it is the first. When a piece of meat or other substance lodges in the throat and prevents breathing, the first-aid giver has only a few minutes to act. A choking victim who cannot talk or cough is usually panic stricken and clutches at the throat or chest. If the victim can breathe, speak, or cough, DO NOT INTERFERE with his or her own efforts to free the blockage.

FIRST AID FOR CHOKING. The **Heimlich maneuver** uses air in the lungs to force an object out of the airway. The purpose of this technique is to dislodge the object by forcing air out from behind the object itself. Applying sudden pressure below the rib cage forces the diaphragm up and compresses the lungs.

The Red Cross recommends a sequence of four back blows and four abdominal thrusts. Support the front of the victim with one arm. Give four sharp blows between the shoulder blades with the heel of your hand. Then administer the Heimlich maneuver with four thrusts.

When using this technique on children, use care in the amount of pressure applied. An infant or very young child should be placed face down over your forearm. Rest your arm on your thigh if necessary. With the heel of your hand apply blows between the shoulder blades. (A larger child may be placed face down over your knees with head lower than the chest.) Pressure on the chest is applied to an infant using two fingers between the nipples.

SHOCK

Shock is a condition resulting from a depressed state of vital body functions. It may be caused by severe bleeding, or loss of other body fluids (as in prolonged vomiting or burns), heart attack or stroke, lack of oxygen, or poisoning. Symptoms include pale, cold, and moist skin. Other symptoms are rapid and shallow breathing, weak pulse, and a vacant stare. The victim may feel faint, dizzy, nauseated, and thirsty. If the victim is breathing, has a pulse, and severe bleeding is controlled, begin treatment for shock. Keep the injured person lying down and, if possible, cover with a blanket or coat to maintain body heat. Raise the feet 20 to 30 centimeters (8 to 12 inches) higher than the heart and

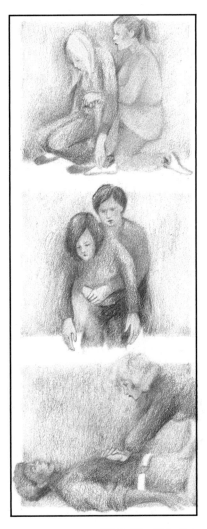

27–6. The Heimlich maneuver. Make a fist with a hand, and wrap the other hand around it. Place the thumb side of your fist against the victim's abdomen, midway between navel and rib cage. Press into the abdomen with a quick upward thrust. If victim is lying down, place both hands on upper abdomen and press upward with heels of the hands.

chest. *Do not* raise the feet if there is a head injury, an unsplinted fracture, or difficulty in breathing, or if such movement causes severe pain. Get medical help immediately. Talk to the victim to help reassure and calm him or her. The stress of fear and panic added to the accident or sudden illness will increase shock. Unless you expect medical assistance to be delayed for more than 6 hours, *do not* give anything by mouth.

INSULIN SHOCK

Diabetes is a condition in which the body cannot efficiently control the production of insulin. Insulin helps convert carbohydrates into usable food energy. If there is too little insulin, too much sugar remains in the blood; if there is too much insulin, there is too little sugar in the blood. In other words, the diabetic in trouble may need two different kinds of treatment. Usually, however, it is low blood sugar that comes on quickly and needs emergency treatment.

Symptoms of insulin shock are excessive sweating, lightheadedness, trembling, impaired vision, slurred speech, and some imbalance. These symptoms sometimes give the victim the appearance of being drunk. Hunger and a high level of irritability may also be present. Give the person sugar or food containing sugar (honey, candy, fruit, orange juice). Call for medical help. If not treated the person may lose consciousness. In this case do a quick check and administer mouth-to-mouth breathing if necessary.

HEART ATTACKS

Emergency treatment for a heart attack victim involves a number of skills. First, you must recognize what is happening. Second, you should be trained and prepared to give cardiopulmonary resuscitation (CPR).

The most frequent first symptom of heart attack is chest pain. The pain is often experienced as a crushing, squeezing, or heavy feeling on the center of the chest. Sometimes it is felt at the top of the abdomen, and the victim may think he or she has indigestion. The pain may travel down the arm and/or up to the jaw. Sweating, shortness of breath, nausea, and sometimes vomiting occur. Help the victim sit or lie down with head higher than chest. Loosen clothes. Call for help, and be ready to describe the symptoms accurately. Give your location. Return to comfort the victim. If the victim loses consciousness, do a quick check. If there is no breathing, and no pulse, the person is in *cardiac arrest*; that is, their heart has stopped. Be prepared to give CPR.

CARDIOPULMONARY RESUSCITATION (CPR). CPR is an emergency procedure that is used with mouth-to-mouth resuscitation when the heart has stopped beating. It is based on the principle of squeezing the heart between the rib cage and the spine to force (or pump) blood throughout the body. CPR should NEVER be performed or practiced on any person who has a pulse, because this may cause cardiac arrest. To check for a heartbeat, place your fingers on the victim's carotid artery, which is found on the left side of the neck. CPR should *not* be used without training. To learn how to perform the techniques of CPR well, one needs supervised practice on mannequins. Training classes in CPR are available in most communities. The Red Cross, various hospitals, and the American Heart Association can provide information about the classes.

Here is a brief description of CPR. First, place the victim on his or her back. Stand or kneel over the victim. If you have given four quick breaths and found no pulse, and no breathing, prepare to give CPR. Find the lowest part of the breastbone. Count up the width of two fingers from that point (the xyphoid bone) and place the heel of your other hand there. Apply firm, rhythmic pressure, depressing the rib cage about 2.5 to 5 centimeters (1 to 2 inches) each second.

27–7. CPR. Find the lowest part of the breast bone. Count up two finger widths. Give chest compressions as shown. CPR must be continued until medical help arrives.

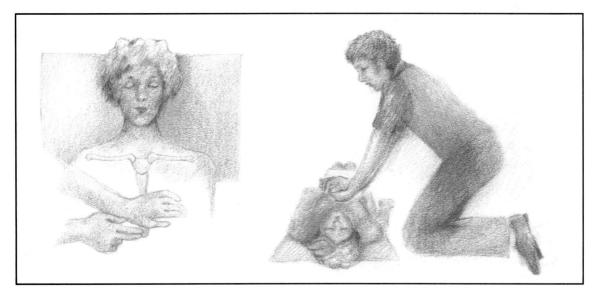

The amount of pressure you apply must be varied according to the size of the victim. Resuscitating a child requires less pressure, and enough pressure could be applied to a baby with the fingers.

The American Red Cross provides the following general directions for deciding when and if mouth-to-mouth breathing or CPR should be given.

1. If a person is not breathing, but *has* a pulse, give mouth-to-mouth breathing.
2. If a person is not breathing, and *does not have* a pulse, CPR is needed.
3. If you have not been trained in CPR, give mouth-to-mouth breathing. The heart may be beating weakly even though you did not find a pulse, so mouth-to-mouth breathing may keep the person alive.

POISONS

A poison is defined as any substance that produces a harmful effect on the body. Poisons can enter the body through ingestion, inhalation, or absorption through the skin or mucous membranes. The first-aid giver is most often concerned with poisons that enter through the mouth. Common symptoms include nausea, vomiting, abdominal pain, burns around the mouth, sweating, abnormal breathing, convulsions, or unconsciousness.

When you know or suspect that a victim has been poisoned, call the operator or 911, or a Poison Control Center if your community has one. Call for medical assistance. Watch breathing closely and, if necessary, apply mouth-to-mouth breathing. Next, identify the poison, if at all possible. Poisons differ in their chemical composition. Some poisons are corrosive; that is, they burn and destroy living tissue. Treatment is somewhat different depending on whether the person has swallowed corrosive or noncorrosive poisons.

FIRST AID TREATMENT FOR POISONING

In all cases, if the person is conscious, he or she should drink one or two glasses of milk (or water if milk is unavailable). For corrosive poisons, which include acids, alkalies, and petroleum products such as paint thinner, oven cleaner, charcoal lighter, kerosene, lye and wax, do the following:

1. *DO NOT* induce vomiting. Bringing the poison back up causes additional burns.

27–8. Common poisons found around the home. To avoid accidents, label poisons carefully. Attach first aid directions. Never keep poisons in a medicine cabinet. Keep harmful substances out of children's reach.

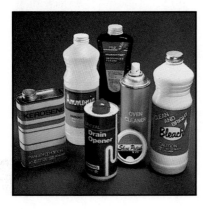

2. When any substance that can cause a chemical burn enters the eye, flush the eye immediately with water and continue flushing for at least 15 minutes.

For noncorrosive poisons including rubbing or denatured alcohol, aspirin, bleach, hair dye, paint, pesticides, rat poison, cosmetics, and detergent, follow these procedures to INDUCE VOMITING.

1. Give 1 tablespoon of syrup of ipecac. Keep the person moving. Ipecac should act within 15 to 20 minutes. Repeat a second time if the person doesn't vomit.
2. If ipecac is not available or if two doses have been taken with no effect, make the person vomit by tickling the back of his or her throat with your fingers.
3. When he or she starts to vomit, make sure the head is in a downward direction. DO NOT USE FORCE. Vomiting often creates panic because a person cannot breathe at the same time.

IN GENERAL: NEVER GIVE LIQUID OR INDUCE VOMITING WHEN THE VICTIM IS UNCONSCIOUS OR CONVULSING.

OTHER FIRST AID EMERGENCIES

FAINTING

Fainting is caused by an insufficient supply of oxygen in the brain. Before a person faints he or she may have such symptoms as paleness, sweating, dizziness, cold clammy skin, and, sometimes, nausea. Lying down will usually prevent fainting. Bending over in a sitting position with the head between the knees will also help to send oxygen to the brain. A person who has fainted should always be kept in a lying position until recovery. Unless recovery is very quick, medical assistance should be obtained. Fainting can indicate more serious conditions.

HYPERVENTILATION

Hyperventilation occurs when a person under stress breathes very quickly and the carbon dioxide in the blood becomes abnormally low. Symptoms include a feeling of numbness or panic, a tingling sensation in the feet and hands, muscle tension, and dizziness.

Calm the victim. He or she needs to build up the levels of carbon dioxide in the blood in order to restore normal breathing. This can be done by breathing into a *paper* bag

27–9. For hyperventilation, have victim breathe into a paper bag for 5 to 10 minutes.

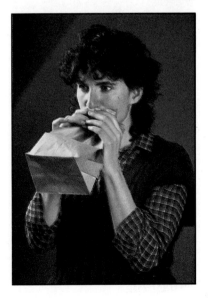

held over both the nose and mouth for 5 to 10 minutes. This causes the person to rebreathe the carbon dioxide (CO_2). Don't worry about lack of oxygen; there is plenty in the exhaled breath. After normal breathing resumes, encourage the person to seek help to make sure the hyperventilation is not a symptom of a more serious condition.

CONVULSIONS

A person having a **convulsion** loses conscious control of nervous system functions. The body may stiffen or thrash about uncontrollably. There are several causes of convulsions, including high fever, epilepsy, and reactions to drugs. You can protect the person from injury by removing all surrounding objects. Don't try to restrain the victim. Call for help at once. *Epilepsy* is a disorder of the nervous system that causes convulsions. These may occur without warning, although some victims can tell when an attack is coming on, and may have time to indicate what assistance they'll need. The attack, called a seizure, can last from 2 to 30 minutes. Most people who suffer from epilepsy take medication to control seizures. Infections in children can also cause convulsions. A rapid increase in body temperature sometimes causes these violent muscular contractions. This seems to be the body's way of reducing the fever. Help to lower the fever by sponging the body down with cool water. Get medical help as soon as possible.

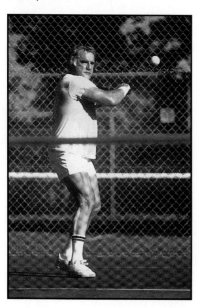

27–10. Heat exhaustion usually results from exercise in a hot, humid atmosphere.

HEATSTROKE AND HEAT EXHAUSTION

Heatstroke usually follows overexposure to the direct rays of the sun. **Heat exhaustion** usually results from exercise in a hot, humid atmosphere. The first-aid giver must be able to distinguish between the two because the treatment for each condition is different.

Victims of heatstroke are in very serious danger because they have lost a great deal of body fluid and their temperatures are very high. Signs of heatstroke are sudden collapse, red face, hot and dry skin, rapid pulse, and labored breathing. There may be muscular twitching. Move the victim to a cool spot if possible. Call for help immediately. Loosen or remove clothes. Apply ice bags or cold cloths to the head. Bathe or spray the body with cold water. The conscious heatstroke victim may be given small, frequent sips of plain water. If the victim is unconscious, check breathing closely. Artificial respiration may be necessary.

Heat exhaustion is usually less serious than heatstroke. A sign of heat exhaustion is pale, moist skin. The person may be restless and weak and complain of dizziness, headache, and shortness of breath. There may be muscular twitching or severe cramps, nausea, and vomiting. These symptoms result from excessive perspiring, leading to a great loss of water and salt. Remove the victim to a cool place. Give a half teaspoon of salt in a glass of water or fruit juice. Keep the person lying down with the head slightly lowered.

BURNS

Burns are classified as **first degree** (reddening), **second degree** (blistering), and **third degree** (charring). They may be the result of fire, overexposure to the sun, or chemical burns.

For first-degree burns, immediately apply cold water or submerge the burned area in cold water until pain decreases. For second-degree burns, immerse the burned part in cold water for 1 to 2 hours. Do not break blisters. Do not apply commercial ointments, especially those containing benzocaine, or home remedies like butter. In spite of what you might have heard, these are not effective and might also cause infection, making it harder for the doctor to treat the burn. If clothing sticks around the burned area, don't pull it off. Cover the area with sterile dressings or compresses, or a clean cloth such as a sheet. Bandage the area gently. Apply an ice pack. This slows the escape of body fluids. Watch for symptoms of shock.

In cases of third-degree burns where there is deep tissue destruction, an ice pack should not be applied except on hands, feet, or face if burned. Cold may intensify the shock reaction. Do not allow the victim to walk. Keep burned feet and legs elevated. If the victim's hands have been burned, keep them above the level of the heart. Arrange for transportation to the hospital as quickly as possible.

The most serious danger with second-and third-degree burns, especially if they cover a large area of the body, is loss of body fluids. Great loss of body fluids produces serious shock. The second danger is infection. A body with burns is extremely open to bacteria. All third-degree burns should be promptly treated by a doctor. Also see a doctor if second-degree burns cover an area over 20 square inches, or if any second-degree burns occcur on the hands or face. Proper medical care can prevent scarring.

27–11. For first-degree burns, immediately submerge the burned area in cold water until pain decreases.

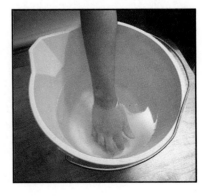

HEALTH TIP

All animal bites should be cleaned with soap and water. If the bite is by *any* animal other than your own pet dog or cat, consult a doctor at once. Non-immunized pets and other animals may harbor the rabies virus. If safety permits, the offending animal should be caught and held for observation.

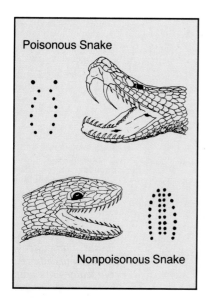

27–12. To determine if a snake bite is from a poisonous snake, look for fang marks at the wound.

FROSTBITE

The ears, nose, hands, and feet are common areas of frostbite. **Frostbite** is an actual freezing of tissue. It may result from overexposure to the cold as well as from being in contact with certain types of chemicals.

Never rub or massage skin that has been frostbitten since this will damage it. Don't give the person anything alcoholic to drink. Alcohol lowers the body temperature. Warm hands or feet gradually in a pan of warm (not hot) water or wrap in a warm blanket. Do not allow the victim of frostbitten feet to walk or move the feet. Keep affected toes and fingers separated with dry gauze or a clean cloth. Apply warm, wet compresses to a frozen nose, face, or ear. Get to a doctor as soon as possible.

SNAKE BITES

Each year about 7,000 poisonous snake bites are reported. Only four species of snakes in the U.S. are poisonous. They are the copperhead, the rattlesnake, the water moccasin, and the coral snake. If you go camping or live in a part of the country where poisonous snakes are common, learn to distinguish between types of snake bites (see Figure 27-12).

If a person has been bitten by a snake, begin the following first-aid measures at once:

1. Keep the victim quiet and be reassuring. Keep the area of the bite below the level of the victim's heart.
2. If the victim has been bitten on the hand, remove all jewelry and ornaments. Clean and dress the wound, and immobilize the extremity.
3. Maintain body temperature, and treat for shock if present.
4. Seek medical help immediately.

If you are within four to five hours reach of a hospital do *not* apply a tourniquet or cut into the bite and attempt to suck out venom. Get the person to a medical facility as soon as possible.

SUMMARY: In a first-aid emergency, control severe bleeding. Then, check the ABCs: airway, breathing, and circulation. Administer artificial respiration or CPR if needed. Move the victim only in an emergency, and then use a stretcher or a flat board. Reassure the victim, keep calm, and send for medical assistance.

CHAPTER REVIEW

words at work

Find the word in the left column that fits one of the definitions in the right column. DO NOT WRITE IN THIS BOOK.

a. abrasion
b. carbon monoxide
c. concussion
d. convulsions
e. fracture
f. frostbite
g. laceration
h. shock
i. third-degree burn
j. tourniquet

1. Freezing of body tissue
2. Violent and abnormal muscular contractions
3. A broken bone
4. A measure used only as a last resort to control severe bleeding
5. A tear wound
6. A scrape-type wound
7. Must be suspected if head receives a blow
8. A depressed state of the circulatory system
9. Charred body tissue
10. A poisonous gas

review questions

1. Define first aid.
2. Why is first-aid training important?
3. List the priorities to keep in mind in case of an emergency.
4. Identify and describe five types of wounds.
5. What is the purpose of a dressing or compress?
6. What is the most serious hazard of wounds?
7. Describe first aid for ordinary wounds.
8. Why are puncture wounds especially dangerous?
9. Name and describe three methods of controlling serious bleeding.
10. Why is the use of a tourniquet only a last-resort measure?
11. Define shock, list the symptoms, and outline a procedure for its treatment.
12. List several causes of respiratory failure.
13. Describe the Heimlich maneuver for relieving a choking victim.
14. Describe in detail the mouth-to-mouth technique for artificial respiration.
15. Outline the procedure for CPR.
16. Explain how carbon monoxide causes asphyxiation.
17. What can be done to reduce the number of cases of accidental poisoning?
18. Outline first-aid measures to be followed in treating a poison-by-mouth victim.

19. What clues are provided by the color of skin of an unconscious person?
20. What would you do for a person who has fainted?
21. Name two serious head injuries.
22. What can a first-aid giver do for the victim of a heart attack?
23. Tell what usually causes convulsions in children and how the child should be cared for.
24. What first-aid measures should be followed in diabetic emergencies?
25. Contrast the first-aid treatment for sunstroke versus heat exhaustion.
26. Tell what the first-aid giver should do for the victim of a bite from a poisonous snake.
27. Classify burns. Outline a first-aid procedure.
28. Describe first aid for frostbite.

discussion questions

1. Discuss psychological reactions and behavior of victims and onlookers at the scene of an accident. What is the role of the first-aid giver in this situation?
2. Discuss the importance of the first-aid giver in time of disaster.
3. Make a list of the common poisons found in your home and discuss first-aid measures for possible victims of these poisons.
4. Investigate the requirements for qualifying for a Red Cross "first-aider" card. What would be the advantages of such training?
5. Discuss any personal experiences that you or someone you know had where first-aid skills were needed.

investigating

PURPOSE:
To learn how to administer the Heimlich maneuver.

MATERIAL NEEDED:
The Heimlich maneuver chart on page 567.

PROCEDURE:
A. Study the Heimlich maneuver in the text and on the chart on page 567.
    1. What are the symptoms of choking?
B. Practice the Heimlich maneuver on another person while they are standing and sitting. Have a third person read the directions to you and watch while you administer the maneuver.
C. Switch places until everyone in your group has practiced the maneuver.
D. Practice the maneuver on yourself.
    2. In your own words, describe the maneuver.

UNIT 8 SAFEGUARDING YOUR HEALTH

HEALTH
CAREERS

EMERGENCY MEDICAL TECHNICIAN

EMTs provide immediate, on-the-scene medical care. They are specially trained to handle all types of life-threatening emergencies. The EMT must quickly determine the seriousness of the problem, and the priorities of treatment. EMTs also transport patients to hospitals, giving them continuous care while on route. To become an EMT you must be at least 18 years old and a high school graduate (or its equivalent). You must also have a driver's license. Finally, you must complete a basic EMT training course. This course covers basic emergency procedures such as controlling bleeding, treating shock, and cardiopulmonary resuscitation (CPR). After 6 to 12 months of basic EMT experience, you can advance to an EMT-paramedic. This requires taking an additional course for at least 500 hours. EMT-paramedics can give more sophisticated emergency care than EMTs. Most EMTs work as volunteers on ambulances. Others use their EMT training during regular jobs as police, fire, safety, or health personnel. For more information, contact the Emergency Medical Division of your state's Department of Health.

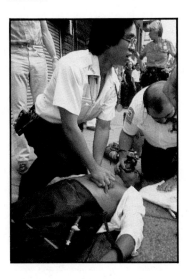

ENVIRONMENTALISTS

Most of us take it for granted that the water we drink is pure, the air we breathe is clean, and the food we eat is safe. Unfortunately that's not always true. Over the past 75 years, the advances of industry have both benefited and harmed our society. The ever-increasing number of environmental health hazards has created a need for a special health professional: the environmentalist. Environmentalists are concerned with all environmental factors that affect our health and safety.

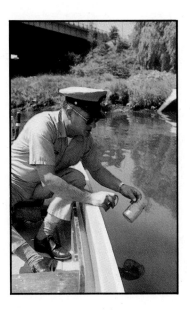

They work in local, state, and federal government agencies and in private industry, and many other places. Some specialize in just one area, such as air-pollution control or occupational health and safety. A four-year college degree in environmental health is your ticket to a beginning job as an environmentalist. If you would like to start planning a career in this field, contact the National Environmental Health Association, 1200 Lincoln Street, Room 704, Denver, Colorado 80203.

PHOTO CREDITS

HRW photos by Katharine Abbe appear on the following pages: 17, 24, 33, 35, 54, 88, and 248. HRW photos by Russell Dian appear on the following pages: 79, 157, 249, 257, 309, 398, 410, and 571.

UNIT 1: p. X (tl) E. M. Bordis, (bl) R. Wheldon/Leo de Wys, (br) Andy Levine/Black Star; p. 1 (t1) Keith Gunnar/Bruce Coleman, (tr) Paul Kennedy/Leo de Wys, (b) Uselmann/Stock Shop.

CHAPTER 1: p. 3 Andy Levine/Black Star; p. 4 John Moss/Black Star; p. 5 Pam Hasegawa/Taurus; p. 6 David Burnett/Black Star; p. 7 B. I. Ullman/Taurus; p. 10 Andy Levine/Black Star; p. 11 Keith Gunnar/Bruce Coleman

CHAPTER 2: p. 16 Granger; p. 19 Jack Fields/Photo Researchers; p. 21 USDA; p. 24 Richard Jeffrey; p. 28 USDA; p. 29 Henry Groskinsky; p. 31 USDA; p. 33 Bruce Plotkin; p. 37 Roe de Bono; p. 40(1) Leo de Wys, (c) Carl Purcell, (r) Will McIntyre; p. 42 Katherine Dudek/Photo News; p. 43 Ken Lax/Stock Shop.

CHAPTER 3: p. 46 Bill Stanton/Int'l Stock Photo: p. 48 Manfred Kage/ Peter Arnold; p. 49 National Library of Medicine; p. 50 M. Rotker/Taurus; p. 55 Intermedics Ind.; p. 56 New York Hospital; p. 57 American Association of Podiatry; p. 62 (t) Focus on Sports, (b1)/bc) Michael Abbey/Photo Researchers, (br) Manfred Kage/Peter Arnold; p. 67 Prof. Dr. J. Keul, Freiburg.

CHAPTER 4: p. 72 Steve Smith/Wheeler Pictures; p. 74 Stock Shop; p. 77 (all) Steve Hoffman; p. 80 Focus on Sports; p. 82 (t) J. Peress/Magnum, (b) Chuck Slattery/After Image; p. 84 Jerry Wachter/Focus on Sports; p. 86(1) David Madison, (r) David Stridel/Bruce Coleman; p. 90 Pam Hasegawa/Taurus Photos; p. 92 Lee Balterman/Sports Illustrated; p. 94 Enrico Ferorelli/Wheeler Pictures; p. 97(t) Leo de Wys, (b) Bruce Thomas/Stock Market.

UNIT 2: p. 98/99 Martha Swope.

CHAPTER 5: p. 100 Richard Hutchings/Photo Researchers; p. 102 Runk/Schoenberger/Grant Heilman; p. 106 New York University Skin Care Clinic; p. 107(t) L. V. Bergman & Assoc., (b) Photo Researchers; p. 108(t) Lester Bergman, (b) Peter Benew/Image Bank; p. 109 Courtesy of Medic Alert; p. 110 New York Botanical Gardens; p. 111 Eastman Kodak Company, Industrial Laboratory; p. 112 Manfred Kage/Peter Arnold; p. 113 James Webb; p. 114 (t) Dick Luria/Stock Shop, (b) Dr. Tony Brain/Photo Researchers; p. 115 Steven Mark Needham; p. 119 Dr. Isabelle Grayson; p. 120 David Madison/Black Star; p. 121/122 American Dental Association.

CHAPTER 6 p. 126 Martha Swope; p. 128 Michael Abbey/Photo Researchers; p. 130 J. Werner/Outline; p. 131 Nina Leen, Life Magazine, © 1964; p. 132 Suki Coughlin/Photo Researchers; p. 133 Figi Miyazuma/Black Star; p. 133 NASA; p. 135 E Weiland/Photo Researchers; p. 136 Bert Bartholomew/Black Star; p. 137 Sepp Seitz/Woodfin Camp; p. 140(t) printed by permission of the Estate of Norman Rockwell, © 1961, (b) Kennedy/The Image Bank; p. 141(b1) Keinger/Photo Researchers, (bc) Fred Ward/Black Star, (br) Andy Bernhauf/Black Star; p. 143 Steve Rutherfauer.

CHAPTER 7: p. 146(t1) Eddie Adams/Leo de Wys, (tc) Rhoda Sidney/Leo de Wys, (tr) Barbara Burns/Photo Researchers, (b1) Edward Lettau/Photo Researchers, (bc) B. I. Ullman/Taurus Photos, (br) Ivor Sharp/Image Bank; p. 147 Andy Levine/Black Star; p. 148 Culver Pictures; p. 149 Enrico Ferorelli/Wheeler Pictures; p. 150 Eric Stein/Black Star; p. 152 Elliott Erwitt/Magnum; p. 153 Courtesy, Karen Gotimer; p. 154(t1) Norris Clark/Int'l Stock Photo, (tr) Jeffrey Reed/Stock Shop, (b) Roger Tully/Black Star; p. 156 Bettmann Archive; p. 159 John Lei/Black Star; p. 160 Ann Hagen Griffiths/DPI; p. 161 Will Stanton/Int'l Stock Photo; p. 162 Magnum; p. 166(t1) Tim Bilder/Image Bank, (tr/bl) Kathleen Foster/Black Star, (br) Andy Levine/Black Star; p. 169(t) Guy Gillette/Photo Researchers, (b) Russ Kinne/Photo Researchers.

UNIT 3: p. 170(l) Thomas Sobolik/Black Star, (r) Earl Dotter/Archive Pictures; p. 171(l) Liss/Liaison, (r) Enrico Ferorelli/Wheeler Pictures.

CHAPTER 8: p. 172 Geoffrey Gove/Image Bank; p. 174 Pat Rogers/Image Bank; p.175(5) Culver Pictures, (b) Turnau/Stock Shop; p. 177(l) Bill Stanton/Int'l Stock Photo, (r) Arthur Tress/Magnum; p. 178 Larry Nicholson/Photo Researchers; p. 180 George Catlin/National Museum of American Art, Smithsonian Institution. Gift of Mrs. Jos. H. Harrison, Jr.; p. 183(l) Stock/Boston, (tc) Andy Levine/Black Star, (lc) Owen Franken/Stock, Boston, (r) L. Albrizio/Image Bank; p. 184 Andy Levine/Black Star; p. 186 David Attie/Stock Shop.

CHAPTER 9: p. 190 Andy Levine/Black Star; p. 192 © Hank Ketchum Enterprises; p. 193 Bettmann Archive; p. 194 Everett C. Johnson/Leo de Wys; p. 195 Ricardo Ferro/Black Star; p. 196 Sygma; p. 197 Mimi Cotter/Int'l Stock Photo; p. 198 Michael Hayman/Black Star.

CHAPTER 10: p. 202 José Urbach/HRW; p. 204(t) Burk Uzzle/Woodfin Camp, (b) Jon Riley/Stock Shop; p. 207 Peter B. Kaplan/Photo Researchers; p. 208 HRW by Richard Haynes; p. 210 Granger Collection; p. 212 Derek Bayes; p. 213 Susan Johns/Photo Researchers; p. 215 Bettmann Archive; p. 217 New York Public Library/Picture Collection; p. 218 San Jose Mercury News/Black Star; p. 220 M. Fennelli/Photo Researchers.

CHAPTER 11: p. 224 Kathleen Foster/Black Star; p. 226 National Museum, Copenhagen, Denmark; p. 227 Granger Collection; p. 228 Bettmann Archive p. 230 and 232 Louis Fernandez; p. 233 Enrico Ferorelli/Wheeler Pictures; p. 237 Courtesy Eldemar Corp, Phoenix, Arix.; p. 240 Barbara Kirk/Int'l Stock Photo; p. 243 (t) Ann Chwatsky/Lew de Wys, (b) Enrico Ferorelli.

UNIT 4: p. 244/245 HRW photo by James Gilmour.

CHAPTER 12: p. 246 Sigrid Owen/Int'l Stock Photo; p. 247 David York/Stock Shop; p. 251 Drug Abuse Information Campaign; p. 252 Yoav Levy/Phototake; p. 253 Carl E. Willgoose, Health Teaching in Secondary Schools © 1977, W. G. Saunders Co., Phil.; p. 258 Carolina Biological Supply Co.; p. 259 Granger Collection; p. 260 C. Gunthur/Camera 5; p. 261 Kal Muller/Woodfin Camp; p. 262(t) Alex Langley/DPI, (b) National Library of Medicine; p. 266 Leonard Fredd/Magnum; p. 267 Rocky Weldon/Leo de Wys; p. 268 National Institute of Mental Health; p. 269(tl) Bill Stanton/Int'l Stock Photo, (tr) Andrea Blumberg/Stock Shop, (bl) C. SeghersII/Leo de Wys, (br) R. Rowan/Photo Researchers.

CHAPTER 13: p. 272 David Attie/Stock Shop-Medichrome; p. 273 Naideau/Stock Market; p. 274 Granger; p. 275(l) J. Albertson/Stock, Boston, (c) John Running/Stock, Boston, (r) Andrew Rakoczy/Bruce Coleman; p. 276 HRW by James Gilmour; p. 281(t) Dianora Niccolini/Stock Shop-Medichrome, (b) Martin M. Rotker; p. 282 Leo de Wys; p. 283 Syd Greenberg/Photo Researchers; p. 286 Ken Lax/Stock Shop-Medichrome; p. 288 Alcoholics Anonymous.

CHAPTER 14: p. 292 American Cancer Society; p. 293 Granger Collection; p. 295(t) Carolina Biological Supply Co., (b) C. E. Herron/USDA; p. 297 American Cancer Society; p. 299 Richard G. Kessel and Randy H. Kardon; p. 300 Martin M. Rotker/Taurus Photos, (inserts) Stock Shop-Medichrome; p. 303 Mary Evans Picture Library/Sigmund Freud Copyrightists; p. 305 HRW Photo by John King; p. 306 American Cancer Society

UNIT 5: pp. 310–311 Lennart Nilsson, Behold Man, Little, Brown & Co.

CHAPTER 15: p. 312 Manfred Kage/Peter Arnold; p. 313 BioPhoto Assoc./Photo Researchers; p. 320 Martin M. Rotker/Taurus Photos; p. 323 Manfred Kage/Peter Arnold; p. 327 Dan McCoy/Rainbow; p. 329 Michael Inderrieden; p. 332 Fred Whitehead/Animals, Animals; p. 333 Wesley Baxe/Photo Researchers.

CHAPTER 16: p. 336/338 Richard Kessel/Tissue & Organs, W. H. Freeman & Co.; p. 342(t) Kaiser Porcelain Ltd., (b) Arthur Sirdofsky; p. 343 Dick Luria/Stock Shop-Medichrome; p. 344 Dan McCoy/Rainbow; p. 346 Dick Luria/Stock Shop-Medichrome; p. 247 John P. Goeller; p. 348 Alexander Tsiaras/Photo Researchers; p. 350 Courtesy, Dr. Self, New York Hospital; p. 351 Burt Glinn/Magnum; p. 353 Michael Phillip Mannheim/Stock Shop-Medichrome; p. 354 Walder Evans/Photo Researchers.

CHAPTER 17: p. 358 Phillip Harrington/Peter Arnold; p. 362 UPI; p. 364 Janeart Ltd.; p. 365 Yale Historical Library; p. 366 New York Hospital; p. 367 Dr. T. Ellis/New York Hospital; p. 375(t) Enrico Ferorelli, (b) Leo de Wys.

UNIT 6: p. 376–377 Dr. Richard Kessel/Tissue & Organs, W. H. Freeman & Co.

CHAPTER 18: Lennart Nilsson/Behold Man, Little, Brown & Co.; p. 382 Dr. Richard Kessel/Tissues & Organs, W. H. Freeman & Co.; p. 383 Manfred Kage/Peter Arnold; p. 387 Tom and Michelle Grimm/Int'l Stock Photo; p. 385 Aldo Tutino; p. 390 Dr. John Campbell; p. 391/392 New York Hospital; p. 397 Martin M. Rotker/Taurus Photos.

CHAPTER 19: p. 402 Carl Roessler/Bruce Coleman; p. 404 Dr. Raymond Fink, U. of Washington; p. 405 Lennart Nilsson/Behold Man, Little, Brown & Co.; p. 409 Loren McIntyre; p. 412 Culver Pictures; p. 414 Focus on Sports; p. 415 Indiana University Medical Center; p. 416 National Lung Association.

CHAPTER 20: p. 420 Lewis Lainey/Black Star; p. 425 Richard Kessel/Tissue & Organs, W. H. Freeman & Co.; p. 427(t) Katrina Thomas, (b) Manfred Kage/Peter Arnold; p. 428 BioPhoto/Photo Researchers; p. 430 Manfred Kage/Peter Arnold; p. 432 New York Blood Center; p. 433 Joel Gorden; p. 434 Richard Jefferies; p. 435 Omikron/Photo Researchers; p. 437 Granger Collection; p. 438 David Brownell.

PHOTO CREDITS

Step 7. Develop and implement a Plan of Action

Work harder in school, take more science and math courses

Look into financial aid, get a part time summer job to save for college

Continue hospital volunteer work

Step 6. Evaluate and rank all choices

1. Doctor   2. Nurse   3. Medical Research Scientist

Step 5. Identify your goals and values

Obedience? Self-respect? Friendship? Money? Responsibility? Service? Status?

My goal: a career in the health field combining my science ability and interest in people

My values: helping people, personal recognition, and job independence

Step 4. Examine probable negative and positive effects of each choice

Service to others, very good salary and job security, independence on the job

Service to others, shorter preparation time, often more patient contact than doctors, job security

Serve others through science, work independently on the job

Costly education, long preparation long working hours, very competitive admission to medical schools

Demanding work, lower pay, unsteady work

Little contact with patients, long preparation, job security often depends on funding

Step 3. Identify all possible choices

Doctor   Nurse   Medical Research Scientist

Step 2. Get as much reliable information as possible

Talk to professionals, including doctors about their jobs

Discuss your talents and abilities with a guidance counselor

Discuss career plans with your parents

Read books and pamphlets about health careers

Volunteer in a hospital

Step 1. Define the decision

Should I become a doctor, or work in another health-related career?

A DECISION MAKING TREE

TESTICULAR SELF-EXAM

If discovered in its early stages, testicular cancer can be treated promptly and effectively. Your best hope for early detection is a simple self-exam.

What are the signs?
The first sign is usually a slight enlargement of one of the testes and a change in its consistency. There is often a dull ache in the lower abdomen and groin and a sensation of heaviness.

When should the exam be done?
Do the exam once each month. The best time is after a warm bath or shower, when the scrotal skin is relaxed.

How do you do the exam?
Roll the testical gently between the thumb and fingers of both hands. If you find any lumps, see your doctor immediately. They may not be cancerous, but only a doctor can make a diagnosis.

BREAST SELF-EXAM

Over 90 percent of breast cancers are discovered first by self-examination. Breast cancers found and treated early have excellent chances for cure.

What are the signs?
A lump or thickening of the breast or discharge from the nipples are usually the first signs of breast cancer. If any of these signs are discovered, see your doctor. Most breast lumps or changes are not cancerous, but only a doctor can tell.

When should the exam be done?
Do the exam once each month, about one week after menstruation. Begin the exam during a bath or shower.

How do you do the exam?

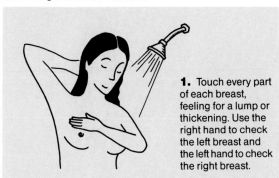

1. Touch every part of each breast, feeling for a lump or thickening. Use the right hand to check the left breast and the left hand to check the right breast.

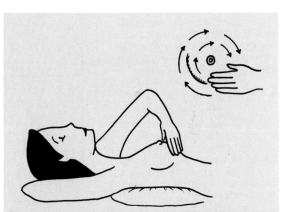

3. Lying down, put a pillow or towel under your right shoulder. Place your right hand behind your head. With your left hand press gently in small circular motions around an imaginary clock face. Begin at the outermost part of your breast for 12 o'clock, then more to 1 o'clock, and so on back to to 12 o'clock. A ridge of firm tissue in the lower curve of the breast is normal. Move in an inch toward the nipple, and keep circling until every part of your breast has been examined. Repeat this procedure on your left breast.

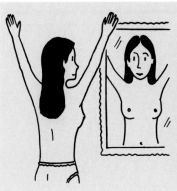

2. While sitting or standing before a mirror, raise your arms high overhead. Look for changes in the shape of each breast, swelling, dimpling of the skin, or changes in the nipples. Then check again with your hands on your hips.

4. Squeeze the nipple of each breast gently between the thumb and index finger. Any discharge should be reported to your doctor

A TOTAL FITNESS PROGRAM

The next three pages outline a total fitness program. Use it as a guideline. Modify it as needed. For best results follow the program three to four times per week, exercising every other day. The number of times you should repeat each exercise depends on your current fitness level. In general ten repetitions is a good starting point.

The Warm-up
(5 to 10 minutes)

1 **Head rolls.** Slowly roll head around first in one direction, then reverse.

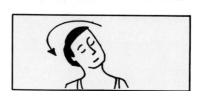 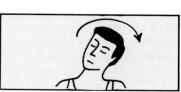

2 **Deep breather.** Rise on your toes while circling the arms inward and upward slowly, and inhaling deeply. At the end of the movement, arms are extended overhead. Continue circling arms backward and downward while lowering the heels slowly and exhaling.

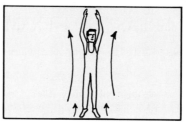 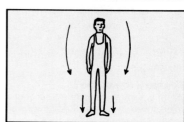

3 **Side stretcher.** Stand with feet slightly apart, and clasp hands behind your head. Bend sideward at the hips to the left as far as possible. Keep feet stationary and point toes straight ahead. Repeat, bending to the right.

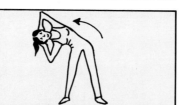 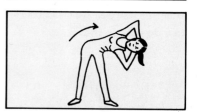

4 **Windmill.** Stand with knees bent, feet spread shoulder-width apart, arms extended sideward shoulder high, palms down. Twist and bend trunk, bringing left hand to the right toe, keeping arms straight and knees flexed. Then bring right hand to left toe.

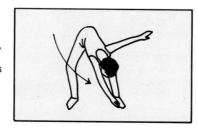 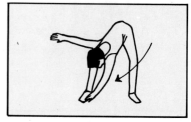

Endurance Phase
(20 minutes)

5 **Jumping jack.** Swing arms sideward and upward, touching hands above head (arms straight) while at the same time moving feet sideward and apart in a single jumping motion. Spring back to the starting position and repeat.

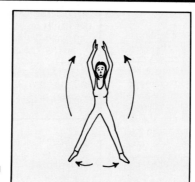 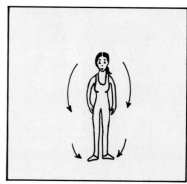

6   **The sprinter.** Assume squatting position, hands on the floor, fingers pointed forward, left leg fully extended to the rear. Reverse position of the feet by bringing left foot to hands and extending right leg backward, all in one motion. Reverse feet again, returning to starting position.

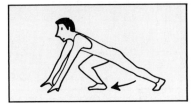
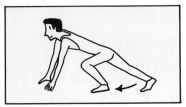

7   **Squat thrusts.** Bend knees and place hands on the floor in front of the feet. Arms may be between, outside of or in front of the bent knees. Thrust the legs back far enough so that the body is perfectly straight from shoulders to feet (the push-up position). Return to squat position, then to erect position.

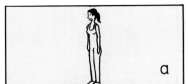
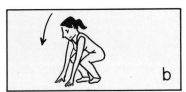
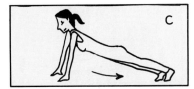
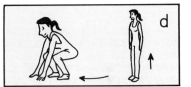

8   **Aerobic exercise** of your choice, such as running, swimming, jump-roping, or aerobic dancing.

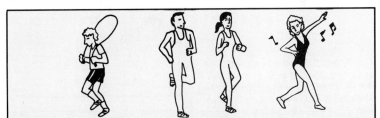

Strength and Flexibility Phase (5 to 10 minutes)

9   **Knee raises.** Lie on your back, knees slightly bent, feet on the floor, arms at your sides. Raise one knee up as close as possible to your chest. Fully extend the knee with the leg perpendicular to the floor. Bend knee and return to your chest. Straighten leg and return to starting position. Alternate the legs during the exercise.

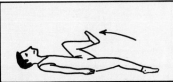
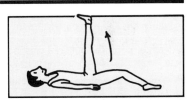
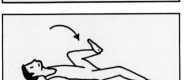
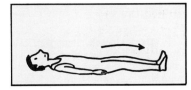

10   **Side-leg raise.** Lie on your side with arms extended overhead and legs extended fully, one on top of the other. With a brisk action, raise and lower the top leg vertically for specified number of counts. Repeat on the other side.

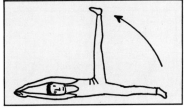
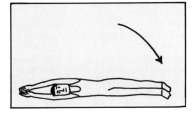

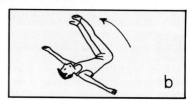

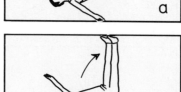

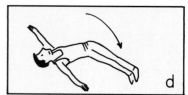

11 **Back twist.** Lie on your back, arms extended sideward, palms on the floor and legs raised to a vertical position. Keeping both feet together swing legs slowly to the left until almost touching the floor. Keep arms, shoulders, and head in contact with the floor. Repeat exercise to the right.

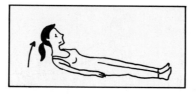

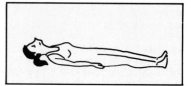

12 **Head and shoulder curl.** Lie on the back with hands at your sides, palms down. Lift head and shoulders off the floor. Hold this position for four counts. Relax, then repeat.

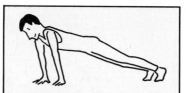

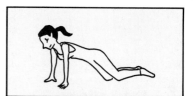

13 **Push-ups.** Boys: Extend your body so that it is perfectly straight. The weight is supported on the hands and toes. Girls: Place knees on the floor and extend body until it is straight from the head to the knees. Bend knees and raise the feet off the floor. The weight is supported by the hands and knees. Keeping body tense and straight, bend elbows and touch chest to the floor. Return to original position. (The body must be kept perfectly straight. The buttocks must not be raised and the abdomen must not sag.)

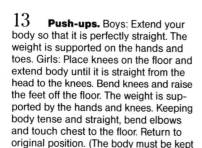

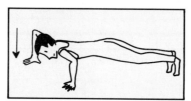

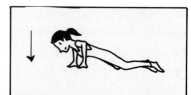

The Cool Down (10 minutes)

14 **Back stretch.** Stand with feet spread apart, arms extended overhead. Bend forward from the hips, knees bent. Swing arms downward between legs. Return to starting position and repeat.

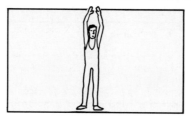

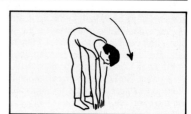

15 **Hip raise.** Lie on your back, knees bent with palms and feet on the floor. Raise your hips off floor as high as possible, keeping your shoulders and feet on the floor. Hold for ten counts. Return to starting position and repeat.

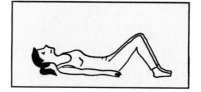

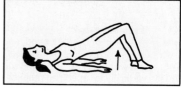

584

COMMON FOOD ADDITIVES

Additive	Function	Additive	Function
Acetic acid	pH control	Hydrogen peroxide	mat-bleach-condit
Ammonium alginate	stabil-thick-tex	Hydrolyzed vegetable protein	flavor enhancer
Arabinogalactan	stabil-thick-tex	Lactic acid	pH control
Benzoic acid	preservative		preservative
Benzoyl peroxide	mat-bleach-condit	Lecithin	emulsifier
Beta-apo-8' carotenal	color	Mannitol	sweetener
*BHA (butylated hydroxyanisole)	antioxidant		anti-caking
BHT (Butylated hydroxytoluene)	antioxidant		stabil-thick-tex
Butylparaben	preservative	Modified food starch	stabil-thick-tex
Calcium alginate	stabil-thick-tex	Monoglycerides	emulsifier
Calcium bromate	mat-bleach-condit	*MSG (monosodium glutamate)	flavor enhancer
Calcium lactate	preservative	Pectin	stabil-thick-tex
Calcium phosphate	leavening	*Phosphates	pH control
Calcium propionate	preservative	*Phosphoric acid	pH control
Calcium silicate	anti-caking	Polysorbates	emulsifiers
Calcium sorbate	preservative	Potassium alginate	stabil-thick-tex
Caramel	color	Potassium sorbate	preservative
Carrageenan	emulsifier	Propionic acid	preservative
	stabil-thick-tex	*Propyl gallate	antioxidant
Cellulose	stabil-thick-tex	Propylene glycol	stabil-thick-tex
Citric acid	preservative		humectant
	antioxidant	*Saccharin	sweetener
	pH control	Silicon dioxide	anti-caking
*Citrus Red No. 2	color	Sodium alginate	stabil-thick-tex
Corn syrup	sweetener	Sodium aluminum sulfate	leavening
Dextrose	sweetener	Sodium benzoate	preservative
Diglycerides	emulsifier	Sodium bicarbonate	leavening
Disodium guanylate	flavor enhancer	Sodium calcium alginate	stabil-thick-tex
Disodium inosinate	flavor enhancer	Sodium citrate	pH control
EDTA	antioxidant	Sodium diacetate	preservative
FD&C Colors:		Sodium nitrate, nitrite	preservative
*Blue No. 1	color	Sodium propionate	preservative
*Red No. 3	color	Sorbic acid	preservative
*Red No. 40	color	Sorbitan monostearate	emulsifier
*Yellow No. 5	color	Sorbitol	humectant
Fructose	sweetener		sweetener
Gelatin	stabil-thick-tex	Sucrose (table sugar)	sweetener
Glucose	sweetener	Tartaric acid	pH control
Glycerine	humectant	Turmeric (oleoresin)	flavor
Gum arabic (Carob bean, Karaya,	stabil-thick-tex		color
Larch, Locust bean)		Vanilla, vanillin	flavor
*Heptylparaben	preservative	Yeast-malt sprout extract	flavor enhancer

* **Try to avoid**

Preservatives help prevent food spoilage from bacteria, molds, fungi, and yeast.

Antioxidants help prevent rancidity or browning.

Emulsifiers help distribute particles of one liquid in another and improve consistency, stability, and texture.

Stabilizers, thickeners, and **texturizers (stabil-thick-tex)** improve consistency or texture.

Leavening agents affect cooking results.

pH control agents change or maintain acidity or alkalinity.

Humectants cause moisture retention.

Maturing and bleaching agents and dough conditioners (mat-bleach-condit) improve baking qualities.

Anti-caking agents prevent lumping or caking.

Flavor enhancers magnify or modify the taste and/or aroma of food.

Flavors heighten natural flavor or restore flavors lost in processing.

Colors give desired color to food.

Sweeteners make the aroma and/or taste of food more pleasurable.

GLOSSARY

A

abnormal personality a type of person unable to function in his or her environment

abrasion a scrape type of wound

accommodation of the eye the action of the eye lens and muscle that focuses rays of light from close objects onto the retina

acne skin conditions that can include blackheads, pimples, and boil-like lumps

acquired immunity immunity developed during a person's lifetime

acromegaly abnormal development, chiefly of the bones of the face and extremities of the body, associated with disease of the pituitary gland

ACTH (adrenocorticotropic hormone) a hormone secreted by the anterior pituitary gland, which influences the adrenal glands

addiction physical dependence on the continued supply of a drug

additive any substance added to foods

adenoids tonsil-like masses of tissues that grow on the back wall of the nasopharynx

ADH (antidiuretic hormone) a hormone secreted by the posterior pituitary gland, which regulates water balance in the body

adhesions bands of tissue that bind the bones in the middle ear

adrenal glands glands located on top of the kidneys, which regulate some of the body's most important processes

adrenaline (epinephrine) a hormone produced by the adrenal gland

aerobics exercises that use oxygen to fuel muscles over long periods of time

agility the ability to change direction quickly while moving at full speed

albumin a blood protein that regulates the amount of water in plasma

alcoholism addiction to alcohol

alimentary canal the tube from the mouth to the rectum through which food travels, is digested and absorbed, and through which wastes are eliminated

allergens certain protein substances that cause inflammation of the mucous membranes

allergist a physician specializing in the treatment and diagnosis of allergies

allergy the reaction of body tissues to an irritating substance

alopecia temporary hair loss

alveoli air sacs in the lungs

ambulatory care a form of treatment in which patients enter a hospital but do not stay overnight

amino acids substances from which organisms build proteins

amnesia a form of hysteria in which memory and identity are repressed

amniocentesis a technique in which some amniotic fluid surrounding a fetus is withdrawn and analyzed for possible genetic defects

amoeba a protozoan

amoebic dysentery a disease of the intestinal tract caused by an amoeba

amphetamine a drug that acts as a stimulant and gives a false sense of mental alertness

anabolism a constructive phase of metabolism

anemia a condition in which the blood is low in red corpuscles or hemoglobin or both

anger a feeling of hostility or rage

angina pectoris cardiac pain associated with coronary heart disease

anorexia a condition in which a person starves the body in order to become thin

anoxia lack of oxygen

antabuse a drug used to prevent drinking by making a person violently ill if he or she takes even a small amount of alcohol

anterior lobe the front lobe of the pituitary gland, which secretes powerful hormones

antianxiety drugs called tranquilizers, they reduce emotional tension and anxiety

antibiotics powerful germ-killing substances produced by molds or fungi

antibodies the immune substances in the blood and body fluids

antidepressant drugs called psychic energizers; their mood-elevating effects combat depression.

antidiuretic hormone (ADH) a hormone secreted by the posterior pituitary gland, which regulates water balance in the body.

antimanic drugs drugs that reduce the severely excited manic state

antiperspirant a substance that closes the pores and reduces or stops perspiration

antisocial personality a type of behavior characterized by a need to dominate others, irritability, defiance, and cruelty

antitoxin a substance developed in the body that counteracts a toxin

anxiety a feeling of apprehension, tension, or uneasiness in certain situations

anxiety disorder a mental disorder marked by an intense and generalized feeling of anxiety that is unrelated to a specific object or situation

aorta the largest blood vessel in the body, which carries blood from the left ventricle of the heart

appendicitis infection and inflammation of the appendix

appendix a narrow tube that extends from the caecum in the lower right-hand part of the abdomen

appetite a desire or craving for food

aqueous humor the watery fluid filling the cavity between the cornea and the lens

arteries a system of tubes of varying sizes that carry blood away from the heart

arterioles tiny arteries

arteriosclerosis hardening of the arteries

arthritis inflammation of a joint

arthropods a group of animals including insects, spiders, and shellfish

artificial kidney a term used for a portable dialysis machine

asbestos a substance related to several respiratory diseases including lung cancer

ascorbic acid (vitamin C) essential for the health of the gums and blood vessels and for the prevention of scurvy

asphyxiation suffocation due to drowning, choking, or heart failure

assertiveness training a form of behavior modification in which people learn how to react to real-life situations confidently

association the ability to draw conclusions from past experiences and to use them in present situations

association areas portions of the cerebrum of the brain concerned with emotion and intelligence

astigmatism a vision defect caused by an irregular cornea or lens

astringent a drying lotion applied to the skin

atherosclerosis hardening of the arteries caused by deposits of plaque

athlete's foot an infection caused by fungi

athletics an extension of physical education programs, which allows a student to develop specialized skills

atrioventricular node a node at the junction of the atria and the ventricles of the heart

atrium an upper heart chamber

attention-getting a type of behavior that draws attention to the person using it

attitude a state of mind used in approaching daily situations

auditory nerve a nerve linking the inner ear to the brain

autonomic nervous system that part of the nervous system that controls the vital internal organs and is not under voluntary control

avoidant personality a type of person who prefers to be alone in social situations

axon the single fiber leading away from the nerve cell body

B

bacillus a bacterium shaped like a rod

bacterium a one-celled organism that may cause disease

bacterial endocarditis bacterial infection of the heart valves or lining, usually caused by a streptococcus bacterium

barbiturates a group of sedative drugs used to depress the nervous system

behavior modification a principle of psychotherapy by which the therapist teaches the patient a new response to an old situation.

behavioral medicine prevention of stress disorders by the application of behavioral learning principles and medicine

Benzedrine an amphetamine that causes excitement and sleeplessness

biceps the muscle that bends the elbow and raises the forearm

bicuspids the eight permanent teeth, two in front of each set of molars, which cut and crush food

bifocals eyeglass lenses that have two different lens prescriptions in one pair of lenses

bile a brownish-green fluid secreted by the liver

binocular vision the operation of both eyes together so that they focus on the same spot

bioaccumulation the increasing concentration of pesticides as they travel up the food chain

biofeedback control of body functions by the use of relaxation techniques and conscious mental control

biotin a B vitamin important in metabolism

blackhead dirt and debris from oil glands clogging and enlarging a pore

blended families families formed when members of two or more families are joined

blood-alcohol content (BAC) a measure of the alcohol concentration in the bloodstream

blood sugar, low a low level of sugar in the blood, which leads to fatigue

boil a large skin inflammation caused by bacterial infection

botulism an extremely dangerous form of food poisoning caused by bacterial spores

Bowman's capsule the microscopic, cup-like end of a kidney tubule

brainstem the lower portion of the brain just above the spinal cord

breathalyzer a machine used to measure the blood alcohol content

bronchi the two tubes at the lower end of the windpipe, which lead to the lungs

bronchial asthma an allergic response resulting from sensitivity to pollen, dust, or other irritants

bronchial pneumonia a lung infection caused by bacteria in the bronchioles

bronchioles branches of the bronchi in the lungs

bronchitis an inflammation of the walls of the bronchi

bronchoscope an instrument used in examining the bronchial tubes for lodged objects

bruises injuries to tissue caused by pressure or a blow

bulimia a condition in which a person binges on food and then purges

bunion an enlarged inflammation at the joint of the big toe

bursa a sac of fluid that underlies muscles and tendons at various points, acting as a shock absorber

bursitis inflammation of a bursa

C

caecum the blind pouch where the small intestine joins the large intestine

calcitonin a chemical regulator that reduces the calcium level of the blood and promotes its deposit in bone

calcium one of the most abundant minerals in the body; necessary for formation of the teeth and bones and for blood clotting

callus a bony deposit around a fracture; the thickening of an irritated area of the skin

Calories units used for measuring the amount of heat supplied by food

cancer a rapid, disorderly growth of cells that becomes a tumor, which crowds out normal tissue

cannabis (marijuana) a plant whose leaves are smoked for their mind-altering effects

capillaries small, thin-walled vessels that carry blood to individual cells

carbohydrates foods that furnish energy

carbon monoxide a poisonous gas that readily combines with hemoglobin and is given off by cars and tobacco

carboxyhemoglobin a compound formed in red corpuscles when carbon monoxide combines with hemoglobin

carcinogens substances that cause cancer

cardiopulmonary resuscitation (CPR) an emergency procedure used when the heart stops beating

cardiovascular system the heart and the blood vessels

carpal one of the eight bones of the wrist

cartilage semisoft, bonelike material, such as that at the end of the nose and in the ears

cataract a condition in which an eye lens has become cloudy or opaque

catatonic schizophrenia a form of schizophrenia in which the patient lies rigid and motionless for hours

cell the unit of structure of all living things

cementum the outer covering of the root of a tooth

central nervous system the brain and the spinal cord

cerebellum that part of the brain lying in the lower back part of the cranial cavity

cerebral hemorrhage the result of a blood vessel bursting in the brain or on its surface

cerebral palsy a group of disabling conditions caused by damage to the central nervous system, which result in lack of muscular coordination and speech disturbance

cerebrospinal fluid a clear fluid in the ventricles of the brain and surrounding the spinal cord

cerebrospinal meningitis an infection of the membranes of the brain and spinal cord

cerebrum the uppermost and largest region of the brain, divided into two halves

cervical vertebrae spinal bones of the neck

chemabrasion a procedure used by a dermatologist to improve the appearance of acne scars

chemotherapy the use of specific drugs to destroy viruses and bacteria within the body and to treat mental problems

chiropodist a person who specializes in treatment of the feet

chloride a mineral found in salt, which maintains proper water balance in the body

cholecystitis an inflammation or infection of the gallbladder

cholesterol a waxy substance produced by the body or found in animal products

choroid layer the second, inside layer of the eyeball

chronic adhesive deafness a condition that prevents transmission of vibrations to the inner ear

chronic disease a disease of long duration, often of a degenerative and disabling nature

chronic pulmonary emphysema a progressive disease of the lungs occurring in middle-aged or older people

chyme food that has undergone digestion in the stomach

cilia tiny hair-like parts of the mucous membrane lining the trachea

ciliary muscles the lens muscles of the eye

cirrhosis a disease of the liver in which tissue changes form by shrinking and hardening

clavicle the collar bone

client-centered therapy a form of psychotherapy that focuses on the client's present attitudes and behavior

cocaine a drug made from the leaves of the coca plant, which is both a stimulant and a painkiller

coccus round-celled bacterium

coccyx four fused vertebrae forming the tailbone at the end of the spine

cochlea the hearing apparatus of the inner ear

codeine a narcotic made from opium and used in cough medicines

cognitive learning the process by which information and stimuli are analyzed and assimilated

cold sore a fluid-filled or crusty lesion in the upper layer of the skin, caused by a virus

colon the large intestine

color blindness an inherited condition found in men; partial color blindness results in difficulty in seeing shades of red or green; complete color blindness results in seeing only shades of gray, black, and white

communicable disease an infection that can be passed from one person to another, directly or indirectly

compensation a mental mechanism that directs efforts toward a new goal when an old goal is unattainable

complex carbohydrates sugars found in starches and cellulose

compress a type of dressing applied directly over a wound to control bleeding

compulsion an unconscious drive that compels an action

concussion a temporary loss of the nervous system's function, caused by a sudden blow

conditioning the use of rewards or punishments in training to get a specific response to a specific behavior.

cones receptors in the eye that give distinct vision in bright light and that function in color vision

congenital heart defect a heart abnormality present at birth

conjunctiva a membrane that covers the white of the eye and lines the eyelids

conjunctivitis a contagious infection causing reddening and swelling of the eyes and eyelids

connecting neuron a central neuron in the spinal cord that passes messages between a sensory neuron and a motor neuron

conscience attitudes that influence conscious decisions

conscious mind that portion of the mind functioning at the level of awareness

constipation a state of difficult and infrequent bowel movement

contact dermatitis a common form of eczema caused by direct skin contact with an allergy-producing substance

contact lenses tiny lenses that fit over the corneas

contraction the shortening and thickening of muscle fibers

controlling reinforcement a form of behavior modification used by therapists that rewards the patient each time an appropriate action is carried out

contusion a bruising of the brain or nerves

conversion a mental mechanism that transforms a struggle in the unconscious mind to a physical symptom in the body

conversion disorder a type of hysterical neurosis in which an emotional conflict is transformed to a physical disability

convulsions violent and abnormal muscular contractions

coordination the ability of muscles and nerves to work together

copper a mineral found in the bloodstream

cornea the clear, circular window in the front of the eye

corneal scarring a scarring on the cornea, which can lead to blindness

corneal transplant an eye operation in which a cloudy cornea is replaced with a clear one

corns hard, thickened area of epidermis

coronary circulation circulation of the blood through the heart

coronary heart disease impairment of circulation to the heart muscle

coronary occlusion clogging of a coronary artery

coronary thrombosis a blood clot formed in a coronary artery

corpuscles blood cells

cortex the outer surface of the brain, kidney, and adrenal gland

cranial bone one of the eight bones forming the brain case

cranial cavity the protective helmet housing the brain

cranial nerves nerves that connect various regions of the brain to different structures of the head

cravat a type of bandage that resembles a necktie

cretinism a disease caused by extreme thyroid deficiency during infancy; results in physical stunting and mental deficiency

crown the part of the tooth that appears above the gum

cryosurgery a procedure used by dermatologists to improve the appearance of acne scars

crystalline lens the convex lens behind the pupil opening to the iris of the eye

CT (computerized axial tomography) a procedure that produces pictures of the human brain far more complete than ordinary X rays

Cushing's syndrome a condition caused by an overactive pituitary gland, in which women between 15 and 35 develop round faces, fatty deposits around the face and neck, and elevated blood pressure

cuspids the large teeth near the corners of the mouth that cut and tear food

customs practices that express social and cultural attitudes, beliefs, and values

cuticle the skin around the nail that forms a hardened margin

cystitis a painful infection of the urinary bladder

D

dandruff normal flaking of the epidermis of the scalp

decision-making skills skills that help a person reach full potential through self-awareness.

dehydration excessive water loss from the body

delirium tremens (DT's) withdrawal symptoms of trembling and hallucination experienced when an alcoholic stops drinking

denatured alcohol a poisonous substance used for industrial purposes

dendrites fibers that carry impulses to the nerve cell body

denial a mental mechanism used to avoid facing an unpleasant reality

dental caries the progressive destruction of the teeth, also known as tooth decay

dentin that portion of the tooth beneath the enamel layer

dependence a physical or psychological requirement for a continuous supply of a drug, also called addiction

dependent personality a type of person who relies completely upon others for a sense of security

depilatories chemical creams or sprays used to remove hair

depressant a chemical agent that diminishes the activity of bodily function

depression a state of sadness and dejection

dermabrasion a procedure used by dermatologists to improve the appearance of acne scars

dermis the middle layer of the skin

desensitization a method used in therapy by which relaxation techniques are used as the patient imagines stressful events

despair a feeling of complete hopelessness

detached retina a condition in which the retina of one or both eyes separates from the choroid layer of the eyeball

detoxification the removal of the drug from an addict's body; the first step in treatment for drug addiction

Dexedrine an amphetamine that causes excitement and sleeplessness

diabetes insipidus a condition in which a person craves water constantly

diabetes mellitus true diabetes, a disease that makes a person unable to use or store sugar

dialysis a method of treatment for acute kidney failure by which the patient's blood is cleansed in a machine and then returned to the body.

diaphragm a sheet of muscle dividing the chest from the abdominal cavity

diarrhea abnormal discharge of loose or fluid material from the colon

diastolic pressure arterial blood pressure maintained between heartbeats

dietary fiber plant matter that cannot be digested

digitalis a drug used to slow and strengthen the heartbeat during heart failure

diplococcus pairs of short filaments of spherical bacteria

dislocation an injury by which the bone ends are moved out of place at the joint and the ligaments holding them are severely stretched or torn

displaced aggression a mental mechanism that transfers aggression to a substitute person when it is impossible to direct the aggression to the person who provoked it

dissociative disorder a type of hysterical neurosis in which a person's memory becomes separated from his or her behavior

diuretics substances that eliminate salt and water from the body

diverticulosis a disease of the colon

Down's syndrome a genetic disorder caused by a

chromosome abnormality, resulting in mental retardation

dreams expressions of the unconscious mind during sleep

droplet infection disease spread by droplets expelled by coughing and sneezing

drug any chemical substance that alters either the mind or the body

drug abuse the overuse of beneficial drugs and the misuse of potentially dangerous drugs

ductless glands endocrine glands that have no ducts and whose secretions pour directly into the bloodstream

duodenum the upper part of the small intestine

duration how long an activity lasts

E

eardrum the circular membrane stretched across the inner end of the auditory canal

eczema a skin disorder resulting in red, swollen, scaly areas, which tend to "seep" a clear fluid

edema swelling caused by water retention

EEG (electroencephalogram) a test that records electrical activity, the so-called "brain waves," of a cerebral cortex

elective surgery surgery that is not immediately essential to save or prolong a life

electrocardiograph an instrument used to analyze heart action

electrolysis a technique used to permanently remove hair

EMG (electromyograph) a tool that measures the electrical impulses of the muscle fibers

emotion a feeling that sparks mental and physical changes in a person

emotional maturity the ability to reason and direct emotions into positive actions

emphysema a respiratory disease by which the air passages of the body are constricted and air flow is reduced

emulsion a milky fluid formed by the action of bile on fats

enamel a white protective layer that covers the crown and neck of the tooth

encephalitis a disease also known as sleeping sickness, which is carried by a tsetse fly and destroys the gray matter of the brain

encounter groups groups in which people are helped to understand how to improve their interactions with others

endocardium a tough membrane that lines the chambers of the heart

endocrine glands ductless glands of the body that produce hormones

enriched foods foods in which vitamins lost in processing have been replaced

environment the complex of factors surrounding an individual or community

envy a mixed emotion combining self-love, anger, and fear

enzymes substances that aid digestion by helping in the breakdown of foods

epidermis the outer layer of the skin

epiglottis a leaf-like lid that partially covers the opening of the larynx

epilepsy a brain disorder that brings on convulsions and loss of consciousness

epinephrine (adrenaline) a hormone produced by the adrenal glands

equilibrium balance

erepsin an enzyme of the intestinal fluid, which converts peptides to amino acids

esophagus the tube leading from the throat to the stomach

estrogen a hormone secreted by the ovaries

ethanol (ethyl alcohol) a form of alcohol found in beverages

Eustachian tube a tube in the middle ear involved in the equalization of air pressure

exhalation the forcing of air from the lungs

exocrene glands glands that secrete their products through ducts to the outside of the body or to the digestive tract

extended family a family that includes other members, such as grandparents, aunts, uncles, and cousins, besides the immediate parents and children

extensor the muscle that straightens out a joint

external respiration the process of breathing by which oxygen is taken into the body and carbon dioxide and water are released

F

facial bone one of the 14 bones forming the nose and nasal cavity, hard palate, cheeks, and upper and lower jaws.

family therapy a form of therapy in which the family and the relationships within the family are examined and treated

farsightedness (hyperopia) a condition of the eye in which the point of focus is in back of the retina

fatigue tiredness

fats foods that yield energy and contain certain vitamins

fear any feeling that stems from a threat to security

femur the thighbone

fermentation the process that produces alcohol by the action of yeast on sugars and starches

fibrinogen a blood protein that works with platelets in the clotting process

fibula one of the two bones of the lower leg

first aid the immediate temporary care given to a person in an accident or with a sudden illness

fission reproduction by cell division

fissure (rectal) a crack in the membrane lining of the rectum

flagella slender, whip-like threads that propel bacilli and spirilli through a fluid environment

flexor a muscle that bends a joint

fluoride certain mineral salts added to drinking water that aid in the prevention of tooth decay

folic acid a B vitamin important in metabolism

follicle a pocket in the dermis containing a hair root

follicle stimulating hormone (FSH) a hormone secreted by the pituitary gland, which plays an important role in the menstrual cycle

fortified foods foods to which an extra amount of vitamins already present are added.

fovea a pit in the center of the retina where distinct vision occurs

fracture a broken bone that is classified as greenstick if fibers only are broken; closed, if the bone does not pierce the skin; and open, if the bone pierces the skin

freckles small patches or spots of melanin

frostbite an actual freezing of tissue

functional disease a disease resulting from the impaired activity of an organ

fungi small, one-celled microorganisms, such as yeast, which affect nails, skin, and hair

G

gallbladder a sac-like structure in which bile is stored and converted

gallstones stones formed in the gallbladder

ganglion a mass of nerve tissue containing nerve cells

gangrene death of tissue caused by reduction of blood supply to the tissue, particularly in the legs and feet

genes the chemical determinants of heredity

gingivitis inflammation of the gums

glaucoma an eye disease in which fluid pressure builds up on the eyeball and damages the fibers of the optic nerve

globulin a blood protein that contains antibodies

glomerulus a twisted mass of tiny blood vessels within a kidney capsule

glottis the opening of the windpipe

glucagon a hormone of the pancreas that changes glycogen to glucose

glucose blood sugar, or the end product of carbohydrate digestion; the body's primary fuel

glycerol an end product of fat digestion

glycogen animal starch

goiter a condition in which the thyroid gland becomes enlarged

gonadotropic hormones hormones secreted by the pituitary gland that cause physical changes in the body during adolescence

gonads the reproductive organs

gonorrhea a communicable venereal disease that can cause blindness and other complications

gray matter masses of nerve cell bodies in the brain and spinal cord

grief a feeling of deep sadness

group therapy a method of therapy in which several people work together with a therapist at the same time

guilt an emotion experienced when something conflicts with the conscience or with self-expectations

H

habits acts that become automatic

hallucinations experiences of sensations with no external cause, usually arising from a disorder of the nervous system or from drug abuse

hallucinogens drugs that produce hallucinations and visions

hangnail a sliver of cuticle that has separated along the edge of the nail

hashish a concentrated form of marijuana

Haversian canals canals penetrating the compact substance of bone

head louse a parasite that lives on the blood it sucks from the scalp

health a state of complete physical, mental, and social well-being

heart failure a condition in which the heart lacks the strength to keep the blood flowing through the body normally

heartburn a disorder in the stomach causing a burning feeling near the heart

heat exhaustion weakness, high body temperature, and collapse due to overexertion in a hot, humid atmosphere

heatstroke a serious condition caused by overexposure to the sun

hebephrenia a form of schizophrenia in which the patient is completely out of touch with reality

Heimlich maneuver a technique used to force out obstructions in the lungs when someone is choking

hemoglobin an iron-containing red pigment combined with a protein substance found in red blood cells

hemophilia an inherited disease in which blood fails to clot or clots very slowly

hemorrhoids enlarged veins in the rectum

hepatic portal veins vessels that transport digested food and water to the liver

hepatitis a severe virus infection of the liver

heredity the transmission of traits from parent to offspring

hernia a tear in the muscle layer of the abdomen that allows the intestine to press through and cause a bulge

heroin a derivative of opium, the most dangerous and addictive narcotic known

herpes simplex a disease caused by a virus; commonly called cold sores

high blood pressure (hypertension) a narrowing of the arteries and arterioles that causes an increase in blood pressure

hirsutism the condition in which excess hair appears where there is usually little growth of hair

histrionic a type of personality that needs constant excitement and attention

hives an allergic reaction recognizable by red, raised areas on the skin

holistic an approach to total health in which the body, mind, and spirit are all key factors

homogenization the processing of milk to break up the fat content

hookworm a roundworm that enters the body through the feet and damages the intestinal tract

hormones the secretions of the endocrine glands

host an organic body upon which bacteria and other fungus plants live

humerus the bone of the upper arm

hunger a desire for food resulting from physiological activity of the stomach

hydrochloric acid a chemical secreted by the stomach glands, which is important in destroying food bacteria and aiding in the digestive process

hydrophobia (rabies) an acute and generally fatal infection of the brain caused by a virus and transmitted through the bites of rabid animals

hyoid a bone that lies at the base of the tongue, just above the larynx

hypertension (high blood pressure) a narrowing of the arteries and arterioles that causes an increase in blood pressure.

hypnosis a form of psychotherapy in which the patient is put in a trance in order to reach the unconscious

hypochondria a form of anxiety in which a person lives in constant fear of disease

hypoglycemia low blood sugar

hypothalamus an endocrine gland located in the brain, which controls automatic functions

hysteria a form of behavior marked by extreme emotional excitability

hysterical neurosis a form of neurosis in which unconscious drives convert to temporary paralysis, loss of speech, or other disorders.

I

idealization a mental mechanism in which the abilities and attributes of others are overestimated

identification seeking to connect oneself with others by adoping the same feelings and behavior

ileum the lower region of the small intestine, approximately 5 meters (15 feet) in length

ilium one of the three parts of fused bones forming the pelvis

immune globulin a blood substance containing antibodies against disease organisms

immune therapy the use of sera, vaccines, and other immune products in treating and preventing infectious diseases

immunity a condition of the body in which a given disease organism cannot produce an infection

impulse a message picked up by a sensory receptor neuron and translated into a signal

inborn immunity a natural resistance to a disease or infection

incision a sharp cut

incisor the four upper and four lower permanent teeth that cut and tear foods

indigestion a term used to describe a stomachache, heartburn, or pain in any part of the abdomen

infection invasion and establishment of infectious organisms in the body's tissues

infectious disease a disease passed by direct human contact

infectious hepatitis a form of hepatitis in which infection is passed by direct human contact

inferior vena cava a vein that carries blood from the lower parts of the body to the heart

infestation the invasion of the body by parasites

ingrown toenail a condition in which pressure on the nail forces it to grow toward the nail base

inhalants drugs that are volatile chemicals and that cause intoxication when inhaled

inhalation the sucking of air into the lungs

initiative the ability to determine an action and then carry it through

inner ear that portion of the ear involved in balance

insertion a muscle attachment to a movable bone

insomnia the inability to sleep

instinct an automatic and unlearned prompting to action

insulin a hormone secreted by the pancreas, which controls the level of sugar in the blood

intelligence the ability to reason and act accordingly

interferon a protein substance produced in cells to combat virus infection

iodized salt salt that contains iodine

iris the circular, colored muscle behind the cornea

iron a mineral found in hemoglobin; a deficiency causes anemia and general weakness

irritable bowel syndrome a disorder in which the bowel contracts suddenly and violently

irritability the response of protoplasm to its environment

ischium one of the three pairs of fused bones forming the pelvis

islets of Langerhans cells scattered throughout the pancreas, which secrete insulin and glucagon

isometric exercises exercises that contract the muscles but do not move the joints

isopropyl alcohol a poisonous substance used in paint thinners, varnishes, and shellac

isotonic exercises exercises for strengthening various parts of the body by lifting or moving weights

J

jaundice a yellow coloration of the skin due to excess bile pigments in the blood

jealousy an emotion that stems from fear and insecurity

jejunum the second region of the small intestine, about 2½ meters (7½ feet) in length

joint the point at which two bones meet

K

keratin a transparent substance manufactured by the epidermis cells of the skin

kidney stones abnormal mineral deposits in the kidneys

kinesthetic sense the sense of muscle pull and position

L

laceration a torn wound

lactase an enzyme in the intestinal fluid that converts lactose to simple sugars

lacteal a vessel containing lymph that collects digested fats in the intestinal wall

lactogenic hormone a hormone secreted by the anterior pituitary gland, which causes milk secretion after childbirth

laryngitis an infection of the larynx that produces hoarseness or complete lack of voice

larynx the upper part of the windpipe containing the vocal cords

laser therapy an experimental form of treatment with light for removing birthmarks and tattoos

learning a relatively permanent change in behavior as a result of an experience

learning disability a breakdown in the way the brain processes information

left brain the part of the brain that controls the right side of the body and most logical thinking

leukemia a disease in which a great excess of white blood cells is formed

ligaments tough strands that bind bones together

liver the largest organ in the body lying just below the diaphragm and on the right side of the abdominal cavity

lobar pneumonia a lung infection caused by one of several types of pneumonia organisms in the respiratory passages

lobes folds in the cortex of the cerebrum

lockjaw (tetanus) a painful disease involving the voluntary muscles of the jaw, caused by a poison of a microorganism, and usually introduced through puncture wounds

longitudinal arch the arch that extends from the heel of the foot to the base of the toes

love a feeling of pleasure and satisfaction

LSD (lysergic acid diethylamide) a hallucinogenic drug (sometimes called acid) that produces visions and pronounced behavioral changes

lumbar vertebrae spinal bones in the abdominal region

lung cancer a disease of the lungs that is significantly more common in cigarette smokers

lymph the clear liquid that enters the spaces between body cells

lymph nodes gland-like structures that make lymphocytes and filter lymph

lymphatic system a division of the circulatory system made of vessels called lymphatics

lymphatics tubes that convey lymph throughout the body

lymphocytes a type of white blood cell that provides immunity against disease organisms

M

mainlining injecting a narcotic drug, usually heroin, directly into the veins

malaria a fever caused by a parasitic protozoan and spread by a particular species of mosquito

malignant tumor a mass of cancerous cells that crowds out normal tissue and absorbs vital nutrients

malnutrition lack of proper food

malocclusion irregularity in the position and bite of teeth, which is correctable by orthodontistry

maltase an enzyme in intestinal fluid that converts maltose to glucose

manic-depressive disorder a type of disorder in which a person is either in a state of extreme excitement or depression and may switch rapidly from one state to the other

mannerisms behavioral habits, such as nail biting and knuckle cracking, usually associated with nervous tension

marijuana (cannabis) a plant whose leaves are smoked for their mind-altering effects

marrow soft tissue in the hollow parts of the bones

mastitis a streptococcus infection of the udder and milk glands of cattle

mastoid bone a porous bone behind the middle ear

mastoiditis an inflammation of the mastoid bone

maximum heart rate the number of times a heart beats per minute when a person has been exercising as fast as possible

medulla the enlargement at the upper end of the spinal cord containing vital centers for control of respiration and circulation; also the inner region of an adrenal gland and kidney

medullary canal an area at the center of a bone's shaft filled with marrow

melanin a dark pigment formed in deep layers of the skin

memory the ability to recall past experiences

meninges the protective membranes of the brain and spinal cord

meningitis an infection of the meninges of the spinal cord and brain

menstrual cycle a one-month cycle assiciated with the production of an ovum (egg) by the ovaries

mental disorder a condition in which a person cannot cope with the environment and cannot get along with others

mental fatigue tiredness resulting from sustained mental activity

mental health an attitude of self-respect and tolerance toward oneself and others

mental mechanisms devices developed to justify behavior; also called defense mechanisms

mental retardation a condition of mental deficiency in certain people

mescaline a hallucinogenic substance with severe side effects, found naturally in peyote but which can be made synthetically

mesothelioma a deadly form of lung cancer

metabolism the process by which the body produces energy

metacarpal a bone in the hand

metastasis the spread of cancer cells to new areas

metatarsals bones in the foot

methadone the commercial name for a synthetic narcotic drug used to cure heroin addiction

methanol a highly poisonous form of alcohol used in paint thinners, varnishes, and shellac

methaqualone an addictive drug that produces a feeling of well-being and calm but can have harmful side effects

microorganism a microscopic living organism

midbrain that part of the brainstem that connects the cerebrum to the cerebellum

middle ear that portion of the ear beyond the eardrum that contains three bones; it carries vibrations into the inner ear and is also involved in equalization of air pressure

migraine the type of headache that appears during a period of emotional strain and is caused by disordered activity of the blood vessels supplying blood to the brain.

milieu (environment) therapy changing a patient's environment to encourage changes in attitudes and behavior

minerals inorganic salts necessary for regulating body activities, forming bones, forming teeth, and so on

mixed nerves nerve bundles containing both sensory and motor nerve fibers

modeling a technique used in behavior modification therapy in which a patient watches a model carry out stressful actions

molars the three teeth on each side of the upper and lower jaws behind the bicuspids, used to grind food

mole a slight overgrowth of both epidermis and dermis containing an excess of pigment

mononucleosis a glandular disease caused by a virus; symptoms include weakness, swollen glands, and general discomfort

morphine a fine, white powder made from opium and used as a painkiller

motivation the driving force behind behavior

motor areas the portions of the cerebrum that control movements

motor neuron a conducting nerve that leads to a muscle

mucous membrane a membrane that forms a protective lining in various body openings

mucus the lubricating substance secreted by the mucous glands

multiple personality a dissociative disorder in which a person's memories and emotions separate into two or more distinct personalities

multiple sclerosis a disease that attacks the outer coating of nerve fibers, resulting in muscle tremors and partial or complete paralysis

murmurs any unusual heart sounds

muscle a mass of fibers grouped together that moves the bones of the body

muscular dystrophy a muscular disease common in young children consisting of gradual and progressive destruction of muscle fibers, which may finally leave the limbs useless

mutagens substances causing hereditary changes that are passed from one generation to the next

myasthenia gravis a disease causing rapid fatigue and weakness of voluntary muscle

myocardial infarction the death of a section of heart muscle due to a lack of blood supply, commonly called a heart attack

myocarditis inflammation of the heart muscle, often during rheumatic fever

myocardium the muscular wall of the heart

myxedema a disease caused by extreme thyroid deficiency in adult life

N

narcissistic personality an egocentric personality that results in behavior that is conceited and arrogant

narcolepsy a condition in which a person cannot help falling asleep.

narcotic a drug designated by the federal government as addictive

nares the opening of the nasal cavities

nasal septum a thin sheet of cartilage and soft bone, which divides the nasal chamber into a right and left side

nasopharynx the upper cavity of the pharynx that lies in back of the nose and above the roof of the mouth

nearsightedness (myopia) a condition of the eye in which the point of focus is in front of the retina

neck the portion of the tooth visible at the gum line

nephritis an acute or chronic bacterial inflammation of the kidneys

nerve impulse a message picked up by a sensory receptor neuron and translated into a signal

nervous system the brain, spinal cord, and nerves of the body

neuritis an inflammation of the sheath around a nerve fiber

neurodermatitis the skin's reaction to stress, which produces symptoms similar to eczema

neurologist a physician specializing in diagnosing and treating disorders of the nervous system

neurons nerve cells

neurotransmitters substances that regulate sleep activities

niacin a vitamin that prevents pellagra

nicotine a poisonous substance in tobacco

night blindness a condition in which there is difficulty in seeing in dim light

nitroglycerine the principal medication used to relieve cardiac pain

nits eggs laid by head lice

nondirective therapy client-centered therapy in which the therapist does not tell the patient how to act and react

normal personality a type of person who views the world in a realistic way

nuclear family a family composed of parents and children only

nucleus the central structure within the cell

nutrient density the ratio of nutrients to Calories in foods

nutrients chemical substances that the body needs for energy, growth and repair of tissues, and regulation of its functions

O

obesity excessive fat; overweight

obsessions ideas that remain with people against their wills

oculist a medical doctor who specializes in eye diseases and vision defects

olfactory nerve the nerve involved in the sense of smell

ophthalmologist a medical doctor who specializes in eye diseases and vision defects

ophthalmoscope an instrument used to examine the interior of the eye

opium a narcotic made from poppies; the parent of a family of powerful narcotic drugs

optic nerve the nerve leading from the eyeball to the brain

optician an expert in the grinding of lenses and the fitting of glasses

organ an arrangement of tissues in a specialized structure

organic disease an illness resulting from a structural disorder

organic mental disorder a mental disturbance caused by a physical illness or injury that affects the brain

origin the immovable point of attachment of a muscle to a bone

orthopedists doctors who specialize in the treatment of bone disorders

ossification the replacement of cartilage with bone and the deposit of minerals in the bony region

osteoarthritis an arthritic condition characterized by bony enlargements of joints

osteomyelitis a term applied to various bone infections

osteoporosis a metabolic disorder of the bone, common in older people, in which the bones become easily breakable

otosclerosis a hearing defect caused by an overgrowth of bone in the inner ear

otoscope an instrument used to examine the ears

outer ear the visible portion of the ear

ovaries the reproductive organs of the female

overload a workout of muscles that exceeds normal demands

over-the-counter (OTC) drugs drugs sold without a prescription

oxidation the process by which oxygen combines with another substance

oxidation the chemical breakdown of glucose to produce energy

oxygen debt oxygen deficiency accompanied by the accumulation of metabolic fatigue substances in the tissues

oxytocin a hormone secreted by the posterior pituitary gland that stimulates smooth muscles to react

P

PABA a sun-block substance that offers the greatest protection against burning and tanning

pacemaker an electronic device inserted under the skin of the abdomen, used to keep the heart beating at a proper rate

pancreas a gland situated behind the stomach, which aids in digestion and secretes insulin

pancreatic juice a substance secreted by the pancreas, which is important in digestion

pancreatitis chronic inflammation and scarring of the pancreas

pantothenic acid a B vitamin important in metabolism

papillae the ridges of the skin

paranoid schizophrenia a form of schizophrenia marked by delusions of persecution or delusions of grandeur

paraplegia paralysis of the legs and lower body

parasite an organism that lives on and takes nourishment from a living host

parasympathetic nervous system a part of the autonomic nervous system

parathyroids four endocrine glands located at the back of the thyroid gland

paregoric a mild narcotic made from opium and used in treating digestive pain and diarrhea

Parkinson's disease a deterioration of the midbrain that affects older people

parotid glands the largest of the salivary glands located in the sides of the face

passive-aggressive personality a behavior in which moods are unpredictable and are generally pessimistic

pasteurization a heating process that destroys bacteria in milk

patch test a test used in determining the presence of tuberculosis by placing a small amount of tuberculin on the skin

patella the knee cap

pathogenic causing disease

PCP (angel dust) a synthetic drug once used as an anesthetic for animals and now a dangerous drug used by humans

pectoral girdle the two shoulder bones

pediculosis an infestation of head lice, which causes irritation and itching of the scalp

peer group people of the same age and interests; people who are considered a person's equals

pellagra a disease caused by niacin deficiency,

which causes rough and reddened skin, sores on the mouth, diarrhea, and possible paralysis

pelvic nerve a nerve that connects the spinal cord in the hip region to the organs of the lower part of the body

pelvis the three pairs of bones that join to support the weight of the body; the central cavity of a kidney

penicillin the first antibiotic; discovered by Dr. Alexander Fleming

pepsin a protein-splitting enzyme in gastric fluid

peptic ulcer an open sore in the stomach or duodenum

perception the ability to receive stimuli such as sight and sound from the environment

pericarditis inflammation of the covering of the heart, often during rheumatic fever

pericardium a fiber-like bag in which the heart rests

peridontal disease (pyorrhea) a disease of the gums, mouth lining, and bony sockets of the teeth, caused by plaque

peridontal membrane the fibrous membrane that anchors the root of a tooth in the jaw socket

periosteum the tough, living membrane covering the bones

peripheral nerves bundles of dendrites and axons grouped together

peripheral nervous system the nerves leading to and from the spinal cord

peripheral vision vision out of the corner of the eye

peristalsis the squeezing motion of the digestive organs that moves food through them

permanent teeth the teeth that replace the primary teeth by the age of six; the adult teeth

personality distinctive personal character; qualities that produce individuality

pesticides chemical poisons used to control insects and other pests

peyote a cactus that yields a hallucinogenic drug substance

phagocytes white blood cells that swarm to an area of infection

phagocytosis the process by which phagocytes devour microbes, thus forming pus

phalanges bones of the fingers and toes

pharynx the throat cavity

phenylketonuria (PKU) an inherited disorder, which, if not treated, will cause retardation

phobia an intense, unreasonable fear of certain things or situations

phosphorus one of the most abundant minerals in the body, which helps regulate many activities of the body cells

physical fitness the ability to carry out daily tasks comfortably with energy left over

pimple a local infection in a skin pore or hair follicle

pinkeye a common, contagious infection of the conjunctiva

pituitary gland an endocrine gland in the brain, which secretes hormones that influence the activities of other glands

planing surgery an abrasive procedure used by dermatologists to improve the appearance of acne scars

plantar wart a deep wart in the sole of the foot

plaque a sticky colorless film formed on the teeth, which destroys tooth enamel and irritates gums; deposits in the blood vessels that cause atherosclerosis

plasma the fluid part of the blood remaining after the living cells have been removed

platelets small cells in the blood that are essential for the clotting of blood

pleural membrane double sacs covering the lungs

pleurisy inflammation of the pleural membrane

podiatrist a person specializing in the treatment of feet

polio (poliomyelitis) a virus infection of the spinal cord and brain

polyunsaturated fats fats that are liquid at room temperature

pons the part of the brainstem that forms a bridge between the cerebrum and the cerebellum

pores small openings in the skin surface

portal circulation circulation through the digestive organs

posterior lobe the back lobe of the pituitary gland that releases hormones

posture the relation of the body parts to one another; general bearing

potassium a mineral involved in maintaining water balance in the body

preconscious mind the part of the mind where memories are stored

prescription drug a drug that can be purchased only with a doctor's written permission

primary teeth (baby teeth) teeth that arrive at about six months of age and after a period of time give way to permanent teeth

processed foods foods that are treated rather than left in their natural state

progesterone a hormone secreted by the ovaries

progressive relaxation a way of reducing body tension from head to toe

projection a mental mechanism by which a mistake or failure is blamed on someone else

proof a term used to express the alcohol content in hard liquor; it is twice the percentage of alcohol

prophylaxis professional tooth cleaning

prostatitis inflammation of the prostate gland

prosthetics the science of designing and fitting artificial limbs

protein an element in food that builds and repairs the body

protoplasm the basic life substance of which all living things are made

protozoan a one-celled animal

psilocybin (psilocyn) a hallucinogenic substance made from a variety of certain mushrooms

psoriasis a skin disease that appears as red, raised skin and silvery scales of dead epidermis

psychiatrists doctors who specialize in mental and emotional disorders

psychiatry a branch of medicine specializing in the treatment of mental illness

psychic energizers (antidepressants) drugs that combat depression and are mood-elevating

psychoanalysis a form of psychotherapy that studies a person's background from birth to the present, concentrating on the individual's unconscious mind and repressed conflicts

psychologists specialists in human behavior

psychosis a mental illness during which the affected person loses touch with reality

psychosomatic pertaining to the relationship between the mind and the body as manifest in disease

psychosomatic medicine treatment of stress disorders through psychology and medicine

psychotherapy a relationship in which a therapist helps a patient become emotionally more mature

psychotic depression a psychosis characterized by an extreme state of depression and dejection

pubic bones one of the three pairs of fused bones that form the pelvis

public health community efforts to combat disease

pulmonary artery an artery that carries blood from the heart to the lungs

pulmonary circulation circulation of the blood through the lungs

pulp cavity the area in the center of the tooth that contains the nerves and blood vessels

pulse the beating of the heart and arteries; it can be felt most easily at the wrist and neck

puncture a piercing wound

pupil the round opening in the iris that allows light to enter

purgatives laxatives that flush the intestine rapidly

pyloric sphincter a valve formed by the stomach muscles where the stomach joins the small intestine

pylorus the lower end of the stomach

pyorrhea a disease of the gums, mouth lining, and bony sockets of the teeth, caused by plaque

pyramids projections of the kidney medulla

pyridoxine (vitamin B^6) a vitamin that regulates growth, skin condition, and muscle functions

Q

quacks a slang term for medical malpractitioners who mislead the public

quadraplegia paralysis of the arms and the legs

quarantine isolation because of suspected infection

R

rabies (hydrophobia) an acute and generally fatal infection of the brain caused by a virus and transmitted through the bites of rabid animals

radius a bone in the lower arm

rapid eye movement (REM) darting of the closed eyes during periods of deep sleep

rationalization a mental mechanism used to avoid facing a loss of self-esteem or to prevent feelings of guilt

reaction formation a mental mechanism by which a person's true motives are kept at an unconscious level

reaction time the time delay in responding to a stimulus

receptors nerves that detect messages of heat, cold, pain, and touch and send information to the central nervous system

red blood cells (red corpuscles) concave blood cells that carry hemoglobin

reflex, simple an involuntary process in which a stimulus causes the passage of an impulse along a nerve to the spinal cord, from which a motor impulse is transmitted to a muscle or gland

reflex arc a pathway for a simple nervous reaction, such as a knee jerk

reflexes very simple inherited behavior patterns

regression a mental mechanism to avoid adult problems by retreating into childish behavior and attitudes

releasing factors substances released by the hypothalamus

REM (rapid eye movement) darting of the closed eyes during periods of deep sleep

renal circulation circulation of the blood through the kidneys

repression the blocking out of memory in order to forget painful experiences

resentment a mixed emotion, combining anger and self-pity

respiration, cellular the exchange of gases between the body cells and the blood stream

respiration, external the exchange of gases between the alveoli and the blood stream

restraint holding back from an action

retina a thin, inner layer of nerves of sight at the back of the interior of the eyeball

retinol (vitamin A) a vitamin important in preventing night blindness

Rh factor several protein substances present in the blood of 85 percent of the population

rheumatic fever an allergic reaction to streptococcus that causes painful swelling and inflammation of the joints and damage to the heart and its valves

rheumatoid arthritis the most serious form of arthritis; characterized by swelling, pain, and stiffness of the joints

riboflavin (vitamin B^2) a vitamin promoting and regulating growth and development

rickets a disease caused by a lack of vitamin D in which the bones and teeth develop improperly

rickettsias microorganisms much like bacteria, which cause Rocky Mountain spotted fever and typhus fever

right brain the part of the brain that controls the left side of the body and interprets the world through patterns, meanings, and emotions

ringworm a fungus condition of the scalp

rods receptors in the eye that register light and darkness and allow for peripheral vision

roentgens units in which radiation is measured

rubella (German measles) an infection that is relatively harmless to children but is extremely dangerous to pregnant women

S

Sabin vaccine a polio vaccine containing harmless living viruses

sacroiliac the joint at which the pelvis meets the sacrum

sacrum the five fused vertebrae of the pelvic region

saliva a secretion of the salivary glands that moistens food as it is being chewed

salivary amylase a starch-splitting enzyme that changes starches to maltose in the mouth

salivary glands glands located in the mouth that play an important role in digestion

Salk vaccine a polio vaccine containing dead viruses

saprophytes organisms, such as bacteria, that digest nonliving food supplies

sarcoma cancer of the connective tissue

saturated fats fats that increase the cholesterol level in blood and become solid at room temperature

scapula the shoulder blade

schizoid personality a kind of behavior that is extremely sensitive to rejection and criticism from others and tends to withdraw

schizophrenia a type of psychosis in which a person has a split personality

sclera the tough outer layer of the eyeball

scoliosis lateral curvature of the spine; "S-shaped" spine

scurvy a disease caused by a lack of vitamin C (ascorbic acid)

seborrheic dermatitis a scalp condition that resembles dandruff but is more serious and more difficult to control

sebum an oil that is a protective covering for the skin

sedatives drugs that slow down nervous activity

seizure a "storm" in the brain caused by sudden electrical imbalance

self-preservation a basic instinct to preserve one's own life

semicircular canals structures found in the inner ear involved in balance

semilunar valves valves located at the openings of the arteries, which force blood from the ventricles into the arteries

sensory areas portions of the cerebrum of the brain that receive impulses from the sense organs

sensory neurons nerves that carry sensory impulses toward the brain or spinal cord

septum the wall dividing the heart into a right and left side

sera substances that give resistance or temporary immunity to disease

serum plasma from which fibrinogen has been removed

serum hepatitis a form of hepatitis that results from a transfusion of contaminated human blood

serum sickness a serious reaction to immune sera from animals

sex hormones hormones produced by the reproductive organs, which cause dramatic changes in physical, mental, and emotional characteristics during adolescence

shaft the slender area at the end of a bone

shingles a disease, caused by a virus, that affects the sensory nerves.

shock a depressed state of the nervous system due to loss of blood

sibling a brother or a sister

sickle-cell trait a hereditary condition in which the red blood cells are malformed and block small blood vessels, ultimately resulting in anemia

sidestream smoke the smoke-polluted air resulting from a cigarette, which causes nonsmokers to become passive smokers

sigmoid colon the lower, twisted section of the descending colon

simple carbohydrates sugars that are found in fruits, vegetables, whole grains, and milk products; also refined sugars

simple goiter an enlargement of the thyroid gland resulting from a deficiency of iodine

simple reflex an involuntary process in which a stimulus causes the passage of an impulse along a nerve to the spinal cord, from which a motor impulse is transmitted to a muscle or gland

sinoatrial node a small mass of tissue in the right auricle from which a heartbeat starts

sinuses cavities in the nasal bones that connect with the air passages

sinusitis an infection of the sinuses

skin the body's protective covering and largest external organ

skull fracture the breaking of the cranial bone

small intestine a section of the alimentary canal extending from the stomach to the colon

smokeless tobacco tobacco that is chewed or dipped

sodium a mineral found in salt that maintains water balance in the body

somatropic hormone (growth hormone) a hormone that is secreted by the pituitary gland and promotes growth

spastic colon a disorder of the bowel in which constipation alternates with diarrhea

species preservation the instinctive response of sacrificing oneself for the preservation of one's group

species specific behavior similar instinctive behavior of all animals in the same species

sphygmomanometer an instrument for measuring blood pressure

spinal column the vertebrae

spinal cord a slender nerve cable that goes from the brain down through the spinal column

spinal nerves the nerves that branch off from the spinal cord between the bones of the spine

spinal tap a procedure by which a doctor inserts a needle between the vertebrae of the spinal column and draws out a small amount of the spinal fluid for analysis

spirillum a bacterium shaped like a twisted rod or spiral

spirochetes organisms resembling both bacteria and protozoa

splint a mechanical support for a fracture

spongy bone bone substance at the joint ends, which is loose and porous

spontaneous combustion fire caused by substances that absorb so much oxygen that they ignite spontaneously

spore an asexual reproductive body formed by a bacterium

sprain an injury caused when a joint is moved too far

sputum material coughed up from the lungs

stapes (stirrup) one of the small bones of the middle ear

stapes mobilization an operation to restore hearing

staphylococcus a spherical bacterium

stereoscopic vision the ability to see depth as well as length and width

stethoscope an instrument used to listen to breathing and heartbeat

stimulants drugs that stimulate the central nervous system and give a feeling of alertness and nervousness

stimuli conditions, situations, or problems that promote a response

stomach a digestive organ and food reservoir lying between the esophagus and small intestine

strain an overstretching or tearing of the muscles; excessive mental tension

streptobacillus filament or sphere-shaped bacterium

streptococcus a group of bacteria with ball-shaped cells arranged like a string of beads

streptomycin a powerful antibiotic substance used in treating tuberculosis

stress response the body's physical and mental reaction to disorder and personal conflict

striated muscle skeletal muscle that has stripes running across its fibers

stroke brain damage caused by a hemorrhage or clot

styes infections of the glands of the eyelids, caused by bacteria

subclavian vein a large vein that joins the left jugular vein in the neck region

subcutaneous layer the deepest layer of the skin

sublimation changing the direction of a basic drive

toward a new goal when the previous goal is impossible to obtain

sublingual glands salivary glands under the tongue

submaxillary glands salivary glands in the angles of the lower jaw

sucrase an enzyme in the intestinal fluid that converts sucrose to simple sugars

sulfa drugs a family of drugs with germ-killing power

sunburn reddening of the skin due to overexposure to sunlight

superior vena cava a vein that carries blood from the head and upper parts of the body to the heart

suture a zig-zag point of two cranial bones

sympathetic nervous system a part of the autonomic nervous system

synapse the gap an impulse must cross in order to be relayed from one nerve cell to another

synergistic effect the reaction that takes place when two or more drugs are taken at the same time

synovial fluid a fluid secreted by the membranes covering the joints of bones

syphilis a sexually transmitted disease that in its third stage attacks the nervous system

systemic circulation circulation of the blood through the body tissues

systolic pressure arterial blood pressure during heart contraction

T

tapeworm a parasitic flatworm that lives in human intestines

tar a harmful tobacco by-product

target heart rate seventy-five to eighty-five percent of the maximum heart rate

tartar a substance on the teeth caused by the accumulation of plaque

taste buds nerve endings situated in the tongue

tear ducts tubes through which tears pass to the eye

tendon a tough strand that attaches a muscle to a bone

tension an emotional state caused by stress

tension fatigue tiredness resulting from stress and emotional pressure

tension headache the type of headache that develops because of stress; it may include increased tightness of the scalp and nerve muscles

teratogens substances that cause birth defects

testes the reproductive organs of the male

testosterone a hormone secreted by the testes

tetanus (lockjaw) a painful disease involving the involuntary muscles of the jaw, caused by a microorganism and usually introduced through puncture wounds

tetany painful muscle spasms

thalamus a gland that relays information between the spinal cord and cerebrum

THC (tetrahydrocannabinol) the active substance in marijuana

thiamin (vitamin B^1) a vitamin that stimulates growth, appetite, and digestion

thiouracil a drug used in treating goiter

thoracic duct the largest of the lymph vessels, which returns lymph to the general circulation through the subclavian vein

thoracic vertebrae the spinal bones in the chest region

thrombosis a condition in which red streaks and soreness develop along a vein

thymus an endocrine gland located under the breastbone and in front of the heart

thyroid gland an endocrine gland located just below the larynx in the throat

tibia one of the two bones of the lower leg

tics twitching of the muscles, especially those of the face

tissue a group of specialized cells

tolerance the body's ability to become used to a drug's effect, thus requiring a larger dose in order to experience the same effect

tone the condition in muscles in which they are slightly contracted even when they are not pulling

tonometer an instrument used by an opthalmologist to measure pressure on the eyeball

tonsillitis an inflammation or infection of the tonsils

tonsils masses of soft, lymphoid tissue embedded in folds at the back of the mouth

torniquet a device for stopping profuse bleeding, especially in an arm or leg

toxin a poison formed by bacteria in living tissues and also in nonliving food substances

trachea the windpipe

tranquilizers drugs used to quiet the nervous system and to relieve anxiety and psychosomatic illnesses

tranfusion the addition of whole blood or plasma to the circulation of a recipient

transverse arch the arch that extends across the foot at the end of the metatarsal bones at the base of the toes

triangular bandage a type of bandage used in first aid

triceps the muscle that straightens the elbow and lowers the forearm

trichina a type of parasitic worm

trichinosis a disease caused by the penetration of the muscles by the trichina, a worm present in certain meats, especially pork

trypsin a protein-splitting enzyme in pancreatic fluid

TSH (thyrotrophic hormone) a hormone secreted by the anterior lobe of the pituitary gland that regulates the size and activity of the thyroid gland

tubercule a lesion in the lungs containing tuberculosis bacteria

tuberculin material containing dead tuberculosis bacteria, used in testing for tuberculosis

tuberculosis a bacterial infection of the lungs and other organs of the body

tubules microscopic tubes in a kidney

tumor abnormal growth of a mass of cells in the body

U

ulcer an open sore

ulcerative colitis a serious disorder in which multiple ulcers develop in the lining of the colon

ulna a bone in the lower arm

unconscious mind that portion of the mind functioning below the level of awareness

uremia a disease in which the kidneys fail to remove waste products from the blood

ureter a tube leading from the kidney to the urinary bladder

urethra a tube that carries urine from the bladder out of the body

urinalysis a chemical analysis of the urine to determine the general state of health

urinary bladder the sac where urine is stored until emptied through the urethra

urine a liquid accumulation from the kidneys consisting of cell wastes, excess salt, and water

V

vaccination protective inoculation with any vaccine

vaccine a substance that gives immunity to a disease

values the personal standards that people live by

valve a flap-like structure in the heart or in a vein that prevents backflow of blood

varicose veins bulging veins in the legs caused by leaking valves

vegetarian diet a diet containing only plant foods and sometimes dairy products and eggs

veins vessels in the body that carry blood toward the heart

venae cavae the largest veins carrying blood from the body to the heart

venereal diseases diseases such as gonorrhea and syphilis, which are spread by contact

venom poison from some reptiles that affects the nervous system

ventricles the lower chambers of the heart; also chambers in the brain

venules tiny veins

vertebrae the bones of the spine

villi tiny, finger-like projections in the walls of the intestines

virus the smallest form of living matter known to cause disease

virus pneumonia a lung infection involving only parts of the lungs

visual purple a pigment in the rods of the eye

vitamin B complex a family of vitamins including thiamine, riboflavin, and pyridoxine, found in liver, whole grains, and meats

vitamin C (ascorbic acid) a vitamin essential to the health of gums and blood vessels and in the prevention of scurvy

vitamins chemical regulators found in food

vitiligo white patches of the skin produced by the absence of melanin

vitreous humor the fluid filling the eyeball behind the lens

vocal cords two bands of ligaments that stretch across the glottis and produce speech

W

wart a raised growth on the skin caused by a virus

white blood cells (white corpuscles) cells involved in combatting disease and infection

white matter masses of nerve fibers in the brain and spinal cord

willpower a controlling force in behavior

wisdom teeth molars that appear between the ages of 18 and 21 and often grow crookedly, thus requiring extraction

withdrawal symptoms physical reactions including nervousness, nausea, trembling, and cramps, which occur when a drug is taken away from someone who is addicted to it

wound any external or internal break in the skin or mucous lining of the body

INDEX

A

Abnormal personality, 203–204

Abrasions, *561,* first aid for, 563–564

Accident(s), automobile, 546–549; classification of, 545–546; firearm, **552;** home, 550–552; occupational, **555**–556; swimming and boating, 552–553

Accident-prone people, 546

Accommodation, of eye lens, *341*

Accutane, 106

Acid rain, 521

Acne, 104–**105;** control of, 105–106; medical treatment of, 106–107

Acquired active immunity, 500

Acquired immune-deficiency syndrome (AIDS), 504–505

Acromegaly, *362*

ACTH (adrenocorticotropic hormone,) *361, 364*

Acute nephritis, 397

Addiction, *see* Drug abuse

Additives, 38–41

Adenoids, *404*–405

Adhesions, and hearing loss, 352

Adolescence, emotions during, 154

Adrenal glands, 359, *364*

Adrenaline (epinephrine), *361*

Adulthood, emotions during, 154

Aerobics, 79–81, 85

Agent Orange, 522

Agility test, 76

Aging, diseases of, 476–477

Agglutination, *430*

Ailments, home treatment of, 531–532; *see also* illness

Air pollution, 520–521; control of, **525**–256

Alanon, 288

Alarm, 174

Alateen, 288

Albumin, *430*

Alcohol, and accidents, 277, 281–282, **283;** decisions about use, 288; drinking patterns, 273–274; and crime, 282; effect on family life, 283; effect on human body, 276–281; mixing with drugs, 277; nature of, 274–275; production of, 275–276; route through body, 278–281; *see also* Alcoholism

Alcoholics Anonymous, 287–**288**

Alcoholism, *283*–286; signs and stages of, 285–287; treatment of, 287

Aldosterone, 364

Alimentary canal, *279*

Allergies, skin, *109*–110; treatment of, 110–111

Allergist, *111*

Alopecia, *114*

Alveoli, *407*

Alzheimer's disease, 477

American Medical Association (AMA) 515, 534

Amino acids, *20;* digestion of, 381

Amnesia, 214–*215*

Amniocentesis, *454,* **455**

Amoebic dysentery, *486*

Amphetamines, *253*–254

Anemia, *434*–435

Anger, 147, *150*–152

Angina pectoris, *461*

Anorexia, *36*

Antabuse, *287*

Anterior lobe, pituitary, *361*–363

Antianxiety drugs, *234*

Antibiotics, *502*–503

Antibodies, 20, *431,* 498

Antidepressant drugs, *234*

Antidiuretic hormone (ADH), *363*

Antigens, *498*

Antimanic drugs, 234

Antioxidants, in foods, 38

Antiperspirant, 104

Antisocial personality, *218*

Anxiety, *149*–150, 207–209

Aorta, *423*

Appearance, 101

Appendicitis, *390*

Appetite, *25*

Arm, bones of, 56

Arm wrestling, 82

Arterioles, *425*

Artery(ies), *421, 425*

Arthritis, 475–476

Arthroscope, *62*

Articular cartilage, 48

Artificial heart, 467

Artificial respiration, 566–567

Asphyxiation, *410, 566*

Association, 134

Asthma, 414

Astigmatism, *344*

Astringent, 105–106

Atherosclerosis, *427* 461

Athlete's foot, 486

Athletic trainer, 97

Athletics, and diet, 42; *see also* Exercise(s)

Atrioventricular node, *424*

Atrioventricular valves, *422*

Atrium, *422*

Attitude, *239*–140; changing, 142

Autoimmune diseases, 504, *505*–506

Automobile(s), accidents, 546–549; protective devices, **549;** stopping distances, 547

Autonomic nervous system, *325*–326

Avoidant personality, *216*

Avulsions, *562*

Axon, neuron, *314*

B

Bacillus, *484*

Backbone, *see* Spinal column

Bacteria, as infectious agents, 483–484

Bacterial pneumonia, 413–414

Balance, and ear, 350

Baldness, 224

Bandages, 563–**564**

Barbiturates, *255*–256

Basic metabolic rate (BMR), 29

Behavior, biological basis of, 128–134; and cultural differences, 242–142; defensive, 191–192; forces affecting, 138–139; and heredity, 127–134; learned, 127–128, 134–138; and social

G

H

nature of, 134; *see also* Learned behavior

Learning disabilities, 137–138

Leg bones, 56–57

Lens, eye, 340–**341**

Lens cells, 341

Leukemia, *435–436, 471*

Life crises, *218–221*

Life cycle, and emotions, 153–155

Life stress scale, 176–177

Life-style, and environmental pollution, 527; and health, 7; and stress, 178–179

Ligaments, *60*

"Light" foods, 43

Lightning, safety during, 556

Liver, alcohol effect on, 280–**281;** in digestion, 383–384; disease of, 392

Lobes, brain, 316

Longitudinal arch, *57*

Love, *148*–149, 163

Low-tar/nicotine cigarettes, 301–302

LSD (lysergic acid diethylamide), *259–*260

Lumbar vertebrae, *54*

Lung(s), 406; alcohol effect on, 280; cancer of, **416**–417, 470, 472; smoking effect on 298–**300;** structure of, **406**–407

Lutinizing hormone (LH), *369*

Lymph, 425–*426*

Lymph nodes, *426*

Lymphatic system, *421,* 425–**426**

Lymphocytes, *498–***499**

M

Mainlining, *263*

Mainstream smoke, *296–*297

Malaria, 489

Malignant tumor, *468*

Malocclusion, *119*–120

Maltose, 381

Manic-depressive disorder, *214*

Mannerisms, *138*

Marijuana, *256–***258**

Marriage, 163–165

Mastoid bone, *351*

Mastoiditis, *351*

Maximum heart rate, *79*

Medicaid, 540

Medical care, choosing proper, 532–539

Medical laboratory specialist, 441

Medical research scientist, 509

Medical specialists, 534–535; communicating with, 536–537

Medical therapy, 234–235

Medicare, 539–540

Medication, taking of, 537

Medulla, brain, *320*–322, *364;* kidney, *395*

Medullary canal, *49*

Melanin, *102*

Memory, *134*

Meninges, *316*

Meningitis, *332*

Menstrual cycle, 363, **369–370,** 371

Menstruation, *368*

Mental defenses, 192–193

Mental disorder(s), anxiety, 207–209; causes of 205–206; classification of, 206; dissociative, 214–215; medical therapy for, 234–235; mood, 213–214; nature of, 204; personality, 216–218; prevention of, 239–240; schizophrenia, 211–213; somatoform, 209–210

Mental health, nature of, 204; problems, history of, 225–227

Mental health services, 236–239

Mental mechanisms, *192;* defensive, 192–199; evaluating, 199

Mental retardation, *137,* **449**

Mescaline, *261*

Mesothelioma, *518*

Metabolism, *365*

Metacarpal bones, 56

Metastasis, *468*

Methadone, *263*

Methanol, *274*

Methaqualone, *256*

Midbrain, *320*

Middle ear, infections, 351

Migraine headache, *328*

Milieu (environment) therapy, *236*

Milk, processing of, 37–38

Mind, levels of, 191–192

Minerals, 18, 23–24; essential, 27

Mismatched vision, *345*

Modeling, *231*

Molars, *117*

Moles, *108*

Monoclonal antibodies, 500

Mononucleosis, *491*

Monounsaturated fat, *23*

Mood disorders, 213–214

Morphine, *262*

Motivation, *138*–139

Motor neurons, *313*–314

Motor skills, 68; exercises for, 83–84

Motorcycle safety, 549

Mountain sickness, 409

Mouth, cancer, 470, 472; in digestion, 381

Mouth-to-mouth breathing, 566

Multiple personality, 215

Multiple sclerosis, *331*

Multiplier effect, *277*

Murmurs, *424*

Muscle(s), energy source for, 64; exercise of, *see* Exercises; and good posture, 68–69; healthy, 66–69; heart, 423–424; kinds of, 62–63; and motor skills, 68; stomach wall, **382;** working of, 63–64; *see also* individual muscles

Muscle cramps, 65

Muscle injuries, 64–65; first aid for, 564–565; prevention and treatment of, 59, 564–565

Muscular dystrophy, 65

Mutagens, *518*

Myasthenia gravis, *505*

Myocardial infarction, *462*

Myocardium, *421*–422

N

Nails, 115; shaping of, **115**

Narcissistic personality, *217*

Narcolepsy, *91*

T

Tapeworm, *486*
Tar, *295–296*
Target heart rate, *79*
Tartar, 118
Taste, sense of, 355
Taste buds, *355*
Tay-Sachs disease, 452
Teeth, brushing, **122;** care of, 120–122; decay, 117–118; and diet, 120–121; flossing, **121–**122; structure of, **116;** types of and arrangement, 116–**117**
Temperance movement, 274
Temperature inversion, **520**
Teratogens *518*
Terminal illness, 478–479
Testes, 359, 363, *368;* cancer of, 470
Testicular cancer, 470
Testosterone, *368*
Tetany, *366*
Tetrahydrocannabinol (THC), *257*
Thalamus, *319–320*
Therapy, *see* Psychotherapy
Thermography, **469**
Thighbone, 56
Thoracic vertebrae, *54*
Throat, cancer of, 470, 472; infections, 412
Throwing, 84
Thymus gland, *366*
Thyroid gland, 359, 364–**366**
Thyrotrophic hormone (TSH), *361*
Thyroxine, *360,* 365
Tibia, *56–57*
Tissues, bone, 47–48, 50
Tobacco, addiction to, 295–296; interaction with drugs, 299–300; social effects, 303–304; *see also* Smoking
Tolerance, *248*
Tongue, **355**
Tonsillitis, *404*
Tonsils, *404*
Tornadoes, safety during, **556–**557
Touch, sense of, 354
Tourniquet, *563*
Trachea, *405*

Traits, inheritance of, 445–*447*
Tranquilizers, *234,* 256
Transverse arch, *57*
Travelers' diarrhea, 387
Triage, 538
Triathlon competition, **77**
Triceps, *64*
Trichina worm, *487*
Trichinosis, *487*
Tubercule, 414–*425*
Tuberculosis, *414*–415, *500–501*
Twins, effects of heredity and environment on, 130
Typhoid, 490

U

Ulcer(s), 180, 391–**392**
Ulcerative colitis, *392*
Ulna, *56*
Ultrasound, 454
Unconscious mind, *191*
United States Department of Agriculture (USDA), 515
Ureters, *393*
Urethra, *393*
Urinalysis, *396*
Uterus, cancer of, 470, 472

V

Vaccination, 500–502
Values, 139–*140*
Varicose veins, *433–434*
Vasodilators, 466
Vegetarian diet, *31–32*
Veins, *421,* 425; blood pressure in, 427–428
Ventricle, 422; brain, *316*
Ventricular fibrillation, *462*
Venules, *425*
Vertebrae, *51*–54
Villi, *383–384*
Viral pneumonia, 414
Viruses, *484–485*
Vision, binocular, *341–342;* mismatched, *345;* problems, 343–344; stereoscopic, 341–*342;* testing, 343; *see also* Eyes
Vitamins, 18, 24; essential, 26
Vitiligo, *107*

Vocal cords, **404**–*405*
Vomiting, inducing of, 571

W

Warm-up, 85
Warts, *107*
Wastes, solid, pollution by, 523
Water, as infection source, 488; as nutrient, 24–25; pollution of, 521, 526
Water safety, 552–553
Weight, control of, 32–37; gain, 37–38; loss, 33–36; *see also* Obesity
Weight gain diet, 37–38
Weight loss diet, 33–36
Weight training, **82**–83
Wellness, 7, 12–13; *see also* Health
Wellness test, 12–13
Wellness Watch, 348, 354, 370, 399, 417, 438, 506
White blood cells, **428**–*429;* as infection defense, 497
White corpuscles, 428–**429**
Windburn, 108
Wisdom teeth, *117*
Work place, pollution of, 525, 526
World Health Organization (WHO), 515–**516**
Wounds, *561,* first aid for, 561–564

X

X rays, as radiation hazard, **522**–523

Y

Youth physical fitness program, 75–76

Z

Zygote, *446*